Radical Healing

OTHER WORKS BY RUDOLPH M. BALLENTINE, M.D.

Diet and Nutrition
Yoga and Psychotherapy (coauthor)
Science of Breath (coauthor)
The Theory and Practice of Meditation (editor)
Transition to Vegetarianism

Radical Healing

INTEGRATING THE WORLD'S

GREAT THERAPEUTIC TRADITIONS

TO CREATE A NEW

TRANSFORMATIVE MEDICINE

Rudolph M. Ballentine, M.D.

Illustrations by Linda Funk

Three Rivers Press / New York

Grateful acknowledgment is made to the following
for the use of previously published material:
Excerpts on pages 44–48 from *Sacred Plant Medicine* by Stephen Harrod Buhner.
© 1996 Stephen Harrod Buhner.
Used by permission of Roberts Rinehart Publishers.
Illustration (page 409) from *Yoga and Psychotherapy*. Used by permission
of the Himalayan International Institute of Yoga Science and Psychotherapy.
Illustration (page 424) from *Hands of Light* by Barbara Ann Brennan.
Copyright © 1987 by Barbara Ann Brennan.
Used by permission of Bantam Books, a division of Random House, Inc.

Published by Three Rivers Press,
201 East 50th Street, New York, New York 10022.
Member of the Crown Publishing Group.

Originally published in hardcover by Harmony Books in 1999.

BOOK DESIGN BY CATHRYN S. AISON

Random House, Inc. New York, Toronto, London, Sydney, Auckland
www.randomhouse.com

THREE RIVERS PRESS is a registered trademark of Random House, Inc.

Printed in the United States of America

Library of Congress Cataloging-in-Publication Data
Ballentine, Rudolph, 1941–
Radical healing : integrating the world's great therapeutic traditions to create
a new transformative medicine / by Rudolph M. Ballentine. — 1st ed.
p.   cm.
Includes bibliographical references and index.
1. Holistic medicine.   I. Title.
R733.B255   1999
615.5—dc21   98-28802
CIP

ISBN 0-609-80484-7

10 9 8 7 6 5 4 3 2 1

FIRST PAPERBACK EDITION

Dedication

to
my mother
*who imbued me with
a spirit of independence*

to
my father
*who taught me to look
at both sides of every issue*

and to
Shri Swami Rama

*who helped me see that
healing is what we're here for*

Contents

Acknowledgments

The vision of healing presented in this book is a synthesis of those of my teachers, especially Swami Rama, though many great and patient others gave me their time and attention. It rests, too, on the written works of pioneers in the fields of holistic medicine and spirituality, many (but not all) of whose books are cited herein. I also must acknowledge that circle of intimates who have helped nurture and sustain the consciousness from which this book could emerge: Lorie Dechar, Neal Fox, Joseph Aldo, Branden Blinn, Collin Brown, Linda Bark, Richard Foltz, Lorinda Rodway, Kai Ehrhart, Thom Namaya, Bill Dennis, and others.

This book also bears the imprint of those who taught me about healing by helping me up when I was broken: Morton Beiser, Irwin Marcus, John Pierrakos, Dorothy McCrary, Carlos Velasquez, and Don Shewey as well as Lorie, Joseph, and Kai. Special thanks go to those who helped me keep my life together during these years of writing: Lorinda Rodway, Neal Fox, Cazibe Tongur, Bob Shrem, Noelle Hanrahan, Ilene Jacobs and my daughter, Rebecca.

I appreciate the many, many hours generously given by those who read and critiqued the manuscript: Tim Cooley, Karen Lawson, Joyce Vassallo, Don Shewey, Neal Fox, Lorie Dechar, Annie Colt, and Jerry Gore; the expert input of my editors at Harmony: Leslie Meredith, who (fortunately) had no tolerance for my meanderings, and Peter Guzzardi, who coaxed me into a final heroic effort at the finish line; and the spirited vision of Carol Mann, my agent, who opened the way for this book to be written, and supported and encouraged me at each step. Ed and Alison Levy helped with critical reshaping in the eleventh hour and Swami

Ajaya, responding to a last minute call for help, kindly offered many hours of patient review and comment in order to set me straight and rescue the soul of the book. Jim Walsh's patient attention to detail as he shepherded this complex book through production at Crown was a gift, as were the skillful work of the design team and Linda Funk's lovingly rendered illustrations.

I also must acknowledge the extent to which this book is a compendium of the many profound lessons taught me by my amazing children and by the sincere and courageous seekers I have been privileged to serve as physician. I also know that this work would be considerably less significant without the input and guidance I received from the realm of Spirit. Lastly, the writing of this book would not have been possible without Pennell Whitney's devoted attention to our four children. I owe her a special debt of gratitude.

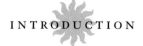

Origins of
a New Vision

Five years ago I presented an integrated system of holistic healing at a conference on "The Interaction of Western and Eastern Medicines," held in Israel. The audience was largely professional, and while I had hoped it would be receptive, the response I got was remarkable. I had left my twelve-year-old daughter outside the auditorium to supervise a table of literature on my work. By the time I had finished the session and joined her, I found her surrounded by eager participants who had snatched up most of the materials, were fighting over what was left, and had pushed forward with such enthusiasm that she was backed against the wall. "I don't think I can do this, Dad," she said, laughing, throwing up her hands in mock surrender. One of the information-seekers explained to me: "This—the integration—was what we thought the whole conference was going to be about. But except for your talk, it wasn't. The Chinese doctors talked about Chinese medicine, the Ayurvedic doctors talked about Ayurvedic medicine and the naturopaths talked about naturopathy. We've already heard that before."

I had presented to that audience a comprehensive vision of medical care—one that brought together the various holistic schools of healing, integrating their insights and skills. The structure of that presentation would become the skeleton of this book, *Radical Healing*. It was an exciting integration—and one that had been a long time in the making. For more than twenty years the search for that wholeness had been my professional—as well as my personal—quest.

* * *

At the end of the 1960s, as I was finishing my residency training at Charity Hospital in New Orleans, my spirit of adventure was being nurtured in the womb of the French Quarter. Psychiatry residents were allowed a certain license, so my local foray into the world of alternative medicine—which at that time meant co-founding a Free Clinic for "street kids"—was regarded with benign indulgence. I became a familiar presence on Decatur Street. Whenever a wild-eyed flower child was found cowering in a corner, suffering the terror of a bad trip, he was turned over to me. I was even invited to speak to the annual AMA convention on the subject of "Drugs and Youth."

But my young patients taught me more than I taught them. They introduced me to vegetarian food, yoga, and herbal potions, and sparked in me a curiosity about the frontiers of consciousness. Having grown up wandering alone through the woods and fields of the rural South, communing with the trees and frogs, this all sounded a familiar chord. When I became disillusioned with the medication-oriented psychiatry that was beginning to dominate the field, my new interests led me to India.

There I met a teacher who inspired me to probe deeper within. He called himself Swami Rama, a sort of generic non-name, equivalent in India to calling oneself "Father John." A free spirit who managed to both embody and convey the boldness of ancient healing traditions, Swamiji encouraged me to look beyond the mind as I'd learned to conceive of it in my psychiatric training. When I began to grasp the power of doing that, and to see how the most profound healing had its roots in a process of radical spiritual unfoldment, I decided to give up the practice of medicine, return to the United States, and simply teach yoga.

But my medical training was discovered by my students, who would approach me with their ailments after class. I explained that I wasn't practicing medicine anymore, but they wouldn't be put off. "I know," they would say, "but if I go to a regular doctor he'll give me all this medicine that throws me off balance, and I'm really serious about yoga. . . ."

Soon I was back in India again, this time to study homeopathy and Ayurveda, techniques for healing that didn't create negative side effects, that were effective because they promoted growth and evolution—mentally, emotionally, spiritually. When I returned to America this time I was full of enthusiasm, determined to set up practice in a new kind of medicine. But the reality awaiting me was sobering. I became acutely aware of how far I had stepped "over the line." In 1973 most people, especially in the medical community, laughed at homeopathy, and no one, it seemed, had even heard of Ayurveda.

Nevertheless, I set up shop in a rented, unfurnished house in a middle-class neighborhood in suburban Chicago. Having no money, I made do with a card table for my desk, a cardboard box for my files, and two borrowed folding chairs, one for the patient and one for myself. Another empty box in the living room, upside down with a cotton shawl over it, served as a makeshift magazine table. Waiting patients were invited to seat themselves on the floor. The only clothes I had were the traditional white homespun kurtas and pajamas that I had brought back from India.

All these eccentricities notwithstanding, my reputation spread. I was, at that time and in that area at least, one of a kind, and those looking for an alternative sought me out. One of them was a rather well-to-do lady obviously not prepared for my odd furnishings and Indian clothes. Though she benefited from what we did and went on to write a positive magazine article about her experience, she was jarred. "He met me at the door," she began her account, "wrapped in a white sheet. . . ."

I was operating way outside the system. I began to feel insecure, concerned about my fringe status—at times frankly fearful of reprisals from the medical establishment. If not for the support of the local community of yoga students and Swami Rama, who came regularly from India to teach them, I might have lost courage. But I had found solid grounding in a healing work that rang true for me in the deepest and most satisfying way I could imagine. It combined harnessing nature's medicinals—plants and other natural substances—with commonsense essentials such as diet, exercise, and cleansing, as well as the most profound principles of spiritual and psychological transformation. Before this, my life had felt fragmented—my allegiances to nature, to healing, and to spiritual pursuits pulling against my training in science, psychology, and medicine, had seemed to scatter me in a half-dozen different directions. Now I was doing a kind of work that was fulfilling to all the many aspects of my being. I could be physician, psychiatrist, herbalist, Ayurvedic practitioner, homeopath, and teacher—all in one.

Patients continued to seek me out—sometimes, it seemed, too many. At times I was overwhelmed. I remember telling one patient in those early years, "I will try to help you on one condition. If you get better, don't tell anyone." I felt I needed more time to study each case, to investigate techniques that might help, and to explore how they might fit together.

But, despite my initial insecurity, over the years the work proved sound. By 1983 I had set up six clinics and trained more than twenty physicians. Meanwhile, holistic medical centers were being opened by others, too, and a growing number of researchers were beginning to document the effectiveness of various holistic approaches. Gradually the distinctive attributes of this new kind of integrative medicine began to become clear to me and I ventured to put them into words. Over the years I've continually strived to reformulate and refine these points.

Radical Healing is built on these unifying concepts; they are the practical essence of a medicine that is simple and universal, rooted in the perennial principle of healing as personal evolution. What follow are these fundamental points. You will see through the course of this book how they undergird a totally new, profoundly effective, and deeply transformative system of healing.

1. Self-awareness

Effective holistic medical therapy depends on self-awareness. This medicine is based on what you pick up by tuning in to inner cues—not on what a laboratory test might tell you. Your lab is your body; experiments going on there constantly allow you to find out what suits you and what doesn't. You make major decisions about your own treatment according to what creates a sense of well-being, what boosts your energy, or what brings clarity of mind.

This new kind of patient, operating on the basis of self-awareness, calls for a new kind of doctor, too—one who is a consultant and guide, a fellow explorer, not one who is distant or assumes an air of omniscience, or who hands you routine prescriptions. Operating from your own awareness also allows you to pick up signals and make adjustments in your life while you are still basically healthy, instead of waiting until you're sick. Remaining relatively healthy and only rarely venturing into illness situates our work in an arena quite different from what is customarily considered the proper domain of medicine.

2. Transformation

Bringing awareness to your body, to its unique reactions and processes, and to its symptoms and strengths, sets you up for growthful insight. For where you founder—precisely where your system begins to break down—provides a valuable clue to what needs to change in your life. Working from the perspective of this process of discovery permits you to approach a health crisis with curiosity instead of fear, and with optimism instead of disappointment. Sickness and health become a major way you learn from life. Although dysfunction and disease point to what you need to work on, they also hold the seeds of your unfoldment. From this point of view, illness is an opportunity for growth and transformation, while "recovery" is only a return to an obsolete status quo. Authentic healing will often involve radical changes in how you live. Old habits and attitudes that supported the development of disease will fall away, to be replaced by new ones that go with a new way of being in the world.

3. Wholeness

One of the things that makes holistic medicine fascinating and fun is rediscovering that the parts tell us about the whole. As we will see, your hand or your face, or even your tongue, can speak volumes about the whole of you, not only your physical state, but your mind, too. (This may be why the hologram has become such a central organizing image in holistic medicine, since it demonstrates how every piece contains the whole.) From the holistic perspective, our suffering comes from forgetting our wholeness. The word "health" comes from the Anglo Saxon *häl,* whence also come "heal" and "whole." Perhaps the simplest definition of *healing* is "to make whole."

Holistic healing requires, however, that the way we achieve wholeness not only makes us more complete as individuals, but also reintegrates us into the whole of nature. The unique value of medicinals made from natural substances is that they weave us back into our place in the body of the earth. But there's an even more profound dimension to the deepest healing: it's also spiritual. The same root that gave us *heal* and *whole* gives us *holy,* too.

The state of wholeness that heals us must be extended to include the spirit, and reconnecting to the whole means freeing yourself from the narrow consciousness of the constricted ego. Letting go the fear and isolation of the narrow ego allows you to open up to a larger sense of who you are, to identify with a more encompassing consciousness—the universal matrix that sustains us, the healing force or higher power of the great spiritual traditions.

From this more complete, holistic perspective, illness is not an interruption of life, but a crucial and valuable effort to reach for more wholeness of spirit. Little pieces of life experience provide the step-by-step progress that takes you along your path of spiritual development. Often it's your health problems—even the small ones—that clue you in to what you need to address, leading you on to increments of the transformation that moves you closer to an identity with the Greater Whole. Such illnesses and ailments are critical components of spiritual life. Crises of the body are ultimately expressions of underlying crises of the spirit.

The Emerging Vision

The above principles are at first suggested and then repeatedly reinforced as one holistic approach after another is pulled into a combined framework. Though these points emerge with compelling clarity as the various schools of thought are integrated, up to now they have gone largely unrecognized because the field of holistic medicine has remained as fragmented as an unassembled jigsaw puzzle. This book aims to show how the pieces of that puzzle fit together and how the whole that results is greater than the sum of its parts.

Each of the great healing traditions has arisen in its own culture to help resolve problems peculiar to that setting, so each—e.g., Ayurveda, homeopathy, Traditional Chinese Medicine, European and Native American herbology, nutrition, and psychotherapeutic bodywork—has its weaknesses as well as strengths. By integrating them, superimposing one upon another in layer after layer of complementary perspectives and techniques, we can arrive at an amalgam that is far more potent and thorough than any one of them taken alone. That's why I've called the integrated approach that results from this synthesis *Radical Healing*.

It's *radical* because, as the philosophies and methods of these various traditions are melded, and the profound principles buried in them become clearer and stronger, an intensity of effectiveness becomes possible. Healing and reorganization accelerate and deepen. Though time is needed at certain stages to absorb and consolidate change, this integration makes spurts of rapid transformation possible. After using a synergistic blend of techniques I recommended, one patient commented, "I've made more progress in three visits than I did in years of psychotherapy."

The word *radical* comes from the Latin *radix,* which means "root." Radical healing tackles the root causes of illness and the hidden impediments to optimal health. These are attitudes and emotional postures embedded in the mind and in the unconscious. They shape the way that subtle energy is organized, which in turn influences what happens in the physical body. Using pharmaceutical drugs to influence biochemical and metabolic reactions is superficial and very limited, compared with treatments that reach down into the deeper levels of human functioning.

Besides its relation to the Latin *radix,* the term *radical* has a less well-known and more technical botanical significance. It denotes the tiniest, hairlike terminals of a plant's root, which extend its action into the depths of the soil, and, by finding and entering cracks and crevices in the bedrock, slowly fracture it and split it open. Some of the beliefs and assumptions about our reality that sustain and promote our suffering are the deepest and most resistant to change. It is those assumptions that can make diseases seem untreatable or "incurable." The *modus operandi* of radical healing is to penetrate the strongholds of human limitation and rend them asunder, opening the possibility of a transformation and evolution that conventional medicine has not ventured to approach. Without that probing thoroughness, that radical intensity, we will not be able to heal the profound disorders that are now plaguing us, individually and collectively.

Besides presenting a new vision of medicine, *Radical Healing* is also intended to anchor that vision to practical, well-proven techniques—such as the use of herbal and homeopathic remedies, exercise, flower essences, and Asian diagnosis—and to offer you guidance in their use. You won't truly *grasp* this new vision of healing until you have experienced its effects yourself. That's why this book has to be, in part, a handbook. Read it, and don't be afraid to try out what you're reading about. By using it you will begin to feel its power.

Using the Power of Holistic Healing for Yourself

You have to do two things to effectively harness the power of holistic healing. First you have to continually cultivate your awareness of the new vision and, second, you have to learn to "do the technical stuff" needed to put it into practice. The interaction between those two generates the magic and the fun. This book is designed to walk you back and forth across the terrain of the different holistic fields and specialties so that you become familiar with their views and methods. It explains the philosophies and practices of each—examining and teaching a variety of practical tools while continually clarifying and strengthening the vision that ties them all together.

The tools used for holistic healing are different from those used in the old kind of medicine. The more frequently used holistic tools, such as simple homeopathic remedies, diet, cleansing techniques, and energetic breathing, foster awareness rather than blur it; they reorganize rather than disrupt your mental and physical processes, bringing out emotions or concerns that are submerged, rather than covering them over and hiding them.

I've recounted a lot of case histories throughout the book. One reason for this is that they're fun. But the chain of narratives also supports a systematic explication of the theory of integrated holistic medicine as well as careful instruction on how to use it. Although you may want to use the book as a reference at a later stage, at the outset it's wise to go through it once from beginning to end. On this first time through, you might want to skim the more detailed sections. The book will take you through a progression of five sections to help get you clear on the mindset and learn enough skills to get started.

SECTION I. NATURE'S MEDICINALS

To begin, we plunge right into what's already "in your face" these days—the mysterious little bottles you see arranged in exotic-looking rows in your local health-food store. These are "nature's medicinals." Their immense (and rapidly growing) appeal stems from the fact that they are fundamentally different from conventional drugs. Instead of disrupting or diverting the chemistry of metabolism, they convey complex informational patterns directly from nature.

These patterns trigger a kind of physiological and psychological reorganization that brings you more into synchrony with the flux and flow of the larger gestalt of which you are a part. This is healing *into* harmony with nature. Though gentle in their action, such remedies can have an impact that is profound and curative in a way you may not have imagined.

By the time you've finished Section I, you will be able to walk into your health-food store or natural pharmacy, recognize the groupings of remedies, and choose the right one when you need it. Working with these remedies is a great entree into holistic medicine: in a sense, natural medicinals start the ball rolling. For example, even before you have learned about subtle energy (*ch'i,* as the acupuncturist calls it), you can experience the effects it has on your body and mind, you can feel it shift. Later in the book you'll come to understand what was going on inside you when this healing occurred, and how it is part of a larger transformative process.

SECTION II. SELF-ASSESSMENT

Natural medicinals and other holistic remedies and techniques are highly individualized—as they have to be, because they are intended to provide for the reorganization and evolution of a certain person who is attempting to move through a specific crisis at a particular moment. Each crisis involves a specific pattern of resistance to change and flow into the future. To make effective use of the holistic tools at your disposal, you must somehow grasp the essence of that resistance or "illness" so you can choose the remedy or technique that fits. There are many systems for doing this—for "diagnosing," so to speak, and each diagnostic approach has its own utility.

Modern high-tech diagnosis is based mostly on mechanical tests of the body's chemistry or tissue changes, which provide lots of detail at that level of function, but pick up information only late in the game. By the time such changes are evident, the disorder has progressed far enough to cause unnecessary suffering. What's more, a conventional laboratory approach lacks the richness of systems of assessment that tap body-mind interactions. Asian diagnosis, for example, looks at the body in a way that clarifies how physical symptoms relate to hidden emotional or spiritual crises. This section helps you begin to think in such holistic terms, and helps you to free yourself from preoccupation with conventional diagnostic labels that can leave you fearful and helpless. In Section II you will learn a range of more constructive options for identifying your problem when you have one—and how to stay out of trouble by providing what your particular constitution requires.

SECTION III. FOUNDATION STONES

When the Karate Kid began his apprenticeship with Mr. Miyagi, he was put to painting a fence. At first he thought this menial work was intended to teach him humility. Only gradually did he come to realize that the motions of the brushes were the same as those he would use in sparring. By then, they were thoroughly programmed in, *and* the fence was painted! The wisdom of the East may sometimes be elliptical, but it is also efficient. Yoga teaches that the processes you learn as you master the physical postures of hatha yoga are the same processes you will later apply to dealing with the much more slippery and elusive mind during meditation.

The same principle holds true in holistic medicine: Exercise, nutrition, and cleansing are important because what you learn by working with them on the physical level can be applied to the less tangible levels of energy and consciousness. Moreover, if you do not exercise, eat consciously, and cleanse your system, you may find the effectiveness of subtler healing techniques blocked. Most failures of holistic healing occur because such obstacles were not addressed. Section III will lead you through the processes of demystifying nutrition, bringing excitement and discovery to exercise, and developing finesse in the intricacies of detoxification.

SECTION IV. ENERGY AND CONSCIOUSNESS

Up to this point in the book you will have focused on working with your body or with natural medicinals and how that work—a shift in diet or an herbal remedy—might affect your energy or your consciousness. But in Section IV we turn the tables. In this section you'll learn how the healing process can be initiated directly from the levels of energy or consciousness. For example, you'll learn to identify and support some of the important energy currents within yourself, or to avail yourself of the services of practitioners who can help you do so.

Holistic techniques for working with consciousness and the mind are most often based on the principles of the meditative traditions, which teach us that a simple shift in awareness can change the entire configuration of energy flow, which in turn reshapes physiologic events, eliminating what had become, or was on its way to becoming, a physical disease. We will see how this healing shift in awareness is cultivated by raising energy from one energy center (called a *chakra*) to another. We also take a close look at sexuality, since it frequently ties up and drains away the energy needed to power a healing transformation.

Working with energy and consciousness requires a suspension of effort and a relaxing into contact with larger aspects of your existence. As you open to these deeper levels of your being and allow them to reorganize and heal you, you come increasingly into alignment and synchrony with your spiritual essence. The deepest healing, which only comes with such a reconnection to Spirit, requires that you traverse the darkest territories of the inner world. Here you grapple with the "shadow" aspects of your being, and discover that personal healing is your contribution to a larger process of healing, one of global proportions.

Ultimately, you will see that your body represents a weaving together of all the themes of holistic work, reminding you of what needs to be addressed next, revealing your spiritual challenges, and providing the ultimate map to guide your healing and growth.

SECTION V. RESOURCES

This final section of the book provides the resources you will need to integrate holistic healing approaches into your daily life. There is a "Self-Help Index" to what works best for common problems; this is a powerful way to experience what you have read about in the previous sections. For the hands-on type, this is the juiciest part of *Radical Healing*. One practitioner, reviewing the manuscript, wrote in the margin, "This alone will be worth the price of the book!" You may think so, too. Even as you are reading, when problems pop up, turn to the back and try the simple, natural therapeutic measures listed. Then read on to understand why and how they worked. To help you get set up, there's also a list of remedies you'll need for a Home Medicine Chest.

Discussions of points footnoted in the text will be found after Section V. This includes references to research studies that support some of the more controversial ideas presented. In previous books I provided point-by-point documentation, which was possible because I was dealing with fairly circumscribed topics, such as nutrition or psychotherapy. In this present work—striving as it does to encompass the whole of so vast a subject—such detail is not feasible. Yet you will often want to ground the concepts in solid evidence. To make this possible, I have offered numerous references to books that deal authoritatively with specific topics.

Many of these books are logical extensions of what you learn here, and will be valuable to your continuing study; they will be found described in the annotated bibliography titled "Guide to the Further Study of Holistic Medicine" in Section V. A brief description of each book is provided so that you can find exactly what you need. Many valuable concepts and techniques not mentioned in the text because of space constraints—such as light therapy, or the psychological aspects of immune function—will be described in these listings, so don't overlook them. Following Section V, there is also a short glossary of esoteric terms you might otherwise stumble over.

Bias and Inspiration

With the benefits of integration so ample, I offer this book as an initial attempt to pull the field together, though that is necessarily a work in progress. I'm sure that a decade or two from now the integrated model will be more evolved. I've emphasized what seem to me the disciplines destined to be key players in the emerging new medicine: herbology, homeopathy, Ayurveda, Traditional Chinese Medicine, and energy work. This choice does not so much reflect wisdom on my own part as it does the expert guidance I had in my training.

I was nudged into the study of homeopathy by Swami Rama, my spiritual teacher and mentor. "If you want to be a good psychiatrist, you're going to have to learn homeopathy," he told me in the early 1970s, when I first went to India. That made no sense at all to me then—in part, probably, because I hadn't the slightest idea what homeopathy was (and even less interest in finding out). However, after several more prods I asked him, "Well, what *is* homeopathy?"

I remember his provocative expression as he explained, "You know the arborvitae tree?" I did, having grown up with one in my yard and having always been attuned to the plants around me. "Well," he said, "it gets a little berry that looks rough—like a wart." I recalled the berries clearly. "In homeopathy," he continued, "you use that plant to treat warts." I laughed nervously. "Why are you laughing?" he asked. I didn't answer. I was shocked by what sounded absurd to my conventionally trained ear, and embarrassed that I had followed him halfway around the world to learn from him.

It was an uphill struggle for Swami Rama, but when he finally got me into homeopathy, I became enthralled. Through casual comments, inspiring anecdotes, and therapeutic suggestions for cases I was treating, Swamiji continued over the years to steer me gently toward the selection of approaches that I now use—though I have also added components on my own. In any case, I believe the foundation is strong: the basic building blocks of this integrative effort are the product of a yogic seer's penetrating analysis and intuitive wisdom, as well as my own broad education, rooted in the twentieth-century West, and in my—sometimes consuming—curiosity and drive to grasp "the whole picture."

At the very least I believe that this book will start the integrative process rolling—perhaps in the broad field of holistic medicine, but certainly for you, the individual reader. By the time you've finished it, you should understand what makes an approach genuinely holistic, and the life-changing potential it then has. You'll know how to choose which such interventions suit your needs and how they can best be combined. You'll have a grasp of where your transformational work might be heading, and you'll be in a position to chart your own way. You'll also have some crucial skills that you can use with the help of the charts and Self-Help Index.

Using the Study Guide offered at the end, you'll even know how to go beyond what this book offers, deeper into the topics of your choice. Most important, you will know how to keep your work with health connected to your unfoldment as a human being, to your discovery of your fullest potential, and to your spiritual evolution. You will have fully assimilated a new vision of medicine. You should, in fact, be ready to approach any challenge to your health the way Sarah, a patient I first saw fifteen years ago, did.

SARAH'S PSORIATIC ARTHRITIS

At the age of twenty-eight, Sarah had swollen joints and she was covered with sores. Despite the toxic medicine she took, her skin was still disfigured by the thick, scaly patches of a psoriasis that was only partially under control and an accompanying arthritis that often left her joints red, painfully swollen, and unusable. What's worse, she felt constantly restless and ill at ease from the side effect of the drug. To top it all off, she'd been told to abandon her hopes of having a child, because the medication was very likely to produce birth defects. At her wits' end, she finally took her sister's advice and came to see me to try a more holistic approach.

Five years later, Sarah had been medication-free for four and a half years. She had two healthy sons, and her joints were fine. Her only traces of psoriasis were minor flare-ups when she didn't eat properly or when she was under a lot of stress. But she'd gotten to this point only after making radical changes in her life. As she changed her diet, her skin cleared. As she discovered how to assert her own strength in relation to her husband, and moved past a lifelong pattern of accept-

ing other people's suggestions that she was weak and ineffectual, her joints grew stronger.

Sarah's illness had led her to make some fundamental shifts. She gave up on finding a magic pill to deal with her illness. She pushed past fear and persisted against all odds. She recovered her own power and confronted issues that had plagued her since childhood. Plunging into a transformative process that was scary—but ultimately rewarded with exhilarating triumph—she made radical changes and got radical results.

THE FUTURE?

A few years ago I was invited by a group of students at a New York–area medical school to speak on homeopathy and Ayurveda. Over the decades I've been asked to address such subjects at some of the most prestigious medical centers in this country, such as, Einstein, Yale, Columbia, and the University of Minnesota, but always by the students for sessions they planned as "extracurricular"—never by the faculty. On this occasion, after I met with the group, they invited me to join them for a gathering of the student body with their new dean. Because he had a reputation for being energetic and progressive, they were enthusiastic. I explained that I really didn't belong there, but they insisted. In our hours of sharing a different vision of medicine we had formed a bond, and they seemed to want to carry this over into the fresh start that the new dean might bring. They assured me, "You don't have to say anything, just sit with us." Unable to resist their enthusiasm, I acquiesced.

The dean finished his presentation, which was energetic and determined, but not much more than business as usual. A student—not one of those who had attended my sessions—raised his hand. "What plans do you have," he asked hopefully, "to offer instruction in other, alternative approaches to treatment?" The dean seemed not to understand. The room fell silent. "Exactly what do you mean?" he asked the student. "Well, like homeopathy, for example . . ." the student explained, his voice still steady and confident, despite the growing tension in the hall.

For a moment the dean said nothing, though his face began to turn red. Finally he said, between teeth that he seemed to clench to contain himself, "We will never teach *homeopathy* in *my* medical school!" He pronounced the word *homeopathy* as though it were both ridiculous and obscene. I wondered how many people in the room knew that I had, only moments ago, finished a talk in this same building on precisely that unspeakable subject. I could feel sweat break out on my forehead, and I began to wish I could make myself invisible.

Meanwhile the student, a senior who was doing clinical work and apparently feeling more self-assured than the lower classman, wasn't willing to let it go at that. "What experience have you had with homeopathy?" he asked quietly. Everyone seemed to hold his breath. This time the dean's face darkened from a bright red to an ominous purple. The student pushed on, his voice still relatively composed, but now both a bit plaintive and slightly defiant. "How could you be so opposed to something that you know nothing about?" he asked.

The dean stood silent for another moment. I wondered if he might have a stroke. The anxiety in the lecture hall was almost unbearable. Suddenly he turned and began to erase the board where he had outlined his prior remarks. When he turned around again, his face had resumed some of its former composure and color. He began to talk about his plans again, as though the preceding exchange had never occurred. In the hour that followed, the students seemed deflated. The optimism they had shown before was gone. I felt saddened and a bit embarrassed—as though I had witnessed an emotional confrontation in a dysfunctional family.

I've since wondered whether academic medicine will be able to assimilate the fresh currents of innovation that are sweeping through this country. I had always expected that it would be the well-trained scientists who would best evaluate and selectively weave together the emerging discoveries and advances of the brash holistic pioneers. But despite some signs that the public's interest in such subjects as acupuncture and nutrition is at last beginning to be acknowledged by the medical establishment, it still lags far behind the cutting edge, mired in its preconceptions and in its ingrained habits of the past. I seriously doubt that mainstream medicine can accommodate an uncompromising application of holistic principles because, in the course of practicing medicine this new way, a number of startling conclusions inevitably begin to suggest themselves. Some of these are radical enough to shake the foundations of the more conventional medical world. For example:

- Healing requires letting go what is familiar and stepping into the unknown.
- Healing may mean challenging belief systems and daring to break taboos.

- Healing is about getting past the ego, though that is what our culture is built on.
- Healing involves reconnecting with lost aspects of oneself—some of which exist in other than our familiar "reality."
- Healing oneself is an indispensable piece of the healing of the whole planet—our darkness is a part of the net that holds us all captive.
- Healing is the purpose of our lives.

It seems unlikely that the Radical Healing envisioned in this book will materialize in the medical centers of today. Maybe a new medical establishment will arise as the old fades. Or perhaps it will be, like our "schools without walls" and the latest "virtual universities," a movement without the buildings or faculties or tenure or the crippling inertia that has so grievously burdened our conventional institutions. In any case, whatever turn of events ultimately shapes this important development, I strongly suspect that it will remain, at least for some time, consumer-driven. In other words, it is the appreciation and implementation of this new approach by people like you that will contribute most powerfully to its full flowering.

So my advice to you is to make use of it. It's quite possible that at some point it will save your life. It's almost certain that at each turn it will *change* your life.

Seize the power. And have fun!

NATURE'S MEDICINALS

Back in 1972, when I began my search for a better approach to health and illness, one of the first books I acquired was *American Indian Medicine,* by Virgil Vogel. I pored over the descriptions of how different tribes used common plants, many of which I had known growing up in the woods and fields of the rural South. I was fascinated by the notion that nature could heal, and I felt in my bones the power of that truth.

By early 1973 I was in Lahore, Pakistan, sitting beside a *hakeem,* a practitioner of traditional Unani medicine, in his indoor/outdoor consulting booth at the edge of a dusty street. Surrounding him were shelves of hand-labeled bottles holding exotic compounds that had been patiently ground in a mortar and pestle. A year later, when I began my training in Ayurveda and homeopathy, I discovered the subtlety and complexity of such natural medicinals and the power they had, not merely to relieve suffering, but to catalyze personal growth and transformation.

After returning to America, I hauled around my kit of remedies and potions, offering them hesitantly and with some embarrassment to friends and patients. Today, nature's medicinals are quite in vogue, popping up everywhere—shiny new versions of those myriad little bottles fill shelf after shelf in health-food stores and even pharmacies. They come from many parts of the world and reflect a variety of therapeutic schools. The most widely available are herbs, homeopathics, cell salts, and flower essences.

Though each of these classes of natural remedies has its own breed of practitioner, a common thread runs through them: they are all lifted from the same living matrix that nurtures and sustains us human beings. As a result, such medicinals tend to convey complex, natural, informational patterns that can be used by the human system to reprogram the body and mind. Because these medicinals come from the larger biosphere, they encourage the kind of personal reorganization and spiritual evolution that is congruous with an overall shift toward a healthier planet. They heal us into a wholeness with Nature.

Though all of the medicinals we will explore here have the capacity to promote change and reorganization, each type provides a distinct therapeutic "angle," with herbs being used most often to affect organ systems, homeopathics for rebalancing the overall "vital force," and flower essences for addressing the dilemmas of the mind. Understanding the principles that govern the use of each class will allow you to learn to use its basic remedies and, if you wish, to stock and apply the home medicine kit detailed in Section V. Meanwhile, your personal experience with the transformational effects of natural remedies will provide a foundation for much of what you'll learn in the rest of this book.

Herbal Traditions

D r. A. came into the Center for Holistic Medicine in New York City looking sallow and breathing heavily. It had been all he could do to get himself there. He was exhausted and sick, but relieved to have made it. "I left the hospital," he said. "They told me not to, but I did anyway. I couldn't deal with all the tests and medications."

Dr. A. was a psychoanalyst of the old school. He had escaped Vienna as the Nazis arrived, and had come to America already middle-aged. Starting over in New York was no small challenge. In order to open professional doors that would otherwise have been closed to a man his age, he simply told everyone that he was ten years younger than he was. With his energy and determination, he was questioned by no one, and he'd become quite successful.

But now, at the age of eighty-six, it was all catching up with him: the cumulative professional responsibilities, the rapid tempo of New York City, and a physical constitution that had never been very strong. Under the stress of trying to maintain the pace of a younger man, all his systems had begun to fail. He was admitted to the hospital with a laundry list of complaints including anemia, chest pain, and a bloated abdomen. Whether it was due to the barrage of invasive tests he was put through there or the side effects of strong medications, he found his strength ebbing alarmingly. So he signed out "against medical advice" and retreated to his cottage on Cape Cod. After recovering enough to travel again, he came in to see me.

I looked at his swollen ankles, listened to the moist sounds in his chest, and said, "You're in heart failure!" His heart was letting fluids accumulate in his lungs and legs. "You've got to go back into the hospital . . ." I began to explain patiently. "Oh no!" he interrupted, mustering more intensity than I thought him capable of at the moment. "I'll die at home first." Hospitalization was out of the question; he'd already done that, he insisted, and it had nearly killed him.

Two and a half hours from the city was the Himalayan Institute, where we did residential holistic therapy programs. We weren't set up for intensive care, but he couldn't remain at home. Soon I installed him there and he started on a holistic program.

By the second day of his stay, I was nervous. Dr. A. wasn't getting any better. His condition was serious, and it was becoming obvious that the diet and exercise regimens we offered weren't going to do the trick. I pulled down my Scudder's textbook of Eclectic Medicine, *published in the 1800s, and studied the various herbal remedies that had been used for heart failure. I didn't dare give him digitalis unless it fit his symptoms precisely. If it did fit, a small dose would turn him around. If it didn't, the dose needed to get results could be dangerous, since foxglove, the plant from which the digitalis leaf is taken, is quite poisonous. Unfortunately, it didn't fit. Digitalis works well when there's a slow pulse, but his pulse was fast. That, along with his bloated abdomen and fluid accumulation, pointed me in the direction of convallaria, the common name of which is lily of the valley.*

"Where can I get convallaria?" I asked our pharmacist. "I can order it," he offered, "but it could take a week or more to get it. And that's if I can find a source. . . ." "I can't wait that long!" I blurted out. Hearing the panic in my voice, Kevin Hoffman, who gathered plants and made remedies at the center, said, "I know where there is some lily of the valley growing wild in the woods near here. I can gather a few bulbs, grind them in alcohol, and within a few hours, the patient can start taking it." And so he did.

I went away for a day, leaving Dr. A. on the convallaria tincture and in the capable hands of the cardiologist on our staff. When I returned, I was a little nervous about what I would find. "Did you hear what happened to Dr. A.?" I was asked as I walked in. "No," I said, turning a bit pale. "He was up all last night urinating, and he got rid of *so* much fluid! He's breathing a lot easier now and feels much better!" Dr. A. had come out of his crisis, and his improvement was steady after that.

When an herbal remedy is correctly matched to the patient, the result can be dramatic. Each plant has its own unique quality. How to harness that uniqueness is what herbal medicine is all about. Herbalists of different traditions have come up with a number of ways of understanding the therapeutic potential of each plant and of matching that to the specific people or states of sickness it will help. Most of what you'll find written on plant medicine will relate to one of the four best-known traditions, the Chinese, the Ayurvedic (from India), the European, and the Native American. Each has its own wealth of insights and approaches, and we'll explore all four, picking up a few of the most effective remedies from each. But the themes that run through all four, how they mesh, and how they seem to blend together will be the focus of this chapter.

Herbalism is a living art, continually evolving, incorporating new discoveries and assimilating older, less familiar traditions as populations shift and cultures collide. The current synthesis is certainly not the first. In fact, what happened in North America a century and a half ago provides some interesting parallels to the conflicts and clashes of value systems surrounding the emergence of holistic medicine today.

The American Eclectics

In the early nineteenth century, the descendants of white settlers in America were mostly farmers and rural folk, closely tied to the land. An independent spirit prevailed, as did a healthy suspicion of reliance on professionals of any kind. Public sentiment often turned against the harsh practices of "regular" physicians, practices such as bloodletting and purges, which were often debilitating and sometimes fatal.

During this period Samuel Thomson, who would become one of the most influential exponents of herbalism in history, grew up on a farm, eagerly picking up from his father and those around him the knowledge of natural medicine prevalent at that time. Some of this came from the folk use of plants brought from Europe, while some of it had been absorbed from the natives of the New World. As a boy of four, chasing cows in the meadow, Thomson discovered the purging effects of lobelia, a Native American remedy for cleansing the bowels, emptying the stomach, and opening the lungs. It was to become the trademark of a whole school of herbal medicine. By eight, he said, "I had a very good knowledge of the principal roots and herbs to be found in that part of the country, with their names and medicinal uses. . . ." The neighbors, "by way of sport, called me 'doctor.'" Family hardships precluded his going away to study medicine, but the ambition never left him. He stayed on the farm, and some years later, when a local physician left Thomson's little daughter to die of scarlet fever, he took his child's case into his own hands. Using steam and warming drinks, he broke the fever and cured her. The year was 1791, and he was twenty-two.

Such incidents brought him a reputation among the local people, and treating the sick gradually became his life. His success was legendary. In 1805 an epidemic, thought to be yellow fever, took half the patients who went to the regular doctors, while he reportedly lost none. But jealous competitors among the ranks of the regulars lay in wait, and when ultimately a patient he had treated died under their care, he was arrested as a murderer. Fortunately the judge was someone Thomson had cured of a serious fever, and he was honorably acquitted of the charge.

As his fame spread, Samuel Thomson became a leader in the movement to put medical care back in the hands of the common man. In 1813 he patented his system of herbal medicine, and began selling rights to practice it for twenty dollars. By 1839, 100,000 people were registered Thomsonian practitioners in this country. That was one out of every 170 people! Despite attempts to discredit Thomson, this groundswell of popular support resulted in legislation that virtually eliminated medical licensure, and put the Thomsonians on a legal par with doctors. According to popular opinion, opening medical practice to everyone, regardless of credentials, was a blow for liberty. But the guardians of organized medicine—the so-called regulars—were disgruntled if not outright frightened, and began to lay plans to recover their dominance.

Meanwhile, in contrast to the majority of the regulars, some physicians sensed the popular interest in natural remedies and, having some inclination in this direction themselves, shifted their practices toward the increased use of herbs. These "botanic physicians," as they came to be known, were the professional counterparts of the Thomsonians, the mavericks of organized medicine in their day. They were open to gentler and more natural approaches, however humble their origins. One of them wrote, "I have not thought it beneath me to converse with root and Indian doctors, and anyone who possessed any valuable remedy, or any improved method of treating disease. The hints and suggestions of experienced nurses and female practitioners have not escaped my notice."[1] That was pretty radical stuff a hundred and fifty years ago!

As the Thomsonians gained legal status and respectability, these botanic physicians, who were initially quite critical of them, began to find them more acceptable. By 1845, the two schools had joined forces and formed the Eclectic Medical Institute. This movement, founded as it was on folk medicine, became a major force for blending the herbal medicine of European origin with the herbal lore of the many different Native American tribes. The Eclectics managed to raise this synthesis to a position of unprecedented prestige and influence.

By the 1880s, the Eclectics had trained more than ten thousand physicians. Eclectic medical schools could be found in a number of major cities, especially in the Midwest. Up to this time, herbal medicine had been very much a rural folk phenomenon. To the well-heeled urban population it was primitive and grounded in superstition. Yet here was a strong professional force, practicing and promoting methods of healing that had come from country folk and Indian shamans—an extraordinary turn of events!

Eclecticism flourished through the late nineteenth century and well into the twentieth. An official pharmacopoeia of Eclectic preparations, published in 1854, went through nineteen editions by 1909. But by the turn of the century, the rising pharmaceutical industry had made significant inroads into the medical field, bringing a new philosophy of "patent" medicines that was financially lucrative. Because the largely herbal medicinals of the Eclectics did not lend themselves to economic exploitation of this sort, their competitors soon outstripped them in power and influence.[2] What's more, it was easier to prescribe the new patent medicines, and so, with the advent in the 1930s of the sulfa drugs, the first antibiotics, the ranks of the Eclectics thinned disastrously. The last of the great Eclectic Medical Schools closed its doors in Cincinnati in 1939.

In many ways the medical scene today is reminiscent of the early 1800s and the drama that played out between the Thomsonians and the medical establishment of that time. Mainstream conventional medicine has become mired in its routines, offhandedly dismissing well-researched and documented advances made by those working in the fields of nutrition, natural medicine, and holistic therapy. Sincere physicians, caught in the inertia of the current system, desperate to help their suffering patients and yet ignorant of gentler alternatives, push the use of harsh treatments beyond the point where they might be helpful. Cancer patients, for example, are routinely pressured to undergo surgery or chemotherapy, sometimes even in cases where there is no clear evidence that those methods will prolong life or relieve suffering.

Meanwhile, as a growing population marches off to the practitioners of alternative care, naturopathic medical schools are springing up around the country to provide academic training in natural medicine. They teach a spectrum of holistic traditions: Traditional Chinese Medicine, Ayurveda, homeopathy, nutrition, as well as herbal medicine. They are, we might imagine, the Eclectic medical schools reincarnated.

This reappearance of schools of natural medicine and, indeed, the larger holistic movement of which they are only a small part, suggest that we are witnessing another resurgence of the deep human need to recover our relationship with the healing power of nature. And once again it involves—as it probably always does—a return to reverence for the therapeutic potential of plants, an appreciation of that peculiar quality inherent in the plant that has the capacity to draw us back into the complex network of interacting forces that we call Nature.

Natural Remedies and How They Work

An herbal preparation is medicinal, but I always feel a bit ambivalent about calling it a medicine. That word is too often used interchangeably with the word "drug." That's why I prefer the term *medicinal.* It makes you pause and open your mind to a different sort of concept, and it's a word that hasn't been worn out yet. Another option, "remedy," sounds a little quaint—conjuring up visions of soda fountains and old-fashioned pharmacies. But it has an appeal, too, since it implies correction rather than covering up. To *drug* someone is one thing; to *remedy,* on the other hand, is a different matter entirely—it carries a sense of "setting right."

Interestingly, the word *remedy* is usually reserved for the more natural agents, such as herbs and homeopathics—and rightly so, I think. In fact, how we use the expressions "to drug" or "to remedy" in casual speech reflects how differently we see the workings of pharmaceutical drugs and natural medicinals. To me, they appear to act in exactly opposite ways.

Drugs are most often chemical compounds (usually synthetic) designed to alter metabolic reactions. They interfere with targeted biochemical processes in your body. This may reduce or even get rid of certain symptoms, but generally this happens through "biochemical manhandling." Drugs set out to wrench around a metabolic reaction, when something in the overall system is trying to make it go a different way. That "something" that keeps pushing to make things go the way they were before you took the drug is usually an outmoded way of functioning. But since it operates on a level of organization higher than the molecular, it is not set right by this approach and continues to push. You may even feel the conflict between the action of the drug and the impulse within you, so that the drug effect feels "foreign."

Often the drug also disrupts other biochemical processes in your body besides the one that was targeted. Therefore, even though your nose is less stuffy (the intended result), your alertness is diminished (interference with pathways in the brain—*not* an intended result). Meanwhile, the disease process remains. Only its full expression is thwarted. That is why conventional medical people today rarely speak of "cure." In fact, to do so is often considered suspect. They talk instead of "disease management."

Remedies are quite different in their action. They are natural substances that are chosen with the intent to *correct* an underlying problem. They prompt and support a "reorganization of the basic operating plan," so that the underlying push toward disorder is eliminated. This is often done by bringing the disorder out so that it is more obvious and can be resolved: your fever may go higher, or your anger may become more blatant. The higher fever may kill off microbes associated with your illness; the anger may sweep your interpersonal issues out into the open, where they demand attention and resolution. As a result, you attain a fuller sense of well-being and vitality, and the energy and motivation to move enthusiastically to the next challenge in your life. To understand how these miraculous results might be possible, we must dig a bit deeper into the basic nature of natural remedies.

Natural remedies are made from any number of substances plucked out of the complex web of nature: leaves, roots, flowers—even mineral deposits or insects. Each such component of the natural world has some basic quality or essence that sets it apart and makes it unique. Analysis of humans also reveals groups of similars, groupings of functional likeness: we have allergic children, adults with slow metabolism or Type A personalities.

In the Western mind, however, classes of plants and classes of humans belong to separate universes. If I asked about a similarity between the daisy and the hyperactive child, I'd be regarded as confused. One of the least known truths of natural science, however, is that there are basic organizational patterns that cut across our commonly accepted categories. A given quality or essence can underlie both the flower and the hyperactive child. This is based on the fact that both are functional components of a larger, encompassing natural order.

We have libraries of books on botany and even more on human physiology and disease, but we have lost all awareness of how these two sciences relate to one another, how their objects of study are parts of a whole. Yet two classes of "cells" in the organism called Nature—a particular plant and a specific person—*can* share a certain pattern of function. When they do, their congruence creates a resonance that can be used therapeutically.

Such patterns may be obvious in the physical appearance of the plant. Their expression in the person, on the other hand, is likely to be subtler, coloring physiological functioning perhaps, or even the way thoughts flow in the mind. For example, the aspen tree has leaves that tremble or "quake" in the wind. Its flower essence is frequently used to calm the anxious mind. Something of the nature of that plant is echoed in the person's neurophysiology and in his or her mental processes. Although this principle is quite foreign to what has until recently been considered scientific thinking, it may become a key element in the science of the future. It is certainly a fundamental part of the medical wisdom of the past.

Let's look at the principle more closely: A bowl is an expression of a circle. So is the edge of a coin or the iris of your eye. Each of these exists in a very mundane, obvious way, but the underlying pattern, the prototypical circle of which they are all examples, exists somehow in a more subtle and less obvious way. That's the "essence" or pattern of which they are all expressions.

This is not a new idea. Plato talked about it. In fact the circle is his example. It's a good one because it's one of the simplest patterns in nature. Most of nature's patterns are more complex. The way I'm functioning at this moment is an expression of some complex pattern that is not my sole property,[3] and is likely to be expressed in other places in nature—in a certain plant or mineral, perhaps. The mysterious similarity between the organizational pattern of a person who is unwell and that of a leaf or root is the key to the power of natural medicine, and the search for patterns in nature that match conditions observed in sick people is the essence of the science of healing through natural remedies.

The plant kingdom provides many opportunities to apply this principle, and many powerful remedies have been developed using this approach. Often the appearance of the plant is enough to tip you off to its possible use. For example, the ornamental dusty miller plant grew in my mother's flower bed when I was a child. I never wondered why it was called that—its surface was white and powdery looking, just like everything in the mill where my father took me to see corn ground into meal. When I heard it was used to treat the cloudy lens of early cataracts, that seemed an obvious choice.

Shepherd's purse, whose little fruit is purselike, is used as a remedy for problems of the uterus, to which it looks similar. *Lobelia inflata,* Thomson's favorite remedy, whose little flowers look like an overinflated sack, is used in asthma, where one can inhale but has trouble expelling the air taken in. In natural medicine the proposition that the structure and appearance of the plant can be a clue to its therapeutic action is sometimes referred to as the Doctrine of Signatures. If the sick person's symptoms reflect his pattern of disorder, we need a plant that will exhibit that same pattern. When the plant is introduced into the disordered person, something "clicks," and a process of reorganization occurs. We call this "healing."

It may be helpful to conceive of this reorganization as occurring first at a level within the body-mind complex that is more subtle than the physical. You might think of this as the "energy level." Just as the acupuncturist's needle will redirect the flow of energy or *ch'i* in a specific channel or meridian, so might an herbal remedy reorganize, in a more general fashion, the overall pattern of energy flow. The result, the energy shift, then has an impact on the physical body and how it functions.

THE SIGNATURE OF A PLANT
AND ITS INFORMATIONAL CONTENT

A wart, for example, is a good illustration of a disordered energy pattern. If we could step back and see the overall pattern of how a person was functioning, where he sent energy and how much, warts might look like little whirligigs of misdirected energy—energy spun off in tangential, unfocused ways—dissipated, lost. Some say that this is related to thoughts that are scattered and distracted with no very productive purpose. We might call them "worries." Perhaps a sense of this prompts our use of the expression "worry wart."

This pattern is also expressed elsewhere in nature. A good example is the arborvitae, the evergreen bush with large, vertically flat networks of needlelike leaves that first introduced me to natural medicinals. In the fruiting season, these bushes produce a strange-looking berry that is rough and horny, like a wart. The homeopathic remedy made from arborvitae that is used for treating warts (Fig. 1) is called *Thuja occidentalis,* after the old botanical name for the plant.

A patient whom I saw many years ago came in quite handicapped by a monstrous wart that covered the entire back of her foot. It looked as though she had dipped her heel in concrete, which had then hardened. Over many years she had been to a variety of doctors, to no avail. She felt discouraged and defeated. I tried several remedies including *Thuja,* but it was only when I went to a very high potency[4] that we got results. She called me, shocked and jubilant. "It just fell off!" she exclaimed. I was almost as amazed as she was.

The beauty and profundity of natural medicine is revealed in the fact that *Thuja* is not simply a remedy for warts, but for the disordered functional pattern that results in warts; this pattern is rooted in the mind. My patient with the heel wart was not only a worrier, but she and her husband and kids (who also had warts) were constantly overcommitted, overworked, and obsessively concerned about the overwhelming minutiae of their typically American lives. (*Thuja* is a commonly needed remedy.)[5]

Though the *Thuja* pattern may represent a disorder in humans, it is a perfectly normal state of affairs in this plant; clearly, the formation of warty berries by the arborvitae tree is not unhealthy. Arborvitae is one of the places where nature appropriately produces warty growth. In some mysterious way, the plant's healthy expression of this pattern is healing to us. Maybe the remedy made from it brings information on how we can integrate, master, and move past that particular organizational pattern.

The resonance between the plant used as remedy and the person needing it may occur on the level of physiological functioning—where the organizational pattern of the remedy corresponds to something that is wrong with your physical body, such as a wart. It can also occur on mental or spiritual levels, like the trembling of the aspen leaf, which corresponds to the anxiety and shakiness experienced in the mind.

This concept that nature may leave its signature on a plant, revealing by its appearance what its healing effects might be, is a part of many ancient traditions. The Chinese and Koreans use ginseng root, for example, as a sort of universal tonic for the human, because, they say, the shape of the root is reminiscent of a man's body. It will often have subroots that look like arms and legs. Westerners who consider themselves scientific

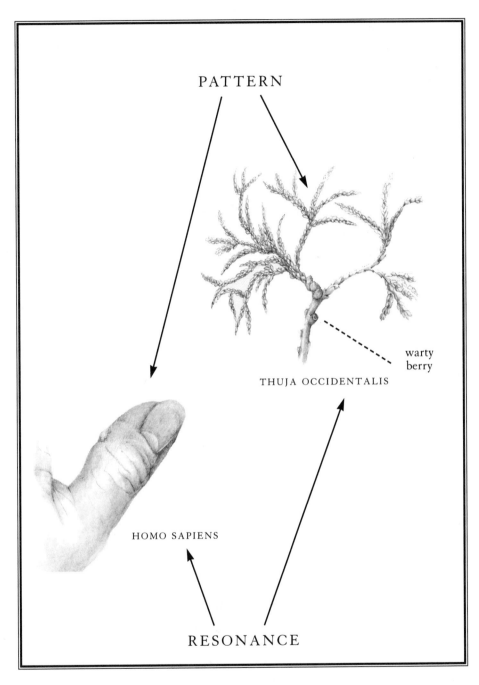

PATTERN

warty
berry

THUJA OCCIDENTALIS

HOMO SAPIENS

RESONANCE

FIGURE 1

might brush this off as a "folk belief"—a sort of superstition that is left to anthropologists to study and classify. Yet so many of the relationships that Asian herbalists have sensed between human health and plants have proven insightful that we should not be too quick to dismiss such ideas.

Medical research has supported the idea that ginseng is an adaptogen, an herb that provides broad-based support to cope with heavy demands and stresses—that is, it has a global effect on the human system. In view of that fact, it may not be outrageous to postulate that this strong a tendency to support the organizational makeup of human beings would affect even the manner in which the plant shaped some of its own structures. With this "human-organizing" informational pattern, it should not be surprising that its root takes on a vaguely humanoid form.

The principle behind this—if we can tease it out—may turn out to be cutting-edge science in the next century. Twenty years ago, physicists began to acknowledge that some of their newest conclusions about the unity and nature of matter had already been articulated by Eastern philosophers thousands of years earlier. Yet the field of biology, upon which medicine is based, has been slow to assimilate the advances of physics. Biologists have still not revised their thinking from its basis in the Newtonian mechanics of a century ago. According to that model, each cell is like a little machine with moving parts, and molecules look like clusters of balls that interact by forming or breaking chemical bonds. Though Newtonian physics might have been just the ticket for stimulating the design of those machines needed to drive the Industrial Revolution, it may turn out to be a bit crude for dealing with biological systems, and even less relevant to grasping how those systems resonate with one another.

Buying Time with Drugs

To update biological science, we might turn to an electronic/computer model to replace the old mechanical one. Here, function is altered by information introduced into the system. Just as a computer operates quite differently when new software is installed, information carried by a remedy reconfigures the "program" that manages the functioning of the organism. This is also more in line with our growing realization that much of illness is related to the mind. Up to now we haven't known what to do with that fact. We could drug the body or the brain, but it simply hadn't occurred to us that we could introduce information—via natural medicinals—that would reorganize the mind and produce a reorganization in the body. Now that our experience with computer technology is making this way of working look almost commonsensical, we find that, lo and behold, herbalists and homeopaths may well have been doing just that sort of thing for centuries.

From this point of view, each natural remedy is an informational package, and the outer form of a plant provides a rough reflection of the underlying pattern of information that it holds. Finding the right informational package for your condition and introducing it into your system at the right time are the keys to reprogramming the disordered pattern you are trying to correct. This reprogramming can take place on the physiological, energetic, or psychological level, or on all levels at the same time. In other words, when something is not running properly, take this little informational package and drop it in. If it is the right information, and if your system is ready to receive it, you experience a sudden shift as everything reorganizes. This very quickly reprograms the troubled area, leaving you running smoothly and feeling better.

Conventional drugs don't have the capacity to do this because they do not affect the level where such reorganization must take place. When you take an aspirin and your headache goes away, it's because the acetylsalicylic acid is blocking certain pain-causing endorphins, not because some repatterning of your mental/emotional or energetic function has eliminated the origin of that chain of events that produced the headache.

Since conventional medications work on the grossest physical, molecular level, any effects they produce higher up are almost always undesirable—creating disruption and disorganization. If we manage to put enough of a drug into the body, we might exert some effect on the mind, but it will almost always be negative.

When I first began my training in psychiatry, I was assigned a very disturbed patient who had just been admitted to the locked ward. I prescribed the customary drug, one similar to that still used today in such situations. To my delight, the patient calmed down and seemed remarkably less agitated. "You seem a lot better!" I enthused the next day. She studied my face for a moment. "Not really," she said. "Before, I was nervous on the outside. Now I'm nervous on the inside."

Suddenly I could see the deep suffering in her eyes. It occurred to me that although her more docile behavior was convenient for me and for the nursing staff, I might not have done her any great service by giving her the medicine. In fact, I might have pushed the agitation to a deeper level, where it was even more difficult for her to bear. That was the beginning of a disillusionment that grew in me until, years later, I was able to work consistently with patients without using drugs.

Though I do not equate drugs with remedies, since they lack the subtle and complex information needed to correct an imbalance, they can sometimes be used to "buy time." It is not possible in every situation to deal with the underlying problem immediately, and in some cases it is not even wise to try to do so. Sadly, the following incident, which occurred during my training, taught me that lesson in no uncertain terms.

> *Dr. G., one of our professors of internal medicine, had recently been taken with the role of the mind and emotions in physical illness. He was a rather abrupt and overly assertive type, and as his new perspective developed into a sort of subspecialty in the medical center, he became infamous for his views. He had strong convictions, and you simply didn't argue with him.*
>
> *On this particular occasion he had just admitted a young woman suffering from severe asthma. Reluctant to follow the customary medical regimen and cover up the evidence of her emotional conflicts, he stood over her in the emergency room—pushing her to share her feelings.*
>
> *Imposing figure that he was, the young woman was no doubt terrified, and her breathing only became more constricted. The result was a sort of impasse—one that, tragically, ended with the patient losing consciousness. All efforts to revive her failed, and she expired.*

Natural remedies can sometimes be quite effective in asthma, even addressing deeper emotional causes, but in dire circumstances it may well be more prudent to use conventional medication for the moment.[6] This will temper the crisis and buy the time needed to search for and implement a course of therapy that is properly reorganizing and genuinely healing. Antibiotics can play a strategic role in critical cases of pneumonia or meningitis, for example, but it is important to remember that the drug has not corrected the basic problem. Too often, once the crisis is over, the physician assumes he has done his job and the patient is sent home with no further advice or guidance.

Actually, when a conventional drug has been used in this way, the real work of healing begins only after the crisis has passed. The patient needs to find out what created the crisis, and to identify and address those issues in the ways we will explore throughout this book—with natural remedies, counseling, or whatever offers the potential to accomplish a healing reorganization. Since the drug has not resolved anything, but only bought time, that time should be used efficiently and carefully, for it is bought at a price.

Conventional medications clutter the delicate ecology of the internal milieu. Aside from the danger that entails,[7] we also pay for their use with the labor involved in getting them out. If used, they will need to be cleared from the body and the undesirable alterations they produced— the drug's side effects—will need to be reversed.[8] All of this requires energy and time, and, if ignored or dealt with by using another medication, will pile layer upon layer of complications over the original crisis. A large percentage of the patients I see have reached a point where they need a period of detoxification to uncover their inherent capacity for thorough healing.

Resorting to a drug to correct a human problem is analogous to dealing with a computer glitch by grabbing a screwdriver or a pair of pliers and trying to rewire its circuits. Only someone totally out of touch with the electronic age would go for the pliers when a few judicious taps on the right keys could modify the operating system and reprogram the malfunction out of existence. Any attempt to tamper with the delicate microcircuits would be absurd. Subtle interventions can produce far-reaching changes, but if you don't know which keys to tap, you might become frustrated, confused, and frightened, and feel like reaching for the pliers.

But we're not machines—not even supercomputers—and finding exactly the right natural medicinal to catalyze a healing reorganization is not a straightforward matter. There are countless herbs, and their effects may range from the subtle down to the purely physical. In order to use a natural remedy successfully, we need a way to capture the essence of its organizational message—to identify its healing potential—so that we will know when to give it. Many traditions have wrestled with this challenge, and each has come up with its own unique approach. Modern Western herbology has focused primarily on the physiologic actions of the herbs it has used.

ACTIVE COMPOUND — OR COMPOUND ACTIVITY?

Current herbalists of the more European schools speak of *febrifuges,* which drive away fever, or *diaphoretics,* which produce sweating. This

focuses attention on those effects of the plant substance that make sense
to the more reductionistic Western mind (see Fig. 2). *Carminatives* promote digestion and reduce gas. A *cholegogue* will increase the flow of bile.
Though the mindset such terms reflect is relatively mechanistic and their
emphasis is physiologic, they are regarded as quaint or "unscientific" to
mainstream physicians, since they draw on an older view of physiology
that differs from that of today's conventional medicine.

But this old-fashioned physiologic perspective is close enough to
orthodox medical thought to allow this system of classifying herbs to be
useful as a "bridging" approach, allowing those trained in academic medicine to begin, at least, to think about the actions of herbs. It served me as
an introduction to the medicinal actions of plants, and provided me with
a familiarity with some of their properties that was a valuable foundation
when I began to explore their subtler effects.

Unfortunately, much of what has been published in recent years by
such Western herbalists has been limited to research data that reinforces
this physiologic approach, and further distracts attention from the capacity of herbs to exert a fuller therapeutic effect. Certainly, herbal preparations can be used in a way that is similar to conventional pharmaceuticals.
When an herbal remedy is not properly selected so that it has a corrective
resonance on the energetic or informational level, it may simply act like
a drug. In fact, some commonly used drugs are plant concentrates, given
in doses strong enough to push far beyond the subtler informational
potential of the plant they're made from. Cocaine and morphine, as well
as digitalis, fall into this category. Though they come from plants, when
they are used as drugs their reorganizational potential as natural medicinals is ignored.[9]

Other common medicines are synthetic imitations of compounds
derived from plants. Our all-time best-selling pain reliever falls into this
category, tracing its history to white willow bark, a traditional European
remedy for rheumatism. In the nineteenth century, salicylic acid (from
Salix, Latin for "willow") was prepared from willow bark, and heralded
as a potent pain reliever. In 1860 it was synthesized, but was distressingly
bitter and had a tendency to irritate the stomach.

Later a new, slightly altered version (*acetyl*salicylic acid) was developed and sold under the trade name Aspirin. It was less unpleasant and
made its original manufacturer, Bayer, prosperous. The financial incen-
tives to duplicate this success story have been tremendous, since nowadays the altered synthetic versions are patented, and if they sell well,

---

EUROPEAN HERBS

Contribution: Rich in:
Physiology   Antidotes to Affluent Living
                                 Nervines, antispasmodics,
                                 blood cleansers, digestives

Celandine (Greater—called *Chelidonium* in homeopathic literature):
Generic liver remedy. The alchemists called it "gift of heaven."
Rheumatism, gout, insomnia, chronic bronchitis (when such conditions are related to liver dysfunction). Tincture in *limited* doses,
e.g., 8 drops in 2 tablespoons of water before each meal.

Chamomile: Calming and soothing to nervous system and digestive
tract. Steep (flower heads), covered, 10 mins.

Fennel: The seed is warming, digestive, and carminative. A favorite
after-dinner tea in Germany, and the seeds are chewed after meals
in India. "Mildest and safest" heating stimulant.

Hawthorn berries: Used to warm and tonify the heart. Considered a
digestive by the Chinese. Tincture is nontoxic (in contrast to many
cardiotonics).

St. John's wort: Recently rediscovered for its use in depression.

FIGURE 2

profits can be huge. Many former plant-derived medicinal standbys have
given way to patentable approximations of the originals. This is unfortunate, since the altered form of the compound will often act in a somewhat
different fashion from the original herbal one, and is liable to produce
toxic side effects. Even aspirin, long thought to be the ideal harmless
medicine, has been found to increase the risk of developing a serious
brain condition called Reye's syndrome.[10]

With isolated compounds, whether chemically altered or not, the
integrity of the informational pattern that the natural plant material car-

ried is lost. The complex and subtle qualities of the intact plant are destroyed when it is fractionated, and precisely that aspect of the herbal remedy which could have the most thorough corrective effect is sacrificed. Yet this has been the fate of many of the herbal remedies found in the U.S. Pharmacopoeia prior to 1941. Even Western herbalists have sometimes fallen into this reductionistic trap. Identifying and using only the "active compound" from an herbal remedy is tantamount to taking the cleverest part of a computer program, transferring it to a disk, and throwing the rest away. Unfortunately, this has been the trend for nearly a hundred years, which may be one reason the Eclectic movement ultimately failed: as herbal medicine moved from forest and farm into the academic world, it lost its soul. In an effort to scrub away its country dirt and dress it up in the trappings of scientific respectability, we lost sight of the reorganizing healing force of the intact plant.

As a result, much of the knowledge that existed in villages and on homesteads never made it to town, but died on the land, along with its practitioners. The same is true of the know-how of Native American tribes—scattered across the vastness of a continent in a rainbow of tribal cultures and languages. In none of these cases was the cumulative wisdom ever formalized or pulled together into a systematized whole. To find a way to characterize the compound effect of the plant and its therapeutic potential, we must look instead to the East. There the plant's full therapeutic potential—physical, energetic, and mental—has been formulated in such a fashion that we can apply it knowledgeably and skillfully.

The Eastern Traditions

The great Asian schools of natural medicine have, over thousands of years, plumbed the depths of herbal medicine and refined their formulations of this ancient science. Perhaps this is because the traditional way of life in that part of the world has remained intimately connected with the rhythms of the land, even while a centralized, semi-academic medical science flourished and advanced. In fact, their more consistent integration with nature may be one of the reasons that the philosophy and science of the East have proven so durable.

This durability is clearly illustrated by the example of Ayurveda, one of the oldest and most comprehensive of the Asian systems. Though we tend to think of Ayurveda as Indian, it is actually the traditional system of medicine indigenous to most of South Asia—India, Tibet, Nepal, Bangladesh, and Pakistan (known there as Unani rather than Ayurveda)—and has influenced many other traditions, Eastern and Western, as diverse as Greek, Persian, and Chinese. In fact, Ayurveda embodies what may be the most extensive herbal knowledge that exists today.

This is probably because it has long been focused geographically on the slopes of the Himalayas, where nearly every climate of the world can be found. There you don't ask whether a plant grows in the area, but at what altitude. From the tropical valleys to the arctic peaks, you can find a habitat suitable for almost any medicinal plant. This setting has provided the raw materials for the development of a highly evolved system of herbal medicine over the last several thousand years.

Western medicine is just beginning to show an interest in such remedies as *gugulu,* a resinous gum valued in Ayurveda for its capacity to clean arteries. Gugulu preparations for the prevention and treatment of heart disease and strokes are popping up everywhere now. In Ayurveda, this gum is often combined with other herbs to focus its cleansing and rejuvenative effects on the organ desired. Myrrh, a similar gum that is sometimes burned as incense, is said to have been one of the precious gifts (along with gold and frankincense, both of which are also important medicines) brought by the wise men of the East to Jesus at his birth.[11]

Myrrh is not only considered detoxifying and rejuvenative, but also has been shown to support immune response by stimulating the production of white cells, as well as by directly killing microbes. Myrrh has been more available in the West, and more a part of European and American herbal medicine, than gugulu. Years ago, when I visited the Clymer Clinic in Pennsylvania, an establishment renowned for its herbal formulas, the physician in charge shared the secret of their success with me: it was a combination of echinacea, goldenseal, and myrrh—a highly effective immune-stimulating preparation that was their herbal equivalent of conventional antibiotics and the mainstay of their practice. I still fall back on it from time to time.

The Ayurvedic tradition holds many secrets of its own, and often we find here more refined versions of what we customarily use in Western herbalism. Valerian, for example, has gained a deserved reputation as a gentle, effective, and safe sedative. It will calm frayed nerves and relax the weary, but it has a tendency to dull consciousness and make one heavy. Its Ayurvedic counterpart, *Valeriana jatamamsi,* provides the same

AYURVEDIC HERBS

Contribution: Rich in:

Taste pharmacology[a]   Rejuvenatives

Ashwagandha: Literally, "that which has the smell of a horse," gives the
vitality and sexual energy of a horse. Major male tonic and rejuvenative. The ginseng of Ayurveda. For general and sexual debility,
exhaustion, aging, loss of memory, weakness. Nurturing, promotes
deep, dreamless sleep.

*Gotu kola (Hydrocotyl asiatica/*Brahmi): Perhaps the most important
rejuvenative in Ayurveda. Revitalizes nerves and brain cells.
Increases intelligence, longevity, and memory. Strengthens the
immune system and adrenals. Also a blood purifier—used for psoriasis by homeopaths. Tea, 2 fresh leaves or grita.[b]

Gugulu: A resin similar to myrrh. A strong purifier and rejuvenator.
Many formulas. Rejuvenative for *vata*[c] ("regenerates nerve tissue")
and *kapha,* only aggravates *pitta* mildly after long use. More for
chronic than acute disorders. Used widely now for arteriosclerosis.

Shatavari (asparagus root): Major rejuvenative tonic for women, as ashwagandha is for men. Rasayana for *pitta* and for the female reproductive system. Promotes fertility. Good food for menopause.

Amla: A fruit that is the basis of many Ayurvedic preparations—e.g.,
chavanprash. One walnut-sized fruit has more vitamin C than a
dozen oranges. A nourishing rejuvenative. One of three fruits in
trifala.[d]

a. See Chapter 6, pp. 191–4, for more on taste pharmacology.
b. A grita is an herbal preparation made in ghee.
c. See Chapter 6 for explanations of the three doshas, *vata, pitta,* and *kapha.*
d. See Chapter 8, p. 306.

FIGURE 3

calming effect while making the mind sharper and more alert rather than dulling it (see Fig. 3).

The origins of Indian and Chinese herbologies are intermingled. Scholars say that the earliest Chinese book on herbs is a translation of an Ayurvedic text that probably entered China from Tibet. But the Chinese gave the use of these herbs a different twist. In the last couple of hundred years, traditional Chinese herbalists have explored and identified the effects of plants on specific organs. To take advantage of their discoveries, however, we must grasp what Chinese physicians mean when they speak of an organ.

ORGAN REMEDIES

The Chinese understanding of physiology is much less purely physical than its Western counterpart. Each organ is associated with a meridian and represents not just a single anatomical part, but a whole sphere of human functioning—mind, body, and *ch'i,* or energy. So when a Chinese traditional doctor says, "This is a kidney problem," he doesn't think only of the pair of bean-shaped organs in the small of your back, but of the fluid balance in the body, the water-based nervous system, your ability to be flexible and yielding in life and relationships, and your capacity to reproduce and perpetuate the "flow of life" into the next generation. Thus, the Chinese word *shen* is far broader and more evocative in meaning than its usual English translation, "kidney."

The complex informational patterns of plants find a congenial context in the Chinese system, where meaningful connections can be made between them and human functioning. When an herbal remedy is given "for the liver," for example, its informational package is expected to play a reorganizing role in a whole orb of functions, psychological and emotional as well as physical. Thus when Long Dan Xie Gan (a gentian and *Bupleurum* root formula) is given to quiet "liver fire blazing upward" or calm "arrogant liver yang ascending," the Chinese doctor assumes that the patient's anger will diminish. Anger is an integral part of such disruptions of normal liver function.[12]

Although Chinese medicine currently has the most highly developed awareness of the therapeutic affinity of herbs for specific organs (see Fig. 4), the idea is neither new nor exclusively Eastern. Paracelsus wrote in 1603, that "the herbs are the organs; one is the heart, another the spleen, etc." This perspective came down through the homeopaths to the

Eclectics,[13] and has been adopted to some extent by modern Ayurvedic writers, probably owing to their contact with Chinese medicine and Western thought. While any plant preparation is possessed of an integrity that will exert general effects on the person who takes it, nevertheless its reorganizing impact may be focused most predominately on a specific organ's sphere of functions and all those aspects of the person associated with it. Here are some of the target organ complexes and the herbs that have a reputation for affecting them in various ways:

Liver Though there are many herbs that act on the liver, the "generic" liver remedy is *Chelidonium,*[14] also known as greater celandine. It's a common weed in temperate areas. Though excess doses can be toxic, eight drops of tincture in a little water before meals can be tolerated for years, and is something I give nearly half of my patients at one time or another, since a "sluggish liver" is so common—as a result of such factors as high levels of environmental toxins.[15] *Chelidonium* has a wide range of applicability, in part because it is cooling, and in the terms of traditional medicine, liver derangements often involve excess heat. Most Chinese herbal formulas for liver problems rely heavily on *Bupleurum,* another cooling and widely effective liver remedy. It is said to be able to "dredge out" old sadness and anger that has been stored in the organs and tissues. There are many other liver remedies, such as dandelion root, but their uses are more specific.

Heart In the case of "Dr. A.," we compared convallaria (lily of the valley) and digitalis (foxglove), two well-known herbal heart tonics, but they are not the most commonly indicated. I was taught that the generic heart remedy is *Cactus grandiflorus* (night-blooming cereus). It is mild, effective, and especially suited to the garden variety of congestive heart failure.[16] It's an ingredient in the "gold drops" carried by German businessmen, which they drip on a sugar cube and pop in the mouth to abort a beginning heart attack. Hawthorn berries *(Crataegus)* are a good choice when there is hardening of the arteries and high blood pressure. When soaked in wine and sweetened with honey, they make a tasty tincture that stimulates digestion as well as warming the heart. (Of course, you can buy the tincture ready-made.)

Kidney/Bladder *Rehmannia* (Chinese foxglove) is the principal herb for nourishing the kidney—which, in Chinese medicine, is responsible for the juiciness of vitality. When this "kidney yin" or *jing* dwindles, we dry

CHINESE HERBOLOGY

Contribution: Rich in:
Organ affinities   Adaptogens

Ginseng: Perfect yang tonic. The adaptogen par excellence Organ affinity: spleen[a] and lungs.

Astragalus (yellow vetch): Immune support—especially against inclement weather and external stresses. Strengthens digestion (in contrast to goldenseal). Treats chronic weakness of the lungs. Energizing effect immediately (ginseng is slow). Organ affinity: spleen and lungs. Tincture.

Fo ti (Ho shu wu, Polyganum Multiflorum*):* Energizes lower centers.[b] Consolidates and strengthens lower back. Rejuvenating—promotes male and female fertility, darkens gray hair, nourishes semen and blood. Tincture.

Rehmannia: Kidney yin support/tonic—therefore for conditions of kidney yin deficiency such as night sweats, thirst, wasting, nocturnal emissions, and kidney deficiency back pains. Clears yin-deficient heat (wasting diseases). Should be combined with digestive stimulants, e.g., cinnamon.

Bupleurum: Pungent, bitter, cool. For a wide variety of liver diseases, including such serious ones as cirrhosis and hepatitis. Usually used in formulas. Strong ascending energy—used to treat organ prolapse and raise sagging spirits.

a. The spleen in Chinese medicine nourishes the entire person.
b. See *chakras,* Chapter 10.

FIGURE 4

up and age, losing our ability to reproduce. So *Rehmannia* is rejuvenative. Unfortunately, it's greasy and hard to digest, so it is rarely used alone, but rather in formulas, with digestion-stimulating herbs like cinnamon, cardamom, or ginseng. Nettle also has a reputation for being nourishing to the kidney, and sarsaparilla is a cooling herb that washes out the whole urinary tract. Sarsaparilla was boiled alone or with sassafras root, then fermented with sugar and yeast for a few hours to make root beer. Juniper berries are one of the best natural diuretics, but are pungent and heating—not so great for the acid, irritable, fiery type or when the urinary tract is highly inflamed. They can be combined with soothing herbs like marshmallow to treat bladder problems.

Uterus/Prostate Blue cohosh *(Caulophyllum)* tones the uterus. It relieves menstrual cramps and is often given as a tincture or in homeopathic form when labor stalls. Shepherd's purse *(Thlaspi bursa pastoris)* is a more cooling remedy for the uterus that soothes and quells heavy bleeding. The most popular herbal remedy now for prostate problems is saw palmetto *(Sabal serrulata)*. Though numerous studies have shown that it can shrink the common enlargement of the prostate that sends so many middle-aged men to the bathroom all night,[17] it often fails. Some herbalists insist this is because the berries used weren't fresh, while others emphasize that the dose must be sufficient (see Fig. 6).[18]

Some of the correspondences between certain herbs and the organs they help were discovered by more than one tradition. Different herbal traditions do share the use of certain herbs (see Fig. 5). A few plants, such as licorice root and gentian, will turn up in the Chinese *Barefoot Doctor's Manual,* in Ayurvedic texts, and in *Culpeper's Herbal* from seventeenth-century England. What keeps these traditions separate is not so much the difference in the plants they use as in the way they choose which ones to use, and when. To select a remedy, you need two things: a way of formulating what is wrong with the patient, and a way of categorizing medicinals according to what they do. This is what makes Chinese and European herbalists look so different. While the European herbalist may describe herbs in terms of more Western notions about physiology, his Chinese counterpart will instead mention remedies for "damp heat" or "to strengthen yin." The Ayurvedic physician uses another entirely different set of concepts. She will talk about emptying the "mucusy accumulations" related to *kapha,* or soothing the firelike *pitta.*

Much of how the Native Americans prescribed their wealth of medicinals has been lost to us. Most of what was picked up by European settlers were simple herbal cures for common complaints, while the widespread practice of using plants in healing ceremonies was ignored. Even today the more obvious herbal treatments are receiving some atten-

OVERLAP HERBS
FROM TWO OR MORE TRADITIONS

Wide use indicates their broad applicability

Ginger: Warming digestive that dissolves mucus. Stimulates yang energy. Excellent for motion sickness. Facilitates rapid absorption and assimilation of other herbs. Contraindications: high fever, bleeding, inflamed skin, ulcers. With honey, relieves *kapha,* with rock candy *pitta,* with rock salt *vata.* Dried is hotter—use fresh for deranged *vata.* Lowers cholesterol and reduces platelet aggregation.

Barberry (Berberis vulgaris): Gouty constitutions. Clears *aama.* Dissolves the stones of high living. Eight drops of tincture every 2–6 hours for acute kidney or gallbladder colic due to lodged stone.

Comfrey (Symphytum): Also called "boneknit." Reputation for healing fractures. Root is nutritive, but cooling and kaphic. Regenerative for lungs and mucous membranes. Leaves are astringent and anti-inflammatory. Leaf juice applied topically to skin cancers.

Angelica: The Chinese variety (*Angelica sinensis* or dong gui) is considered one of the primary herbs for all sorts of female disorders related to blood, menstruation, and pregnancy. A similar reputation in Native American circles, though less so among European herbalists.

Licorice: Used to improve the flavor and harmonize the effects of many herbal formulas. Quite effective in peptic ulcers—but side effects due to glycerrhizin, a cortisone-like compound. Deglycerrhizinated licorice (DGL) is often used when high doses are desired.

FIGURE 5

tion, but the ceremonial use of herbs is generally dismissed as superstition—or, at best, as having a placebo effect—that is, of creating an expectation of results that then may occur. The possibility that the informational essence of the plant's complex nature might, through the process of the ceremonial experience, be conveyed to the person needing help has hardly been considered.

Native Americans and Plant-Spirit Healing

Like the Indian and Chinese systems of herbology, the Native American approach is grounded in a way of seeing the world that is unfamiliar to most of us. The English phrase "respect for the earth" is often used to describe the consciousness of indigenous Americans, but it fails to reflect the gulf that separates their reality from ours. Animals, plants, stones, and the sky were as full of complexity and information for Native Americans as our newspapers, television, and books are for us. Moreover, these natural phenomena knit Native Americans together with the forces that shaped them in a way that we have forgotten is possible. From stars and leaves they read signs that correlated with the stirrings in their bodies and souls, and they grasped the integrity of the whole from a perspective that is not comprehensible to the intellect alone.

Grounded in such a worldview, the use of plants would necessarily be a very different process from merely readjusting physiology. It would entail communicating with the essence of the plant, using its rich significance to help weave your own existence back into a synchronous interplay with that complex web within which it is embedded. Stephen Buhner is a contemporary herbalist who has immersed himself in Native American traditions. Taking a cue from his book, I've used usnea, a lichen that grows on trees throughout North America, to treat chronic bronchitis. It recalls for me the Doctrine of Signatures. If you picture a tree turned upside down, it resembles a lung, its leaves like alveoli where gases are exchanged, and its branches corresponding to bronchi. There, distributed along the surfaces of those branches in a way that would parallel the linings of the bronchial tubes, is the gray-green lichen usnea.[19] It is a highly effective antibiotic, more active against some bacterial strains than penicillin.[20]

Buhner discovered, after sitting with plants for some years, that he could slip into a kind of half-waking, half-dreaming state during which the spirit of the plant "spoke" to him. He describes his communion with usnea; as he sat contemplating the lichen, his vision softened, and colors seemed enhanced.

> The feeling tone of usnea, usually subtle, increased in intensity of its own accord until I felt myself lost in it, my normal sense of personal boundaries dissolving. At that moment the plant appeared to me as a youngish man, hair curled and growing like the plant itself. He smiled and told me that usnea's primary function in the Earth's

ecosystem is to heal the trees; that it acts as an antibiotic for the lung system of the planet; and that its effects in humans are only a by-product of its intended effects for the trees. He went on to tell me that usnea is specific for infections in any lung system. He left, and I gradually became aware of my surroundings again, waking from the state I had entered.[21]

On another occasion he encountered angelica for the first time. Its large stalk stood nearly six feet tall. Crowned by softball-sized seedheads, it exuded a presence that stopped him in his tracks. Pausing to sit beside it, he sensed such a quiet dignity and maturity of spirit that he spent an hour absorbing its essence. By the end of this visit with angelica, he was, he writes, "struck by the feeling of 'femaleness' and strong purity of spirit that the plant emanates. It is a shy plant, rarely in great abundance. It is a plant of water—always growing near a water source. . . . It is clear that the plant sits in balance between Heaven and Earth." Rising up to carry the spirit energy between these two realms is its powerful broad stalk, which, if cut, reveals an open space within.

Some time later, Buhner introduced a troubled young woman to the plant. Fragile and unsettled, she had been diagnosed with a borderline personality disorder. She was in the midst of a divorce and in the throes of rage. She felt herself empty inside, hollow. When taken into the forest to a colony of angelica plants, she stopped, drew a deep breath, and visibly steadied, her usual tremor ceasing. Her eyes lost the rigid and fixed stare that had characterized them before. Buhner shared with her what he knew about angelica, and suggested she ask the plant to come into the empty place within *her*. When she did so, her body straightened and the lines of her face softened. As she opened her eyes again, she said, "For the first time I don't feel hollow and alone inside."

We don't know exactly what has transpired in such a healing experience. Did the young woman absorb some sense of a new way of being in the world from the gestalt of the plant? Or did the presence of the angelica plant act as some sort of catalyst that enabled energetic and/or spiritual infusions to come through Buhner from subtler levels that we don't comprehend? Whatever it was, this process of entering into communication with the spirit of a plant—or of a stone or an animal, for that matter—is an ancient and universal one.

The interrelations between plants and animals provided another rich dimension of the Native American's experience of the living nexus which held him in place. Osha, for example, *Ligusticum porteri,* which is another powerful antibiotic, has a deep connection to the bear. Bears will roll around on the plant and cover themselves with the scent. Males have been observed digging up the root, which they then offer to the female during courtship. The bear will chew the root into a watery paste and spray it over its body. The herb is active against parasites.

Osha tincture is strong-tasting and potent. I've often seen it knock out a cold or flu quickly. But, like the bear, it is a power to be reckoned with. Buhner says that if you sit in meditation with osha, "do not make the mistake of focusing on its [delicate] leaves and flower seeds. Its life and power is in the root. . . . let your mind travel down along its stem under the ground to where osha lives. There you will see it like a bear, curled in its den. When you call on osha to become your plant ally, you must have your own 'warrior' energy available.

"You do not beg osha to come and be with you. You ask it from a place of strength and power. When osha knows you are a warrior too, it will be with you and help you. People who are struggling with their own internal demons, who are trying to develop their own warrior strength— for those who fight with the darkness within—I give them osha. You must be willing to become a person of passion and strong feelings to work with osha. You must allow your rage and power to come out, to draw the line in the sand and say, 'No more. No further.' Osha goes to the root of the matter. It is a plant that helps those who are going through destructuring. It understands the stripping-away process necessary to deep transformation. It is for those who struggle to learn the truth of the bear."

In the Native American tradition, each animal is the embodiment of a specific consciousness. To find his way through the inner world, especially through those sticky places that relate to suffering and disease, the healer needed to be familiar with many of those animal allies so as to be able to access the inner space that would help in healing. The bear is a significant medicine animal because it knows about plants. To enter the inner space where your consciousness is congruent with that of the bear provides an inroad to the spirit of medicinals. Shamans go to that place, and the bear shares that space. Its herbal savvy is legendary in many cultures.

There is a story about a village on the American continent long before the Europeans came:

An old man who was covered with sores and smelled entered the village. He was very ill, and he had no possessions or food. Coming to the first lodge in the village, he asked the people there, "Will you help me? I need a place to stay and something to eat. I'm very hungry."

The people drove him off, afraid he would infect their children. They didn't want such a sick old man in their lodge. He went from lodge to lodge, and each time he was driven off. Sick and in despair, finally the old man came to the one remaining lodge in the village. Set apart from the others, it was sheltered under the branches of a great tree.

The old man approached and called for help. Seeing that he was sick and in need, the woman who lived there helped him into the lodge. She fed him and gave him her place to rest. He ate, then sank onto the bed, where he fell into a deep sleep.

The next day the man felt better, but was still too weak to go home. He ate and rested. Upon waking the following morning, however, he was much worse. The woman applied what knowledge of healing she had, but to no avail. Each day the old man became sicker and sicker. At last, having done everything she could, the woman knew the old man would die. He knew it, too, and lifting his hand, he called her over.

"I was told in a dream from Spirit," he said, "that there is a certain plant that grows in the forest that can heal me. Spirit told me to tell you of it." The old man described the plant exactly, saying, "Go and fetch it." The woman went into the forest, found the plant, and picked it with prayers and ceremony. When she returned, the old man told her of further prayers and ceremonies to use during the preparation of medicine from the plant. She followed his instructions, and after he took the potion, the old man improved. Each day he grew stronger and stronger.

But before too long, he began to fall ill again. The woman tried all the healing methods she knew of, but again it was to no avail. The old man only got sicker. Again, when he was on the point of death, he called her over and told her of a second dream from Spirit about a plant that could heal him. Again she did as he said, and again he was healed.

This happened over and over again for a year. In the end, after taking the final plant into his body, the old man grew well. He did not get sick again. Eventually he rose from his bed and went to the door.

He turned to the woman and said, "Spirit told me that there was one in this village who was to be taught how to heal the people.

I was sent to find you and teach you all I knew of healing. I have
done so."

And, turning once again, the old man went through the door of
her lodge and into the light. The woman ran to the door and looked
out. As the old man entered the forest, he turned into a huge bear.[22]

Only by immersing ourselves in the natural world can we begin to
feel of its potential and understand its logic and order. Even though the
thinking this story represents takes a giant step beyond what is usually
considered rational and scientific, much of our most intimate and sensitive of probings into the nature and meaning of healing have likely been
rooted in such an age-old sensibility. European herbalism may be physiologic in its current emphasis, but its earlier knowledge of plants was
grounded in pre-Christian earth religions.[23] Even Ayurveda, codified as
a system of medical treatment, has roots in the ritual use of herbs
described in the *Atharveda*[24] millennia ago.

It is probable that people have always tended to see the actions of
plants as physical and medical in a restricted sense on the one hand and,
on the other, have stretched to reach for the more encompassing spiritual
significance of what the plant might offer. The Native American tradition, though much of it is lost, may be our best way of gaining a sense of
the sacred in herbal medicine, because of its vision of a living Earth and
its reverent partnership with other life forms.

The perception of the plant as sacred and as possessing spiritual
power is, I think, the special offering of the Native American herbalism
to us, just as the modern European school elucidates the physiology of
herbs and Chinese herbology teaches us the relationship of specific plants
to organ complexes. In the world of natural medicine today, increasing
numbers of practitioners are following more than one tradition. We seem
to be moving rapidly toward a universal school of natural medicinals that
will capitalize on the strengths of all the healing traditions.

Each of the great schools of herbal medicine, for example, has
focused on a specific type of remedy. Ayurvedic medicine excels in the
area of rejuvenatives, such as ashwagandha and chavanprash, while
Chinese medicine is especially rich in adaptogens and remedies that
tonify such as ginseng, astragalus, and fo ti.[25] As a result, these Eastern
traditions offer a wealth of herbs for maintaining strength and vitality
even into the later years of life.

The European school has surpassed the others in exploring the use of

NATIVE AMERICAN HERBS

Contribution: Rich in:
Ritual Use   Antimicrobials

Echinacea: Herbal antibiotic; detoxifies/cleanses blood and lymph; activates white cells; less depleting than goldenseal. Vatic—combine with licorice or marshmallow. Needs to be taken every 2 hours in acute conditions. Tincture.

Goldenseal: Herbal antibiotic; clears GI tract of yeast and bacteria. Detoxifies. Removes yellow mucus. Can weaken digestion. Tincture or caps.

Osha: Potent herbal antiviral/antibacterial. Destructuring/stripping away for deep transformation. Good for cough, indigestion, and early ulceration in stomach/duodenum. Tincture.

Lomatium dissectum: Antiviral. Specific for chronic fatigue. Best to use the "isolate" (drops).

Usnea: Lichen that grows on tree branches. For lung conditions—individual and planetary. Tincture.

Saw palmetto: Reputation for prostate—but must get 160 mg. of liposterolic extract (85–95 percent fatty acids and sterols) twice daily (= 20 g. berries!) Also used for impotence, frigidity, and catarrhal respiratory problems due to cold and deficiency.

FIGURE 6

plant remedies to antidote the effects of overly affluent living: nervines, antispasmodics, blood cleansers, and digestives. Celandine *(Chelidonium)* for the liver is an example, as are barberry *(Berberis)* for stones and hawthorn for arteriosclerotic heart disease with high blood pressure. If you are faced with the consequences of a rich diet, you might look at a European herbal guide. If it's a natural antimicrobial you need, think of the Native American school, rich in herbs that can replace antibiotics. Besides usnea, osha, echinacea, and goldenseal, there are a number of others that are extremely valuable (see Fig. 6). Synthesizing the different herbal traditions yields a complex, multifaceted approach that offers the best of many. For the first time, a truly planetary herbology is beginning to be available.

When you're troubled with aches and ailments, reaching for an herbal remedy is not merely a way to escape annoying symptoms. It is a step toward returning to a healthful and sane relationship to the world you inhabit. To heal is to make whole, and part of our wholeness is our connection to the plant life of the planet. We are tied to the world of plants by an inextricable interdependence that is expressed on all levels. Plants provide us with food (either directly or indirectly, through animals), we depend on them to absorb and convert our exhaled CO_2 to the oxygen we require, and, perhaps even more important, they express the energetic and spiritual themes that knit us into a coherent and cohesive fabric of life forms—the planetary whole of which we are a part. Using plants as medicine is simply a means of reasserting that connection and revitalizing our participation on all levels.

Though recent attention has focused mostly on a purely medical or physiologic approach to herbs, the subtler psychological/spiritual impact they might have may emerge as their more significant potential for supporting profound and thorough healing. While one way to gain access to this is through the Native American approach, another is to bring out the "spirit" of the natural substance through a special process called *potentization*. In the next chapter we will explore medicinals prepared according to this principle.

Homeopathic Remedies
and Cell Salts

When I studied Ayurveda in India, I lived with a professor at the College of Traditional Medicine in Lucknow. Like many physicians who teach, he also had a private practice. In the courtyard of his home, he kept an herbal garden and a small hut where the man who made his medicinals worked. Sometimes the preparation of remedies was a laborious process. On one occasion, from my second-story window I watched the compounder grinding a powder in his mortar and pestle for hours. The next day he was at it again. Finally, I asked what was going on. My host told me about *pipali,* a sort of tree pepper, which, he said, had to be ground for eight days in order to produce a remedy that would, without fail, cure asthma.

Later I saw a Himalayan yogi pass a jar of apple cider around a circle of his students, instructing each to shake it for as long as possible. This, he explained, altered the iron in the juice, so it could be more easily assimilated and the product used as a treatment for anemia. Such elaborate preparation is also needed for other remedies besides those made from plant sources alone. Ayurvedic physicians combine minerals with herbs and seal the mixture in clay containers, which are buried in a smoldering fire, and left to bake for months. When unearthed, the pot is broken open and more herbs are added, and it is sealed again and returned to a fresh fire. This process is repeated hundreds of times. The resulting *bhasma* is highly regarded as a "purified" medicinal; even when made from a toxic ingredient such as mercury, it is both harmless and very beneficial.

It is thought that such a procedure augments the healing properties of a substance and decreases any usual adverse effects. The substance seems to be lifted to a higher level—its informational or reorganizational capacity is amplified, while its physical, material aspects are diminished. It's as though we are extracting the *essence* of the substance—that subtle formative pattern that underlies its existence—the same essential quality that can trigger a restructuring of our minds, energy, and bodies. In some schools, this is referred to as *potentization,* the process through which the healing potential is brought out.

Knowledge of this principle forms the basis of several types of European medicinals, too. One of these is the homeopathic remedy, which begins as a liquid solution and is taken through a series of steps involving shaking or *succussion* to potentize it. Homeopathic remedies are derived from plant, mineral, or animal substances—just about anything found in nature. Another potentized remedy is the cell salt, which is made by grinding one of several specific minerals to amplify its therapeutic essence so that it can be used to reorganize and rebalance metabolic processes in certain tissues of the body.

Harnessing the Therapeutic Essence of Minerals: A Primer on Cell Salts

Also known as Schuessler salts, after the German physician who developed them, cell salts are gentle, completely harmless, and quite effective in a wide range of acute and chronic problems. They are also one of the simplest, safest ways to begin to experiment with natural medicine. You can learn the basic principles of their use in a few minutes; in fact, by the time you finish reading the next few pages, you should know enough to get started.

Cell salts are created by triturating, or grinding, one of the mineral compounds naturally present in the body. Nowadays this is done with a machine that imitates the motion of a mortar and pestle. One of the cell salts, for example, is *Natrum muriaticum,* which means sodium chloride or table salt. It's great for runny noses and eyes when the discharge is thin and watery like seawater (which, of course, is essentially salty water). This makes it a useful remedy for hay fever, at least in those cases with watery nose and eyes.

You can't just use salt off the table, however. To make the remedy, you must grind the salt with lactose (milk sugar), whose sharp crystalline structure makes it particularly valuable for this process. One part of salt is ground with nine parts of lactose. This yields a one-to-ten preparation and would be designated *Natrum mur* 1x (the *x* deriving from the Roman numeral ten). The grinding is done thoroughly, usually over a period of an hour, after which one part of the resulting mixture is ground again with another nine parts of lactose. That procedure is repeated six times in succession. The result is *Natrum mur* 6x.

Though it's possible to do this at home, it's a lot easier to buy these remedies already made at the store. In your natural pharmacy or health-food store you will see the little bottles of cell salts lined up on the shelf: *Natrum mur* 6x, *Calc phos* 6x, etc. Alongside them you may see other remedies—*Belladonna* 12x or *Pulsatilla* 30C. Don't get confused. These are *homeopathic* remedies. Historically, homeopathy developed separately from the school of cell salts, though both originated in Germany at around the same time. Homeopathic remedies are often prepared on a centessimal scale, i.e., one to 100 instead of 1 to 10 like the cell salts. Hence the designation "30C"—it's been diluted (homeopaths say *potentized*) 1 to 100 thirty times. The cell salts are almost always triturated to 6x.

The idea behind grinding the mineral six times in succession to make a cell salt harks back to our notion of amplifying the subtler, informational content of the mineral. Unlike the preparation of their Ayurvedic counterparts, making the cell salts also reduces the amount of the original material with each step. But, despite the decrease in the amount of the mineral, the more you grind it, the closer you get to its essence. Ultimately the serial trituration results in a remedy that functions quite differently from the simple substance itself. Calcium, for example, can be taken as a supplement, but often it's not fully assimilated or well used by the body. But *Calc fluor* 6x seems to reorganize the metabolic reactions related to particular aspects of calcium metabolism so that they move along in a more optimal way.

If, for example, you develop a laxness in the walls of your blood vessels, the veins in your legs may begin to bulge (varicose veins)—as might those around the anus (hemorrhoids). Liver problems can also contribute to hemorrhoids, and constipation to varicose veins, but if their main cause is weakness of the connective tissue itself, then the problem is likely to show up in more than one spot—both hemorrhoids *and* varicose veins, for example—and perhaps hernias as well. This is when a cell salt—in this case *Calc fluor*—will help. *Calcarea fluor* (or calcium fluoride) is found in the elastic fibers throughout the body. When the biochemical processes involving this compound are out of balance, the connective tissue loses its elasticity.

Sagging structures will result—dropping of the uterus or bladder, for example, or loss of tone in the skin. Or disorders of the opposite extreme can begin to appear: hard, lumpy knots such as bone spurs, or fibrous nodules in the breasts. Or both can occur—the excessively loose *and* the excessively tight. *Calcarea fluor* can slowly restore the balance of these biochemical or cellular or tissue processes. Because of this effect on all tissues of a certain type, these mineral remedies have also come to be known as "tissue remedies" or "tissue salts."

Calc phos (calcium phosphate) addresses a different set of body tissues. It is invaluable for promoting healthy mineralization of bones and teeth. I've seen countless toddlers given *Calc phos* during their difficult teething months calm down and sleep better. They seem to develop stronger teeth, too. In this case I usually depart from what is customary with the cell salts and use the 3x—only triturated three times in succession. This takes us back down a bit more toward the material level, and might be thought of as more of a "tonic" than a remedy. The same is true of *Ferrum phos* (iron phosphate) in cases of anemia. Though it is customarily used in the 6x as a tissue salt, the 3x seems to work best as a tonic for supporting the production of red blood cells.

Dr. Schuessler worked with those minerals present in the tissues in substantial quantities—not only calcium, sodium, and iron salts, but also those of magnesium and potassium. In the late nineteenth century, these were the only minerals known to play a role in human biochemistry.[1] The discovery of the role of trace minerals, such as zinc and selenium, came much later, well after the turn of the century, when we had developed the technology required to detect and measure much tinier amounts of an element. The use of low potencies—3x or 2x—of these trace minerals to promote their utilization, or of 6x's as additional tissue remedies, are fields of therapy still awaiting exploration.

Therefore, in the traditional Schuessler system there are only twelve salts (see Fig. 7). These are compounds that already exist in the body, not foreign substances. They are simply potentized forms of those mineral compounds naturally present in the tissues, and as such, they serve to catalyze in some fashion the biochemical reactions that involve those compounds. By so doing, they reorganize the way the tissue functions, lifting those tissues out of their pattern of dysfunction so that they begin to function properly. The trick is to identify which tissues need this little nudge, and then match them to the appropriate cell salts.

THE TISSUE OR CELL SALTS
(ALSO KNOWN AS SCHUESSLER OR BIOCHEMIC SALTS)

Abbreviation	Usual Designation	Full Latin Name	English for Compound
CF	Calc fluor	Calcarea fluorica	Calcium fluoride
CP	Calc phos	Calcarea phosphorica	Calcium phosphate
CS	Calc sulph	Calcarea sulphurica	Calcium sulfate
FP	Ferrum phos	Ferrum phosphoricum	Ferric phosphate
KM	Kali mur	Kali muriaticum	Potassium chloride
KP	Kali phos	Kali phosphoricum	Potassium phosphate
KS	Kali sulph	Kali sulphuricum	Potassium sulfate
MP	Mag phos	Magnesia phosphorica	Magnesium phosphate
NM	Nat mur	Natrum muriaticum	Sodium chloride
NP	Nat phos	Natrum phosphoricum	Sodium phosphate
NS	Nat sulph	Natrum sulphuricum	Sodium sulfate
Sil	Silica	Silicea	Silicic acid / Silica

FIGURE 7

KEY TO UNFAMILIAR LATIN TERMS

KALI ——— Potassium ——— { KM, KP, KS }

NATRUM ——— Sodium ——— { NP, NS, NM }

FERRUM ——— Iron ——— FP

MUR ——— Chlorine ——— { NM, KM }

FIGURE 8

Don't be put off by the Latin names. They have been kept so that the remedies are not confused with the crude, unprepared chemical compound. *Calcarea* is calcium, *Kali* is potassium, and *mur* is chloride, as in *mur*iatic, i.e., hydrochloric, acid (see Fig. 8). People also sometimes find it hard to grasp the nature of cell salts because minerals seem pretty abstract compared to herbs that we may already grow or cook with. To grasp the essence of minerals, think about large deposits of them and what role they play in nature. Calcium, for example, is most obviously present as limestone (calcium carbonate), and is the crust of the Earth. Calcium remedies often deal with structural issues like the strength and resilience of bones and connective tissue. Sodium is primarily found in the sea and relates closely to water. Silica is sand, grit, glass.

Sulfur, on the other hand, is the major constituent of brimstone—which conjures up images of heat, fire, and bubbling, boiling eruptions. It is given in the higher potencies (as a homeopathic remedy) for those who are warm-blooded, hotheaded, who babble on philosophically ad nauseum, and are unkempt. Their lives seem to be a chaotic eruption of disorder—as are the itchy skin eruptions that often cover their bodies.

I once had a roommate who fit the bill perfectly. Our sofa gradually became piled with magazines and newspapers he had left open, alternating with plates and food scraps from snacks he'd nibbled while watching TV. Like an anthropologist, you could go through layer after layer, cataloging what he had eaten or read over prior days. Finally, out of desperation, one morning I gave him a dose of *Sulphur* 200C. Since he'd seen me before for medical problems, he didn't question the remedy (though he didn't know what it was—or particularly care). I came home that evening to find that he'd cleaned the whole house—for the first time ever!

Such potencies as 200C and higher address the subtle psychological expressions of the essence of a substance such as sulfur. Even in a lower potency, such as 6x, we see this same nature expressed—only in a more concrete way. Sulfur corresponds to the outward-moving physiological processes, with bubbling up and throwing off.

Now you can begin to figure out which cell salts do what (see Fig. 9). Each is a combination of two basic minerals. If you understand the essence of the individual elements, you can see how they might combine to produce a joint effect. *Natrum* (sodium) is the extracellular ion, and it attracts water. (Remember how salt in the shaker gets wet on humid days?) Sulfur helps move things from the inside out—it is an exterioriz-

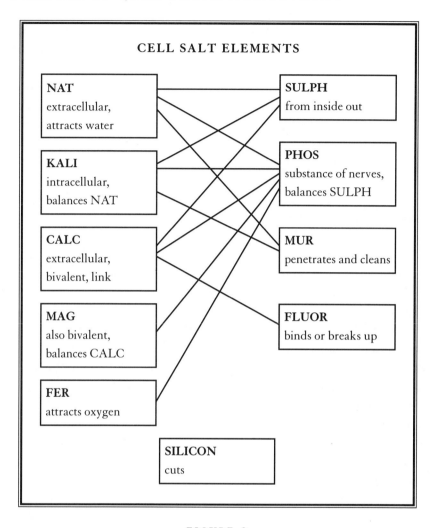

FIGURE 9

ing element. *Natrum sulph,* the combination of the two, therefore picks up water and removes it from the body. When people suffer from humidity or dampness, or they have a lot of trouble with the kidneys and bladder, with water retention and swelling in the hands and feet, *Natrum sulph* is called for.

When my eighty-five-year-old grandmother complained to me about swollen ankles, I gave her *Natrum sulph* 6x. After she had taken it for a couple of years, the swelling in her lower legs, ankles, and feet diminished dramatically. It is often thought that such problems are an unavoidable part of aging or that it is necessary to take diuretic drugs. Those drugs may force a temporary diuresis (release of fluid from waterlogged tissues), but are known to be hard on the kidneys, which usually, by the eighth or ninth decade of life, will have already lost much of their reserve capacity and will be struggling just to keep up with normal demands.

Instead of harsh diuretics, the kidneys of an older person need gentle, restorative support, which *Natrum sulph* 6x (especially when combined with *Kali mur* 6x) seems to provide. The therapeutic effect of the salts is very gradual. In such chronic cases, one will need to take them for six months to two years before the problem is eliminated. Eventually, after tissue function is thoroughly reorganized, you can see and feel the results, which usually last even after the remedy is stopped.

Tissue salts can be used for acute ailments, too. How to do so is perhaps easiest understood if we look at the salts in terms of their use in each of the stages through which an acute inflammatory process typically goes:

1. *Ferrum phos* 6x. This corresponds to the initial stage of inflammation, where there is redness, heat, and often pain. It is especially good for fevers and hemorrhage. Most of the parents of my pediatric patients now know to reach first for the *Ferrum phos* 6x instead of Tylenol or aspirin when temps go up. "I gave FP 6x as soon as I realized he had a fever, and it went down . . ." You can remember that *ferrum* means "iron" and think of a red-hot iron. Of course, it is the iron in hemoglobin that attracts and holds oxygen atoms, which in turn transform the bluish venous blood into a bright red. Red tissues, where blood has rushed in, or actual bleeding, call for *Ferrum phos.*

2. *Kali mur* 6x. The cell salt I prescribe most. It's used in the second stage of inflammation, when there is a white or grayish mucus. By this time the fever has passed and we have mucus congestion. So Mom (or Dad) switches to KM 6x. Potassium is the major intracellular ion, and *Kali mur* helps protect the integrity of the cell against viral invasions— including almost every cold and flu, as well as more serious viruses. I've heard that when smallpox used to sweep India, health workers would go from village to village ahead of the epidemic, handing out *Kali mur* 6x. Where this was done, it is said, the epidemic passed over, or there were only mild cases.

Nine times out of ten, if you do not know what else to do for common colds or flus, take *Kali mur* 6x and vitamin C and you will feel much better. In the course of my nearly thirty years as a holistic physician, the combination of vitamin C and *Kali mur* 6x has become for my patients the equivalent of "Take two aspirin, go to bed, and call me in the morning." Mostly they don't call, and if they do, they're almost always a lot better.

3. *Calc sulph* 6x. The tissue salt used when there is yellow mucus. This corresponds to the third stage of inflammation, where the process has settled in and there are signs of dead white cells that have come into the site to clean up and to combat any microbes that may be growing in the inflamed tissue. *Calc sulph* 6x cleans out the infection, making it very useful for situations like sinus trouble (at least in those cases where the telltale yellow mucus is produced.) Any cold, cough, or vaginal inflammation with this kind of discharge also calls for *Calc sulph.*

Most acute problems will involve one or more of the stages of inflammation. Often *Ferrum phos* and *Kali mur* are given together, when there are red, inflamed areas but also gray or white discharge. Sometimes *Calc sulph* and *Kali mur* are both given, as in chronic sinusitis or bronchitis.

4. *Mag phos* 6x. Often the pain that is experienced during an acute ailment comes not so much from the inflammation itself as from spasm and cramping. Where there is inflammation, tissues may be sore and tender, and muscles around the affected area will often tense up and hurt. Calcium and magnesium are known by nutrition buffs to be the answer to muscle cramps. The problem is, they may not be used well. Poorly utilized calcium can build up in the tissues, causing a new set of problems. The tissue salts won't do this.

Calc fluor and *Mag phos* 6x (magnesium phosphate) promote proper use of calcium and magnesium and are wonderful for pain due to cramps and spasms. They are very important in backache, and even *Mag phos* alone is often soothing in cases of menstrual pain. It is a great boon to tired parents with colicky babies, and it can even take the edge off the bronchospasm that results in wheezing. While it cannot produce the deeply reorganizing and potentially curative results in asthma that the higher-potency homeopathic remedies can, it will often provide symptomatic relief. With colic and irritable bowels, *Mag phos* 6x is often combined with *Natrum phos* 6x, which is the cell salt that addresses problems of gas and bloating.

There's even a tissue salt for anxiety and depression. Potassium is the main ion inside the nerve cells, and the bulk of the organic constituents

MAJOR TISSUE OR CELL SALTS

Calc fluor	Too loose/too tight: nodules and hernias
Nat mur	"The washerman": watery discharges
Nat sulph	"The dryer": edema/urogenital problems
Nat phos	Gas and gynecological problems
Fer phos	First-stage inflammation, fever
Kali mur	Second-stage inflammation, gray/white mucus
Calc sulph	Third-stage inflammation, yellow mucus
Mag phos	Spasm and cramps (anywhere)
Kali phos	"Nerve weakness," heavy-heartedness
Calc phos	Teething

FIGURE 10

of nerve tissue are phospholipids (compounds of phosphorous and fatty substances). So it's not surprising that *Kali phos* 6x (potassium phosphate) would be helpful in cases of nervousness or of weakness and exhaustion (the old term *neurasthenia* meant "nerve weakness"). Schuessler, in his original treatise, says that *Kali phos* 6x "cures states of depression of the mind and of the body." He also adds "hypochondriac and hysterical ill humor" and nervous insomnia. I give it for a heavy feeling in the chest ("downhearted").

This is a brief rundown of the main tissue salts. They cover a broad range of complaints and are very safe. With the little you have gleaned from these few pages and the use of the charts and tables here (see Fig. 10), you should feel comfortable trying them. The dosage is the same for all of them: dissolve three little tablets under the tongue four times a day. They are totally nontoxic and harmless, and if you are patient and persistent, you may be pleasantly surprised at the results.

MINERALS VERSUS HERBS

We might stop here and compare the tissue salts with what we learned earlier about using herbs. Minerals have an energy very different from that of plant preparations. They are inorganic, inert. "Dead" might be too strong a word, but in fact "stone cold" is an expression we use when all life has departed. Given as crude substances, i.e., as inorganic supplements, minerals can crowd the molecular environment. This may produce some shifts in biochemical reactions, but it's not likely to result in any real reorganization. To accomplish that would require more information, and to bring out their informational content we will need to raise them to a higher potency.

If we take that process to a very high level, for example the two-hundredth step, as we did with the *Sulphur* I gave my friend, the remedy will operate on a very subtle organizational level. His effusive messiness was a psychological issue, so the higher potency addressed it; we will deal with such homeopathic preparations in the next part of this chapter. If the potentization is more limited, the action will be closer to the physical. At the 6x, which is what the cell salts are, what we produce is a remedy that works on the organization of physical structure, that of the cells and tissues.

Herbs, in contrast to minerals, are organic—alive. They already have the informational complexity of a biological system, even without the homeopathic potentizing procedure. Although we do make homeopathic potencies from herbs, herbal remedies, even in nonpotentized form, carry a pattern of energy that corresponds to certain living systems. Their organization has a sort of coherence and shape that is organic, or organlike. That's why some herbs have the special affinity for specific organs that we saw earlier.

If you think of mineral remedies—cell salts—as working in a horizontal fashion, affecting the structural components that run through many organs in the body, then you might visualize herbs as exerting their effect more vertically, tending to affect selectively one or more organ systems. Thinking of minerals and herbs in this way may allow you to better appreciate their complementarity, and understand how you can use them together. You can take *Kali mur* 6x for congestion and *Ferrum phos* 6x for fever at the same time you are taking echinacea (as an herbal tincture) to boost your immune system. That way, you're coming at the problem from two directions. If you add vitamin C, you've got a third angle on it, and you're almost sure to get results. Commonly indicated combinations of this sort will be found in the "Self-Help Index" in Section V.

The Homeopathic Principle

You've probably heard more about homeopathy than you have about cell salts. It gets more press, since homeopathic treatment has the power to produce a more profound reorganization in the person treated. Though homeopathy shares with the system of cell salts the use of potentized preparations, homeopathic remedies are prescribed according to a different, more rigorously scientific principle than that used to select cell salts.[2]

Ancient Ayurvedic scriptures describe two approaches to treatment. One is based on a principle of contraries: if you have a fever, do something that will cool you down—sponging with cold water, for example. The other is the homeopathic (*homeo* meaning "same," and *pathos* meaning "suffering"). This approach is based on the principle of similars—in which you deal with a fever by wrapping yourself up and drinking something hot so you will begin to sweat and the fever will "break." According to Ayurveda, both principles are valid, but in some situations, the homeopathic approach is much more effective.

For example, the homeopathic treatment for frostbite would be to apply something cold, while a strictly allopathic (i.e., working according to the principle of contraries) approach would be to use heat. Abrupt heat, however, will only cause pain and aggravate the problem: If you jolt a frostbitten hand by putting it in hot water, the subtle energy will only retreat even farther from the hand, and the frostbite will worsen. You might think of frostbite as a situation in which your subtle energy has been shocked out of the afflicted part. You want to coax back that energy by conveying information about what sort of adaptive response is needed. Beginning with something cold and slowly bringing the temperature up, you gently encourage the body to marshal an appropriate response to the icy insult it has sustained.

The homeopathic principle has not been totally ignored by conventional medicine. An immunization or vaccine applies a sort of "like cures like" strategy, using the same microbe that causes a disease to convey information that will prevent it. Allergy inoculations are also homeopathic in a way, since they give the patient the substance to which he or she is allergic, in order to diminish allergic symptoms. Conventional medical researchers have trouble explaining why this works. The usual interpretation is that when dilutions of the offending substance are used, this causes a gradual "desensitization." But without acknowledging the homeopathic principle, it doesn't make much sense that one exposure would sensitize and another *de*sensitize.

From a homeopathic point of view, however, allergy shots make perfect sense. We are coaxing the body into a more appropriate response to the allergen. As a matter of fact, results are even more impressive when we use a process similar to that described for preparing cell salts: that is, the substance one is allergic to is put through a process of potentization. For homeopathic remedies it's usually serial *dilution*—shaking or "succussing" it with a mixture of water and alcohol. This procedure is repeated, using a small amount of the first solution with more water/alcohol mixture until it's been done a number of times (thirty seems to work particularly well). With this preparation of the offending substance, symptoms can be suddenly and dramatically reduced. I have seen many patients who react to ragweed get immense relief by taking ragweed pollen prepared this way (*Ambrosia* 30C).

The concept of immunization could be updated and refined by reframing it in terms of an information model. If we do that, we may discover that it's not necessary to use such large doses of the microbe to create or support immunity. A tiny bit might do the job. To help the body deal with an inflammatory process, we might make a potentized preparation of the microbe involved. Let's take the example of cellulitis—a condition that involves a spreading red inflammation around an infected wound or sore. In this sort of case it is usually streptococcus that is involved, since it has the peculiar capacity to infiltrate the spaces between the cells and produces this characteristic pattern of infection. I have seen a preparation of streptococcus, raised to the 200th dilution/potency, resolve the tender, hot, red swelling of cellulitis within hours. The same principle can be applied to a variety of illnesses. Here's such a case:

Agnes was eighty-two and a respected spiritual teacher. She was poised, articulate, and charming, but she wasn't well. She had bronchiectasis, a condition that sometimes results from chronic bronchitis. The walls of the bronchi, due to repeated bouts of inflammation, are weakened, enlarged, and begin to accumulate mucus. It's as though the normally narrow bronchial tubes become bulging pipes. Bronchiectasis is very debilitating and considered incurable because the bronchi have dilated so much that mucus pools in them, providing a perfect place for bacteria to grow. This, of course, leads to more infection and tissue damage, especially if the bacteria present, such as Pseudomonas aeruginosa, *has a special propensity to destroy bronchial walls. Unfortunately, the green mucus that Agnes was coughing up was a telltale sign of* Pseudomonas.*

Multiple courses of antibiotics had served only to subdue the bacterium temporarily. But fungal toxins, which is what many antibiotics are, also debilitate the immune system. So each time the crisis recurred, she felt weaker. Ordinarily energetic, she was in the midst of writing a book, but this illness was getting in her way. She asked tiredly, "What can I do? I've been to so many doctors, and all they do is give me more antibiotics. There has to be something else." She had started echinacea as an immune booster, and I added Kali mur 6x *and* Calc sulph 6x *for the mucus and purulent sputum. I knew that wasn't going to be enough to knock out the* Pseudomonas, *however, so I suggested she try to locate a homeopathic preparation of it.*

Ten days later she called me. She had used the herbal tincture and the tissue salts. She was feeling better, and the congestion was less. But she couldn't find the potentized Pseudomonas. *She said, "It makes sense to me. I want to take it. What can I do?" I answered, "Make it yourself." Without hesitation, she replied, "Tell me how."*

So I did: "First, you collect some of your sputum. This is better than a pure culture of Pseudomonas *anyway, because it will contain whatever bacteria happen to be growing in your bronchi. We don't know what else is in there. Mix one part of the stuff you cough up with ninety-nine parts of an alcohol/water solution. It should, for best results, be 87 percent grain alcohol and 13 percent distilled water. But don't get hung up on that. If you can't find anything closer, just use*

vodka. Shake your mixture and pour some into a glass test tube, fill-
ing it about half-full. Shake this ten or twelve times. Then empty it
and refill it again half-full with your alcohol/water mixture. What
remains on the inside of the tube will be about one one-hundredth of
what you pour in—so you have roughly a 1-to-100 dilution. Keep
emptying, refilling, and shaking. This is called serial potentization.
Do this thirty times and you have the 30C. That's what you take, a
drop two or three times a day."

She made up her potion, and when she began taking it, a lot more
mucus came out. Then it began to diminish. When improvement
stopped, she made a second remedy and took it. After several months,
she was remarkably better. There was no more green stuff, and the
amount of mucus had decreased dramatically. The cough was essen-
tially gone, she had more energy, and she had gotten her book off to
the publisher. And she was off all conventional medications.

So you *can* make your own. I've been looking for an article I read a
long time ago in a dusty old homeopathic journal. It was from back at the
turn of the century, about a nurse who went to New Zealand—one of the
earliest Europeans in that particular region of the country. There were no
doctors and no medicines. She provided the only medical care available to
the settlers. Fortunately, she'd taken a course on homeopathy and she had
a couple of bottles of wine. So, using the wine, she made her own remedies
from whatever she found lying around that the natives said was poison.
She would find out the symptoms of the toxic substance and use that as a
guide to when to give it: If she was dealing with a stinging, swollen
inflammation, she would make a remedy using the local bug that caused
stinging, swelling inflammation. Eventually, she had a whole practice built
up with her own native homeopathy that she developed in New Zealand.
Homeopathy is a very practical system, one that is open to your own creative interpretation and adaptation. By preparing a homeopathic potency,
you can introduce into the human system a healing message based on what
that particular substance is all about in the context of nature.

First Aid, Nature's Way

When you undergo physical trauma, you have an inner reaction as well
as the mechanical response of your physical musculoskeletal apparatus. If

you're hit over the head, for example, you may raise your arms in defense and your head may be pulled between your shoulders turtle-fashion, but that's not all that happens. Something inside also recoils. I was made aware of this many years ago when I was treating a young man for shoulder pain. As we tried to untangle the origin of his difficulty, he mentioned an auto accident he had been in some time before. On a hunch, I gave him *Arnica,* the supreme remedy for trauma. He came back a few weeks later, looking much better. "Now I realize," he said, "that all this time I've been, in some way that you can't see—and that I wasn't quite aware of—scrunching my shoulders up, just the way I must have at the time of the accident. I had never stopped." Now that he had released that subtle tension, his shoulder pain was gone.

Arnica montana is a plant that grows on the slopes of the Alps. Its German name, *Fallkraut* (*Fall* = accident; *Kraut* = herb), attests to an ancient awareness of its value to the unfortunate climber. As a trauma remedy it is unsurpassed. There seems to be something in its essence that is instrumental in reshaping the subtle body after it has been knocked askew by a physical insult. The Swiss make a tea from the plant, and now you can get a pleasant, non-greasy ointment made from it, which is wonderful for rubbing into sore, aching muscles.

But *Arnica*'s most dramatic effects are seen when it is potentized homeopathically. Raising it to the 200th potency seems to bring out its capacity to act on a higher organizational level in the human being. Sprains, strains, and contusions heal in a fraction of the time they would otherwise require when you use *Arnica* 200C. Each year I am amazed that no NFL team doctor has discovered *Arnica*. (Maybe one has by now.) I have always felt confident that the first team to appreciate its value would easily win the Super Bowl.

The power of *Arnica* is further reflected in the story of a patient who came to me with a number of vague miscellaneous complaints.

Jerry was a young man who had been born with club feet, and had to be operated on as a child of two. In taking his history, I was struck by the vividness of the picture he re-created from so long ago—of a stark, isolated hospital room and his feeling of being an abandoned little boy there. This was in contrast to his otherwise bland, neutral demeanor. Besides that, his feet stuck out—both in the sense of being held in an awkward position and because his oddly shaped corrective shoes called attention to them. You simply couldn't meet him without noticing his feet—they always seemed to be interposed between him and whomever else he was with.

Not knowing what else to do and feeling that it can never be wrong to address what is stuck in your face, I decided to give a remedy for the trauma of the surgery he'd had so long ago. I gave him a very high potency of Arnica—10M. This is carried through the dilution/potentizing process 10,000 times. Often the very high potencies will go deeply into the mind and emotions to deal with the roots of a disorder.

The next week, Jerry called me and asked what I had given him. "Was it some kind of sedative?" he asked. I assured him it was not. "It really knocked me out. I slept nearly two solid days." He seemed brighter after that. I felt he had let go some deep tension he had been carrying most of his life. And now when you meet him, you no longer notice his feet. They are where feet are supposed to be, and just blend in naturally.

The right remedy brings on a kind of relaxation and release—a feeling of well-being that is like a soothing balm to the body and mind. It's as though we register: "Energy rearranged, information now available for restoration of balance and order. Smooth sailing ahead." Often that means releasing the cumulative tension that we have carried as we tried to keep ourselves functioning despite a skewed organizational pattern.

Though *Arnica* is the generic injury remedy in European herbal and homeopathic traditions, it is not the only one. The Chinese use a patent herbal remedy called Yunnan Paiyao (which means "Yunnan White Medicine," manufactured in the province of Yunnan) that greatly relieves the pain of trauma and speeds healing. It is based on tienchi ginseng. Both this remedy (herbal) and *Arnica* (in homeopathic potency) are very useful after surgery. Tienchi (sometimes called pseudoginseng) is also what the Chinese reach for to stop hemorrhage.

When my youngest son suddenly developed an alarming nosebleed, I ran for a brown paper bag, tore off a piece, and folded it so it would fit under his upper lip. When I was a kid, pressing upward with such a device would usually stop a nosebleed, at least temporarily. But this time it seemed to do nothing, and as he stood over the bathroom sink, all I could do was grab ever larger handfuls of tissue to soak up the blood. I didn't have time to get out a book and begin to look for a homeopathic remedy. Instead, I found a little vial of Yunnan Paiyao and dumped a capsule's worth of powder in a hastily filled cup of water. "Here! Drink this," I ordered, lifting up the wad of tissues enough to get the cup to his mouth. He did, and within less than ten seconds he had removed his makeshift compress and was dabbing confidently at his nose. The bleeding had stopped, and—even when he blew his nose and rubbed it—there was no further blood.

Yunnan Paiyao is used for all sorts of hemorrhage. It can be sprinkled right on a bleeding wound. The European equivalent is yarrow. When I have cut myself and the bleeding wouldn't stop I have gone in the yard, grabbed a feathery sprig of yarrow (*Millefolium,* so called for the thousands of little divisions of the leaf), chewed it into a wad, and stuck it in the wound. Both the bleeding and pain stopped almost instantly. Homeopaths use a tincture of *Millefolium* to quell all kinds of hemorrhages, from nosebleed to bleeding bowels or hemorrhoids. Plantain leaves, another common lawn weed, are also useful for cuts. When my daughter had a laceration that gaped, she decided to experiment by covering it with lightly crushed plantain leaf rather than having stitches. We bandaged it and waited two days—almost afraid to unveil the results. What we found then was a line so fine that it was barely visible. I can't say there was no discomfort, however. She had complained that it seemed "too tight"—as though it were drawing shut.

Plant remedies seem to be able to affect the way tissues heal by exerting an energetic effect that is both subtle and powerful. The following story is one that sticks in my mind because it leaves such a vivid image of how the remedy works. A friend's cat had been in an accident that had broken both lower front legs. The fractures were severe and the bones were displaced at odd angles. My friend made an awkward attempt to splint the legs, but this met with little success. In hopes of providing some help, he lay slivers of comfrey root along the leg before bandaging on the makeshift splints, since he was aware of its reputation in supporting bone healing. (One common name for it is "boneknit.")

He felt pretty hopeless about the situation until about an hour later, when he heard the cat let out a sudden yelp. When he found her, both front legs were extended in front of her—rigidly straight. They went on to heal, he reported, with perfect alignment. Generations of homeopaths have used *Symphytum* (comfrey) in the lower potencies (6x or

12x) or even in a tincture as an herbal remedy to speed the healing of fractures.

Other herbal remedies prepared homeopathically have more specific uses for trauma. *Calendula* is for lacerations. *Ledum* is for puncture wounds, which include punctures by needles (injections) or by the stinger of a bee—or even by the proboscis of a mosquito! *Ledum* 30C can greatly relieve the itching and discomfort of such insect bites. *Hypericum* (St. John's wort) is the homeopathic remedy used for nerve injuries. It has a great affinity for the nervous system. The herbal tincture has been used extensively in Germany for depression—and is currently being "discovered" in the United States. The homeopathic potencies (usually the 30C) are used for trauma to the nerves. This could be a pinched nerve (with pain from the neck into the shoulder), or it could be a blow to nerve-rich tissues like fingers or coccyx (see Fig. 11).

To explain how such remedies work, the old homeopaths spoke of the "vital force." They recognized that the pattern of energy flow can become deformed, and each type of trauma has its own peculiar way of doing that. The sensation during and following a puncture wound—if you ever stepped on a nail while barefoot, you will remember—is quite different from that which accompanies the blow from a blunt instrument.

Since the vital force is misshapen in a specific and characteristic way by the particular trauma it suffers, the remedy that corresponds to that "deformation" will straighten it out. When you take *Arnica* after a bruising fall, you may feel the distortion in your energy body just melt away. Healing can occur very rapidly once that distortion is gone. By contrast, it's very difficult for healing to take place if energy is withdrawn from a part of the body. We might say today that, as the remedy is working, a sort of unconscious guided imagery occurs that accelerates the healing. On some level, perhaps, we are picturing the part restored and whole, functioning normally. A homeopath would add that such mental images are related to the vital force moving back into the traumatized part of the body. An acupuncturist might say the imagery is associated with restoring *ch'i* to the injured area. In any case, this energy or "force" brings the vitality for health and healing.

First aid and home remedies give you the opportunity to try your own hand at this healing business and appreciate personally the commonsense foundation of it all. It may seem pretty abstract to talk about homeopathy being based on the Law of Similars and conventional or

HERBAL AND HOMEOPATHIC
TRAUMA REMEDIES

Remedy	Used for	Preparation	Dosage
Arnica	the "generic" trauma remedy	30C, 200C (best); ointment applied topically	3 times a day
Yunnan Paiyao	general trauma, hemorrhage	powder or capsules	as needed
Calendula	lacerations	tincture, salve, 30C	as needed
Ledum	puncture wounds (including insect "bites")	30C	3 times a day
Hypericum (St. John's wort)	nerve trauma	30C	3 times a day
Millefolium (Yarrow)	bleeding wounds	fresh herb on wound	acutely, bandage on
Plantago (Plantain)	minor gaping cuts	leaf around cut	acutely, bandage on
Aloe vera	burns	leaf cut open, laid on burn	acutely, bandage on
Symphytum (Comfrey)	fractures	12x	2 to 3 times a day

FIGURE 11

allopathic medicine following the Law of Contraries, but when you're faced with a child with a high fever, you have to make a choice. Do you give her an aspirin and a cool bath to bring the temperature down, or do you use a homeopathic remedy, bundle her up, and hope the fever will break? Right about there it stops being merely philosophical.

The Homeopathic Method: Will the *Real* Scientific Medicine Please Stand Up?

Homeopathic medicine takes this principle of treating like with like and runs with it. If coffee leaves one wide awake and wired, what do you do for someone who can't stop his busy mind long enough to sleep? You give him potentized coffee. In fact, I have found *Coffea* 200C to be a very reliable remedy for insomnia—*if* you have the characteristic hyperalertness that goes with coffee. If you're restless but drowsy—not wide awake— forget it; *Coffea* won't help. The higher you go with the potentization process, the more important it is to match the symptoms accurately, or you'll get no results. In order to uncover the picture of what a remedy will treat, homeopaths have spent the last two hundred years cataloging what natural substances will do when given to healthy persons.

The symptoms produced when a normal subject takes an active herb is called a "proving." Belladonna ("deadly nightshade"), for example, in its crude or herbal form, will dilate the pupils and flush the face. This is the reason for its name, which means "beautiful lady." Clever courtesans would swallow tiny amounts from a jeweled medicine box to make their eyes deep and limpid and their cheeks rosy. But if they took more than a little, they would wind up with a pounding headache. Belladonna is toxic. So when you complain to a homeopath of a pounding headache and you also have a red face and dilated pupils, you'll most likely get a dose of *Belladonna*.

Though numbers of lovely ladies in bygone times have offered us what amounted to countless informal "provings" of belladonna, the use of *Belladonna* in clinical homeopathy today is much more sophisticated and is based on many carefully controlled provings using the potentized remedy. In contrast to the plain herb, the potency will produce subtler effects, such as those that are psychological. These are exhaustive, double-blind studies in which some "provers" are given *Belladonna* and others a placebo. Even by the late nineteenth century, enough of this data had been compiled to publish a hefty volume of provings cataloging the symptoms of *Belladonna*. The practice of homeopathy is based on such data.

Here's how it's done: After the substance is given to a healthy person, he or she carefully records the symptoms that result. These symptoms are sorted and ranked. Symptoms that occur repeatedly are considered strong indications for that remedy. The pattern they form is its profile or "symptom picture."

Sepia, for example, is the ink of a type of squid, long used as a pig-
ment in paints. Dreamy artists absentmindedly moistening their brushes
with their mouths may have developed the common darkness of mood
we often associate with painters as a result of ingesting sepia. When given
in potentized form to provers, *Sepia* produces a sagging tiredness and a
depressed demeanor. When someone complains of that same pattern of
symptoms, you give them *Sepia*. In other words, what causes the symptoms in a healthy person will cure them in one who's sick (see Fig. 12).
This is a very simple, straightforward principle, and there is no theory
involved here. It is pure, empirical science.

When Hahnemann articulated the basic principles of the homeopathic method in the late eighteenth century, he was intent on establishing a purely scientific medicine. He expressed his disdain for the
"regular" doctors on the one hand, with their bloodletting and violent
purges, and the herbalists on the other, with their Doctrine of Signatures,
which he felt was much abused. (One's fanciful imagination, he maintained—and there was a good measure of truth in what he said—could
lead one to see the "signature" of whatever might be convenient!) He
wanted instead an approach to treatment that was clear, concise, and free
of the problems that plagued most of medicine.

OF PROVINGS AND PROOF

One of those problems is the thorny issue of diagnosis. Though we
will delve into the intricacies of diagnosis in the next section of this book,
it is worth saying here that a number of studies have shown that conventional medical diagnoses are frequently in error.[3] Unfortunately, choices
of drugs or surgery are based on those diagnoses. Moreover, both the
diagnosis and its treatment are subject to changes in perspective—hence,
much of what was done a decade or two ago has since been discredited.
The awkward task of moving from a questionable diagnosis to an equally
questionable (though currently fashionable) medication is avoided when
one follows rigorous homeopathic principles.

When a single homeopathic remedy, developed and prescribed on the
basis of provings, is matched to a particular disorder, we essentially eliminate the need for diagnosis. It is the symptom picture observed in the
patient that dictates the choice of the remedy. The picture we are treating
has emerged in double-blind provings of the remedy. It has been shown
again and again that when the remedy is given to a patient who has

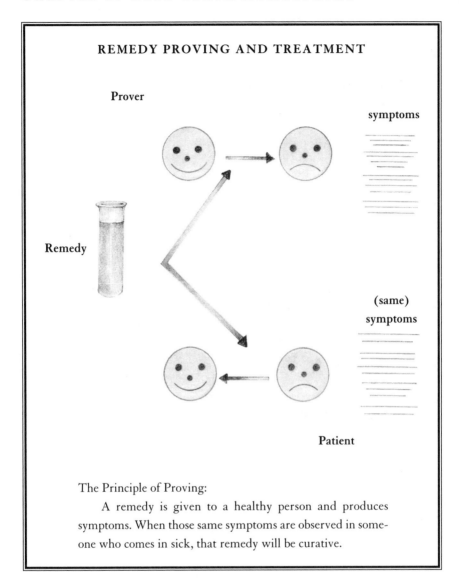

REMEDY PROVING AND TREATMENT

Prover

symptoms

Remedy

(same)
symptoms

Patient

The Principle of Proving:
A remedy is given to a healthy person and produces symptoms. When those same symptoms are observed in someone who comes in sick, that remedy will be curative.

FIGURE 12

symptoms like those arising from the provings, resolution and reorganization will result. This is straightforward and empirical (see Fig. 13).

Despite this, you will hear mainstream professionals say that homeopathy has not been proven, that it is not scientific. What should really be said about homeopathy is that it is not conventional; it is not following currently familiar patterns of drug use. In fact, it is quite thoroughly scientific—not only in the sense that it is solidly based on empirical reason-

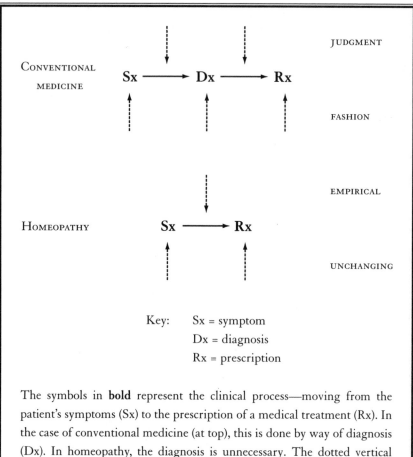

Key: Sx = symptom
       Dx = diagnosis
       Rx = prescription

The symbols in **bold** represent the clinical process—moving from the patient's symptoms (Sx) to the prescription of a medical treatment (Rx). In the case of conventional medicine (at top), this is done by way of diagnosis (Dx). In homeopathy, the diagnosis is unnecessary. The dotted vertical arrows in the case of Conventional Medicine indicate unreliable influences on the clinical process, i.e., judgment and fashion.

FIGURE 13

ing—but also because many studies have been done to investigate its effectiveness.

In 1991 the *British Medical Journal* published an extensive review article by a group of researchers in Holland on the efficacy of homeopathy. Those researchers had gone back and pulled out all the literature published in reputable medical journals on the subject, planning, it seems, to lay this issue of homeopathy to rest once and for all. They found 107 clinical trials that had been published. Seventy-seven percent of those trials showed that homeopathy worked. So they evaluated the methodology used, to see how carefully the trials were conducted. They expected to find that the studies that showed homeopathy to be effective would be the ones most sloppily performed—not good science. Instead, to their surprise, they found that in a clear majority of those more rigorous studies, homeopathy proved effective. They commented, "Based on this evidence we would be ready to accept that homeopathy can be efficacious, if only the mechanism of action were more plausible. . . ."[4]

And there's the rub. The evidence is there, but it is ignored because of the difficulty we have in accepting that nonmaterial remedies can heal. The implications of that proposition are so mind-boggling that most mainstream medical scientists, with their stubbornly materialistic orientation, simply do not want to hear about it. The principles demonstrated by homeopathy will throw into question that majority of our scientific assumptions, which are based on the primacy of matter. Rather than open this Pandora's box, the medical scientist simply thrusts his head in the sand and dismisses homeopathy altogether.

This resistance is not new. It has been in evidence since the rediscovery of the homeopathic principle by Hahnemann in the late eighteenth century. The early successes of homeopathy were not embraced by the conventional medicine of that day, either. In 1813, for example, when the remnants of Napoleon's defeated army drifted back from Russia, bringing typhus with them, an epidemic broke out in Leipzig that gave the emerging homeopaths an opportunity to test their method. By that time they had two remedies that seemed to cover the symptoms of the disease: fever, pain, and debility. One of them, however, *Rhus tox* (poison oak), was characterized by restlessness. (If you've ever had a bad case of poison oak, you may remember the extreme restlessness that accompanies the rash.) The other remedy, *Bryonia,* had shown in its proving a quite opposite tendency: provers wanted to lie down, not move, and be left alone. If bothered, they could be quite irritable.[5]

During the epidemic, these early homeopaths simply applied one of these two remedies—*Rhus tox* or *Bryonia*—depending on whether the patient was restless or wanted to lie still. This was a rather primitive approach to prescribing, but it worked. Out of 183 treated, only one elderly patient died,[6] although in those days typhus usually killed half of those afflicted. This created quite a stir. Similar dramatic results followed in the 1830s, as cholera began to plague Europe.[7]

When the cholera epidemic reached England, it provided another opportunity to compare homeopathic treatment with the conventional methods of the day. Regular allopathic medicine yielded a mortality rate of 59 percent compared to only 16 percent for the homeopaths.[8] When these statistics were collected, the information was so startling that a medical commission was sent to the London Homeopathic Hospital to check the records. Though the data were duly verified, it was decided not to make them public, and the facts were not released until a hundred years later.

STRETCHING THE MEDICAL MIND

Lest we be scornful of such suppression of information, we should acknowledge that the homeopathic pill is a hard one to swallow. Not literally, of course. In fact, it's a pleasant-tasting little pellet of milk sugar. But the concept is one to choke on. Our fixation on the world of matter makes it difficult to grasp the idea that a nonmaterial medicinal could be of any use, and with homeopathic remedies above the 12x, there is no *substance* left. After that many serial potentization steps, there is, statistically, only one chance in a million that even *one molecule* of the original material from which the remedy was made is left. There's nothing there. There's information there, but there's no *thing* there.

This is why scientists, with their limited conceptual repertoire, discounted homeopathy and concluded *a priori* that it was absurd. This is in contrast to herbal medicine, where researchers can feel comfortable with the idea that it might work if they can identify the "active ingredient" and understand its action the way they understand a drug. But there's no way you can stuff homeopathy into a materialistic paradigm. It won't fit, and the dyed-in-the-wool materialist can only insist stubbornly that it can't work. Never mind that people get better—even get well—after they take the remedies, it simply *can't work!* This is, of course, where we cease to be scientific—when we shy away from observations that don't fit our notion of how things should be. The true scientist, by contrast, delights in the "aberrant observation," the event that can't be explained by current theory. He senses that it's the key to tantalizing discoveries that lie just over the horizon. It's the doorway to a new world.

But we don't always remain true to the spirit of science. More often we get stuck in the comfort of the familiar—however boring and counterproductive that may become. We don't want to be jarred loose. It's the same mentality as the first person to experience Bell's telephone. "Where is he? There's no one here, and yet I hear a voice in my ear!" It was too much of a stretch. Mark Twain, with his concrete Missouri stubbornness, refused to buy homeopathy. He said—and we can picture him shaking his head—"It's the soup made from the shadow of a pigeon's wing."

I was hard put to believe that there was anything to it myself. After I began practicing homeopathy and prescribing remedies to my patients, I still clung to some skepticism—the residue, perhaps of my allopathic medical training. When patients told me they got better from the remedies, I would ask, almost surprised, "You did? Are you sure?" So when my teacher suggested a deep-acting remedy he felt was especially suited to me—*Calcarea mur* 1M, I was not expecting much.

I went to the pharmacy I had set up in the utility room next to my kitchen, and put a drop of the remedy on a dab of powdered lactose and let it fall under my tongue. I didn't make it halfway across the kitchen before it occurred to me that perhaps I should sit down. There was no chair, so I sat on the floor. Then it struck me that it might feel even better to lie down. I did so, and lay there on the floor, staring at the ceiling. I felt strangely wonderful. Subtle currents seemed to be moving inside me—in a way that was pleasant, yet totally unfamiliar. Getting up seemed not only overly ambitious but altogether unreasonable. I was very content to lie quietly and stare overhead.

In the morning my assistant found me still lying there, staring at the ceiling, where the light was on. This bit of nothing I had ingested had totally reorganized my energy body. It wasn't that I was disabled; it was simply that moving was such a radically new experience that I was overwhelmed by the prospect. So I had just lain there all night. After that experience, I was a complete believer. I am sure that remedies had had an effect on me before this incident, but if they had, I had not been tuned into their action. I had to be hit over the head to really get it.

It's less difficult to believe today. Intelligent stuff is finally beginning to be written about homeopathy.[9] Water molecules have the ability to shape themselves around each other and around other molecules in very complex ways. The intricate assemblage that results, researchers are now beginning to suspect, might carry a wealth of information. When we shake our bit of sulfur, for example, in a tube to make a homeopathic remedy, perhaps the alcohol that is mixed with the water in some way facilitates the imprinting of information about the sulfur onto that water. This might explain why it is that by the time we've finished, we have a highly charged solution with lots and lots of information, even though nothing remains of the original sulfur from which the information was derived.

This is the most promising perspective to date on how the homeo-pathic remedy might have its amazing effects. But the truth is that, at least for now, this theory remains a matter of speculation. Nevertheless, the fact that the remedies do indeed work is indisputable. The evidence on that is in, and the method for harnessing this healing power has been well articulated and is quite simple: (1) pin down the patient's symptom picture, and (2) match that to the symptoms of the remedy (that come from provings).

Choosing a Remedy

When Hahnemann started his work in the Prussia of the late eighteenth century, the provings that had been done were easy to remember. The first ones were done on his family, and the information was shared with the handful of his colleagues who were using the new method. But as time went on, the volume of data grew until it became difficult to keep track of it all. Thereafter the results of the provings were cataloged in a single volume listing the tested remedies alphabetically, organizing the growing number of symptoms each remedy had produced during the proving tests. This book evolved into the homeopathic Materia Medica. (Herbalists had their Materia Medica, too.)

If a patient came in with swollen neck glands, a physician of Hahnemann's time might suspect that the best remedy would be *Mercurius* (mercury), since swollen glands are a prominent symptom that emerges in its proving. Actually, Hahnemann's group knew this already, since mercury was the cortisone of his day—given in almost every disease when nothing else worked—and there were plenty of people walking around with various degrees of mercury poisoning—again, impromptu provings. They had swollen glands, swollen gums that bled easily and bad breath. But to prevent him from confusing it with other remedies that also have swollen glands as an indication, now the physician could find all the symptoms of *Mercurius,* including those brought out or con-firmed by more-formal provings: e.g., night sweats, but feeling worse, not better, from the perspiration; sensitivity to both heat and cold (like a thermometer!). All these symptoms would be found well organized in the Materia Medica. When a patient came in with such a picture, *Mercurius* could be selected with confidence and easily confirmed.

Eventually, however, the homeopathic Materia Medica became so voluminous that using it to choose remedies was impractical. Hahnemann's *Materia Medica Pura* (1826, 1828) had been two volumes, but T. F. Allen's *Encyclopedia of the Materia Medica,* published in 1887, was ten. You couldn't pore through thousands of pages of symptoms in search of a single one!

To facilitate the process, homeopaths came up with a sort of cross-reference. This was an alphabetical listing of *symptoms* (the Materia Medica being an alphabetical listing of *remedies*). Under each symptom were the remedies that could be used to treat it. If you saw swollen neck glands, for example, you would find a listing under that heading of all the remedies that produced in their provings (and were therefore used to treat) swollen neck glands. (There are seventy such remedies in current editions—though *Merc* is still one of the most prominent.) This reference work with remedy names grouped under symptoms was termed a "repertory" (from the Latin for "list")—the process of selecting a remedy being "repertorization." Thus were born the two basic reference works on which the practice of homeopathic medicine has been based: the Materia Medica and the Repertory (see Fig. 14).

Though there are now lots of simpler (sometimes too simple) books for sale in health-food stores to help you use homeopathic remedies, you can still occasionally find an old-fashioned Materia Medica or Repertory. You may even run across copies of Boericke's little *Homeopathic Materia Medica with Repertory*—the pocket manual that contains both. This was what homeopaths carried with them on house calls for nearly a hundred years. When my sister first sought out a homeopath, twenty years ago, she found herself in the office of Dr. Franklin Cookingham, a former surgeon who had converted to homeopathy and who was, at the age of ninety, still one of the best prescribers around. While she was delighted with the effects of the remedies, she wanted to know about his book. "He pulls this tattered little book out of a drawer, and all the time we're talking he's flipping madly through it. Finally, he slams it shut, throws it back in the drawer, and says, 'Here's what you should take.'"

That was Cookie's Boericke—frayed from decades of use, but as indispensable as ever. Such books are still used, but nowadays the laborious data-processing involved in remedy selection is, as you might guess, moving to an electronic medium. A computer can search the provings of thousands of remedies to see which one might have produced the exact symptom pattern in question—and do it in a matter of seconds.

This promises to revolutionize the practice of homeopathy, making it more available to people who don't have the advantage of an experienced prescriber. But because the process of finding the remedy is not merely

MATERIA MEDICA SAMPLE

BELLADONNA
(Deadly Nightshade)

Belladonna acts upon the nervous system, producing active congestion, furious excitement, twitching, convulsions, and pain. It is associated with hot, red skin, flushed face, glaring eyes, throbbing carotids, delirium, restless sleep, and neuralgic pains that come and go suddenly. *Great children's remedy.* No thirst, anxiety, or fear. Belladonna stands for *violence* of attack and *suddenness* of onset.

Mind. Delirium; frightful images; *furious;* rages, bites, strikes; *desire to escape.* Loss of consciousness. Disinclined to talk. Changeableness.

Head. Pain; fullness, *especially in forehead. Pain worse light, noise, being jarred, lying down.*

Face. Red, *bluish-red,* hot, swollen, shining.

Eyes. Pupils dilated. Eyes feel swollen and protruding, staring, brilliant; conjunctiva red; *dry,* burn.

REPERTORY SAMPLES

EYES

CATARACT—Calc. c.; *Calc. fl.; Ciner.; Euphras.;* Kali m.; Led.; *Nat. m.; Phos.;* Puls.; Sep.; *Sil.; Sul.*

CONJUNCTIVA—**Discharge, creamy, profuse**—*Calc. s.; Nat phos.;* Nat s.; *Puls.;* Rhus t.

Granulations, blisters or wartlike—Thuja

Hyperemia (redness)—*Acon.;* Ars.; *Bell.; Nux v.;* Rhus t.; Sul.; *Thuja.*

LOOK—CONDITION—Sunken, surrounded by blue rings—*Ars.;* Phos.; *Staph.*

Whites of, yellow—*Chel.;* Dig.; Merc.; Nat. p.; Nat. s.; Sep.

EARS

DEAFNESS—HARDNESS OF HEARING—Remedies in general: Arn.; Bell.; Calc. c.; Calc. fl.; Calend.; Dig.; Ferr. p.; *Kali m.; Phos.;* Puls.; Sep.; *Sil.*

CAUSE—Catarrh (mucus in eustachian tube, middle ear)—Kali bich.; *Kali m.;* Kali s.; *Puls.,* Sep.; *Sil.*

FIGURE 14

mechanical, programmers are still at work trying to get the computer to do the kind of conceptual matching of symptom picture to remedy that comes naturally to the human mind. There are certain abstract qualities, for example, that, when seen in a patient, call strongly for a remedy. If you can pick out this *leitmotif* and give the remedy it suggests, the whole symptom complex may suddenly improve.

A case in point is the bearlike withdrawal of *Bryonia*. If one is really adamant about being "left alone" (and if most of the other symptoms are listed as emerging in the *Bryonia* provings), then that's the remedy that will very likely trigger a healing shift. This mood or flavor of the picture is of more importance than the specifics of where pain might be located or which organs are not functioning properly. The intuitive process of identifying the overall picture by stepping back and getting a feel for the patient is also what makes homeopathy fun. It's like learning to scrutinize yourself whimsically until you glimpse the caricature of your weaknesses that the remedy represents.

Once the common remedy pictures are fixed in your mind, they are not really hard to peg. Folks without medical training often excel at seeing the remedy patterns in people, since they don't have so much prior programming to get past. Though there are literally thousands of remedies listed in the current repertories, there are only a few that are often used, and many of them are quite easy to grasp. Their personalities are unmistakable. Here are some examples you might find entertaining as well as useful:

> **Arsenicum.** Arsenicum album is arsenic. Titillating rumors had it for years that the Queen of England carried a little black box with her that contained arsenic. And she did—it was among the remedies in her portable homeopathic kit! Arsenic was used in times past by aristocratic grande dames to bleach their hands so they looked refined and elegant. Its connection with old lace comes as much from that as from the fact that the lady's supply might occasionally be raided to do in an unwanted spouse.
>
> The person needing *Arsenicum* is meticulous about his or her dress, vain in the extreme, and stingy with what he or she has. Drinks are taken in tiny sips, and even the diarrhea will come out in small amounts, though the patient may feel totally depleted and weakened by it. Giving even a little of anything to the world leaves the *Arsenicum* patient exhausted. Despite their stinginess and self-centeredness, they are often beautiful, sensitive, creative

people. The huge, dark, easily frightened eyes of the shy *Arsenicum* child are unforgettably appealing, but the elderly *Arsenicum* adult may be depleted, drawn, and bitter.

I was once flown to the bedside of a wealthy lady of advanced years who refused to go to the hospital for her bleeding ulcer. When she sent the delivery boy back with a glass of carrot juice because it cost fifty cents more than she thought it should have, I began to suspect that Arsenicum *might help. As I sat in her Park Avenue apartment through the night, watching her take her water in tiny sips from a silver cup, I gained more confidence. When she terrified everyone by vomiting dark blood, I felt my career was on the line—but then, as I saw her main concern was not her dire illness, but the risk of staining her elaborate lace night jacket, I was finally convinced and gave her a dose of* Arsenicum album *200C. Within a few hours she was much better, and her ulcer cleared up dramatically.*

Pulsatilla. This is the windflower—so called because it flops around with the wind, a characteristic it owes to a lack of silica ("grit") in its stem. *Pulsatilla* is the caricature of our cultural (rather weird) idea of "the feminine." Weepy, changeable, timid, craving sympathy, and highly emotional; it has been said that if *Pulsatilla* is not born a blonde, she will bleach her hair. Of course, the patient doesn't have to be blond—or even a female for that matter. In fact, one of my first experiences with this remedy was treating a man in India where I was doing intensive yoga practice.

The ashram was being remodeled, and one of the construction workers knocked on my door and asked me for medicine in a remarkably whiny and pathetic voice. His head was wrapped with a cloth, and he looked pitiable. I forget his complaint, but I was so struck by how he resembled the Pulsatilla *picture that I gave him a dose. The next day I inquired after his progress, wondering if he was still sick at home. "He's right there," said one of the other workers—pointing to a vigorous, strong man who was striding past. I would never have recognized him.*

Nux vomica. If Pulsatilla is a cartoon woman, *Nux* is the equivalent man. Irritable and driven, he is the quintessential workaholic. No matter how overcommitted, he always takes on more. We picture him, lean and dark-haired, his collar loosened as he fumes over his desk—working late, as usual. Often sullen and fault-finding, when he picks up the phone he answers curtly or snaps orders. He lives on coffee and cigarettes, though his acid stomach is not at all happy about it.

When my friend Justin came in from a hectic day, complaining of a headache and irritable stomach, I popped a dose of Nux *under his tongue before he could bite my head off. A few minutes later he looked calm and relaxed. "My headache is gone!" he exclaimed. Many of today's working women, caught as they are between the demands of two absurd gender roles, find that* Nux *in the evening for their end-of-the-day irritability and exasperation, and* Pulsatilla *in the morning for their feeling of helplessness at the prospect of facing another day, will make their lives at least tolerable.*

These classic remedy pictures are easy to recognize. You will find them simple to prescribe for common, everyday problems in yourself and your friends and family. They are safe—so it won't hurt to try. But homeopathy is not always a matter of such obvious matches. Sometimes the selection process is more creative.

On one occasion I came home to find my wife upset by our middle son's intractable cough. "He's been coughing and coughing and nothing I've tried has helped. You're the doctor. Can't you *do* something?" I was exhausted from teaching and traveling, but I got her point. Too tired to take out the books and start a systematic repertorization, I decided to lie down beside him in the bed. "This way I can soak up the essence of what is going on with him," I rationalized, giving in to the caress of the futon. I was soon drifting, but my nagging sense of responsibility, the cough of the unhappy little boy beside me, and my wife's hovering anxiety combined to keep me from totally losing touch.

She stuck her head through the door. "And he isn't urinating. He drinks and drinks but doesn't pee." I nodded and began to set sail again, borne away by the marvel of how mothers keep track of such things. Encompassing the scene, my free-floating consciousness suddenly lit up: *Spongia!* One of the classic remedies for loose cough. It's made from natural sponge. Can soak up tons of fluids without a problem—of course he hadn't urinated! Much to everyone's surprise, I sprang from the bed, fully alert, and fetched him a dose of *Spongia* 30C. Within an hour his cough was gone and he was sleeping soundly.

Of course, the choice of a remedy may not involve such poetic imagery, and inspiration of this sort isn't always to be had. When it's not, we can fall back on the mechanics of repertorization. As an example, let's say I'm given three clear symptoms:

1. Mrs. Levy, an elderly woman, has some tightness in her breathing. It's not severe, and she's never had asthma, but it sounds like wheezing.
2. Her face is paler than usual, with a bluish cast.
3. Much to her embarrassment, she's passing a lot of foul gas.

When I look in the repertory under "Asthmatic breathing in old people," I find seven remedies, among them *Arsenicum, Carbo veg,* and *Sulphur.*

Under "bluish face," I find a long list—it includes *Arsenicum* and *Carbo veg,* but not *Sulphur.* So I drop *Sulphur* (see Fig. 15).

The foul gas narrows it down one more step: I find *Carbo veg* under that, but not *Arsenicum.*

Carbo veg looks like it should be the right choice. So I flip through my Materia Medica to *Carbo veg* and, reading it, I ask her, "What would help you breathe better?" She replies, "I keep wanting to be fanned, but then I get cold and want to be covered up!" Though that seems at first paradoxical, I see that it's a characteristic symptom of *Carbo veg,* so my remedy choice is cinched.

Sometimes the poetry comes *after* the choice: In this case I find myself remembering that *Carbo vegetabilis* is charcoal—incompletely combusted plant material. *Incomplete oxidation* is the theme of the case: the digestive fire is low, so the food burns inadequately and ferments, causing bad gas. Oxidizing poorly, the patient is cold, unable to keep her body heat up, and yet craving oxygen. Inadequately oxygenated, the blood is more like that of the venous than the arterial circulation, so her face is bluish. I reflect on how savvy mountain climbers carry a vial of *Carbo veg* 30C, to help them cope with the lower oxygen levels at high altitudes, and I feel both a deep satisfaction at the poetic logic of it all, and a solid confidence that the remedy will provide significant help.

So that's the method. Look up the symptoms in the repertory and see which remedy appears under all (or most) of those symptom listings. Then read about that remedy in a Materia Medica and see if it sounds right. If it does, give it. If more than one remedy appears under most of

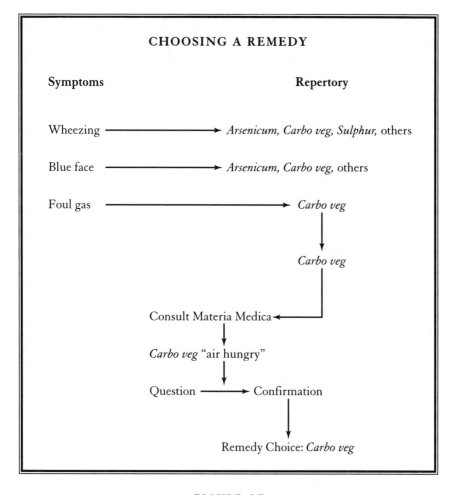

CHOOSING A REMEDY

Symptoms	Repertory

Wheezing ⟶ *Arsenicum, Carbo veg, Sulphur,* others

Blue face ⟶ *Arsenicum, Carbo veg,* others

Foul gas ⟶ *Carbo veg*

Carbo veg

Consult Materia Medica ⟵

Carbo veg "air hungry"

Question ⟶ Confirmation

Remedy Choice: *Carbo veg*

FIGURE 15

the symptoms, read each of them and see which one sounds most like the picture you're seeing in this sick person.

FROM "CLASSICAL HOMEOPATHY" TO "COMBINATION REMEDIES"

Mrs. Levy is flushed with gratitude. "The remedy you gave me for my asthma helped so much! Can I give some to my son? He has asthma, too." I explain that the remedy really isn't for asthma—it's for *her.* Until people get the hang of the homeopathic perspective, they are often perplexed. "You mean there isn't a homeopathic remedy for asthma?" As a matter of fact, there are a hundred remedies listed in standard repertories that have wheezing or asthmatic breathing in their provings. Which one we give depends on what other symptoms are present. Then we select the remedy that corresponds to that total picture. To use the homeopathic method properly, we have to know more than one symptom. Are there also headaches? Pain in the legs? Even the asthma should be further characterized—what makes it better, what makes it worse. Is it aggravated by change in seasons, is it prompted by humid weather? Do gastrointestinal upsets bring it on? It's only with detailed, accurate information that a repertorization can be done effectively.

It takes some time to learn to be a homeopathic patient. One needs to be aware of what's happening to him or herself—to be sensitive to internal events and sensations, and to report them clearly. Even though most of us have a burning desire to put all our cards on the table and tell one person our whole story so we can feel whole again, generally we're quite hesitant to do so. We've all been trained to go to a doctor for a specific problem and limit our discussion to that. Otherwise we may find ourselves chided: "I'm a dermatologist. I think you'll need to see a gastroenterologist to deal with that."

But the most effective homeopathic prescribing comes from putting the complete picture together so that you can pinpoint the precise informational package, i.e., the specific remedy, that will reprogram the entire system and move it to function better. I've seen many cases of asthma clear up almost magically when the correct remedy could be found. Practitioners who focus on finding the single most effective remedy often refer to themselves as doing "classical homeopathy." That means one remedy at a time, carefully selected, and usually given in a fairly high potency (200C and up). This work is demanding but substantial and can be of great value. That is not to say that it is the only kind of homeopathy you'll find out there. There are many other versions and they can be useful at times, too.

For example, all the way at the other end of the spectrum of homeopathic variants are what are sometimes called "combination remedies." You will see these on the shelves of health-food stores with names like "Allergy" or "Cough" or maybe even "Asthma." Sure makes it seem easy, right? No hassling with looking up symptoms and agonizing over choices. To make such a magic little formula for asthma, we might combine into one pill the top six or eight remedies that have shown wheezing most strongly in their provings. We would use low potencies—2x or 3x.

Combination remedies capitalize on an important principle in homeopathy: the higher the potency you use, the more precisely the remedy must correspond to the total symptom picture, or it won't do anything. High potencies—200C and up—should be given only when the subtler symptoms, those which have to do with the overall organization of the system and those which have to do with the mind and emotions, also fit accurately. On the contrary, the lower potencies will often act when the fit is very imperfect. Even when only one or two of the strongest symptoms correspond, there will still be some therapeutic effect. Herbal remedies are, in this sense, the "lowest potency," and can often be prescribed on the basis of a single specific symptom.[10]

So the combination remedies are a sort of "scattershot therapy," analogous to what conventional doctors will do with "broad spectrum" antibiotics: When it is not possible to find out exactly which microbe is present (or when one doesn't want to bother trying), doctors prescribe an antibiotic that will wipe out a broad range of microbes. Unfortunately, broad-spectrum antibiotics also destroy normal microorganisms in areas like the intestinal tract. Combination homeopathic remedies do not generally have this sort of downside. Their main shortcoming is that they act rather superficially—if they act at all. Sometimes they don't do anything much, though often they will reduce the severity of the symptoms and occasionally they will even provide dramatic relief. But rarely will they provide any significant, long-lasting improvement.

Nevertheless, they're easy to use and free of side effects.[11] Such a large number have been developed and tried out over the years that some formulas have evolved that are quite effective in a limited way. For many practitioners and consumers, the use of these combinations is an easy and palatable first foray into the world of homeopathics. Therefore, while the combination remedies should not be disdained or discounted, it is important to acknowledge how very different they are from single-remedy, high-potency "classical" prescribing (see Fig. 16).

When we are aiming for deep-acting, curative treatment, we will usually do best to fall back on the empirically based, solidly scientific process of Hahnemann's original homeopathic method. Here the procedure is clear. We evaluate the whole person—mental and emotional as well as physical symptoms—and we carefully match this to the symptom patterns that have been established by the provings. When we've got the remedy pinned down, we give one dose at a fairly high potency (200C or higher). Then we wait. At least, if we are going to follow this classical method rigorously, we wait. The remedy needs time to act.

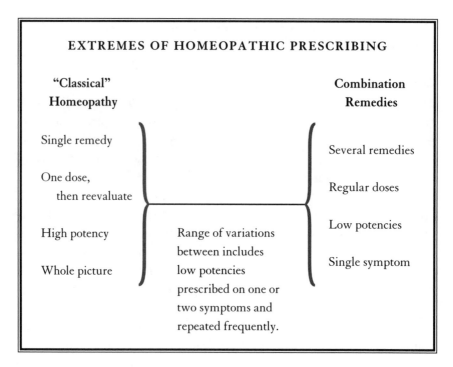

EXTREMES OF HOMEOPATHIC PRESCRIBING

"Classical"   Combination
Homeopathy   Remedies

Single remedy
                                                     Several remedies
One dose,
    then reevaluate   Regular doses

                        Range of variations   Low potencies
High potency   between includes
                        low potencies   Single symptom
Whole picture   prescribed on one or
                        two symptoms and
                        repeated frequently.

FIGURE 16

Dosage in Homeopathy:
"How Often Do You Take It?"

Allowing the remedy time to act is no small challenge, given our human impatience and fear. The classical homeopath of the last century would often refuse to make a second house call for days, despite the entreaties from frantic families, because he feared that their desperate pleas for action would pressure him into repeating the remedy or trying a new one prematurely. I have often resorted to "blank powders" (placebos)—not only so that the patient will feel that something is being done, but also so that he or she will continue to give the remedy permission to act and to observe its effects. Most of us, trained as we are in the ways of allopathic medicine, cannot really get it through our heads that a single dose of a remedy might act for days or weeks.

We get confused about how often to take the homeopathic remedy because we automatically apply what we've done with drugs. Drugs are given repeatedly to cover something up. When a relatively high potency of a homeopathic remedy is given, an informational message has been

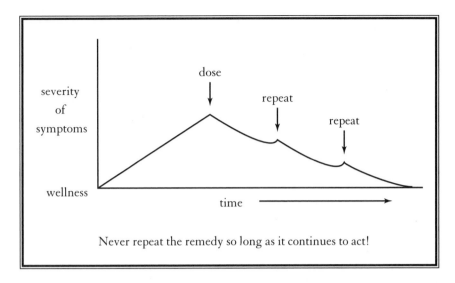

severity
of
symptoms

dose

repeat

repeat

wellness

time

Never repeat the remedy so long as it continues to act!

FIGURE 17

introduced. We need to let it be assimilated. As long as it is working, leave it alone. Don't repeat the remedy. If you stop getting better and start getting worse again, *then* it is time for another dose (see Fig. 17). Let's say it one more time: *Never* repeat a high-potency remedy as long as it is continuing to act. If you do, you may well interfere with it. I have seen patients getting better who take another dose too soon and find themselves in a rapid reversal. If you keep repeating the information, you are no longer informing, you are nagging! All you get then is resistance.

This is generally not so with herbal remedies. They are usually given with regularity. Their informational content has not been sharpened and amplified through the potentization process. It's a softer message, and requires repetition. The same is true with tissue salts or low-potency homeopathics and combination remedies. Though these remedies have been potentized to some degree, this is of a quite different order from a 200C. A 30C preparation might be considered to be of intermediate potency, and is the potency you most often will find for sale in your neighborhood health-food store or in an up-to-date pharmacy. Based on these principles, we can establish a table of durations—how long different potencies need to finish their action (see Fig. 18). These very rough approximations are not to be applied rigidly, since remedies vary in their depth and mode of action, and some will need more time than others, even when given in the same potency. But the guidelines are still useful,

CLASSIFICATION OF NATURAL REMEDIES

Type of Remedy	Potency	Usual Dose
Herbal	none or very low	2–4 times a day
Cell Salt	6x	4 times a day
Acute	6x–30C	2–3 times a day or as needed
Chronic	30C–200C	1–3 times a day (30C) every fourth day (200C) or as needed
Constitutional	200C–1M and higher	wait at least 4 to 10 days
Flower essence	not potentized (usually)	4 times a day

FIGURE 18

and even if someone else is prescribing for you, they will help you know what to expect.

The average person doing homeopathy at home will be using 30C potencies. Let's say you've suddenly come down with a fever. You feel hot, but you're not sweating. There's a certain sense of anxiety—of impending doom—out of proportion to what is probably a minor illness. All these symptoms point clearly to *Aconite*. What you have in your home kit is *Aconite* 30C. How do you handle the dose schedule? You could go one of two ways:

1. You could say, "Hmm. . . . 30th potency, three times a day," and take it every six or eight hours until you were better. Then stop.

2. You could apply the rigorous homeopathic method, give it once, and, after six hours or so, reevaluate:

   a. Are you better? If you are, are you still improving? If so, give the remedy free rein, let the improvement continue, and don't repeat the remedy.

   b. If, on the other hand, there is no improvement, or if improvement has clearly stopped or you're actually worse, then it's time to reevaluate. Maybe a different remedy is needed. Even if the *Aconite* was the correct choice, it may have done what it could do, and the result may be a new constellation of symptoms that call for an entirely different remedy.

This latter method is the most precise and accurate way of doing homeopathy. When things get muddled, you can always drop back to this careful, systematic approach and find your way out. The higher the potency you use, the more desirable it is to follow the rigorous method. But it is also a lot of work. When homeopathy is done on this basis exclusively, it becomes quite time-consuming for the prescriber. This could mean weekly—or even more frequent—visits to a practitioner, an expensive proposition. Such an approach can quickly put homeopathic treatment out of the reach of all except the most wealthy.

Therefore, homeopaths use shortcuts to simplify the business of remedy choice. The most extreme example of this is to violate the basic spirit of homeopathy and give a remedy on the basis of a disease diagnosis. Here I might say, contrary to all we've established about the fundamental method of homeopathy, "the remedy for asthma is *Arsenicum*." Of course this is not true, since more than a hundred remedies have asthmatic breathing in their provings, but if we get ten cases of asthma in our office this week, four to six of them may respond to *Arsenicum*, at least to some extent. Though this is nothing compared to what careful prescribing can do, by the standards of conventional medicine, it ain't bad. A 50 to 60 percent rate of improvement with no risk of side effects is quite good, in fact, and in some situations, the results of such an approach can be even better.

One of the best examples is *Kali bichromicum* for sinusitis. Sinus inflammation and infection is such a strong, consistent aspect of the proving of *Kali bichromicum,* and the picture it produces—thick, stringy mucus and pressing pain at the root of the nose—is so similar to the type of sinus problem prevalent currently, that probably upwards of 80 percent of cases of sinusitis will respond to *Kali bichromicum.* Of course the other 20 percent need a careful study of the homeopathic repertory. So a practical way of approaching sinusitis clinically (since it is not a life-threatening condition) is to start with *Kali bichromicum,* and if it doesn't do the job, then undertake a repertorization.

The use of a remedy for a disease, though it flies in the face of homeo-pathic rules, is a common practice. Homeopaths even have a name for remedies used this way; they call them "specifics." *Kali bichromicum* is a specific for sinusitis, *Coffea cruda* for insomnia. Though the classical pre-scriber, who adheres strictly to the rule of single dose of a single remedy prescribed on the basis of a thorough evaluation of all symptoms, may see red if you mention specifics, chances are there are times when he or she also leans in this direction—albeit discreetly and inconspicuously. It may be merely that when you mention sinusitis, he flips immediately to *Kali bichromicum* in his Materia Medica and reads it first to see if it will encompass all your symptoms, instead of starting with an impartial repertorization.

Another shortcut is to prescribe repetition of the remedy. This is fre-quently done with a specific: I was taught that *Kali bichromicum* 200C should be taken every four days for chronic cases of sinusitis. This is also done in other cases where the remedy is being used for a chronic disorder that is deeply ingrained in the person's habits of functioning. I have given my youngest son *Sulphur* 200C each week for years, and watched his will-ingness to wash his hands or take a bath slowly increase! Again, this is an obvious violation of the "rules"—which say, "Never repeat the remedy without ascertaining whether its action is exhausted. . . ." Inappropriate repetition can produce provings, and such a shortcut should be used only on the recommendation of a trained practitioner; some remedies bear repetition while others do not. Where repetition can be of most value is with what are commonly referred to as "constitutional remedies."

What's Your Constitutional Remedy?

What we've dealt with so far is mostly the treatment of conditions that are a departure from your customary way of functioning. You get a fever or you start wheezing, and you say, "Something is wrong! I'm sick!" But other problems from which you suffer may be so much a part of the sta-tus quo that you may not even notice them. Or, if you do, you may sim-

COMMONLY USED HOMEOPATHIC REMEDIES

Arsenicum   restless but weak and exhausted; fearful, selfish; burning pains better from heat; thin excoriating discharges

Belladonna   flushed face, dilated pupils; near delirium, headache worse from sudden movement

Bryonia   just wants to be left alone; everything worse from motion; mucous membranes all dry

Carbo veg   incomplete oxidation; weak digestion, bad gas; cold sweat, craves air

Merc sol   swollen glands, thick indented tongue; copious sweat that fails to relieve; sensitive to heat *and* cold

Nux vom   ill-tempered adrenaline junkie; stomach irritated by stimulants; miscellaneous ailments from stress

Pulsatilla   weepy, changeable, contradictory; chilly but better outdoors; rarely thirsty; copious bland discharges

Rhus tox   restless but stiff and painful on starting to move ("the rusty hinge"); worse cold or wet

Remedies sometimes used as "specifics"*:

Ambrosia   hayfever (runny nose, sneezing, itchy eyes)
                  (this is potentized ragweed)

Coffea cruda   insomnia (racing thoughts, hyperalertness)
                  (this is potentized coffee)

Kali bichromicum sinusitis (pressure at root of nose; thick, stringy mucus)

*See page 91. While these remedies are sometimes—contrary to all principles of homeopathy—used for the disorders mentioned, this shortcut will only work if the disease has the characteristics noted in parentheses. (That brings it into alignment with the provings.)

FIGURE 19

ply say, "That's just the way I am." These are constitutional disorders. Sometimes they nag at us enough that we go in to the doctor and say, "I've had this problem all my life, but it's bothering me so much now that I have to do something about it!" In evaluating such a case, the skilled homeopath may set aside any acute complaints—and even some longer-term ones—to focus instead on the constitutional "soil" from which those problems arose. She will look not only at the very long-term "all my life" symptoms brought up by the patient, but also observe characteristic features of the person that he or she might never have identified as symptoms at all.

For example, people with a *Calcarea carb* constitution are often large-framed. *Calcarea carb* is limestone. To the homeopathic constitutional prescriber, the crust of the earth, which is predominantly limestone, is its skeleton. The whole earth is one big, hulking *Calcarea carb* body. So, when a big, hulking *Calcarea carb* body walks into your office, you give potentized limestone and it will often make an astounding difference: Weight may be shed with little or no change in habits of diet and exercise. Cracked skin on the heels and fingertips closes up. The patient's tendency to overgrow and burst out of his or her limits is at least mollified.

What goes on during this transformation? We might theorize that through the action of the homeopathic preparation of calcium carbonate, some subtle attunement between the individual and the whole of nature is adjusted. Perhaps a realignment with the overall complex of natural forces allows the ego to give up its need to be huge and hulking in favor of the contentment of participating in the hugeness of the living Earth itself. In any case, things do change, and often the person taking the remedy loses weight. (This does not mean that *Calcarea carb* is a specific for obesity; it will help a person lose weight only when the whole picture of the *Calcarea carb* constitution is present.)

Homeopathy takes the material substance and raises it to "a higher octave" by bringing out its subtler aspects and using them therapeutically. When the picture formed by these subtler effects is matched to the constitutional nature of the patient, profound changes in life patterns can occur. The remedy cannot impose a foreign or dysfunctional pattern on you, unless it is given in error and repeated many times. Such a result, called a proving, would end when you stop taking the remedy (at worst it would need to be antidoted). What the remedy *can* do, however, is bring into evidence patterns of functioning that affect you strongly, but have operated outside of awareness. The action of the remedy then helps

FREQUENTLY USED CONSTITUTIONAL REMEDIES

Calcarea carb   large-framed (limestone), limp hands (oyster), fearful

Natrum mur   stoic, suffers alone; headaches/eye problems, craves salt

Sepia   sad, sagging, loss of libido and feelings for family

Staphysagria   sexual excess/preoccupation; urogenital problems; explosive suppressed anger

Sulphur   messy, the "ragged philosopher"; warm-blooded and hotheaded

Sometimes considered constitutional:*

Arsenicum   selfish and vain; burning pains better with heat; beautiful and artistic

Nux vomica   irritable workaholic, runs on stimulants; digestive distress

Pulsatilla   weepy, symptoms and feelings very changeable; better outdoors

*Some would say a *Nux* "type" may still have a *Staphys* constitution.

FIGURE 20

you move toward resolving the buried issue, so that the energy that had been invested in it and the energy that had been used to keep it out of consciousness become available.

Sepia is a powerful constitutional remedy, especially useful in those who are dragged out, weary, and depressed—*if* they fit the whole *Sepia* picture. Other constitutional remedies we have touched upon are *Sulphur* and (one that is grossly underutilized) *Calcarea mur. Staphysagria* is one of our most valuable and frequently indicated constitutional remedies. It corresponds to hypersensitivity to criticism, suppressed anger, and sexual preoccupation. *Staphys* patients often crave tobacco or ice cream, and are often ravenously hungry even when full. Their teeth tend to stain, and as they age, their gums retract—making them noticeably "long in the tooth." They are given to bladder infections and prostate problems, and their unexpressed explosive anger is so palpable that they are always on edge. Have you ever felt that undefinable but intense discomfort when a fingernail scrapes audibly across a blackboard? Have you ever had a paper cut? It's that sort of retracting, agonizing irritability that permeates the life of the *Staphys* type. Sound familiar? Sometimes fighting the angry frustration of a rush-hour traffic jam, I ponder the ethics of putting *Staphys* 200C in the water supply. . . .

A few of the remedies that we have described as useful in acute situations are also sometimes considered constitutional remedies. *Nux vomica* for the stressed-out workaholic is one of those, as is *Pulsatilla* for those who are weepy, changeable, and hyperemotional. Some would call these remedies for "types" rather than constitutions—there is not total agreement on the use of such terms in homeopathy. I would tend to say, "He's a *Nux* type, and will need it from time to time, but his basic constitution is *Staphysagria*" (or whatever it might be). There are, however, a few constitutional remedies that are widely recognized as being commonly indicated and very powerful. *Calcarea carb* is one of those. *Natrum mur* is another (see Fig. 20).

You can eat table salt and it won't give you any therapeutic effect. You can take the tissue remedy made from it and it will affect a whole set of tissues in your body. But if you take the homeopathic remedy *Natrum mur,* raised to a higher potency, it can correct constitutional imbalances—overall patterns of physiological functioning, psychological and emotional conflicts, and even feelings of spiritual disorientation and confusion. A good example of this involves a man who came to see me because he was suffering from severe headaches.

> *Dr. D. was a widely respected physician who had tried everything to relieve his headaches, including a great deal of pain medication, which had given him an ulcer. I recommended that he learn meditation and relaxation techniques. These helped a little bit, but his headaches persisted. I had given him homeopathic remedies from time to time and he had taken them, not because he gave them any credence at all, but rather, I suspect, to humor me. He liked me and*

thought that I helped him in other ways—to look at what was happening in his life and to support his work with meditation. He would come in every few months to reflect on where he was. But one day it suddenly struck me that he was a Natrum mur *patient. All the hallmarks were there: his depression, his awesome intellect, his very private manner. Of course,* Natrum mur *is one of the sovereign remedies for headaches; they are very prominent in its provings. You may have found that out already—by suffering a pounding pain behind the eyes after too many salted nuts or oversalted popcorn.*

So I gave Dr. D. the Natrum mur *in a high potency just as I had given other remedies, and he took it with the same routine attitude. But a couple of months later he called me and said he urgently needed to speak with me. Before he could get his coat off, he had launched into a rather puzzled description of his recent experience. He explained that since his last visit he had been going through a period of "intense self-examination. I come home and I don't want to read, I don't want to watch television, I just want to sit," he mused. "It's as though I'm reviewing and reassessing my whole life. It's not as though it's something I decided to do," he went on in the same baffled tone. "It's more like I feel some inner urgency to go through this self-examination process."*

"And what I have come to realize," he continued, "is that I'm depressed." *He had never been able to see that before. He was eager to share the many and profound insights he had arrived at over the preceding two months. I was delighted by his breakthroughs, and deeply impressed by what the remedy seemed to have accomplished. But I was also curious about his headaches. For the first time he hadn't mentioned them. Finally the physician in me pushed the more patient psychiatrist aside and blurted out, "But what about the* headaches?"

He looked up as though I were interrupting. "Oh, the headaches. I don't have them anymore." This was the news I had been looking for so long. I ignored the fact that he didn't seem very excited. I was jubilant. "Hey, that's great! They're gone? Your headaches are cured? That's fantastic!" I wanted him to share my sense of victory. "It's not that they're cured," *he began to explain. I was crestfallen. Maybe he had gone back on heavy doses of painkillers. Now it was my turn to be puzzled. "What do you mean?" I asked. "Oh, it's just that during this period of intense self-examination, I realized what it is that I* do

*that causes the headaches. So I don't do that anymore. But if I did, I'm
sure they'd come back. So I wouldn't say they're cured."*

I wanted to say, "That's what *I* mean by 'cure'!" But I didn't. As he
resumed his sharing of the new perspectives on his life, I reflected on the
power of the remedy. He had accomplished a great deal in the past
months, totally on his own. I never knew what he had done that caused
his headaches—and that he no longer did. He didn't seem to want or
need to share that. This was his work, his achievement—one that would
be considered remarkable if it could be attained in years of psychotherapy. Then I understood what Swami Rama had meant when he said, "If
you want to be a good psychiatrist, you will need to learn homeopathy."
A therapeutic tool that brings into awareness the cause of your illness,
and supports your capacity to choose not to do that anymore, is a radically
curative treatment.

As we see in this case, the use of a deep-acting homeopathic remedy
given for chronic or constitutional purposes is not just a way of getting rid
of troublesome symptoms; it is an opportunity for important and strategic reorganization. I am often exasperated by the patient who returns not
having taken the carefully chosen remedy. "I thought I would just ride it
out. I wasn't in such discomfort that I couldn't stand it. So I decided I
could make it without taking the medicine."

That's a reasonable attitude when faced with conventional drugs.
Sometimes sweating it out is part of getting past the entanglement with
undesirable medications. We avoid them because we don't want to suppress the root problems, we don't want to complicate the situation with
side effects, we don't want to interfere with nature's own push toward
resolution and healing. But the homeopathic remedy, when properly prescribed, is nature's ally. Taking it is an opportunity not to be missed!

The remedy supports a healing reorganization. The symptom picture may be seen as a request for the information needed to set such a
process in motion. One who is ill, or one who is constitutionally off, is one
who is in search of the key that will unlock a new way of being. I am frequently surprised by the way patients return after a period of time, as
though asking for another dose of a remedy. I haven't seen Mrs. K. in six
months, let's say. I wonder why she's here, since she has only the vaguest
of complaints. As I look back at her record, I notice that six months ago
she had a dose of *Calcarea carb* 1M. On closer questioning, I learn that
after that her energy was great for four months or so. Recently she's not

quite as enthusiastic about her job. Some of the *Calcarea carb* limpness is coming back into her life. She needs another dose. On some level she knew that, I suspect, and came in.

Miasmatic Treatment

But sometimes it doesn't work. There are cases in which the most carefully selected acute or even constitutional remedy fails to act. Or the remedy helps briefly, but repeated doses do nothing. Here is a pattern I've seen many times:

> *Michael's asthma has responded sometimes to* Arsenicum *and at other times to* Natrum sulph. *We have gone up gradually in potency with both, and now, even in 1M and 10M, there is no further benefit in following them, even though the symptoms still fit. Reviewing his history, I see that Michael had had several episodes of "nonspecific urethritis" earlier in his life. This is a urethral inflammation very similar to gonorrhea, but without the bacterium considered characteristic of the disease. He also has frequent bouts of sinusitis, and his asthma is not infrequently accompanied by bronchitis—two other mucous membrane disorders. Moreover, his wheezing is worse at dusk and better at the seashore. And he is always in a hurry.*
>
> *All these are symptoms of* Medorrhinum, *so I give him a dose of that remedy in the 1M potency. After that the asthma clears, and returns only in a much-diminished form months later. Now it responds quickly to* Arsenicum *or* Natrum sulph.

In such cases *Medorrhinum* is given to address a level of function even deeper than what we've called constitutional—even though it does not fit the details of the patient's symptoms as closely as does *Arsenicum* or *Natrum sulph*. This may appear to be a departure from the straightforward application of the empirical method of homeopathy, and as a result, some homeopaths take issue with it. For them the principle is clear: fit the remedy to the symptoms, and give it—no theorizing, no fancy ideas. But the fact is that sometimes the most painstaking application of the method fails, and Hahnemann himself was the first to notice this. After some years of practicing the new medicine, he observed that diseases that had appeared to clear up would return. Because this happened so consistently, he began to suspect that in such cases there was some underlying pull toward the state of illness—a sort of undertow that operated beneath the calmer waters he had been dealing with in treating the sick. He called this underlying derangement a *miasm*.

The word *miasm* dates back to a time when diseases were attributed to the evil vapors that permeated a locale. Malaria, for example, was thought to develop in certain damp, unhealthy, swampy areas called "malarial miasms." Today we would laugh and say that malaria is caused by a parasite, which is in turn carried by mosquitoes. It may be hasty, however, to dismiss too quickly what was felt to be a meaningful concept. There may be value in viewing the energy and condition of a location as creating the tendency to disease—and the mosquitoes and protozoa as mere intermediaries in the physical aspects of the process. In any case, Hahnemann took the miasm concept of his day and elevated it to a subtler level. His miasmatic swamps were in the mind and in the organizational structure of the "vital force" or energy level of the person—a certain hidden mindset or energy state that allowed disease to take hold.

To Hahnemann, the miasms were the common denominator in all chronic disease. Their presence, their characteristic ordering of thought, energy, and physical function, were responsible for the recurrence of diseases that became chronic. As a twentieth-century Western physician and psychiatrist with training in Eastern philosophy and medicine, I see miasms as the manifestation of unconscious belief systems and archetypal psychological structures that furnish the underpinnings of our thoughts and ideas.

Many of the values and beliefs involved at this level, such as those surrounding the importance of material possessions, are so widely held that we rarely if ever question them. Others—for example, concepts about the primacy of linear time—even provide the rough outlines of what we assume to be "reality." What is important to note here is that such assumptions, while they attune us to the group mind and gear us to function with relative comfort in society, may also place stringent limits on our freedom to change, evolve, and heal. More specifically, they shut off certain directions in which our consciousness might move, and do so in such a way that it has a strong impact on our spiritual life. For example, if I do not believe that there is a universal consciousness I can participate in, I am not likely to allow myself to experience it.

Such beliefs and assumptions, though operating outside awareness, play a powerful role in shaping our patterns of thought and the way we direct and circulate subtle energy in our bodies. While a more superficial rearrangement of energy—or even thought—may result in the temporary resolution of disease, it is easy to see how the miasmatic foundations of function might reassert themselves and repeatedly bring a disorder back into being. Hahnemann's genius penetrated the veil of social norms to reveal the underlying roots in consciousness that feed the recurrence of chronic disease. Even more important, he was able to pinpoint the remedies that can free us from certain of these patterns.

PSORA, SYCOSIS, AND SYPHILIS

Hahnemann identified three basic miasmatic patterns underlying chronic illness. Those three patterns, when left uncomplicated[12] and free to express themselves in their purest form, tended to manifest as three familiar diseases. The first was scabies, colloquially known in times past simply as "the itch."

Here the expression of the disorder was focused on the skin—its effects being the most visibly obvious of the three, but the least serious. The prototypical expression of the second miasmatic pattern,[13] which he called *sycosis,* was gonorrhea. This miasm produced disorders of the mucous membranes, the linings of the passageways that lead into the body. Sinusitis and bronchitis (like Michael's, above) as well as mucous colitis, vaginitis, and middle-ear congestion are common under its influence, and gonorrhea is an oozing of the mucous membrane of the urethra. The third miasm, *syphilis,* whose classic manifestation was the disease we call by the same name, destroyed the innermost aspects of the body (see Fig. 21).

The diseases associated with the syphilitic miasm involved the most vital structures, the brain, the heart, the bones—and, like syphilis itself, would often entail erosion and destruction of those organs. We might wonder what is being said in the language of disease by each of these miasmatic processes—what their progressive withdrawal of vital force from the body might tell us about the mental and spiritual state of the person affected.

Sulphur was Hahnemann's primary remedy for *psora,* the first miasm. It reflects the ragged philosopher who rants on restlessly and has rough, irritated, itchy skin. It was the remedy I gave my messy roommate. While there are other anti-psoric remedies, *Sulphur* is the most commonly needed. *Thuja* was Hahnemann's initial remedy for *sycosis,* the second of the three. It was a remedy for warts and for people caught up in a life of

HAHNEMANN'S MIASMS

Miasm	Prime target area/ prototypical disease	Classic symptoms	Major remedies	Pathologic process
Psora 1°	skin/ scabies	itch	*Sulphur* (*Psorinium*)	deficiency
Sycosis 2°	mucous membranes/ gonorrhea	warts, catarrhal discharges	*Thuja* *Medorrhinum*	excess
Syphilis 3°	central nervous system/syphilis	ulceration	*Mercurius* *Syphilinum*	destruction (erosion)

FIGURE 21

overextension and excess. The literal meaning of *sycosis* is "fig-wart disease." In addition to the oozing of the mucous membranes, disease language perhaps for the inclination to overdo one's interactions with the world, warts are little whirligigs of overdone tissue, and are another hallmark of *sycosis. Medorrhinum,* the other major remedy for sycotic disorders, is made from the urethral discharge of a patient with gonorrhea.

Despite this close connection between gonorrhea and the miasm *sycosis,* they are not identical. For Hahnemann, the kind of disease that developed in a human body became a sort of marker or indicator of the condition of that particular person's system. He had no way of knowing that someday these diseases would be considered infectious. Our fixation on the microbe as the cause of disease makes it hard for us to grasp Hahnemann's concept of miasms.

At the risk of distorting it a bit—but to make it more understandable to us—let's put his intuition into more modern medical terms. Let's say the microbe (which Hahnemann didn't even know existed) growing in the body reveals the state it is in. The body is a medium that will grow one or another microbe, depending on its condition. Imagine a microbiologist who has a box of petri dishes that will grow only one specific bacteria, but has lost the label and doesn't know which bacteria they are used to grow. To identify them, he plants a variety of bacteria on one. When he sees which one grows, he knows which culture medium he has in the plates.

Our microbiologist is clever because he reversed the usual procedure; instead of smearing the culture plate with a throat swab, for example, to find out what's growing in your throat, he inoculated it with known bacteria to determine what the unknown culture medium was. Thinking in terms of miasms involves a similar reversal. The miasmatically affected body is, like a culture plate, the soil the germ grows in. Finding the gonococcus or the scabies mite thriving in a patient showed the homeopath which miasm was present. This is confusing for those of us who are used to thinking of the germ as the *cause* of the disease. The concept of miasms approaches disease from a perspective that might be considered more spiritual, since causality is seen as operative on a higher or subtler level, not merely physical. The organizational state of the system creates vulnerability to microbial growth. And it's on that subtle organizational level where the high-potency homeopathic remedies work.

Mercurius was Hahnemann's remedy for the third, or syphilitic, miasm. Mercury is known to have an affinity for the nervous system, and a profound, toxic destructiveness. Other heavy metals are used to address this deep miasm also, for example, lead *(Plumbum)* and gold *(Aurum)*. Another potentized preparation of diseased tissue was developed, this time from the chancre (the initial ulcer) of syphilis; under the name of *Lueticum* or *Syphilinum,* it has become a mainstay in the treatment of this miasmatic state.

> *Kenneth consulted me for help with a "weak digestive fire," nervousness and tension, and a condition of the eyes called* keratonconus *which involves a conelike distortion of the cornea. "But* fear *is the main problem," he added. Now thirty years old, he had been alcoholic for seven of those years, and had been treated for Lyme disease and multiple allergies. I noted on my examination of him: "A dazed look in his eyes—as though in shock. Speech almost mechanical." The undercurrent of terror created a feeling tone that I have come to associate with the syphilitic miasm—his eyes were literally "bugging out" with fear. I was not surprised that his nights were troubled by violent and "surreal" dreams. He mentioned that he had been washing his hands compulsively, a symptom that emerges strongly in the portrait of* Syphilinum. *I gave him a dose of that remedy in the 1M potency, and his demeanor changed. The fear dissolved, to be replaced by anger—long repressed and ready to work through.*

In this case the erosion of structure was more in the mind than in the physical organs—as evidenced by the alcoholism and the terror. A few weeks after the remedy, the terror had evaporated from Kenneth's face and he seemed more "in his body." In my years as a psychiatrist I never saw psychotherapy move so quickly to resolve issues or to bring new ones to the fore. As we will discuss later, it is my experience that the deeper we probe into this concept of miasms, the more we will understand about how diseases of body and mind relate to our alienation from the spirit— and the more leverage we will have to heal both.

The miasmatic perspective is not an easy one to grasp; it may feel obscure and mysterious at first. But in the field of healing we have often been at a loss for words to deal with those spheres of human function that include the unconscious assumptions and beliefs that shape our diseases.[14] And since to my knowledge there is no other concept quite like this in any other medical system, throughout this book I will use the term *miasm*—both in a generic sense and to denote one of the three classic miasmatic positions described by Hahnemann.

Flower Remedies

Though I am still continually awed by the profoundly reorganizing effects of homeopathic remedies, I feel uncomfortable prescribing them unless I can find a couple of solid physical symptoms to "tie them down." If all I can see are psychological and emotional issues, I will turn instead to another wondrous realm of natural medicinals, the flower remedies.

I often start classes on flower remedies with a description of Blackberry. If you have ever tried to pick blackberries, you know it's tricky. The vines are covered with sharp spines. The biggest and most succulent berries always seem to be a little deeper into the tangle of brambles. You work your way in edgewise so you can reach a bit further. Then suddenly you realize you can't move. The long branches of the blackberry plant are wrapped all about you, and each has thorns that curve back in toward the plant. No matter which way you move, some of those thorns dig in deeper. You are stuck. The essence of the blackberry flower is used as a remedy for those who are at a point in their lives where they feel stuck—unable to find a way to move. Whether it's a job or a relationship one feels stuck in, the flower essence blackberry supports the effort to disentangle oneself from the situation.

Perhaps the most valuable aspect of the homeopathic remedy is its ability to have a therapeutic effect on the mind and emotions, promoting the process of personal evolution. To enable it to do this, we potentize the natural substance—often a plant—to bring out its subtlest effects. Another way is simply to make the remedy from the most subtle part of the plant—the part that naturally corresponds to the mind—the flower. If you think about the flower and how it relates to the plant, it is analogous to our nervous system on the physical level and to our consciousness on a more subtle level. The flower is the blossoming of the plant—the emergence of its true nature. The complexity, beauty, and uniqueness of the plant is made manifest in the flower. Similarly, with us it is our consciousness, our awareness, that is our flowering. A disorder in your consciousness can often be helped with a remedy from the flower that corresponds to it.

Fuchsia is a familiar potted plant, usually hung on porches or by windows, where it spills its dramatic blossoms of purple and pink in a dramatic display. As a flower essence, it's used when genuine emotion is repressed and overflows as hyperemotionality or psychosomatic ailments. I chose it for Bob, who was seeing me for his high blood pressure, and who had violent and melodramatic dreams about authority figures he couldn't confront in real life. Though he was happy-go-lucky on the surface, the anger he held in was manifest in his tight blood vessels. After taking Fuchsia flower essence for a month, he remarked that he felt more spontaneous in his communications, quicker to express his honest feelings.

You may not always be familiar with the flower—or discern its therapeutic effect even when you do recognize it. As I was coming out of a painful divorce, my ex-wife, who was living next door, immediately remarried, creating a new family constellation that left me feeling obsolete. I found myself withdrawing, unable to assert my conviction that what I had to offer my children was important. In the flower essence repertory I ran across the following: "The soul lesson of Penstemon is reminiscent of the biblical story of Job, where unusually harsh or severe life circumstances test the soul's uttermost faith and tenacity. . . ." Though I did not recall having ever seen penstemon, and couldn't even find a picture of it, the description rang a bell. As I took the essence, I immediately began to emerge from my feelings of self-pity and discovered new strength and resilience.

Man has probably used flowers for their healing energy since the earliest prehistory. Australian aborigines availed themselves of the flowers' benefits by eating them whole—or, if they were inedible, by sitting amid a clump of the plants while they were in blossom in order to absorb their healing effects. Most likely, many of our customs of wearing flowers, bringing them into the sickroom, or using them in ceremonies and rituals date back to a time when we were more open to the informational messages they convey, and more attuned to how specific flowers can resonate with specific states of mind and emotion.

We owe the modern approach to the use of flower essences in large part to the efforts of Dr. Edward Bach, who pioneered a system of remedies made from flowers he found in the countryside outside London. His original remedies are still widely used today, and are the ones you will most often find in most health-food stores. Their popularity all over the world has stimulated the development of essences made from flowers in many regions (see Fig. 22).

Dr. Bach was a respected homeopathic physician who decided in 1930 to abandon his medical practice. He had come to feel that the process of matching the homeopathic remedies to the symptom picture was too difficult for most people, and he wanted to find a simpler system. Immersing himself in nature, he observed flowers and arrived at correspondences between specific flowers and certain psychological and emotional states. Aspen, for example, is a remedy made from the flowers of that tree. As I mentioned earlier, its leaves tremble with the slightest movement of the air. Its flower essence is used to treat nervousness and anxiety.

THE FLOWER ESSENCE EXPLOSION

Name	Number available
Alaskan flower essences	48
Hawaiian tropical flower essences	50
Australian bush flower essences	50
Bloesem remedies, Netherlands	19
Desert alchemy, Southwestern United States	26
English essences (Bach)	40
Flower Essence Society (California)	96
French Deva flower essences	64
Himalayan flower enhancers	34
Pacific essences (wildflowers)	24
Orchids of the Amazon essences	20
Perelandra (vegetable garden) essences	26
Siskiyou flower essences (Japan)	11+
Andean flower and orchid essences	10

FIGURE 22

Anyone who has ever tangled with a holly bush might be able to figure out the use for its flower essence. The red berries and shiny leaves are
attractive, but the holly leaf is surrounded by barbed tips that curve under
and in. Unlike blackberry, if you reach for the berries, you're not caught.
You will escape, but you may be clawed mercilessly in the process. Holly
is for people who are nasty and vicious.

My first experience using flower remedies was with Holly essence. A
woman came in with her daughter, without a doubt the nastiest teenager
I'd ever met. She was constantly picking on her younger sister, who frequently looked as if she had just been verbally and emotionally lacerated
by her older sibling. Everyone in the family suffered from her sarcasm and
her biting tongue. Her mother was going crazy and begged for help. I had
just been introduced to flower remedies myself and was quite skeptical,
but didn't know what else to recommend. With little expectation that they
would do anything at all, I gave her Holly drops and sent her home.

A month later, the mother came back. "This is a miracle," she confided, her eyes large with astonishment. Her daughter was totally transformed. She had become considerate and courteous instead of snapping
at everybody. She was even kind to her younger sister. I was as surprised
as her mother, and from that moment on began to study flower remedies
with growing respect and interest.

Perhaps you are already ticking off a list of candidates for Holly
drops. In fact, Dr. Bach considered it one of his two most widely needed
remedies. The other was Wild Oat. As our vernacular suggests, wild oat
has to do with inability to focus or make commitment. Those wild oats we
sow sometimes become an unending prelude to an eternally postponed
settling down. Wild Oat is the generic remedy for such a state, while
Holly is the generic remedy for all the negative, hateful impulses of the
inner being that keep it separate from a loving unity with humankind.

It is, I think, no accident that "holly" means "whole" or "holy," and is
used at Christmas to mark the coming of the Messenger of Love, for Bach
noted that within the complexion of each flower was not only a dark and
troublesome struggle—for example, between hater and hated—but also
the seeds of its resolution. That which seems our most grievous weakness
is not really a defect, he might say, it is merely life's offer of an opportunity to grapple with an issue. It is our chance to address a polarity, grow
in wisdom and serenity, and acquire a strength that we lacked before.
The Holly patient has a unique capacity for love, tolerance, compassion,
and an open heart. It is the personal experience of coming to terms with

his own tendency to swing into a polarized position of anger, envy, suspicion, and hatred against some other or others that can move him past it (see Fig. 23).

The flower essence gently supports this process. The pattern inherent in the blossom holds the answer to the particular riddle that life is presenting you at the moment. Flower essences are your allies in the struggle with polarities. Each polarity involves taking a position that expresses one side of an inner conflict, and projecting the other side out into the world, where it becomes an adversary. While that splits you apart, it also brings what was buried into view. This provides the possibility of discovery, insight, and resolution—the very processes which will take you another step along your personal path.

For Bob, who took Fuchsia, it was getting past the quandary of whether to squelch his emotions or to release them in a smokescreen of overreaction and melodrama. Underneath the polarization was the simplicity of genuine feeling. During my divorce, it was the opportunity to step out of the dichotomy of victim and victimizer and rediscover my strength and uniqueness. The use of these remedies has been called "soul therapy," since it is the task of the soul to embrace the paradox of polarities. There is a deep, soulful insistence, springing from the inner recesses of our being, that we live through certain roles: hater and hated, monster and victim. For the soul's journey it is indispensable to experience the tension between such divergent human tendencies in order to bring fully into play what has been obscure and troubling (see pages 462–65).

Although flower essences are similar to high-potency homeopathic remedies in that both reach deep into the realm of the psyche, there are definite differences. The action of the homeopathic remedy ties together the mind and the body in a network of reorganizing activity. The pattern that is adjusted extends from the physical beyond the mind to reintegrate levels below with the higher spiritual intent. This has a way of bringing the mental and physical back into true alignment with the Higher Self.

The flower essences, by contrast, act primarily on the mind, emotions, feelings of the emerging self—the maturing child—the part of us that must experience to grow. This is the being who's on the path, the human who's subject to error, the searcher who must learn from life's struggles what the Higher Self already knows (see Fig. 24).

Though the flower remedy does not have a direct impact on the physical level, it can still be helpful with physical symptoms. When the underlying emotional issues can be cleared up, physical difficulties will

A BOUQUET OF FLOWER ESSENCES
(Use Them!)

Flower	Patterns of Unbalance	Resolution	System
Aspen	tremulous anxiety	fearless grounding in love	Bach (English)
Blackberry	unable to act	decisive will	California
Dandelion	tense, tight body	effortless ease	California
Fuchsia	body expresses suppressed emotion	genuine feelings	California
Goldenrod	inviting ridicule	confident individuality	California
Holly	anger and hate	love and compassion	Bach
Olive	wearied by long struggle	reconnection to strength beyond	Bach
Penstemon	self-pity, feeling persecuted	inner fortitude	California
St. John's Wort	nightmares, vulnerable psyche	light-filled awareness	California
Star of Bethlehem	trauma or shock	calmness and serenity	Bach
Walnut	tied to the old	open to the new	Bach
Wild Oat	aimlessness, uncertainty	focus and determination	Bach

FIGURE 23

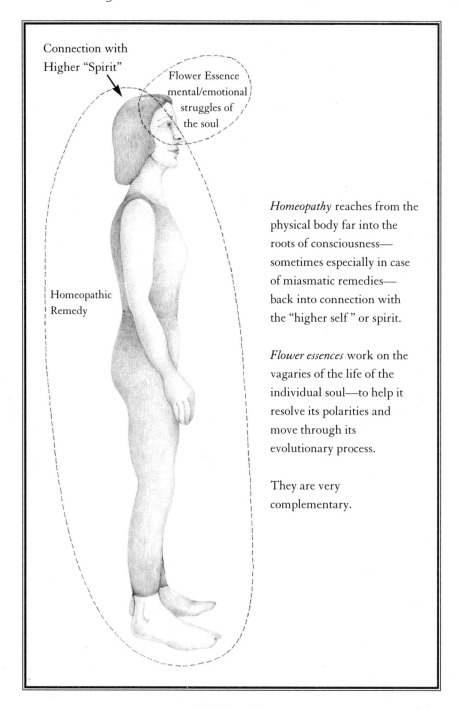

Connection with
Higher "Spirit"

Flower Essence
mental/emotional
struggles of
the soul

Homeopathic
Remedy

Homeopathy reaches from the
physical body far into the
roots of consciousness—
sometimes especially in case
of miasmatic remedies—
back into connection with
the "higher self" or spirit.

Flower essences work on the
vagaries of the life of the
individual soul—to help it
resolve its polarities and
move through its
evolutionary process.

They are very
complementary.

FIGURE 24

often melt away. With less psychological conflict to distort and misdirect the flow of subtle energy, the basis of the physical illness is diminished.

Working on such subtle terrain, and lacking a direct tie-in to the physical, flower remedies may seem outside the realm of medicine. Certainly they have been totally ignored by conventional physicians. While homeopathy is routinely discounted, denounced, or ridiculed, flower essences are simply unknown. I used them for many years without talking about them. I could defend homeopathy in the context of medical science, since it has a clear, empirical foundation that is essentially unassailable, but flower remedies were another matter altogether.

Their use is *not* based on provings. There were no controlled studies demonstrating their effectiveness.[1] Dr. Bach came up with his connections between personality and flower while sitting in the woods! Flower remedies are made by floating the blossoms on a bowl of water that is placed in the sun for several hours. The flowers are then removed and the water is mixed with brandy as a preservative. *This* is what is used as a remedy—something of the essence of the flower has permeated the water, it is said. Try explaining that to a hospital staff!

I used them hesitantly at first, then, as I saw results, with increasing confidence. Little cues supported my growing conviction that they were powerful. One was the look in a fourteen-year-old's eyes. I had been treating him for asthma for years. He had responded gradually to homeopathic remedies, but he was troubled by tension in his body. The muscles in his back were very tight. "He holds everything *in,*" his mother commented. Not wanting to disrupt the action of the homeopathic remedies, yet eager to address what was bothering him, I decided to use a flower essence. I gave him Dandelion, which is used for those tense, overstriving doers who "overform" their lives "beyond the natural capacity of the body to sustain such intensity."

When he came back the next time, much improved, he dropped his shy and hesitant manner for a moment. Looking me straight in the eye, he asked me pointedly, "Have you *always* had these drops?" I felt validated for my choice at the same time I felt chided for not having given him the remedy sooner. Kids don't care about scientific proof; they just want help. All the drugs in the world with tons of studies to back them up (and countless side effects to plague the user) are of no interest to them. A gentle, effective remedy is an obvious thing to do. Why hadn't he gotten it sooner? The answer was my fear of not looking "scientific," and I felt duly humbled.

Although the science behind the use of flower remedies is not to be found in research laboratories at the typical medical center, it is nevertheless quite sophisticated. It is a different sort of science, one that draws on the most ancient techniques for delving into the wellsprings of intuition, and the most futuristic concepts of information theory and subtle energies—as well as a meticulous study of classical botany. Let's look, for example, at how flowers are evaluated for their healing potential:

1. One must familiarize oneself with the unique botanical details of the plant's form and function and its peculiar characteristics (how it responds to weather, for example).
2. One clears the mind so that it might be receptive in an open and neutral way and so that insights will not be contaminated with personal issues and mental static. This closely parallels traditional methods of preparing for and entering meditation.
3. One might envision the shifts in form that occur as the plant moves through its life stages—from sprouted seed to roots and leaflets, to maturity and flowering and ultimately to fruit and involution.
4. Finally, the "personality" implicit in all this must be allowed to take shape as a sort of image (much as Buhner "saw" usnea). One might then enter into dialogue, or even merge empathically, with that image in order to sense the state of mind, emotional tone, and characteristic habits of psyche that would correspond to it and might respond to it therapeutically.[2]

For example, we might imagine that Dr. Bach, contemplating the olive tree, was struck by its gnarled trunk, its worn, twisted tenacity, the way in which its fruit can shrivel and dry, yet still retain its flavor. He was led to prescribe it for those who are weary and have exhausted their reserves. Olive branches have long been a symbol of peace and harmony. Olive essence, he felt, would bring peace to the tired mind and strength to a body exhausted by suffering.

When we enter this realm of inquiry, we are opening ourselves to a new way of *knowing*. Though my years of training in conventional medicine prompt in me endless doubt and skepticism, there are moments when I realize that there is a vast world of lucid perception where discovery works according to different rules. When Galen, my middle son, was seven or eight, he fell into the role of family "goof." His older brother was the leader, his younger the baby. Galen himself, by and large a quiet and patient sort, was often simply ignored—lost in the shuffle. He protested this neglect by playing the fool—doing stupid things that resulted in his siblings calling him "Idiot!" and saying things like, "Oh, you're such a dope. Go away!" It was negative attention, but it *was* attention. I was dismayed and stumped. No amount of discussion seemed to stop this little family dynamic from running its repetitive course.

When Galen was not inviting abuse, he loved to roam the fields and woods. I had taught him a bit about the wild plants nearby. Along about that time he began to bring me sprigs of goldenrod. "Can you make a remedy from this?" he asked. I answered offhandedly, "Sure. *Solidago* is what homeopaths call it, it's used in some cases of kidney disease." This didn't really seem to satisfy him. A few days later he brought me another piece and asked the same question. I said, "You asked me that before, remember?" But that didn't seem to register, either.

Though I had used the Bach remedies for decades by then, I had only recently begun to discover the California flower essences. One afternoon while studying their descriptions, I ran across Goldenrod. "For those who create barriers to social contact through repulsive behavior, or who have a need for negative attention," it said. "Promotes positive individuation."[3]

I probably sat a long time with that book in my lap, staring off into the distance. My mind was having a hard time "wrapping itself around" what had happened. I slowly came to realize that there was a level of awareness and communication here to which I'd been totally oblivious. And as I watched the flower essence work its magic, my son steadily outgrowing his problem, it became obvious that this sphere of non-ordinary reality could hold immense potential for the advancement of healing work.

But flower essences will gain recognition only as they are used and more people experience their effects. The usual way to get your feet wet is by using a combination Bach essence that he called Rescue Remedy.[4] It's used for emergencies, and is a composite of five flowers that cover shock, panic, impatience, desperation, and the tendency to lose consciousness. It is helpful in almost any acute situation, from stage fright to physical trauma. It is not a replacement for homeopathic *Arnica,* however, since its effects are focused on the mental/emotional state, not on the direct return of vital force or subtle energy back into body parts, as is the case with *Arnica.*

One of the five flowers in Rescue Remedy is Star of Bethlehem, which is a generic remedy for all *psychic* shock—i.e., any event that is traumatic to mind and emotions, from bad news to a serious physical blow. Used alone, it focuses on disorganizing effects of shock, while the five-flower formula generalizes the effect to cover all emergency situations.

Many flower remedies come to mind that I would be hard put to do without. I must at least share my enthusiasm for Walnut, which is the generic Bach remedy for supporting changes and transition. While the California essence Blackberry is specifically for those who feel stuck because they have trouble connecting with their will, Walnut, like most of the Bach essences, seems to have a wider scope of application. It's useful in all sorts of shifts and comes in handy for many diverse situations— from the breakup of a love affair to jet lag. Any time I cross more than a couple of time zones, I carry a bottle of Walnut. It helps you let go of one time frame and enter another. But it's even more valuable for major life changes. Dr. Bach said that Walnut is a remedy "for those who have decided to take a great step forward in life, to break old conventions, to leave old limits and restrictions and start on a new way. This often brings with it physical suffering because of the slight regrets, heart-breakings, at the severance of old ties, old associations, old thoughts. A great spell-breaker . . ."

I have wondered whether a small vial of Walnut drops might be marketed with this book, to help us as we try to break out of the old way of thinking about health and illness and move on to a totally new approach.

Concluding Thoughts on

Nature's Medicinals

Flower essences can be used to deal with dilemmas of the mind at the same time a homeopathic remedy is acting to reorganize the overall vital force. Dr. Bach, when he initiated the modern flower essences movement, found the use of flower remedies particularly appealing precisely because they could be combined with other forms of medicine.

In my own practice, I most often begin with cell salts, since their indications are quickly evident and they seem to prepare the system for accepting the more profound reorganizing affects of the high-potency remedies. After some months of therapy, however, it's not uncommon for me to have a patient taking cell salts, organ remedies in the form of herbal tinctures or Chinese formulas, homeopathics in higher potency, and even flower essences to boot—though the orchestration of all these different inputs can require considerable attention. If they can be properly coordinated, their synergism can produce remarkable and rapid results.

These remedies all have a reorganizing effect, but each has its primary impact on a different organizational level: flower essences addressing mental and emotional issues, homeopathics repatterning the "vital force" or overall energy body, cell salts readjusting at the tissue level, and herbs having a special affinity for the organs (though their gestalt or spirit can resonate with the whole person, too).

Because they work on distinct levels (see Fig. 25), you may, for example, simultaneously take *Mag phos* 6x and *Natrum phos* 6x for your intestinal spasms, *Chelidonium* for your liver, *Calcarea carb* as a constitutional, all the while using Walnut as a flower essence to help you adjust to your new job.[5] I find it best to phase them in, one level of treatment at a time, providing time to observe and integrate the effects of each before adding the next. The Self-Help Index in Section V may offer you the guidance

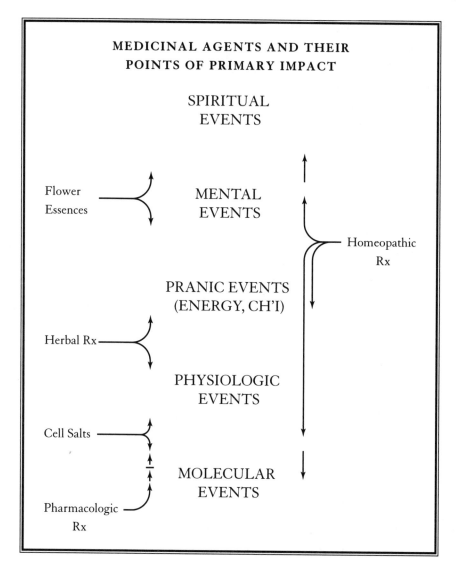

FIGURE 25

you need to begin to put together a multilevel program for dealing with any health challenge you might be facing.

Though the specific kinds of medicinals we have focused on in this first section are only a few of those being used to harness the healing power of nature, they are some of the best established and most evolved. They strike major chords in the emerging symphony of new medicinal approaches. Understanding them should provide a framework for making sense of others.

How the medicinal therapies of the future will be combined, and what treatment will look like fifty years from now, we can hardly imagine. Certainly the healing properties of herbs will play a major role. Homeopathy also seems a prime candidate to capture a central place in the medicine of the future, as its scope and power are finally comprehended.

Many researchers who are at the forefront of the field—particularly in Germany—are exploring the therapeutic use of sound, color, and the direct input of energy-pulsed information. Electronic devices can create tailor-made messages to restore optimal functioning. Although this is exciting and futuristic work, something about it seems otherworldly. It conjures up images of space stations, cold metal surfaces, and artificial life. While such approaches may have their place, it is possible that our healing needs, at least in part, to involve the recovery of a healthy relationship to the pulsing life of our own planet.

Medicinals based on natural substances not only move us past our personal crises but initiate a reconnection with the planetary gestalt or "group soul" that is necessary for the healing into wholeness of our fragmented world.

The principle by which homeopathic remedies and these other natural medicinals work is elegant. By connecting me, as a disordered being, with patterns that exist in nature, they pull me back into the integrity of that natural order, restoring me to my place as a functioning component of an intricate system. They re-empower me to celebrate my uniqueness as an indispensable contribution to the whole. And they bring me back into synchrony with the harmonious orchestration of nature.

Our resonance with the remedy reminds us of where our creativity can flower, of where we belong in nature. It puts us back in our place, so to speak, as both a humble part of the whole and a powerful agent of our own individuality. By putting a drop of a remedy in, the flow is reopened where before it was closed off. A healing force is allowed to rush through our being, energizing us from its source, sustaining our vitality and powering the unfoldment of our purpose in this life.

The healing force on which all our therapeutic work is ultimately based is seeking to move through us and reconnect us to the whole. This force can gradually nudge us toward the point of comprehending the greatest paradox of all: *By being fully integrated into the whole, we are most completely empowered to be totally unique.* As we grasp this mystery, then we are healed. That may, in fact, be the simplest formulation of what true healing is all about.

nize it carefully. In fact, to prepare yourself to use holistic healing successfully, you will need to grapple with the whole question of exactly what diagnosis *is*.

It is important to uncover the worldview that is at the root of the conventional diagnostic process. You want to learn to identify clearly and regard warily the mindset that regards disease as an "other" and an enemy to be defeated—rather than as valuable information about yourself that you can use to speed your journey toward healing and wholeness.

If you can step clear of diagnostic pitfalls, you will be able to use your remedies more freely. You'll also be at liberty to move on to other, more holistic systems for assessment—methods less permeated by fear and projection. Using them, you will learn to read what your body and its imbalances tell you about yourself, which will contribute to your process of discovery and growth. You can also be more accepting of your quirks—studying them to appreciate your constitutional type and your unique needs, rather than seeing them as alarming evidence of pathology. Before you finish this section, you should have pinned down your type, and be ready to use this to identify which foods to eat or which kind of exercise is best for you. But first, diagnosis.

SELF-ASSESSMENT

With natural medicinals you may search for an herb to "boost the immune system" or a tissue salt to quell inflammation, but there's no talk of strep throats or influenza. As a result, the next time you have an illness, you may find yourself in a bind. You have in mind a homeopathic remedy that seems to fit. But there's this *diagnosis* that you have been labeled with—and it sounds serious. Suddenly you're faced with an uncomfortable choice: holistic or conventional treatment? The holistic approach makes sense and holds the promise of a gentle and thorough healing. But the conventional route *seems* safer—and maybe this is "too important to take chances with."

As a holistic clinician, I regard The Diagnosis as the major obstacle to enjoying the fruits of radical healing. It's a wall. If you can scale it, a new world opens up. If you remain boggled by it, you will be severely limited in what you can do. I don't mean that conventional diagnosis is worthless. There are times when caution is called for, and situations—like that of Dr. G. and his asthma patient in the last section—in which appropriate holistic care has not yet been developed or is not readily available. You should not ignore diagnostic information, but you should scruti-

The Meaning
of Diagnosis

When I pick up the *ICD.9.CM,* the international diagnostic classification for medical personnel, with its 1,500 pages of diagnostic codes that are entered on insurance forms, I am truly awed by the huge gulf that separates the old way of thinking about diagnosis from what seems to me to be the promise of the future. Day-to-day medicine, in hospitals and clinics across the earth, is still heavily invested in the concept of pathology and disease. The disease-oriented mindset is dominated by a fear of being attacked—by microbes or by cancer, for example. This psychological space of fearful suffering that we have created, within which exist our hospitals and our doctors' offices, reflects attitudes that run through the entire fabric of our society. Operating from fear, the very act of diagnosing sabotages the effort to heal.

Reaching for a suppressive medication for even a cold or mild cough may miss an important opportunity. The small but significant reorganization that emerges from a "minor" illness may serve as a strategic step forward in your personal transformation. Whether you take an analgesic for a headache or an antidepressant for those darker times, you are thwarting an inner demand for reassessment and change. When you ignore your body's many smaller calls for attention, you build up a growing inner urgency that almost inevitably will lead to a major illness or crisis of some sort. By using the tools in this book, however, you can make each little ailment the occasion for an insight and an internal shift, a small step along your personal path to a deep and radical healing.

Let's start with a common problem, a garden-variety case to cut your teeth on. Watch how we think diagnostically as we consider this patient's situation:

Adrienne telephones me with a tight chest and a cough. She is rest-less, has no fever, and is bringing up a bit of yellow mucus. I ask a few questions, but she's pretty clear that "that's all that's wrong," and doesn't seem in the mood to be interrogated at length. On the basis of this skimpy information, we need to make a decision about what to do for her.

What catches my attention, first of all, is the yellow mucus, which suggests that an inflammatory process is going on in Adrienne's bronchi, and that bacteria—of a type that don't usually grow there—are involved. They are being knocked out by white cells, some of which die and accumulate in the mucus, making it yellow. The tight-ness in the chest sounds like bronchial spasm. It's apparently not severe enough to come across to her as wheezy, so it probably wouldn't be called asthma, though we don't know what it might sound like if one were to listen with a stethoscope.

Responding directly to this information, we can prescribe a simple program: Kali mur *6x for the congestion and* Calc sulph *6x for the yellow-colored mucus, plus* Echinacea *to support her immune sys-tem. These simple medicines will probably help, but adding a homeo-pathic remedy that fit the picture would double the odds that we'd get results.*

Actually, I'm working at an advantage. I know Adrienne, and based on my memory of her meticulous grooming and her artistic inclinations, Arsenicum *flashes on my mental screen. It's a major remedy for wheezy breathing, and it's often marked by burning pains. She has had a sore throat, she says, "sort of burning." "Did you try anything to soothe it—a drink, hot tea or cold water?" She had. Hot drinks seemed to help.*

Burning pains relieved by heat is a peculiar symptom, characteris-tic of Arsenicum. *"Take a dose of* Arsenicum album *30C. And," I add, "limit your diet to things that are light and easily digestible—soups, rice, steamed veggies."*

We've done two different assessments here. The first came out in physiological terms—bronchospasm and mild bronchitis—and led to cell salts and an herb. But then we did another kind of analysis, in which we looked for a remedy picture and came up with a homeopathic prescrip-tion. We aren't always so lucky—but since we were this time, this case serves nicely to demonstrate how we can analyze a situation from two entirely different angles.

That's not the whole story with Adrienne. She had come in two weeks before with a chronic, strange sort of pain in her foot. Underneath that there seemed to be some reluctance to decide which direction to move in her life—where to step next, so to speak! Though she had before given the impression of being supremely confident and well established in her professional work, I pointed out in that session what this symptom seemed to be saying. She was a bit taken aback. Her face registered an initial suspicious surprise, and then her voice dropped. She confided, "I *have* been thinking of other work. The truth is, my job is *not* so stable. In fact, there's talk of eliminating my position...." As she left that day, she'd paused, looked back at me, and said, "Thank you for seeing me the way I really am."

Two weeks later she has tightness in her chest, so I figure I should be careful not to suffocate her with more than she is ready to deal with. So I don't bring up any of those issues today. Instead I treat her very simply and supportively with the low-potency homeopathic remedy, tissue salts, and herb. And she seems reassured. The *Arsenicum,* however, will increase her capacity to deal with the larger issues that she is facing—the issues about life direction that had surfaced earlier. It will loosen some of her fearful self-centeredness. This is the beauty of the holistic approach; the symptoms portray the pattern she is stuck in, and to resolve that sets her up to go to the next step. My teacher would have said, "She is asking for a dose of *Arsenicum.*" The symptom picture expresses the need for reorganizing information that will enable her to move on.

Even when the acute remedy doesn't play a role in resolving the deepest underlying issues, it may be dissolving some of the resistance to dealing with those deeper issues, clearing the way for them to be more easily resolved at a later time. My friends and colleagues seem impatient with me at times because I'm such a stickler for the minutiae of minor ailments. Probably they seem so important to me because, as a psychiatrist, I've learned to see the critical importance of all the little pieces of insight and understanding. Eventually they all add up to the big "Aha!"—the experience that culminates in a powerful healing.

Whether or not you can use the experience of an illness constructively will depend to a great extent on how you see it from the outset—the concept of it that you carry in your mind. A number of very different scenarios can unfold in the process of arriving at such a concept or diagnosis. The first, perhaps most common, and certainly the most insidious, involves simple relabeling.

1. Diagnosis by Renaming

My friend Sally is flushed. She looks anxious and a bit flustered. "What's going on?" I ask. "I'm not feeling too great," she says. "I went to see my doctor because I had a sore throat. I got worried that maybe it was something serious." She pauses, as if for dramatic effect, and lowers her voice. "He said I have pharyngitis."

Though she is obviously impressed, I'm not. "But, but—" I begin to sputter—too exasperated to stop and explain calmly that *pharynx* is simply Greek for "throat" and *-itis* is a suffix meaning "inflamed." "That just means you have a sore throat! And you already *knew* that!" She looks at me blankly, as if to say, "What are you talking about?"

Sally wasn't given information that might clarify what was happening in her throat. Input like "Your throat is probably sore from the irritation of the postnasal drainage I can see dripping down the back of it" might have been helpful—it would have crystallized the doctor's understanding, and offered the patient a chance to ratify the doctor's hypothesis: "Yes. I think that's it! When the pollen came out, I felt the drip start down the back of my throat. It was the following day that my throat got really sore." The doctor thus confirms what he thought—or not—and the patient gets the benefit of the doctor's expertise in furthering her own understanding of what is happening to her and of how it fits into the process of her life.

But Sally had experienced a very different interaction between her doctor and herself. She had been given a simple *diagnosis by renaming.* This relabeling communicates to the patient not information or insight, but rather the message "You are not in charge of this situation." Renaming is, in effect, a *ritual* use of words. It formalizes a specific kind of relationship between the doctor and the patient. In an almost magical way, it transforms the doctor into the *knower* and *doer,* and the patient into the more passive *receiver.*

By pronouncing mysterious medical words, the doctor asserts his knowledge, power, and dominion. If the patient accepts the complementary role, a sort of hypnotism might ensue: "By virtue of this ritual, you are now in control, Doctor. I am a helpless and passive recipient of your powerful interventions. By using a term that is not of my world, you have removed this transaction from the realm of what is knowable to me. I will accept your recommendations unquestioningly. If I were to show doubt or reservations, you would be justified in being indignant—for I would have violated this covenant that we are now agreeing upon."

Seventy-two-year-old Margaret sat before me squirming with discomfort. She wanted to get off Mevacor, a drug given to lower her cholesterol, but she was clearly ambivalent. Maybe afraid *would be a more correct word. The Great White Father—or at least the father in the great white coat—had handed down his verdict. Could she risk going against that? "Well," she said, shifting around in her chair again and holding her handbag in her lap as though it were her only anchor in this most epic battle of medical philosophies, "My doctor says I should take it."*

If this other guy was "her doctor," who was I? To say that I was miffed by her choice of words would be an understatement, and yet I understood her dilemma. After a lifetime of faithfully following the pronouncements of medical orthodoxy—and of feeling that it was one of the few solid, reliable touchstones in a world of growing uncertainties—she was now faced with the prospect of rebelling. It wasn't easy. As an elderly woman, she was taking a stand against the world of male authority. Was she putting her life at risk? If she stopped the Mevacor, would she have a heart attack—as "her doctor" had implied?

Yet she was sure that it wasn't agreeing with her. In some way that was difficult to articulate, it didn't feel right inside of her—she had a tiredness and heaviness since she had started the medication. Those feelings began to lift when she skipped a few doses. This firsthand information was a clear signal from her own body. Which was she to obey—her own sense of truth, or the judgment of the powerful man in the white coat? I think what tipped the balance for her was an off-hand remark made by the doctor at her last visit. He had said casually, "You seem to be doing so well on one tablet a day, why not take two?"

Though this comment was meant to be upbeat and supportive, Margaret didn't take it that way. She had been working very hard to improve her diet and to exercise. She thought that the improvement he had found in her blood cholesterol had been the result of these efforts, and she'd hoped, I think, for some acknowledgment of this. Instead, this official in the white coat not only credited the medication (indirectly claiming credit for himself), but seemed to advocate an unnec-

essary additional dosage as well. I think his attitude represented an extreme of medication-mindedness that went too far for her. She had to declare her independence. And she did.

Margaret stopped the Mevacor. It was a great act of courage. And she felt better—physically, I think, from the elimination of the medication from her system, but also, and more important, psychologically from having taken back her power as the architect of her own destiny. She sat straighter and acted more decisively about her health matters. She was in the driver's seat now.

Most of us are drawn, at one time or another, into the seductive comfort and security of giving over our care to the impressive and well-established world of conventional medicine. This is not surprising. At those moments when we are sick, when we are most vulnerable, that world is most appealing with its promises of power, reliability, and protection. Psychologists speak of regression at the time of illness—a phenomenon I first learned about when I was a sophomore in college and came down with a sort of flu.

I felt achy, feverish, and confused. My roommate came in from class to find me packing my suitcase. "Where are you going?" he asked. "Home," I mumbled. "I don't feel well. I'm going home." Never mind that home was 250 miles away and that I didn't have a car or any idea of what public transportation was available on this day or at this time. All those considerations were too rational for me at that moment. I was sick. I felt miserable. It was clear to me that I needed to go home.

Reason and my roommate finally prevailed, and I was persuaded to go to the Student Health Service. But I remember the strong feeling of wanting to fold myself in the arms of parental protection and omniscience—the same impulse that often drives us into the apparent security of reputable hospitals and well-appointed clinics.

In some instances, taking refuge may actually be a valid move toward genuine healing. At times, it is important to acknowledge and simply be with your feelings of helplessness and powerlessness in the face of an illness that you might have been struggling with fruitlessly for so long. At times you simply need to say, "I'm sick. I give up. I need help."

Yet acknowledging your helplessness and accepting that you are in the midst of a major dilemma is only the initial challenge—the first step into the process of healing. You must go on to other steps, dig deep within yourself, find new resources, and come to grapple creatively with the illness at hand. If you linger too long in the Lotus Land of the passive patient and the omnipotent doctor, you might find yourself in serious trouble. Deepening physical pathology, compounded by the side effects of medications, surgery, and an increasing entanglement in a complex medical system where being a patient can become a way of life are some of the risks you run when you tarry there.

If you find yourself repeatedly drawn to this passive role, if you find its appeal irresistibly seductive, your best bet is to respond to this tendency with curiosity and observe it with interest. Though getting stuck there is a danger, seeing that it has a pull for you provides valuable information. It may be evidence of an unconscious attraction to a regressive scenario of reunion with an idealized and impossibly Good Mother.[1] This basic psychological stance can underlie many disorders, both emotional and physical, and working with it—whether by means of remedies or energy work or directly with the mind—is a fundamental aspect of holistic healing.

So even when letting go is useful in the treatment process, in order to move on in your healing you will need to evolve out of the passive/recipient stage, and take charge of yourself. This is an important step toward the spiritual attunement that might be considered the ultimate goal of healing.

The ideal health practitioner will be alert to the need for a passive period of rest, but will be watching for the recovery of sufficient strength that might signal that it's time to initiate a process of cooperative work. Unfortunately, most clinicians are not sufficiently mature or well enough trained to be capable of such a range of responses, and often they continue to follow their routine—so that if you want to change gears, you have to change doctors.

In any case, the renaming ritual has little to do with diagnosis in the literal sense of the word. It is not an effort to throw light on the patient's trouble. In fact, it is not, in the truest sense of the word, a diagnosis at all. It is, more accurately, a non-diagnosis.

ANOTHER PITFALL WHEN YOU GO
THE RENAMING ROUTE

Diagnosis by renaming not only transforms the roles of doctor and patient. It also often creates a *new* player in this drama: the Disease. This is another aspect to the magic of conferring a Name. The very act of bestowing the name implies the existence of an entity that will receive that name. "What do I have, Doctor? I just want to know what it is." We are like children who want to know the name of the monster. Although the unknown and unnamed make us anxious, naming can too. It conjures up an image and that image takes on a reality that has its own power and that also inspires fear.

Arnie Mindell is a psychologist who helps people move beyond that fear. I had an opportunity to experience his work, and here is the scene I encountered:

> We are in a huge conference room. Sixty people, mostly psychotherapists, are in a large circle that takes up most of the room. After a brief demonstration, we each choose a symptom. Mine is a cough that I have had for four years on and off. First, he says, describe to your partner what this symptom does. I move my hand up the underside of her upstretched arm. I am digging and pushing. This is the way the impulse to cough feels as it moves up my chest. "What does it look like?" asks Arnie. "A mole," I reply instantly. There was no doubt this thing burrowed up my chest like a mole. "Give it a name!" "Malicious Mole," I dubbed it.
>
> But Arnie didn't stop there because simply naming the symptom and conferring upon it an independent existence would leave us with an external, unintegrated enemy—something to fear and be assailed by endlessly. He goes another, crucial step: "Now," said Arnie, "ask this being what its message is to you." My Malicious Mole was urging me to be aggressive, to roar my agony and my indignation when I was pushed around. So I did. Now my monster had become my ally. It was there to remind me when I forgot to speak up for myself. No longer a split-off source of suffering and attack, it was a friend—a part of myself that fought for me.

Diagnosis by renaming—without the further step of analysis and integration—can create an entity outside yourself that can victimize you. So when the patient asks me, "Do you think I have arthritis? My doctor said I have arthritis," she is *not* asking whether she has inflamed joints. That is, of course, all that the term means in a literal sense: *arth* = joint, *-itis* = inflamed. Rather, she is asking whether there is a disease somewhere, separate in a sense from her, that has attacked her: "Do you agree that I am now a victim of this entity called 'Arthritis'—is there a Disease that has taken hold of my body?" If I respond, "Yes, you have arthritis," with the intention of saying, "Yes, your joints are inflamed," this is not what is communicated. Instead, she hears, "Yes, you are now subject to this thing that we call the Arthritis Disease." She may then accede to that and live out a long and tragic course of deterioration and pain. Or, if she's strong enough, she might fight back: "Well, I don't believe it!"

But if I say, "No, I don't think you have arthritis," she'll most likely be relieved: "Oh, thank you, Doctor!" I have said, in effect, "No, I will not conspire with this effort to give over your power to some imaginary external entity that will systematically destroy your joints and progressively cripple you. Instead, I stand beside you as an advocate who believes that you can heal your body, and that it is under your ultimate control." No wonder if she thanks me!

I might have said, "Yes, it's arthritis. Let's see what this arthritis has to say to you." In that case, my aim would have been to get her to listen to this entity's message to her and to integrate it back into herself as a positive, contributing aspect of her consciousness. But, unlike my Malicious Mole—an entity *I* invented—"Arthritis" has a long history of playing on this stage, and my patient is likely to get stuck there. Ideas about disease are so prevalent, and they take on such an immediate legitimacy and power, that I am loath to give them life. Once created, the Arthritis monster may well get out of hand, and my patient may leave my office clear that the Arthritis is a reality, but vague about my efforts to help her integrate it back into her consciousness.

We all need to be alert to such pitfalls along the way of "diagnosis by renaming." It is easy to slip into such thinking without realizing it. Maybe this sort of diagnosis shouldn't be termed "diagnosis" at all, a word that literally means "through knowing" (*dia* = through, *gnosis* = knowing). When we create an unintegrated entity outside ourselves by renaming, when we create the disease "arthritis," for example, or "asthma," this is not a way of "knowing." In any case, it's certainly not the kind of "knowing" that is likely to result in healing.

In Eastern thought, "to know" has several possible meanings. One, to know through names, is notoriously subject to deception and confusion. The other, knowing by direct connection or empathic fusion, is regarded as part of the "Royal Path" to enlightenment and wisdom. It is this second sort of knowing that the practitioner of meditation aims to master. It involves an obliteration of the separation between subject and object. The Sanskrit term used for this process is *samyama*—"to become one with."[2] This sort of knowing is the essence of healing or "making whole again"— since it can bring back together the parts of the whole that were separate.

But the common practice of diagnosis by renaming, and the resulting creation of a separate entity or "disease," has quite the opposite effect. It is a refusal to know (in the sense of being one with); in fact, it is a way of not knowing by putting the cause outside ourselves. Maybe instead of *diagnosis,* "through knowing," it should be called *diaschizis,* "through splitting" (*dia* = through, *schizis* = splitting, as in *schizo*phrenia). For in this case we deal with our suffering by splitting off the cause—projecting it outside, making it something separate and distinct that we are not responsible for and cannot control.

This sets us up to be victimized by the entity we have created. *It controls us.* To separate from it is to give it power; to become one with it, to absorb it, is healing. You can't really succeed by "fighting a disease." Instead you must move with it—as in kung fu. Become one with it. Engage it in a process of *samyama.*

So the act of diagnosis, as it is commonly employed, is essentially formalizing a socially condoned paranoia, one which may mask a deep-seated societal schizophrenia. That may sound extreme, but when the Berlin Wall came down Anna, one of my patients, fell apart.

> *Anna was the daughter of minor nobility in Lithuania at the onset of the Second World War. Because one of her parents was half Jewish, the estate was broken up by the Nazis then confiscated by the Russians. She was separated from her family and suffered terrible privation as a young girl, picking her way through the devastated streets of Berlin, taking shelter where there was a kind hand, and giving birth as a young teenager to a child that was taken away from her. She eventually found her way to America, where she established herself as an artist. I had thought that she would be overjoyed when the Wall came down and the hostilities ended. Instead she was decimated. She sat before me with collapsed shoulders and a fallen face. "So what was the meaning of all those years of suffering?" she asked plaintively.*

Hatred of Communists had been a powerful organizing force for all of us. As a teenager I won a declamation contest for a stirring (and thoroughly paranoid) speech about the threat of Communist infiltration in our society. Remembering that diatribe a few years ago, as I was drawing up a program for an upcoming Yoga Congress, I was prompted to assign myself the title "Learning to Live Without the Enemy." How could we make this transition with the Communist bloc dissolving—where would we put the fear and suspicion? What or who would become our new "paranoid object"? I have since wondered how much of the brunt of this shift has been borne by our diseases—a ready target for the fearful sense of lack of control and power in our lives. To what extent have our "Disease Entities" replaced our political foes? How far is it, internally, from the Cold War to the War on Cancer? As a psychiatrist, I was taught that the economy of the mind is such that it will seize upon a substitute in a totally different realm of our lives as long as it is able to serve the same functional role.

How we can work with this tendency to split and to project as part of our individual and collective healing will be an important facet of working directly with the mind, which is the subject of the last part of this book. Until then, it will be important to consider "The Diagnosis" as it is commonly used: as quicksand—a dangerous territory in which to venture. This does not mean that the diagnostic process itself is without potential, but that it is possible to investigate diagnostically in a more useful and constructive fashion.

2. A Better Diagnosis

A diagnosis that contains new, useful, and clarifying information about what is going on in our bodies is a diagnosis in the real sense of the word. It is an attempt to decipher the presenting picture so that it can be better understood. Remember Adrienne, who complained of tightness in her chest and yellow mucus? Unless she has a good deal of knowledge of how the body works (which unfortunately is unusual), telling her that there is an element of bronchospasm is probably helpful to her—tightness in the chest might well have meant muscle tightness in the chest wall, as far as she knew, but bronchospasm tells her that the tightness is in the airways, not in the muscles of the chest. That the yellow mucus is a sign of a bacterial process may also be valuable information for her. Moving from "tightness in the chest and yellow mucus" to "mild bronchospasm and mild bronchitis," even when translated into colloquial terms, is useful.

In fact, maybe that's a good test of a diagnosis: if you can translate it into "normal English" and it throws new light on the situation, then it's a useful diagnostic label. By contrast, the diagnosis of "pharyngitis" does not convey new information—unless I didn't know that my throat was inflamed and that was discovered incidentally as part of an examination.

Physicians are often faced with a choice of whether to venture forward into meaningful investigation or to back up into the safety and ease of an essentially meaningless diagnosis.

> *Eula, a fifty-year-old heavyset Dominican matron came in with hives. She was covered with large welts. They were angry-looking, it seemed to me, and obviously itched. She was desperate. "What's going on with me?" she demanded. Here was a good opportunity to beat a hasty retreat and cover my tracks with diagnostic renaming. "It's urticaria," I could say, or, if I wished to look like a first-class derma-* tologist *(which would have been pushing it), I might have said* angioneurotic edema. *Both those terms simply mean "hives," but I could follow with a treatment: "I would recommend diphenhy-dramine." Sounds pretty impressive, but I was out of the habit of this kind of medicine, and besides, I didn't know* why *she had hives. My usual curiosity (often my best ally) led me to want to find out.*
>
> *"I don't know what's going on," I admitted, feeling predictably awkward and inept as I confessed my ignorance—despite the con-scious decision I had made to take the course of least comfort. "Maybe you're reacting to something you ate." She hadn't eaten anything unusual, she said, but she was on a medication for high blood pres-sure. Although she'd been on it for a while, levels can build up, I rea-soned, as can sensitivity to a foreign chemical in the body. Moreover, she'd been having other attacks of hives, it turned out, though this was one of the most severe.*

I looked up the blood pressure medication in the *Physicians' Desk Reference.* Sure enough, under "Adverse Reactions, Skin," I found urticaria. "Maybe you're going to have to stop this medication," I began. "But what about my blood pressure?" she interrupted. I looked at her. In the years since I'd seen her last, she had abandoned her previously whole-some diet, had fallen into the habit of regular cocktails and wine, and had gained at least twenty pounds. "Maybe it would be better to control your blood pressure by cleaning up your diet and exercising," I suggested.

After perfunctory objections, she acknowledged the wisdom of this course of action, and within a couple of months she had lost the weight, her blood pressure was down, she was off the medication, and the hives were in abatement. A little bit of detective work can throw light on the process that has led to the patient's problems, and is an important part of the diagnostic investigation. This is where laboratory tests can be invaluable. They can validate the physician's conclusions. They can also convince the otherwise skeptical patient that there is something going on in his or her body that needs attention.

Matthew's mother brought him in because he'd been diagnosed with "attention deficit disorder." Having seen me for over twenty years, she came to me first rather than immediately accepting the necessity of medication. But her son was a disaster. His skin color was an unhealthy gray. He was jittery and scattered. He couldn't sit still or concentrate—and he was infinitely resourceful in finding ways to cover this up or to blame someone else for his mistakes and omissions. "My teacher's a dope," he began, and launched into an exhaustive catalog of what one might guess were accurate observations of his math teacher's faults and foibles.

But Matthew's mother, a teacher herself, was long since wise to his diversionary tactics. She pulled out an essay he'd done on Gandhi for me to see. What I found was a scrawl that looked like the product of a child several years younger and many points lower on the IQ scale than Matthew. "The diet of the typical Indian," it began, "consists of a large prestige [sic] of grains. . . ." His use of words was as off the wall as his blaming attitude, and his sentences were disjointed in a way that showed up on paper more clearly than in his staccato verbal blasts.

Despite a painful awareness of what teenagers tended to eat (having two at home myself), I was still horrified by his diet record: ice cream sandwiches and pizza were the staples, though favorites like French fries with catsup and a glazed doughnut or hot chocolate with Cool Whip also figured prominently. Then there were those places where you could tell that his mother had stepped in and tried to intervene. There you'd find listings such as "three small frozen tofu chocolate-and-vanilla sandwiches"—an ice cream substitute loaded with sugar and of dubious superiority to the real thing. He also had, every other day or so, something that might loosely qualify as real food: a turkey sandwich or eggs for breakfast.

Not surprisingly, he complained of stomachaches—and rather severe ones at that. "They're pretty much always there. And my energy is really low," he says. "I feel exhausted most of the time."

It was obvious to me that diet was playing a pivotal role here, but he tossed off all my suggestions with the same facility he showed in

*dismissing his teachers and his mother. As far as he was concerned, it
seemed, this was a conspiracy to make his already impossible life even
more miserable. The little pleasure he got out of his day—a piece of
pizza or a bit of ice cream—we now wanted to take away. After a
visit or two with little progress, I decided to suggest a stool test. "Let's
see what might be causing your stomach pains." I proposed. He went
for it.*

*At the next visit I handed him a copy of the report. "The '4+' shows
that you have an overgrowth of yeast in your gut." I observed. "Is that
the normal amount?" he asked. "No, this is the highest level the test
can show. You have a severe invasion of* Candida *in the intestinal lining." He was daunted. "Well, what does that do?" he asked nervously.
"It irritates your intestinal tract and causes abdominal pain," I
explained. "It also interferes with your steadiness and grounding
because when your colon is irritated, full of gas, and painful, it's hard
for you to feel stable or anchored on the earth. You can't sit still and
think clearly, because you feel disrupted at your very core."*

*This changed his attitude totally. He began to negotiate. "So what
can I eat?" "What kind of pizza can I have?" "What kind of ice
cream can I have?" As I dodged those questions, he slowly began to
get the picture. Finally he asked, "You're not saying I have to give up
ice cream and pizza?!" "I'm not saying you have to give up anything.
I'm just trying to help you see the relationship between what you're
eating and how you feel—the pain in your belly and the tiredness and
the trouble you're having focusing in school." And he said, "I can't
give up pizza and ice cream." And I said, "Well, maybe not. Then
you'll have pain in your abdomen and you'll have trouble focusing
and you'll be exhausted most of the time." He looked away. As if to
himself, he mumbled, "I can't give up ice cream. . . ."*

But he did. He did it on his own initiative, and he was quite proud of
what he'd done. As he dropped most of the junk food from his diet, his
appearance changed dramatically. He came in with color in his face, and
he began to grow in height. Meanwhile his ability to sit and study
improved remarkably. "I can't get him to stop reading and go to bed!" his
mother said, laughing. Not surprisingly, his grades jumped from C's and
D's to A's and B's. One might call it "the magic of the lab test."

Here's where lab tests can be most helpful—to clarify the physiologic
process. The information about what is going on in your body is made

objective—it is removed from the realm of doctor-patient interpersonal dynamics. It is not what you are being told to do, what an invasive authority is pushing on you that you might be inclined to defy, it's simply information that was collected in a neutral, objective laboratory. You can use it any way you wish. And if you want to feel alert and energetic and calm, you may find yourself using it in a simple and direct way to change your habits.

So laboratory tests have their pros and cons (see Fig. 26). On the positive side, they can make facts already known to the clinician believable to the patient, as they did for Matthew. But laboratory investigation should offer more than psychological impact. It should throw additional light on what is happening physiologically. Besides the stool test, I will often request a hair analysis to look into the trace mineral status of the person, and sometimes do an ELISA/ACT, which is a food sensitivity test, to understand what is happening in the intestinal tract.[3]

Though helpful at times, such tests also have a distinct disadvantage. They tend to reinforce the prevailing materialistic bias. The lab test conveys the message that answers are to be found in the molecules of your blood, or the structures of your organs, or the bacteria growing in your tissues. Illness is seen as molecules and cells gone awry. Any mental or emotional suffering is the result of physical causes. Pulling our thinking toward the material and away from the causal role of the mind and emotions, the mystique of technology blinds us to more important aspects of reality.

LAB TESTS

Pros:
- make facts believable to patient

- *may* throw new light on the situation

Cons:
- hypnotize/draft us into medical power structure

- reinforce a materialistic bias

FIGURE 26

Unfortunately, the practice of medicine today is dominated by such testing, and laboratory machines have come to function unconsciously as the rattles and incense burners in what amount to clinical rituals that bolster the "religion of medical science." In the presence of these "power objects," we fall under the sway of the high priests of medical orthodoxy and begin to function as passive recipients of its treatments, its predictions and its world view.

Most of us don't need further reinforcement of this materialistic orientation. We've long since gotten it thoroughly ingrained in our thinking that the cause of illness is physical. What we need is to explore the opposite perspective—the role that consciousness plays in shaping what happens to our bodies. That's the dimension we bring into play to attain a third type of diagnosis.

3. The *Best* Diagnosis

Mrs. M. was nearing the limits of her patience. She'd made the mistake of asking my opinion of what caused the pain in her knees. This had taken us from too much meat and sugar in the diet and questions about dental hygiene to, ultimately, reflections on how consciousness organizes the body's functioning to produce illness or health. If I could help her position herself to see her problem from a radically different angle, perhaps she could get beyond it. The first step was to see that causality is not limited to the material realm. While Western science assumes that causes operate on the physical level, other systems of medicine disagree. Eastern thought has always held that matter is secondary.

As I explained to Mrs. M., Western science is based on the belief that consciousness arises from matter, awareness being a product of physical processes occurring in the nervous system. By contrast, from the Eastern perspective, consciousness shapes the physical world.[4] Looking at illness from this point of view might change everything. If it is true that human consciousness creates the world of physical phenomena, perhaps, as the yogis say, the realm of suffering we create is ultimately *maya* or illusion. Mrs. M. snorted derisively at this idea: "Well, *my* pain is no illusion."

"Of course not," I heard myself reply empathetically. And yet I immediately regretted that reflexive response. From a certain Eastern spiritual perspective, that's exactly what our pain is—an illusion, grounded in a conviction that we are helpless. When we can see the way in which our habits and attitudes affect our bodies, then we are free to change that. What was before perceived as pain is now decoded as information about what we need to change.

But, looking at Mrs. M. hunched over her painful knees, I could tell that this line of reasoning wasn't going to go over very well with her. Indeed, there was a certain no-nonsense attitude about her that ruled out abstract philosophical discussion. I could see how her stubborn insistence on the "normality" of the physical world had her trapped in a place where her pain was inescapable. She could continue to hang on to her "commonsense" attitude—but at a high price.

When westerners first started going into China in the 1960s and returning with stories of anesthesia by acupuncture, many observers thought this would shatter our rigid attitudes of materialism and the primacy of material causality. But today, though acupuncture is practiced throughout the Western world, medical scientists continue to search for a physical explanation of its efficacy, rejecting the concept it's based on— that the movement of *ch'i* or energy determines much of how the body works. Our culture has an intense resistance to accepting the power of the nonmaterial, a prejudice in keeping with our focus on the acquisition of possessions and other material aspects of life. Many of the spiritual traditions of the world concur that we are in one of the Earth's periodic epochs when materialism is dominant.

THERAPEUTIC INPUT ON VARIOUS LEVELS

Some years ago, I was the guest of Dr. Sukhdev, a very affluent and successful Western-trained physician in Kanpur, India. A kind and generous man, whose life revolved around his clinic and his extended household, he graciously made space in his home for me to have a room to myself—an unheard-of luxury even among the well-to-do in the India of a quarter-century ago. Each day I went with him and his nephew, also an M.D., to observe how they practiced medicine. Since I was living in India in order to learn about Ayurveda and homeopathy, I was baffled by my host's total acceptance of the harsh side effects of the antibiotics and steroids he so lavishly prescribed to his patients. He did not dismiss alternative treatments completely, however. He confessed that when his daughter had had a case of severe eczema that failed to respond to the treatment offered by a dermatologist colleague of his, he had taken her to a homeopath who had cleared it up immediately. He could therefore understand why I might be interested in investigating homeopathy—but he hadn't the slightest interest in doing so himself.

Staying with us was a young lady, Sister Saroj, who was the adopted niece of the Sukhdevs. Her family had disowned her because she had abandoned the ways of orthodox Hinduism to embrace the precepts of a quasi-Christian sect of naturopaths founded by Vinoba, a follower of Mahatma Gandhi. Sister Saroj's mission involved walking from village to village in the rural outback of India, bringing naturopathic teachings and care to the masses. She was a being of radiant love.

When I came down with a cold and cough (the masonry houses were dank and cold, unheated for the short winters), Sister Saroj prepared me a *tulsi* drink, made from milk, turmeric, ginger, and the holy basil culti-vated in the courtyard garden. On the other hand, a painter who was working on whitewashing the house came to consult me when he began to cough. He had heard that I was a homeopath. Though I had only begun to learn, the remedy I prescribed him was as effective for his cough as Sister Saroj's was for mine.

It was only a few days later, however, that I got the full picture of the spectrum of medical traditions represented in this varied household.

> Sister Saroj and I were drawing up in a rickshaw to the walled compound that constituted the residence of the Sukhdevs. But our entry to the house was blocked by a long line of people, waiting to confer with a seated figure on the corner. "What's going on?" I asked Saroj. "Oh, it's the mali," she explained, using the Hindi word for "gardener." He was an elderly, kindly, and very wise-looking old man who tended the garden for the household and always seemed to have a warm smile for everyone. "In the evening he has hours for his clien-tele." Our mali had a reputation as a very effective healer. He pre-scribed mantras for those who were sick. Although Dr. Sukhdev attended lectures by Swami Rama on meditation and mantra, he lim-ited himself to using the most material and, in a sense, grossest of the physical medicines, while what seemed to me the most potent and refined healing techniques remained in the hands of the humblest member of the household.

From the point of view of Eastern wisdom, intervening in the phys-ical activity of molecular events is crude. It is, as we mentioned in the first section of this book, like trying to reprogram your computer with a screwdriver. The higher you go up the scale of functional levels, the more subtle and the more strategic your point of intervention, the more leverage you have. The mystery of the East has always revolved around that paradox: the most subtle and delicate is the most powerful. Western boxers could not fathom how Chinese martial artists could defeat them by studying the fine details of breathing and thought. Scientists still scratch their heads and refuse to believe their eyes when yogis make objects move without touching them.[5] Medical researchers continue to insist that "there is no evidence that homeopathy works," even though there are scores of studies published in their own journals demonstrating the efficacy of the remedies.[6] By maintaining—against all evidence to the contrary—that only the material can work, we tie our own hands and eliminate a whole spectrum of healing methods that offer hope and help to those who need it desperately.

Deepak Chopra has aptly called this attitude "the superstition of materialism." The stubborn insistence that something is true when it flies in the face of the evidence is not scientific, and has all the characteristics of a superstition. We freeze ourselves in the past when we force science to defend and preserve the beliefs and worldview of a century ago. Radical Healing will need to be based on a radical science—one that refuses to bow to fear and prejudice. It must apply uncompromisingly the methods of true science—to make unbiased observations and to search relentlessly for the truth—however it may differ from what we have been accustomed to thinking. Healing of the magnitude needed in order for this planet to meet its present challenges will require a no-holds-barred, totally fearless curiosity. This means a willingness to examine ourselves as well as the world around us and to step past the all-too-human tendency to cling to what is familiar and reassuring.

Because current medicine presupposes that the ultimate cause of what happens is on the physical level, Mrs. M.'s arthritis is thought to be something that begins in her joints—or at least somewhere in her body. If we look carefully, we find that this assumption—considered so self-evident in current scientific discourse that it's not worthy of mention—has no proof to support it. When we subject it to scrutiny, it becomes apparent that it is part of a belief system that has both shaped and distorted our biological sciences.

Basic biology courses teach that the process of evolution arose in a colossal planetary soup, where molecules bounced and bumped and, through random motion, merged to form complex proteins and nucleic acids. Out of this primeval brew appeared, after many eons, the first single-celled organism. This in turn, again by chance and after a long expanse of time, combined with others to produce a multicelled organism. And so the process went for millions of years along a Darwinian path of evolution. This scenario assumes no consciousness prompting this evolutionary process—the assumption having generally been that consciousness arose later. As multicelled organisms combined and formed larger conglomerates, eventually animals complex enough to manifest something we would call intelligence resulted. In other words, this perspective reflects the prevailing conviction that consciousness is an effect, not a cause.

I suspect this little story of bubbling soups and random connections has a powerful impact on our thinking and even shapes a certain spiritual orientation. It serves us, perhaps, as a sort of creation myth, expressing our belief in the primacy of matter—a cultural bias that has colored the entire structure of our "science" and of our medical thought. The assumption that consciousness is secondary to physical structures has created a huge schism between the physician who is working with medications, molecules, and surgical repair, and the priest or psychotherapist who is working with consciousness and spirit. Part of our challenge in applying the holistic approach is to reintegrate these two aspects of healing. Meanwhile, in the doctor's office and in the hospital, it continues to be assumed that in order to influence the course of events—to have a therapeutic effect—we must have input on the material level (see Fig. 27).

To intervene higher, at the level of thought, for example, is assumed to be relatively ineffective. This is the area of outcome, not of input, so it's natural to be pessimistic about treating illness with a therapy that works on subtler levels. Anything you might do there would be overpowered by what's going on down on a more fundamental physical level. If you wanted to affect the mind substantially, then you would give chemical medications—that would be intervening where it counts. Or you would give antibiotics—after looking on the physical level for the causal microbe.

But if we decide to shift our perspective and restore consciousness to the position of playing a causal role, an immense new field of possibilities for intervention arises. At the same time, we will need to reassess many of our conventional notions—to take just one example, our concept of infection.

The "germ theory" has been the linchpin of twentieth-century medicine. Success with infectious diseases paved the way for a golden age of

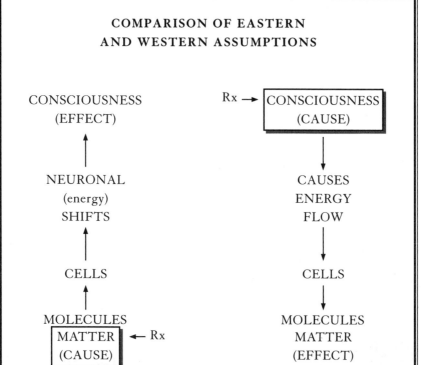

**COMPARISON OF EASTERN
AND WESTERN ASSUMPTIONS**

Of course, both schools of thought acknowledge some degree of causality from both mind and matter. The intent of the diagram is to highlight the difference in emphasis: Though the traditional Eastern physician taught that food and medicines were important, he saw their actions as more than physical. The modern westerner, on the other hand, is more likely to say "mind over matter" as a sort of jest. "Rx" indicates the logical focus of therapeutic input in each approach.

FIGURE 27

pharmacotherapy. Miraculous results with antibiotics in the early part of the century intoxicated us with a vision of the conquest of all disease through the use of such drugs. The infection model was especially seductive, for it not only jibed with our materialistic slant on life, but also provided us with the luxury of a perfect object for our paranoia. The malevolent microbe was the pervasive culprit behind every disease and would be vanquished by the "magic bullet" of antibiotics. Cancer, however, along with a host of other degenerative diseases, has refused to yield to the germ/drug approach. Apparently we have not found the key to relieving human suffering. By killing off the microbes, we may have merely uncovered the deterioration in function that allowed them to grow in the first place.

When the foundations of the germ concept were being laid in the late nineteenth century in conventional medical circles, the homeopaths pooh-poohed the whole idea. Little microscopic beings growing in the body? Nonsense, they scoffed. Of course, time proved them wrong. There *are* little microbes growing in diseased tissue—often. But in most cases we still do not know to what extent they *cause* the disease, or to what extent they are opportunists, growing in a weakened system. Medicine has tended to ignore this question, but it seems ripe for reconsideration.

My own hypothesis is that microbes are present in virtually every case of diseased or disordered tissue, but are more often a by-product of the disorganization than a cause of it. Interesting research by Virginia Livingston and others reveals convincing evidence that there are microbes associated with cancer.[7] Other researchers claim success in treating arthritis with antibiotics,[8] which suggests that microorganisms flourish in diseased joints. Both of these are diseases that have been considered to have nothing to do with infection.[9]

I suspect that we will eventually come around to the idea that most diseases involve disorder on multiple levels, and that the proliferation of bacteria, fungi, or viruses is merely one (physical) manifestation of a multilevel, complex disturbance. If that is true, then virtually every disease will be found to have a typical psychological picture, a distinctive energetic derangement,[10] a well-defined metabolic or biochemical expression, and a characteristic microbe that tends to grow. Which of these levels is playing the more "causal" role might vary from case to case—or even from moment to moment in the same case.

When we eventually learn to handle the matter of diagnosis with the subtlety and intelligence that such complexity demands, to refrain from simplistic formulations, and to acknowledge the role each level plays, the way we manage an illness will look very different. We can only imagine how that might work. In fact, it might be helpful to envision such a system, so let us follow a hypothetical patient through the medical adventure he might experience when a truly multilevel approach is used:

John sits before a holistic medical consultant, looking quite fit and trim. You would think he didn't belong in a medical facility, except for a slight darkness about his otherwise cheerful demeanor. "I've had a strange feeling in the pit of my stomach for weeks, maybe longer," he begins to explain. "It's not so much a pain as a sense of weakness or dissonance. My mind keeps feeling drawn there, as though something's wrong—like my center point is giving way, or something." He ends with hesitation, but his consultant reassures him that such perceptions should be taken seriously. She proceeds with non-invasive tests that reveal a small tumor of a malignant nature in the pancreas.

John does not respond with a sinking feeling or with panic. He does not feel overwhelmed with images of dying. "Such a condition," his consultant informs him, "is easily treated with a special dietary regimen and electromagnetic beams of a carefully calculated frequency." However, he and his consultant agree to defer such treatment, choosing instead to leave the tumor there so it can be monitored as an indicator of what is happening on other levels. "Though the treatment would have no negative side effects," his consultant explained, "it is still in a certain sense intrusive. We can learn so much more by waiting to see if the tumor will recede on its own as you make changes in your life and in the mental/emotional sphere."

To plan the program that he will undergo, they first do an inventory of his habits, environmental stresses, relationships, and preoccupations. "What turned up," the consultant explains as they bend over the test reports together, "is evidence of exposure to dieldrin, a toxic pesticide. The main residues seem to be in the liver and pancreas." They also find that his recent dietary pattern is not one that agrees with his constitution—again, stress on the pancreas. But, wondering why he would gravitate toward foods that disagreed, they begin to suspect and find evidence of anger—expressed only indirectly by forcing on his body food that it didn't really want. "What would you think," the consultant asks, "of doing a sort of exploratory session of move-

ment and imagery to see if anything comes up that would be a clue to the source of the anger?"

During this session, powerful, threatening images of the aunt who raised him arise and coalesce with impressions of his fiancée. John is intensely uncomfortable during this process, especially in the pit of his stomach. The discomfort reaches a climax with explosive rage. Though he is able to partially express this, he comes out of the session shaken, and with the awareness that it is still largely unresolved. "I want you to take a dose of Iris versicolor 1M. This will help to break the pattern of the rage being expressed through the pancreas, and the fear of the illness being beyond your control." In addition they decide on two flower essences: Fuchsia, to bring into awareness and expression repressed emotions that tend to cause physical illness, and Scarlet Monkeyflower, which lends the courage to face anger and powerlessness. He will begin these in several days.

Three months later, John is again sitting across from the consultant. "There've been some rough times with my fiancée," he confides. "For a while it looked like it was off. But after I really blew my top a few times, something changed. I think I realized that it was not her I was really mad at—it was my aunt. She can be so irritating in exactly the same way. And yet it's funny, some of her good qualities also began to remind me of my aunt, and I began to remember how kind she was to me at times. I guess raising me was an incredible challenge for her." Now his relationship with his fiancée feels more realistic and comfortable.

As he has let go toxic feelings, a parallel process has been encouraged in his body by following a regimen of distilled water and colonic irrigations to encourage the excretion of dieldrin. Acupuncture and an herbal compound have been used to support the liver during the detoxification. He has had weekly sonograms, which showed an initial enlargement in the mass, but then a subsequent shrinking. Six months later, the tumor is gone.

John no longer has the strange feeling in the pit of his stomach. Moreover, his relationships are more rewarding, and he has noticed an increase in energy, as well as a sharpened sense of intuition. In fact, he is considering a career change, planning to leave the job where he was exposed to the chemical and which he had for some time disliked. He has recently developed an interest in feng shui and the role of subtle energy in architectural design.

Though this case is fictitious and futuristic, we are very close to being able to provide this level of thorough healing for ourselves now. The main obstacles to our bringing together all the tools and techniques needed to do so are our embedded beliefs about the nature of reality, and the shape they give our thoughts and actions. These unconscious under-pinnings of our assumptions are the miasmatic foundations of both our illnesses and the unhealthy systems we have developed to deal with them—systems that in many ways serve to sustain the state of disease.

To begin to step out of these preconceptions and to capture the multi-dimensionality of the human condition so we might offer the *best* diag-nosis, we may need to incorporate some of the features of older traditions such as that of homeopathy with its concept of miasms, or that of ancient Asian systems such as Ayurveda or Traditional Chinese Medicine, which are holistic by design. These approaches are organized to encompass the many levels of functioning and to reflect the complex interaction that exists. We will explore them in the next two chapters, but first, let us take a final look at the question of diagnosis.

4. Even Better Than the Best?

Thus far we've looked at three varieties of diagnosis. To summarize:

- Diagnosis No. 1—that done by renaming—is not of much help, except to allow you to experience (only temporarily, one hopes) a feeling of helplessness and surrender.
- Diagnosis No. 2—a "better" diagnosis—is that which gives you new information and understanding of what is going on in your body.
- Diagnosis No. 3—the "best" diagnosis—is that which connects the physical with the energetic and mental.

But even this third and "best" diagnosis may not be good enough. To deal most effectively with your health challenges and to maximize your capacity for healing, you need to get past the tendency to focus exclusively on what's wrong. While it is essential to identify clearly the patterns you are trying to free yourself of, you remain limited and trapped until you can get beyond those confining patterns and begin to see your potentials and your strengths.

A few years ago it occurred to me that, as a physician, I had become an expert on defects. I could see them quite accurately, much better than most people I knew. You might have called me a "defectologist"—a good one, no doubt, but situated fixedly in a mindset that was cognizant only of faults and failings. That was my focus.

As we shall see in the next chapter (and throughout this book), there is good reason to regard our physical characteristics as revealing our inner conflicts—all that is "wrong with us." But as a result of making this my exclusive focus, I was depressed by the people I saw around me. Their pathologies seemed overwhelming—so much to fix and so little time. Of course I was nothing more than a pile of defects myself, and no matter how hard I "worked on myself," I constantly seemed to discover more that was amiss.

I began to make a shift when I participated in a gathering called "The Body Sacred." One of our goals was to reexamine attitudes toward ourselves and our imperfections. It was a much-needed antidote to my focus on negatives. The group's intent was to consciously transmute conditioned responses to our bodies, reframing our perceptions so we could see our unique characteristics as assets rather than liabilities.

Wide hips and heavy thighs, for example, might be attributes reminiscent of the classic figure of a fertility goddess, rather than signs of a failure to live up to the standards of rail-thin advertising models. A caved-in chest is pulling away from intimacy, but it can also be a celebration of the sensitivity that leads to that withdrawal. I began to see the possibility of looking at human "defects" from a totally different angle—to see them as perfect ways to deal with an imperfect world, as evidence of our participation in a larger healing agenda. What we call our imperfections might be considered ways we have embodied bits and pieces of the group mind and the conflicts of the collective unconscious. By taking on some part of the negativity of the planet, we can transmute it with joy and love, making of it something positive. Each of us, with a certain quota of that darkness, can collectively heal the whole, of which we are each a part.

As I came to understand that planetary healing—the correction of the ecological crisis and the relief of widespread human suffering—would be accomplished as each one of us heals her or himself, defects seemed less damning and more like the essence of "character"—more like evidence of what each of us had volunteered to heal. I thought of organic produce: those apples with the marks and the dimples, those were apples with flavor. I had long since begun to see their beauty and prefer them to the tasteless perfection of the chemically produced commercial ones. Could I do the same with humans, even with *myself*?

Though for the present we may still find ourselves relying on disease language much of the time, we need to be working toward the creation of "a healing space." This will be a space where we can see our common participation in a great effort to heal and be healed, a place where we can feel safe because we know we are all part of a shared process. It will be a place where we can rediscover connection and support, and focus on our strengths rather than bemoaning our defects.

More than isolating and judging some aspect of yourself to reach a diagnosis, such a space is concerned with seeing the meaning and significance of that detail in a larger pattern—some greater gestalt of which you are a part. From this point of view, my quirks and foibles are uniquely valuable, as are yours. There's room for my peculiarities as well as yours. In fact, we are incomplete if any one of us is missing.

From this perspective, we might see the "informational content" of remedies in a new light. Remembering the arborvitae and its use in the treatment of warts, now we can see *Thuja,* the remedy made from it, as holding the secret of how "wartiness" can be used in nature in the most productive and constructive way. Rather than helping you get over this mode of functioning that warts are evidence of, *Thuja* becomes your teacher. It is an expert on how to do it best, so you can be fully worthy of your warty state in the best of all possible ways: to "work it" to the hilt, to use it creatively and to build on that foundation so you can move on.

Healing is, by its nature, a knitting together, a restoration of wholeness. It requires that we see and accept lovingly all parts of ourselves. Our ability to contain more, to expand our identity, to accommodate the multifarious aspects of ourselves is the basis of healing. When we see our quirks as defects, we undercut the integrative impulse. Every acknowledgment of a symptom needs an enlarging affirmation to follow, so we don't tighten the trap of limitation around our necks.

A SHIFT TO THE POSITIVE

Louise Hay's little book *Heal Your Body* is a bible to many who are treading the path of holistic healing. It lists common disorders alphabetically and, alongside them, what she considers the most common psychological and emotional attitudes and postures that correspond to the disease mentioned. Indigestion, for example, reflects "gut level fear . . . griping and grunting." Though her lack of medical credentials and the tone of missionary zeal that leavens her gatherings of enthusiastic followers has made her the object of derision among some, to me her little book is a gold mine. Countless times it has confirmed my own impressions of the underlying mental state that had given rise to a disease. Not infrequently, it went on to put a finer point on what I had suspected. In other cases it opened new doors, leading me to look at the situation from a fresh and more productive angle.

The book also has a third column besides the Problems and the Probable Causes of a psychological and emotional nature, a parallel listing of "New Thought Patterns." Alongside the problem "Arthritis" we find "resentment the probable cause" (and are advised to look also under "Joints," which are said to represent "Changes in direction in life and the ease of these movements)." Third-column new thought patterns are "I now choose to love and approve of myself . . . and see others with love," and "I flow easily with change." These are what are otherwise known as affirmations. For a very long time I simply ignored them, feeling that they were a bit hokey—too New Age-ish and Pollyanna-like for me. Only during my recovery from being an inveterate defectologist have I come to appreciate their value.

I find that those who get their minds set on their defects are the ones who fare most poorly in their struggle for better health. Those who brush off dire diagnoses with a positive attitude seem to shed diseases as a duck sheds water. Take Ellie, for example, who had come in to work on her bone density. In her late fifties, she wanted to avoid osteoporosis, but didn't want to use the usual drugs. She was energetic and attractive and basically, she felt, in excellent health. What fascinated me about her was that sixteen years earlier she had been diagnosed by a top New York neurologist as having multiple sclerosis.

> While abroad, Ellie had come down with a high fever. Her body had reacted violently to something—maybe it was the tampons she had used, she speculated. It was a strange sort of sickness. After the acute episode was over, she discovered she had lost her sight in one eye. She sought the best of specialists, and extensive tests were done. Finally she was informed of the results. "You have a severe demyelinating disease. It's multiple sclerosis, and it's progressive."
>
> I looked at her. She certainly didn't look or act like someone with MS. "What did you do?" I asked.

"I thought, well, if I do have this, they can't do anything about it. So why put myself in the hands of these cold, negative people?"

Instead, she found an acupuncturist who had been trained as an M.D. and who told her, "I can say with everything in my heart that you don't have MS." He gave her seven treatments. After that he said, "I think you're fine."

"And since then?" I asked.

"A year later my eye bothered me again—the one that had sent me to the doctor in the first place. So I went back to the acupuncturist. After two more sessions it cleared up. I've been fine for the last fifteen years."

I was stunned. It was one of those lucid moments when I could see how much the mind shapes our destiny and our attitudes.

"All those dire predictions and elaborate tests," I was musing out loud.

"Yes," she said. "It was grueling—not to mention expensive! The doctors' fees alone added up to nearly a thousand dollars, and that was more than a decade ago. And, since I'd just come back from Europe, I didn't have any insurance."

I whistled softly, thinking about the immense amount of money we pour into creating negative expectations—a sort of expensive, high-tech form of voodoo.

"Were you able to manage?" I asked.

"Yes," she answered, "I was." She paused for a moment, her eyes downcast, apparently remembering that time in her life.

"I paid the doctor," she sighed, then she looked up with a twinkle in her eye. "But I didn't buy the diagnosis."

5

Body Maps:
Techniques for Self-Diagnosis

*M*r. *Decker walks into my office with a flourish, and seats himself.*
He is a successful businessman who exudes confidence. Having
recently developed an interest in holistic medicine, he's been struck by
the wisdom of doing some preventive work. He begins to describe the
symptoms that have concerned him but I realize vaguely that I am not
hearing his voice. I am totally taken by what his face is saying. What
grabs my attention most forcefully are the bags under his eyes. For a
man in his mid-fifties they are enormous, and that screams "kidney
problems."

A vertical line between his eyebrows—deeply etched and with
edges that look almost swollen—is thought in Asian diagnosis to sug-
gest liver dysfunction. Hmm. Liver and kidneys. Not unusual. In fact,
rather typical of the general population, though less typical of the
patients that I see. They are generally more conscious of the habits
that lead to overburdening the organs of detoxification. Mr. Decker
also has a dark, ominous-looking raised spot on his left cheek. This is
a point where the lung area intersects a strip corresponding to the
large intestine—and something unhappy is going on there.

That makes a full house of excretory problems: large intestine, kidneys, liver, and lungs. Then I notice the cleft in his chin. Here the signal
is not quite so clear—though the cleft is deep enough to demand attention. What does it mean? A series of associations flash through my mind:
Critical developmental stages—sides of the fetus uniting—contempora-
neous knitting together of the face and the heart. Septal defects, mur-

murs, probably mild—or maybe not even structural, maybe only a functional discoordination. Then there's the connection of the chin area with sexuality. This mélange of impressions floating, as yet unconnected, awaiting the emergence of a pattern around which to coalesce.

Oriental face-reading: Can a well-trained doctor take such stuff seriously? Is it science or superstition? It seems to me that it probably *was* superstition—or at best an intuitive process—but that it is beginning to make scientific sense in a way it didn't before. Newer ways of thinking may be elevating the status of Asian diagnostic techniques from primitive to highly evolved. The principle here is fundamental to the holistic approach. If a small part reveals the secrets of the whole, then we have a basis for discovering much about ourselves that can contribute to healing and transformation.

The Holographic Face

Our understanding is frequently limited by our conceptual models. Something "doesn't make sense" if we can't envision it, if we have no image that will accommodate it. Early machines offered a model for nineteenth-century concepts of how the body worked, and later the thermostat provided a basis for understanding metabolic feedback mechanisms. More recently, in a similar way, the advent of the hologram has offered a new template for conceptualizing how the parts of living systems reflect the whole, and how each individual system is itself part of a greater, encompassing natural order.

The hologram is produced by a technology that captures and displays an image through the use of lasers. The laser is simply a projector or gun that emits a pulsed, coherent beam of light. Normally a light source will radiate in all available directions, but the laser beam is "super focused." In a hologram, the image of an object is created on a photographic plate by using two separate laser beams that hit the object from different angles. The "photograph" thus produced can then be used to re-create the image in three dimensions, so that the viewer may move around it and observe it from many angles. This suggests that the hologram is capturing more information about the object than a conventional photograph.

Secondly, it is organized in such a way that information about the whole is distributed throughout the "photograph." You can look at the photographic plate and see nothing until it is reconstituted, which is done by subjecting it to twin laser beams fired at it in the same way as was done to create it. But what is amazing about this two-dimensional plate is that if you take any small part of it—a corner, let's say—that piece alone can be used to reconstitute the whole image. Every piece contains the whole. The degree of resolution or detail that results from such a small piece of the photographic record will be lower than if you used the whole thing—that is to say, it might be a bit blurry—but the entire image will be there.

This holographic principle is stimulating scientific thought with an intriguing new metaphor. Older models led to a "reductionistic" attitude: examine an object, reduce it to its parts, and study each part separately. Approaching living systems in that fashion will yield lots of detailed information about the parts, but little understanding of how they fit together. The holographic metaphor implies that each piece contains the essence of the whole. Each cell in the body, for example, would somehow embody the quality or carry a tendency to manifest the form of the whole—as cloning research has discovered. Each animal would carry something of the formative essence of the whole planet—and even of every planet of the universe.

This represents a radical departure from our fragmented, analytical thinking of past decades; it gives us a very different frame of reference for studying the integration of living systems and their interrelationships. Never again will we be able to dismiss the rain forest as simply a source of rare tropical lumber or as potential grazing land for beef cattle. Our most advanced science now sees that rain forest as the lungs of the planet—and each individual's respiratory apparatus as a reflection within the human body of that larger biological breathing entity that serves the Earth as a whole.

This perspective gives us a new appreciation of ancient traditions such as face diagnosis. The notion that the shape of the ear might tell us something about the nervous system or kidneys of a person, or something about his personality, suddenly doesn't seem so preposterous. In fact, it now seems a likely possibility. Why *wouldn't* it reflect information about the whole?

Meanwhile, thoroughly trained physician that I am, I set aside my hypotheses about Mr. Decker, try to ignore what his face seems to be yelling at me, and set about to collect the more conventional information that doctors are taught to gather. By the end of the hour-long evaluation,

I wind up with the diagnoses that I might have had at the outset by simply looking at his face. A Western-style physical examination and medical history have provided confirmatory evidence of problems with the liver and kidneys and a likelihood of stagnation in the colon. Though I suspected all this at the outset, now I am "sure." I have satisfied my reductionistic medical programming as well as confirmed my intuitive impressions.

I personally find the combination of the reductionistic and the more holistic intuitive diagnostic approaches reassuring. I need both. Unfortunately, there is not much of a balance of the two in the medical world that most of us encounter. Hospitals and clinics rely almost exclusively on the maddeningly narrow data that emerge from laboratory tests and cursory examinations. Holistic practitioners, in growing numbers—though still in the minority—are delighting in the recovery of their intuitive faculties, though often with an eagerness that outpaces their training or preparation.

Problems also arise when clinicians carry over their reductionistic attitudes and assumptions to the use of holistic diagnostic techniques. We cannot, for example, take a specific mark or crease on the face and draw definitive, reductionistic conclusions from it. We can't say, "Aha! Cleft chin! You have an atrial septal defect. And let's see, the cleft is 3 mm deep; therefore the defect in the wall between the two chambers of the heart is 3 times 0.8, or 2.4 mm wide." Mixing methodologies in this way yields results that are obviously absurd.

Instead, remember that one of the characteristics of the holographic image is that re-creating it from only a fragment of the record will yield a picture that is of poor resolution—that is blurry. We will get a sense of the whole—but we won't get reliable information on details. If you want details on one little part, take a conventional photo of that part and blow it up. If you want details on the heart, do conventional sonograms or angiograms and look at the specifics. Another feature of the holographic approach, however, is that the more chunks of the record you bring into play, the clearer becomes the reconstruction of the image. So we can look at the face, the hands, the body, the ears—any number of parts of the person that have been studied by traditional medicine—and allow all the impressions to blend together to form an image of growing clarity. In this chapter we will look at some of these body parts, how they have been "mapped" over the centuries, and how to read them, so you have several to combine.

The Tongue: Instant Update

Maureen is a retired office worker who comes to see me because of her eyes, which are red and irritated. They burn, and all attempts to treat them, including the ministrations of an ophthalmologist, have failed. Her tongue is also an angry red, and leads me to think in terms of an "overheated liver." She is frustrated with her husband and has felt trapped for years.

The tongue is a sort of litmus or indicator of what is going on in the body, dramatically showing the general state of the person through its color, texture, shape, and coating. A fiery red tongue suggests excess heat in the system. It will tend to be seen in those who have a fiery constitution, are prone to fits of ire, and tend to get acid stomachs and high blood pressure. These are the people the Ayurvedic physician would term *pittic,* and the Five-Element Chinese diagnostician would call Fire types. The skin of such folks will also have a flushed or plethoric look—they are the red-faced souls one sees in the street. But it is the tongue that will literally look as if it's hot and overheated (see Fig. 28).

A cold system, by contrast, will be reflected in a pale tongue. Lack of color suggests weakness and lack of vitality—not enough fire to run the engine. If the pale tongue is also wet and coated white, it suggests that the

---

TONGUE DIAGNOSIS I

COLOR	SIGNIFICANCE
RED	EXCESS FIRE
PALE	LACK OF VITALITY (Cold)
PURPLE	CONGESTION OF BLOOD (Sluggish Circulation)

(see also TONGUE DIAGNOSIS II, Chapter 6, Fig. 51)

FIGURE 28

system is not up to burning the food and has accumulated a mucu_ of unprocessed substance.

One time my teacher stopped my mother in the hall and said, "Your tongue is black. You should take *Chelidonium*." Her tongue didn't look black to me, though its coating did have a darkish cast to it. "How did he know my tongue has been sore?" she asked. A dark coating on the tongue is associated with conditions of toxicity, and it's the liver that is primarily responsible for the detoxification of so many of the substances that can poison the body.

A sluggish, overburdened liver is also reflected by irritation and irregularities along the edge of the tongue. Standing in front of a mirror, extend your tongue. Put the full tongue out, but don't strain. Allow it to relax just slightly. Now focus on the edges. If they are scalloped or serrated, like a bread knife, that means that your teeth have left an imprint. Perhaps your tongue has been unconsciously retracted, creating a partial vacuum in the mouth which actually draws the edges of the tongue close and more forcefully against the teeth. When the scalloped edge is found on a swollen tongue, Chinese physicians tend to think of problems with the spleen.

A purple tongue means stagnation. Blood not circulating freely is inadequately oxygenated and therefore not bright red. Sitting at the computer one morning, I noticed a heaviness in my stomach—as if there were a stone there. When I looked at my tongue, it was purple. The center, corresponding to the area that is often connected with the digestive system, was raised. It was, if anything, even more intensely purple than the rest. "Stasis in the gut," my mind registered. Then it occurred to me that I hadn't exercised in two days. "I should've known that," I thought, feeling a bit impatient with my own failure to recognize what was happening. No exercise, no digestion—and no wonder the food just sits there. After twenty minutes on the trampoline, my tongue was less purple. But that wasn't enough. I was too far behind with my activity, and it took a forty-five-minute session at the gym to return my tongue to its normal bright pink color. I could understand how, after long years of sedentary living, patients might come in with deeply purple tongues that brightened only many months after resuming exercise.

The appearance of the tongue can be echoed, in a less dramatic way, in the face and hands: purple coloration suggesting stagnation, dark spots of color showing toxic accumulations, and a paleness or sunken look, suggesting deficiency—of energy or blood or moisture. Dehydration will be

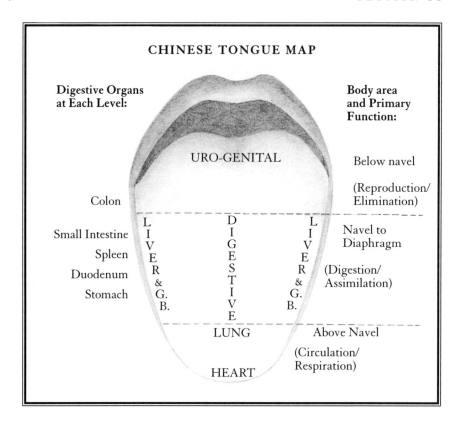

CHINESE TONGUE MAP

Digestive Organs
at Each Level:

Body area
and Primary
Function:

URO-GENITAL

Below navel

(Reproduction/
Elimination)

Colon

Small Intestine

Navel to
Diaphragm

Spleen

Duodenum

(Digestion/
Assimilation)

Stomach

LIVER & G.B.

DIGESTIVE

LIVER & G.B.

LUNG

Above Navel

(Circulation/
Respiration)

HEART

FIGURE 29

seen in a dry, shiny tongue, and the skin of hands or face will look parch-mentlike. When pinched, it forms a "tent" that is slow to drop back into alignment with the rest of the skin.

Chinese doctors have made the most detailed study of the tongue. They make a distinction between the body or "substance" of the tongue and its coating, or "moss." The tongue material or body is what has color and shape, and indicates something about the general condition of the person. The moss is said to be more directly related to the digestive process. It's considered to be a sort of "smoke" that results from the cooking of the food that occurs in the stomach and duodenum, and through the action of the spleen. If the stomach and spleen are weak, there will be little or no moss; if they are strong, it will be substantial and firm. Too much moss, or discoloration of it, reflects the accumulation of "matter" in the system that needs to be thrown off. A thick, greasy-looking moss suggests excess mucus or waterlogged tissues.

Though there is not total agreement on how the areas of the tongue correspond to the organs they might be associated with, there is a consensus that the layout of the tongue corresponds roughly to that of the body. The upper part of the body is represented by the tip and the lower part of the body by the back or base of the tongue (see Fig. 29). This regional division connects the rear third of the tongue with the organs of excretion, the middle third with the digestive organs (lying between the navel and diaphragm), and the third of the tongue that forms its tip with the cardiorespiratory organs (heart and lungs) in the chest. The sides of the middle third relate to the liver (and gallbladder).

Face Maps

Our faces are on display for the world to see. As you might expect, the face has been studied by a number of traditions and schools. Probably the most detailed and extensive is the Asian, which uses at least two major approaches to mapping the face for medical diagnosis.

The first considers that regions of the face relate to general functional systems of the body (see Fig. 30). The upper face, not surprisingly, is related to the nervous and mental functions of the person. The middle area of the face, that which extends across the nose, is connected to circulatory activities. The lower third, which encompasses the mouth and chin, is an indication of digestive and reproductive aspects of the body.

In the other major mapping of the face, particular points or areas are associated with organ complexes of the sort described by Chinese medicine (see Fig. 31). This is closest to our Western reductionistic expectations, so we grab these eagerly, delighted with the prospect of using them to surprise everyone with our magic knowledge! Yet there is no indication that the Chinese used this map with the same mechanical attitude that we might. In fact, traditional Chinese physicians approach such clues in a global, general fashion that allows them to overlook specific inaccuracies and failures. In a way that baffles the Western student, the Chinese doctor will say, "Yes, that corresponds to the intestine—but no, in this case there doesn't seem to be anything wrong with the intestine."

And apparent contradictions are inevitable. If the middle region relates to circulation, but the chin reflects heart problems, how do we deal with that? What's more, there are other maps, too. The meridians, used

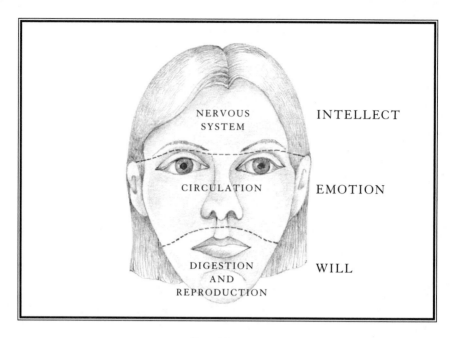

FIGURE 30

in acupuncture and shiatsu, often end or begin in the face (see Fig. 32). The bladder meridian, for example, crosses the forehead just to one side of the midline and comes to an end at the inner corner of the eye. "But the forehead was supposed to be nervous system and the middle of the face circulation and excretion," our linear "left brain" frets. To use this tool properly, we must grasp it with a looser grip. To use these maps fruitfully, we seem to need to be able to let them flow together, with both contending and corresponding streams of influence canceling and intensifying one another until a picture begins to take shape.

And sometimes it doesn't. At least not at my level of expertise. That's why I am happy to have alternative angles from which to examine a case. When the face doesn't "speak" to me, I may look at the hands. Or I might study the symptom picture to find the homeopathic remedy that corresponds to it and see what that tells me about the totality of this person. If one language or perspective doesn't work, let's try another.

But the face and hands—and the tongue, too—are readily available and laden with information. We may as well have a go at them. Besides, reading body maps is fascinating. A major part of the intrigue is that the body reflects not only the state of the internal organs but also, true to our holographic model, that of the mind as well.

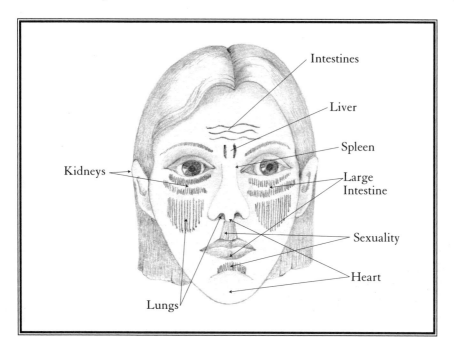

Intestines

Liver

Spleen

Kidneys

Large
Intestine

Sexuality

Heart

Lungs

FIGURE 31

Over the millennia, developing alongside the systems for reading physical health from the body, yet relatively independent of them, have been traditions of deciphering the personality,[1] the tendency to certain behaviors and even life events. For example, looking back at Fig. 30, the top third of the face reflects intellect, the middle third emotion (circulatory functions, including the heart), and the lower third your strength of will (how decisively you take in and digest the challenges of life). Oriental face readers might quickly surmise that the guy with the domed cranium is an "egghead," while his friend with the prominent lower jaw and chin strong-willed, as well as having an "ironclad stomach" (and sometimes an unruly sex drive).

Such correlations are not always obvious or simple. A nose with a cleft tip was considered an indication of a person who is suspicious and timid and who is difficult to get along with. Meanwhile, the Asian health practitioner says that the cleft nose indicates that the heart is beating in a discoordinated fashion or that there is a murmur. We are left to ponder how the timid person who lacks "strength of heart" might be given to disorders of the physical heart, and how that might have to do with a troubled integration of the right and left aspects of his or her

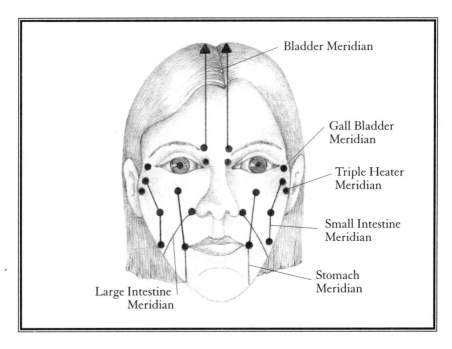

FIGURE 32

being. The right side of the body (and left half of the brain[2]) corresponds to the rational, analytical side of our thinking, as well as the assertive and proactive aspects of our behavior. The left side of the body reflects the more intuitive and receptive. Isn't the coordination, the knitting together of these parts of ourselves, a necessary foundation for the hearty and robust personality?

These are the reveries of the holistic physician. The overlay of different frames of reference, and the correspondences and questions that emerge, are an endless chain of fascinating hypotheses that often, surprisingly and gratifyingly, lead to unexpected but very practical prescriptions.

The Hands: Palmistry, Pulses, and Reflex Points

The face may be the most fascinating and information-packed part of the body, but it is also notoriously given to deception. The mask we wear is an intentional, if subconscious, effort to hide what the face might reveal. From contrived expressions to makeup, humanity has shown endless ingenuity in trying to cover up the messages the face is prone to broadcast.

But the hands are more honest. We may wear gloves—and in a more formal time it was only proper—but when they come off, the story the hands have to tell is clearly evident. The shape of the hand is what strikes us first. I am still astonished by the dramatic differences among the many hands that are extended to me when I meet new people. Some are damp, small, and nearly formless, seemingly hesitant to declare themselves. Others are large, square, and almost wooden, suggesting the angular construction of a table or a homemade chair. And then there are those that are hot and oily, full of fire and determination. To grasp such a hand is to feel invaded by the insistent intention and impatience of its owner.

These latter are the hands of the Fire type. The shape of the hand recalls a flame, with the fingers showing a subtle tendency to veer off in different directions, like the points of a flame licking upward. The broad, chunky hand with stubby fingers is earthy and indicates solidity and stability—the sign of an unshakable personality, one you can lean on. In the next chapter we will go deeper into these constitutional types and how the shape of the body and its parts reveals the type.

The shape of the fingers is also an expression of certain aspects of the person. Sitting on a plane once, I fell into a conversation with the man next to me, primarily, I have to confess, because I was fascinated by his hands. The fingers were long and elegantly shaped. Their graceful movement was telling me something, but I couldn't figure out what. Finally I asked him, apropos of nothing, whether he played the piano. He didn't, but it turned out he was a lawyer—a professor of law, in fact. As I came to learn, long fingers are found on those who are fond of details and who retain and arrange them with care and attention. One of my colleagues constantly amazed me with his ability to recall the smallest medical details of this disease or that. And his fingers were half again as long as mine! My stubby fingers betray my difficulty in hanging on to particulars. I am nearly always focused on general principles. My passion and aptitude is for how it all fits together, and I find myself looking to others to fill in the needed richness of specifics.

The color and shape of the nails is a constant meditation on the confluence of nutritional deficiencies, health problems, and personality traits. White spots on the nails, for example, suggest an excess intake of sugar and often a resulting lack of zinc. Homeopaths say that they also hint that the pattern of energy organization of the person calls for *Silica,* which is characterized by weakened resistance and "lack of grit." Traditional hand-readers regard such white specks as "the first warning of delicate

nerves . . . a *beginning* of the loss of vitality." Confronted by a hand with
white-spotted nails, I am left to contemplate how these different perceptions fit together and apply (or not) to this person before me.

MEDICAL PALMISTRY?

The study of the palm, long regarded as mere superstition, takes on
an intriguing new potential when we begin to think in holographic
terms. When a friend went with my teacher, Swami Rama, to a reputed
palmist in Nepal, they entered incognito. He read her palm first, then
asked to see Swamiji's. As soon as it was opened, the palmist gasped and
fell to the floor in the traditional gesture of respect. "I have waited all my
life to see a palm like this!" he said reverently.

Like the face, the palm has been mapped in various ways. The most
common is according to its major lines—traditionally known as the head,
heart, and life lines (see Fig. 33). Palmists examine the heart line for evidence of the emotional life, the head line for signs of intellectual and creative capacity, and the life line for indications of vitality and longevity.
Traditional Asian healers view the heart line and the area of the palm it
transects as related to the circulatory and excretory systems, the head line
to the nervous system, and the life line to digestion and respiration. The
fate line, running up the center of the palm from the wrist, is sometimes
thought to be an indication of general health. When it's deep and clear, it
suggests a firm commitment to one's path in this life.

The palm has also been mapped by reflexologists—those who work
therapeutically by applying pressure to the soles or palms. Not surprisingly, from the point of view of our holographic model, there are dis-
agreements on which points relate to which organs; but there is also a
substantial degree of consensus. Fig. 34 represents some of the more commonly accepted point connections. As in the face, acupuncture meridians
in the hand provide a third mapping. Each finger serves as a point of ter-
mination for one or more meridians. The dotted lines in Fig. 35 represent
the meridians that traverse the back of the hand (not the palm).

The hand also comes to the attention of the traditional Asian physician because it's where he feels the pulses. Accurate pulse diagnosis is considered by most Ayurvedic and Chinese doctors as the pinnacle of
accomplishment in clinical assessment. Volumes of information might be
offered by a *vaidya,* an Ayurvedic physician, after he stands quietly for a
few moments concentrating on what his fingertips tell him about the subtleties of the patient's pulses. How accurate can this be?

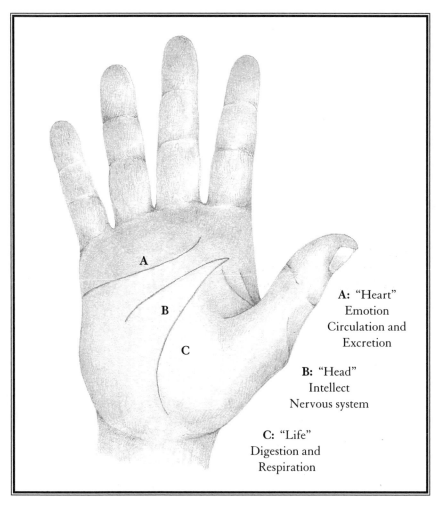

A: "Heart"
Emotion
Circulation and
Excretion

B: "Head"
Intellect
Nervous system

C: "Life"
Digestion and
Respiration

FIGURE 33

The tale is told of the Indians who set out to debunk a prominent Ayurvedic physician's reputed acumen at pulse diagnosis. It is said that in those days the art had reached such heights of evolution that the most accomplished vaidyas could do pulse diagnosis without even touching the patient. This was a crucial skill, since the wives of the Mogul rulers were not to be seen or touched by other men. To satisfy the stringent rules of Islamic propriety, the traditional physicians had learned, we are told, to read the pulse by holding a silk cord that was attached to the wrist of the lady as she lay behind thick, concealing drapes.

On this particular occasion the conspirators had arranged a consultation that was the usual in every respect but one: the silk cord that

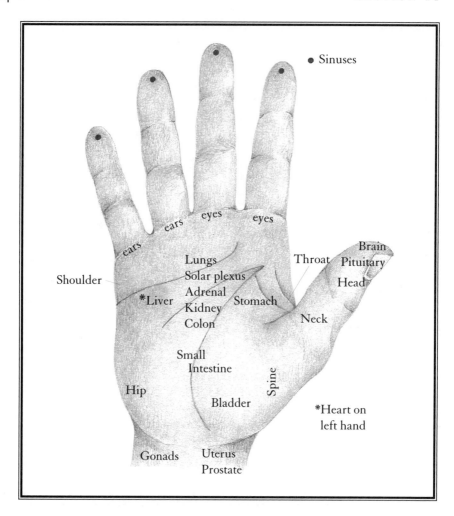

FIGURE 34

ran behind the curtains was attached to the foreleg of a cow. The famous physician arrived, seated himself, and took up the cord. His face became quiet and focused. Soon, however, it was marred by a growing frown. Finally he opened his eyes. He looked flustered and embarrassed. "I'm having great difficulty with this," he confessed. "I cannot get a clear picture of Her Highness. The only thing I can say with certainty, and I know this sounds odd"—he paused, mortified to have to make such a recommendation to a member of the royal fam-ily—"is that it is necessary for this patient to be on a very restricted diet, a diet of nothing but . . . grass."

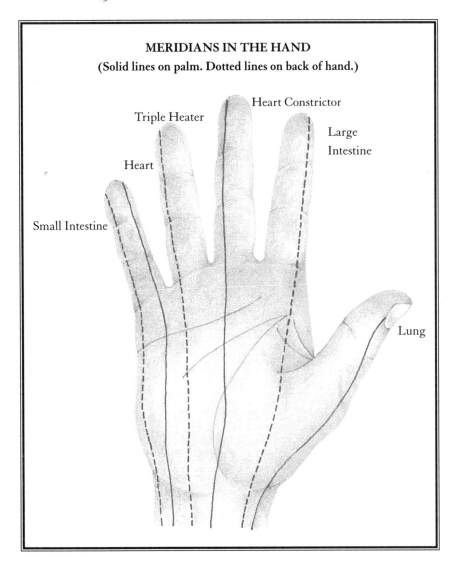

MERIDIANS IN THE HAND
(Solid lines on palm. Dotted lines on back of hand.)

Heart Constrictor

Triple Heater

Large
Intestine

Heart

Small Intestine

Lung

FIGURE 35

What is charming about this story is that it manages to acknowledge both our disbelief and the mysterious accuracy of pulse diagnosis. That's a conflict I've wrestled with endlessly. Consider how it's done: The three first fingers are placed on the radial artery of the right wrist, for example. You can do it on yourself. With both palms facing up, bring your left palm against the back of your right wrist. Curve the fingertips around until they find the artery, placing the middle finger on the bony prominence. The forefinger is said to assess the lungs and large intestine while the finger alongside it, the middle finger, taps into the stomach and small intestine (see Fig. 36). "Now," my Western science-trained mind taunts, "*how* exactly can one segment of a small artery, only *millimeters* from another segment, reflect the functioning of a totally separate organ system?"

Yet I've seen it work. I've seen skilled practitioners hold the wrist, concentrate quietly for a few minutes, and talk perceptively about what's going on inside the person before them. In fact, I've even done it myself. What the story of the cow brings up for me is a long-standing suspicion that what is going on with pulse diagnosis is not limited to receiving information through the fingertip. Might it not be that concentration with the finger placed on a point we have come to associate with a specific organ helps us tune in intuitively to that organ and access subtle perceptions we might otherwise ignore or discount? In other words, the focus on the pulse may turn on our intuitive "radar" and direct it toward each part of the body in turn.

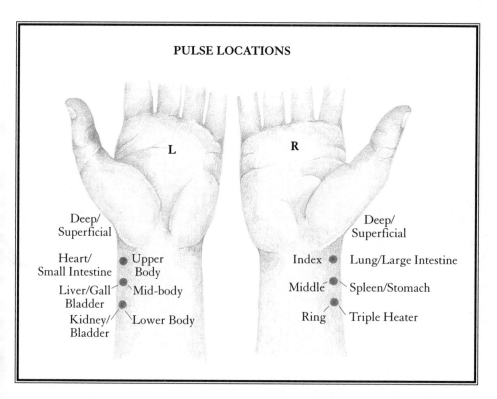

FIGURE 36

However, the idea that there is indeed some degree of correspondence between the particular point on the artery and its associated organ is supported by the fact that different traditions have come up with point-to-organ connections that are similar. For example, the distal (farthest from the heart) pulse on the right monitors lung and large intestine in the Chinese system, while it is said to reflect *vata* in the Ayurvedic. *Vata,* the airy and "spacey" aspect of our functioning is considered by the Ayurvedic physician to be expressed primarily through the colon and lungs (see Fig. 36). Although this similarity could be attributed to the historical cross-currents of influence between the two traditions, I find it difficult to discount the notion that there is some inherent connection between that particular point on the artery and the lung/large intestine complex of functions.

And this is in keeping with our holographic model. If points on the tongue have connections with parts of the body, then it is logical to think that different points on the artery might also have intricate and detailed correspondences. This doesn't mean that other ways of tuning in to the target organs and functions are not also operating—the sense of smell, some collection of observations we've made about the person's psychology and family background, or any number of other cues that we as clinicians have learned to process subconsciously and add into the pot as we hold the wrist. Certainly our more intuitive faculties are also likely to come into play here and enrich our perceptions.

In fact, I suspect that intuition often plays a role in many diagnostic procedures—including those that appear to be quite "objective." This might even be true of high-tech testing in the most up-to-date hospital. Let's say an X ray, for example, "needs to be read by the radiologist." He pops it onto the screen, rears back in his chair, ponders a bit, and says, "I think it's benign." "He's the best," the referring internist says. "I'll take his word for it."

DEVELOPING THE INTUITIVE

Sometimes it's the first glance at a face when you might get a "hit" of a perception of a color—a dusky look, or a redness that becomes less noticeable when you settle into a conventional social or professional interchange with the person. That brief window of opportunity to perceive a bit more might actually dip into the intuitive—the color you pick up at that brief moment might be not physical but energetic. The "color" of the energy of the person is something we usually tune out; it's not part of the world we have been socialized to include in our seeing. This "aura" can be a source of useful diagnostic information, if one has the openness and the patience to cultivate his or her sensitivity to it and to develop a thorough grasp of the connections between different colors or qualities and the states they are associated with.

I first heard of "reading auras" in the 1960s and figured there was something to it, since the energy state of the person is certainly a key to how he or she functions. Light is one form of energy—and that subtle light would be something that we could either glimpse or miss entirely. Therefore, though most of us have grown up trained to tune out any perception of that aspect of the world around us, I was willing to believe that some people managed to hang onto vestiges of the ability. I also suspected it was true that, as Swami Rama had suggested, those perceptions are liable to get mixed in with our own projections—what is going on with us or what we expect or fear or want.

Attending a conference, I was with a group in a darkened room where we were led through a sort of guided meditation. During the process, I sat up and looked across the room at the person who was guiding us. Her head was surrounded by a soft blue light. I started to rub my eyes, assuming they weren't focusing properly. Then I realized, "Oh, this must be what people call an 'aura.'" Once I accepted that it could happen to me, I found, when sitting with patients trying to tune into my sense of what they were about, that I sometimes entered a state where this could be seen.

If you want to explore this realm of diagnosis, have your subject sit where there is a plain, preferably white background, and look at him or her with your eyes not focused directly on the face. You, too, may find that you have been vaguely aware of a sort of halo, or light, in such situations, and that you have habitually refocused your eyes to eliminate it—assuming, as I had, that it was a sort of visual distortion.

Radical healing is based on enhanced self-awareness, and that enhancement comes from bringing into full consciousness what was previously on the periphery of your field of attention. That field is often defined culturally: although an Indian child is more likely to be socialized to notice and integrate memories from other lifetimes, a Western child usually is not. Healing of a radical nature often requires breaking down socially imposed taboos to bring into consciousness what before had been dismissed or ridiculed.

The Language of Disease

We read body maps to discern energy flow, to see the state of internal organs, and to monitor emotional and psychological processes going on underneath the surface. We can also read the effects of disease on the body. By determining the inroads it makes, the manner in which the body is altered by its processes, you can infer something about the connection between the body and the spirit—how successfully the spirit is engaged with the body to carry out its life's agenda. The way I do this is to read the miasms as they are reflected in the disorders of the body. Like Ayurveda or Traditional Chinese Medicine, this is a way of understanding the pathology of body and mind. Unlike conventional modern diagnosis, however, the concepts used in these older systems encompass body, mind, and energy, and their connection to the realm of spirit.

The diseases of homeopathy's first miasm, *psora,* are functional, that is, they don't generate structural change. Most typical are rashes on the skin that are red and itch. The fundamental mindset, the mental/spiritual posture that this miasm expresses, is one of being distracted from your deepest and most authentic inclinations by the appeal of what you see others doing—in other words, of *itching* to do what isn't really you. For a whole host of reasons—including a fear of assuming the power that is yours—you resist your special destiny. You come to see your own path as less compelling, despite deeper impulses that would push you toward it. The grass may seem vastly greener where others stand, and what they are doing may appear more exciting.

Such attitudes create a strong desire to operate from outer rather than inner directedness. While in this psoric state, you resist that inclination, but you are *burning* to give in to it, and your energies are so caught up in the struggle with yourself over whether to do so or not that they are not available for such functions as digestion or assimilation, and you are therefore increasingly subject to deficiencies. Your nervous system also suffers, and you experience anxiety and functional disorders of organs such as the heart—paltitations or panic attacks, perhaps. But the most prominent manifestation of the pattern is on the skin, which itches and burns. On the microscopic level, you might find the scabies mite (though often you won't).

Because it's the most superficial of the miasms, the tissues of the body affected are those that are embryologically of ectodermal origin, that is, those that develop from the layers closest to the surface. This includes the skin and nervous system.

The diseases of the second miasm—*sycosis*—begin to reach *into* the body, affecting mucus membranes, which are the linings of the passageways that connect inner and outer. These are the openings through which you interface with the world, and their oversecretions and excess discharges express a behavior pattern of overconsumption and overdoing. Just as the physical process has taken another step in this second miasm and moved into the body, the mental stance has also taken a second step and plunged into the seductive indulgences the psoric resisted. Because this "going for it" is prompted by outer cues and not by your authentic, innermost impulse, however, it's cut off from the inner sense of fulfillment that would turn it off when you've had enough. So there is ceaseless overdoing—too much eating, too much activity, too much reading, too late at night, too long. The structural disorders that develop also express this process. They are diseases of overconstruction—cysts and tumors, warts, excess body hair, obesity.

The homeopaths spoke of the diseases of the third miasm, *syphilis,* as erosive, eating away the structure of the body: ulcers, loss of bone mass, and degenerative diseases of the nervous system (see Fig. 37). They saw these diseases as destroying the vital organs and the vital capacities. But that is disease as "other." If we step out of such a position of projection and splitting, we will see that the body's structure is deteriorating in syphilitic diseases because we have withdrawn the energy and intent from it.

The body is a vehicle that constitutes itself around our purpose, our direction, and our actions. Each body is uniquely designed to serve as a medium for the experiences of its specific owner in order to move through his particular life's agenda. If he abandons that agenda, his body will begin to disintegrate. It is the "city of life"; when we withdraw the population, it falls apart, like a ghost town. The erosive processes tell us that we have moved out.

The miasmatic perspective helps us see that a disease process is a sequence of events that follows partial or total disengagement from the body. If we watch a disease scenario unfold and decline to take responsibility for it, we might attribute to it a life of its own, give it a disease name, and fear it—or even declare a war against it, as in the case of cancer.

Cancer is a combination of all three miasms. It has the psoric foundation on which is superimposed the sycotic overgrowth and, finally, the erosive syphilitic tendency to eat away normal structures as the over-

PHYSICAL SIGNS OF THE MIASMS

Psora	Sycosis	Syphilis
Surface	Penetrating	Destroying
Inflammation	Oozing	Erosion
eczema	bronchitis	bone loss
itching	growths	ulceration
nosebleeds	gout	Alzheimer's disease
bur.	vaginal discharge	polio
> eruptions	< dampness	< night
Hypofunction	Hyperfunction	Dysfunction
Atrophy	Hypertrophy	Dystrophy
Weakness	Overactivity	Ataxia
Inhibition	Expansion	Destruction

> = better from, < = worse from. *Atrophy* here is meant to indicate withering from disuse, without any structural change, while *dystrophy* means essential components are destroyed. *Ataxia* is a lack of coordination seen in neurologic diseases.

FIGURE 37

growth invades and destroys.[3] The following story confirms what we might surmise from a miasmatic analysis of the disease:

> *I am standing beside a friend in a huge treatment room occupied by a mammoth nuclear accelerator, used for the radiation treatment of cancer. He is director of this clinic, but he shakes his head and smiles wryly. "I look forward to the day when this is a museum," he says. This expensive and dangerous therapy was not, he observed, very effective. "But your results are good," I replied, aware of the reputation of the center. He laughed. "Our secret is more low-tech."*

"When I began this work, decades ago," he explained, "I hired my wife, who was a social psychologist, to help patients manage their personal lives when they left the hospital." After some years of her handling this end of the work, he began to notice that she sighed and said, as certain patients were discharged, "Doesn't look good." Those cases would relapse and succumb to the disease. With others she voiced optimism, and again, her forecasts were accurate. At first they regarded this as a coincidence, then as a weirdly uncomfortable curiosity. But as one of his wife's assistants began to show the same capacity for predicting outcomes, my friend became intrigued. "Whatever it is you're picking up, it must be crucial to recovery from this disease," he told them.

So, like some sort of psycho-detectives, they watched themselves watch the cases, and studied their own reactions. After several years of careful analysis, it finally became clear what they were seeing, and it was surprisingly simple. Almost everyone, they observed, who came to the center with cancer was facing a life that he felt was unbearable. Sometimes it was a difficult marriage, in other cases a job that was stifling. If, during the course of the illness and hospitalization and the disruption of life that accompanied that, something shifted, allowing the patient to return home to a different situation, he recovered. If it didn't, and he went back to the same impasse, the disease continued its relentless course and he did not survive. Cancer was a ticket out of an intolerable life.

Of course, it was the social workers who were making the connections, since they were aware of the details of each person's circumstances. My friends shifted their focus after that, putting their energy into identifying what had stagnated and become oppressive for their patients and helping them deliberately change it. At that point their statistics began to improve.

From a miasmatic point of view, the patient had already left, so the body was undergoing the predictable process of self-destruction. Reconnecting with one's original intent for this life, and reorganizing the context of it so that it seems possible to fulfill that intent, brings the spirit and body back into synchrony. Then the destructive process comes to a halt, producing what we consider a "miraculous" remission.

It may seem risky to adopt such an attitude toward a grave disease like cancer, and it does require courage to assume that stance. Yet not to do so means to cast yourself in a role characterized by fear and victimhood, which is even riskier. Nevertheless, consciously addressing miasmatic distortions and influences is something new. Homeopaths dealt with this level of disorder quietly, giving their remedies and watching for subtle evidence of deep change. But the path of radical healing outlined in this book grounds itself in self-awareness. For the fullest transformative emergence from dis-ease, it will not be enough to be the passive recipient of even the most expert and holistic of therapies. You must be consciously involved in the process of understanding, integrating, and restructuring.

Nose Maps and the Breath

It's curious how holistic approaches to healing cluster around a focus on sensing subtle energy. Self-awareness always runs up on the breath—when you turn your attention inside, that's what you'll find happening. Mapping the inside of the nose has uncovered an exotic intersection of physiology, the energy of emotions, and shifting currents of air.

Freud pioneered this work, collaborating with Wilhelm Fleiss to experiment with reflex points in the inner nose. Though I had completed a very analytically oriented residency in psychiatry, I had heard only the vaguest mention of this research until I met Dr. Maurice Cottle, a Viennese-trained physician who had been involved with the development of the electrocardiogram. He recalled with a sense of irony how the test was ridiculed when it was first proposed. I think this prepared him to look with a jaundiced eye on the attitudes of the medical profession toward his own work, and to shrug off their prejudice.

A specialist in diseases of the nose, Dr. Cottle had devised a diagnostic machine that he called the rhinomanometer. It was equipped with a trochanter or tube that was put against the nostril, and while one breathed through this, it measured the pressure exerted by the stream of air.

The day I arrived for our first meeting, I entered the room to find him seated by the machine. Apparently a patient had just left. He didn't look up. Instead he merely muttered, "Sit down," and handed me the trochanter. "Put that in your right nostril and breathe," he ordered.

I briefly considered explaining that I was not a patient, that I was a physician who had come to learn of his work, but his tone was the sort you didn't argue with, so I did as I was told. Still he hadn't looked at me, so intently was he watching the squiggly lines as they emerged on the graph paper. "Now do the other side," he commanded. I did.

When the recording was complete, he ripped the paper off the machine, lay it across his knees, and studied it eagerly for a brief moment. Then he looked up at me and smiled. "Now I know who you are—all about you, in fact! And I won't forget."

I was hooked. Each week I made the trek across North Chicago to sit with Dr. Cottle, gradually coming to understand his work. He could, it seemed, derive a tremendous amount of information from breathing patterns. Those patterns, he felt, were modulated by the rhythmic swelling and shrinking of the tissues lining the nose—tissues that are erectile, like those of the nipples, penis, and clitoris. Specialists like Dr. Cottle had always known that sexual overstimulation could produce a dramatic nasal obstruction as the lining became over-engorged, a condition known in the profession as "honeymoon nose."

In early explorations of the erotic, Freud and his collaborator Wilhelm Fleiss, who was an ear, nose, and throat specialist, became fascinated with the relationship between sexuality and the details of nasal engorgement. They found reflex connections between certain spots on the turbinates (the conch-shell-like formations inside the nasal cavity) and specific organs. Shrinking and numbing one spot with a tiny drop of cocaine, for example, would immediately stop menstrual cramps, while the swelling of another point corresponded to peptic ulcer disease. Their work ran into a roadblock when Fleiss's attempt to excise a chronically swollen area in one patient resulted in a disastrous hemorrhage. But the curiosity their discoveries stirred up led to decades of work by other methodical German scientists and a detailed map of the inner nose with its corresponding organs. This had just begun to emerge when the entire line of research came to an abrupt halt with the beginning of World War I.

Dr. Cottle felt that where the air hit during the flow of breath through the nose, nerve endings were triggered and important reflexes set off. If these were disrupted, the associated internal organs could be adversely affected. He identified one respiratory pattern that involved a clearly observable delay before the intake of the next breath. He called this a "mid-cycle rest." It usually came after a long exhalation, like a sigh. Then there was the interruption, as if the subject lacked the motivation to take another breath, and waited to do so until prompted by the discomfort of having insufficient air.

This pause was an indication of depression, Dr. Cottle said. It was also seen in patients with heart disease—just before they had a heart attack. When he presented his conclusions to a group of fellow rhinologists, a colleague stepped forward from the audience to be tested, and was found to have precisely the pattern described. Those present smiled indulgently, assuming the presenter needed to rethink his hypothesis. But a few months later the physician who had volunteered succumbed to a fatal coronary while standing on the podium at another professional conference.

His theory was to get further—even more personal—confirmation. Some months later, Dr. Cottle was demonstrating to a patient what a normal tracing should look like. He casually picked up the trochanter, stuck it in his own nose, and breathed. What he saw on the paper was a clear mid-cycle rest. A month later he was in the ICU, having survived a mild heart attack.

What I learned from my time with Dr. Cottle was invaluable, but eventually we parted ways. He thought a mid-cycle rest was a sentence to heart disease, that breathing was involuntary and beyond our control. I believed it could be retrained. I knew that the *swara yogis* made a career of the voluntary control of the breath. Though they might disagree with his conclusions, they would not be surprised by Dr. Cottle's findings. They even maintain that the "shape" of the current of air, as it emerges from the nostril,[4] reflects the tone of your thoughts as well as the physiologic "gear" you have in force at the moment. If that current was shaped by the shifting patterns of engorgement in the inner nose, then Dr. Cottle had discovered the physical basis of what the yogis did.

From the yogic point of view, however, the physical changes—the filling of the linings of the nose with blood—were usually secondary. They might reflect shifts in thinking patterns, for example, the subtle being generally more powerful than the gross. In other words, maximal leverage comes from "within"—where our awareness is the key to what happens with the body.

SELF-AWARENESS AND HOLISTIC DIAGNOSIS

Currently, a curious thing is happening in medicine. Diagnostic technology has been sailing ahead of therapeutic know-how. The investigation of gross material changes is beginning to lose ground to the detection of subtler changes—the changes that precede the development of clear structural damage or actual physical disease. A couple of decades ago, we could confirm the diagnosis of a heart attack only by X ray or EKG. Now we are able to pick up the obstruction of the coronary arteries that will lead to it. With technology like that of Dr. Cottle's, or like the electroacupuncture testing of meridian weakness that is being pioneered today in Germany,[5] we may soon be able to forecast even the *tendency* to collect plaque in the arteries.

Already I see patients who have been told, essentially, to come back when the disease is further along. "Then we can do something." Many patients aren't willing to wait, and begin to look for healing techniques that can be used earlier in the course of the "natural history of the development of the disease" (see Fig. 38). Doctors also are beginning to feel the frustration of having their hands tied until matters reach a point where no solution is very satisfying. Why must we wait until bypass surgery is necessary? Such physicians, the equivalent of the botanic physicians of the last century, are "pushing the envelope" and experimenting with the gentler, subtler methods of holistic medicine, which are so perfectly suited to intervention before structural change has occurred.

The key to a truly holistic medicine is to shift not only the focus of our attention from the gross to the subtle, but also our vantage point—where we stand to look. The person needs to be viewed from where he or

---

THE HEALTH-TO-DISEASE SPECTRUM AND WHICH DIAGNOSTIC AND THERAPEUTIC APPROACHES ARE APPROPRIATE AT EACH STAGE

Holistic techniques excel   *Conventional techniques applicable**

high-level wellness	good health	"not feeling well"	"diagnosable" illness	critical illness	terminal illness

all tests normal		blood tests abnormal	X-rays, etc., show structural damage

*Although currently holistic techniques are not available for this aspect of medical care, that doesn't mean they would not (or will not) be preferable.

FIGURE 38

she can be seen best—inside. A score of precision-minded specialists sur-rounding you can never see the complete picture the way it can be seen from the perspective of your own inner awareness. The eight blind men who debated the nature of the elephant—one holding the trunk and say-ing it was very like a snake, another the leg, insisting it was more like a tree, and so on—might have more productively asked themselves how the elephant experienced himself. The artwork produced by psychotic patients often portrays clinicians poking and probing from the outside, while fearfully avoiding any sincere attempt to grasp the internal world of their patients as they themselves experience it.

Though all of us may feel some reticence about immersing ourselves fully in our own experiential inner world, that is precisely where the cen-tral switchboard is. No one on the outside can ever grasp the intercon-nectedness of all our many thoughts, feelings, energy shifts, and physical sensations the way we ourselves can. The ultimate diagnostician is the inner observer. Even with all the space-age electronic equipment and mind-boggling ingenuity available, nothing will ever replace the elegance and simplicity of lucid self-awareness. It's only there where all the intro-spective and external information can be coordinated with an authentic sense of what we need and where we need to go.

Self-awareness is the fulcrum of holistic medicine and healing (see Fig. 39). It very decisively "puts the patient back in the driver's seat." A health-care provider will find it difficult to write a patient out of the pro-gram if the patient is pulling it all together and making critical decisions. The process of true healing is first and foremost a matter of insight, understanding, and reorganization—often accomplished in profound ways that are deeply felt but that defy verbal articulation. Generally the way such a result can be brought about most effectively is for the person who's going through the transformation to be in charge of the process. Skilled and sensitive healers can make a huge difference, but in the final analysis, they are only assistants.

Yet, as we step into this driver's seat, we find ourselves ill prepared to take the wheel. Organizing our perceptions of the inner world is a project that most of us who were raised in a modern Western context have had lit-tle acquaintance with. Eastern traditions, on the other hand, have millen-nia of experience and insight to offer, and Western seekers have been quick to pick up their lingo. Hosts of yoga students and meditators now talk casually of chakras or *ch'i,* and have to, because there are no compa-rable terms in our reductionistic, materialistic language. We have precise

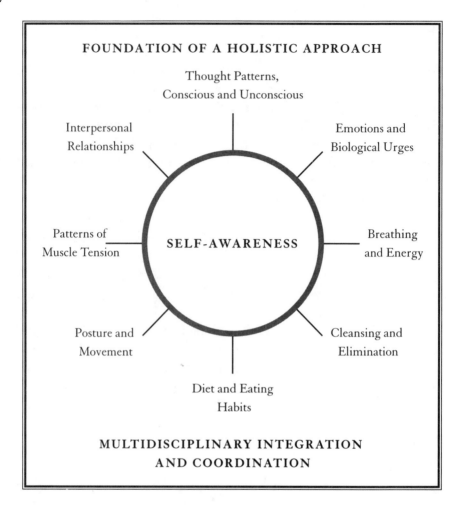

FIGURE 39

words to pinpoint physiologic functions and anatomical structures, or to detail psychological processes. But we have no concepts or terms that refer to both of them simultaneously or that could help us knit them back together into a comprehensive, operational *whole*. Perhaps, given enough time, we could evolve concepts and a vocabulary of our own to deal with such matters. But why wait when there are already several that can be plucked ready-made "off the shelf," and that are time-tested and, seemingly, both concise and accurate?

In the next chapter we will look at such conceptual frameworks, some of which have been around several thousands of years and seem currently to be making a comeback.

6

Multilevel Diagnosis and Constitution: What's Your Mind-Body Type?

Look in the mirror. What do you see?

- In what basic and important ways are you different from others?
- When you learn of a new healing technique, how do you decide whether you are a person whom it could benefit?
- What "type" are you?

In your holistic view of yourself, you want to be aware of more than the physical. You want to look simultaneously at the physical, the mental, and the "energetic," that intervening level which bridges the body and mind. This will make your observations considerably more complete, but it will also make them more complex—and sometimes more difficult to grasp or to formulate.

When we try to apply our Western diagnostic labels in a more enlightened way, aiming to encompass these other levels of being, too, they just don't make it. An ulcer is an ulcer. We can elaborate by saying it was caused by "unresolved dependency needs that have led to hyper-secretion by the duodenum," but it sounds strained.

And it is. As a result of the history of our system of medicine, there's a gap here. In such a case we are lifting from one side what was conceived of as a purely physiologic diagnosis: an ulceration in the lining of the intestine. Then we are reaching way over into the field of psychology to pull out a complex of emotional inclinations and attempting, with great effort, to tie the two together. The result is bound to be suspect—both by the physically oriented doctors who described the ulcer and by the psychologists and psychoanalysts who formulated this understanding of a certain emotional state. It's a stretch.

Without terms comprehensive enough to span these various levels, we are left with delimited labels and the fragmented view of reality they imply. We are in a bind. One solution to this dilemma is to look to Asian systems of medicine. Though they often lack the detailed physical quantification and the preoccupation with material minutiae that we expect, they are possessed of a different sort of sophistication. They understand that a whole being is body, mind, and spirit. In the ancient and highly evolved cultures of the East, holism was a given. The systems of medical practice and the thinking underlying them were based from the outset on a view of the human that acknowledged the many levels of his being. When we turn to them, there's no schism to bridge; the traditional medical terms of Asia are comprehensive in their fundamental meanings.

Approaching this Eastern perspective, we encounter two distinct traditions, that of India and that of China. The acupuncturist, practicing Traditional Chinese Medicine, and the Ayurvedic practitioner, using herbs and exotic cleansing treatments, seem to be totally different. But underneath, they are more similar than you might have thought.

Many years ago, during introductory training in acupuncture, I attended a class on the history of Chinese medicine. The instructor flashed on the screen what was considered the oldest surviving acupuncture chart. It was of an elephant, and the points were labeled in Sanskrit. Much of what we think of as purely Chinese or strictly Indian may, in fact, have arisen from the interplay between the two. If not siblings, they are certainly cousins. If you dig deeply enough, you find enough commonalities to suggest that they evolved from the same roots. Chief among those is their use of the concept of "Five Elements."

These Five Elements are the key to understanding much of Asian medicine, and will provide a foundation for a system of constitutional types. As you understand your type, you will be enabled to provide more skillfully for your particular needs and work more successfully with your uniqueness.

The Five Elements in India and China

The Tantric[1] philosophy of ancient India and Tibet bases its cosmology on the Five Elements. In a core body of writings known as the *Shivagama,*

Shiva, the dancing god with the graceful, androgynous body, is explaining to his adoring lover, Parvati, the origin of the universe. Parvati embodies the *shakti* or power of the goddess and of the earth. Shiva brings to bear the consciousness of the heavens that blends with that *shakti* to create human life. The goddess poses to him, as the bearer of that consciousness, the ultimate questions: How did the universe come forth? How does it continue? What sustains it?

Shiva explains that all we see and know emerged from a blending of the Five Elements or *tattvas*. They are the subtle bases of all that is physical and energetic—or even mental. To grasp their emergence from the void and their swirling confluence is to understand the very essence of nature and of ourselves. By patiently studying these Elements, he claims, the accomplished yogi comes to grasp how they relate to the breath, and can deliberately shape events and even physical objects through the management of his own currents of internal energy. In the late 1960s, Swami Rama was invited to the Menninger Foundation so that scientists could study someone with such yogic abilities, or *siddhi*s, as they are termed in Sanskrit.

> *Seated in the lab with a pencil suspended before him by its center, he was challenged by the researchers. "Can you make it turn, simply by concentrating on it?" He thought he could, and as he sat focusing, the object began to rotate. Perhaps because his face was close to the object and he was muttering a* mantra *to focus his consciousness, or perhaps because he had made such a point of explaining that breath was the yogi's handle on the blending of the currents of subtle energy that give rise to the phenomena within and around him, some of the researchers were suspicious.*
>
> *The idea that the subtle might control the physical was not an option they considered. He'd said such things were done with the breath; they concluded he'd blown on the rod. So they rigged a new setup—a mask he was asked to wear to prevent his exhalation from deflecting the object. It moved anyway.[2]*

To understand how this is done, the yogis say, you must probe the underpinnings of the physical world. You must search for the field where the most primordial hints of manifestation first appear out of nothingness. This is *Akasha,* or Ether, which, Shiva explains in the *Shivagama,* "is the initial and least tangible of the Five Elements, although it is really still nothing. But it *is* the very essence of potential. It is pregnant emptiness—the possibility of being. It is the first 'Element' to emerge from the utter void."

Though empty, this *Akasha* or Ether is considered the medium through which sound is transmitted. That is why a "seed sound," or *mantra,* when chosen to resonate with your essence, is thought to have the potential to reconnect you with your source. To the Tantric master, you have your origin in this Akashic realm, and it was some simple sound that initiated your unfurling into manifestation. That sound, if you concentrate on it, has the power to lead you back, deep into that point of universality and unity whence you came. There, according to the yogis, all phenomena originate. When you tune into that subtle current of energy, you participate in the shaping of events in the energetic world—which in turn shape physical events.

Shiva goes on to sketch out the Tantric view of the evolutionary process that leads to the appearance of the world as we know it. "From *Akasha* spin out swirling masses of gaseous matter. This is the second Element, *Vayu* or Air. These orbs then combust, forming heat and light and giving birth to the third Element, *Tejas* or Fire. After that," he continues (and I am paraphrasing liberally), "residues condense and pool, and lo, there appears moisture, the fluid, liquid Element that was called *Apas* or Water. Finally comes the last step, crystallization and solidification occur and we have the *terra firma,* the Earth or *Prithivi.*"

If modern astronomers and physicists don't exactly quote this—or even study it—one could easily think they did, so striking is the parallel between this vision of the origin of our phenomenal world and our most up-to-date ideas about the "Big Bang" and the beginnings of our galaxy. A few physicists are beginning to suspect that the clear intuition of the yogi—who had explored his own unconscious and cleared away his tendencies to distortion—might have reached profound levels of understanding and a comprehensive grasp of the makeup of the universe eons ago.

It may not be too sweeping to say that the Tantric concept of the Five Elements resonates with our most fundamental sense of what the roots of reality are. In fact, the Five Element theory taps into a basic truth that seems to run through many traditions. Native American cultures talked of the Elements—and in much the same way. A magazine cartoon, some years ago, showed two lab-coated researchers huddled over a printout coming from a giant computer. "It says the universe is made up of Earth, Water, Fire, and Air!" one of them exclaims to the other.

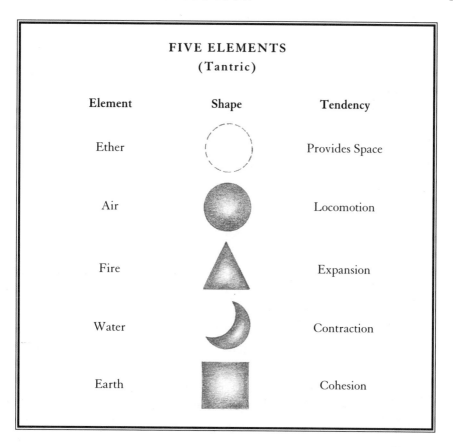

FIVE ELEMENTS
(Tantric)

Element	Shape	Tendency
Ether		Provides Space
Air		Locomotion
Fire		Expansion
Water		Contraction
Earth		Cohesion

FIGURE 40

We will leave Shiva's narrative here, though he goes on to reveal the nature of inspiration and expiration and how the knowledge of the breath "is a jewel in the crown of the wise." This knowledge, he says, "is the subtle of the subtle, it excites wonder in the world of unbelievers." It certainly did among the researchers at the Menninger Foundation. To the *swara* yogi, who is attuned to the subtle currents of energy, the secret of his mastery of himself and the universe lies in his attention to these currents and in learning how to blend with them through conscious breathing. "In the flow of the breath is the wisdom of the Scriptures." We might call this applied spirituality.

Working experientially with the breath, and watching things shift within and around you, is quite different from the sort of spiritual pursuit that involves abstract discussions by theologians. It's also more relevant to that process of internal reorganization we call *healing*. We will return to a careful consideration of breathing techniques and their application in the last section of this book. But at this point let's look back at our discussion of the principles of natural remedies. Reaching up into subtler realms to attain a point of leverage is also what the manufacture of homeopathic remedies is all about. Repeated processing through serial dilution and potentization gradually shifts the remedy from the material plane toward the Akashic or ethereal. It becomes a sort of seed message, like a mantra. By progressively diminishing its matter, and by "unearthing" its subtler essence, we uncover the core of its structuring tendency, the most concise expression of an organizational form. Just as a mantra, when skillfully chosen, helps to reshape, refine, and streamline our consciousness, so the remedy helps to restore simplicity and resilience to our energy organization by throwing off those encumbrances of nonessential, burdensome, and disabling habits and tendencies that lead to disease.

THE CHINESE VERSION

While the Indian version of this "reality base" constitutes a map of our origins in pure consciousness and plays with our connections to it, the Chinese version is much more practical and is more grounded in everyday life. We might say the Five Elements in Indian thought are vertical—reflecting the way we connect with the Infinite. The Chinese Five Elements arrange themselves, by contrast, in a horizontal circle—with an emphasis on mutual interplay and on how they interface with the world around us (see Fig. 41). But the two schools still have much in common.

The Chinese philosopher, like the Indian, concluded that there is an "earthy" aspect to the human that provides substance and stability, and that lends us steadiness and solidity. This Earth Element is the nurturing mother; it is taken up as we digest and assimilate food. When parenting figures early in life don't manage to extend the tender, caring input that "bonds" the infant to this incarnation, then the Earth Element will be deficient. The child may grow up to have weak or unreliable digestion and problems with bonding and boundaries.

The watery part of us that gives fluidity and flexibility is also related to nurturance. While the Earth Element has to do with bonding, boundaries, and grounding, the Water Element provides the "juice" that plumps us up and flows through us. Picture a bowl of dehydrated food on a camping trip. The dry crisps as they emerge from the package are all Earth Element. Now add water and observe the transformation. Since

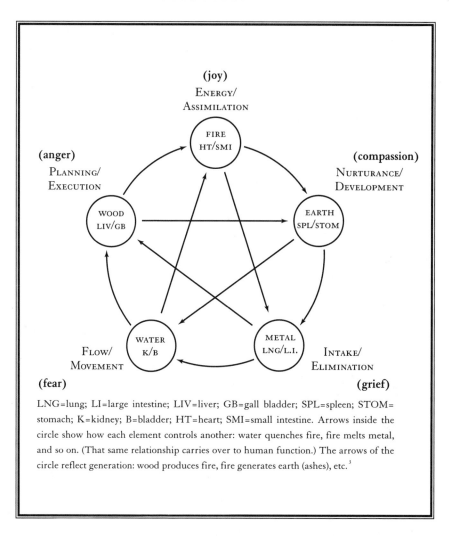

LNG=lung; LI=large intestine; LIV=liver; GB=gall bladder; SPL=spleen; STOM= stomach; K=kidney; B=bladder; HT=heart; SMI=small intestine. Arrows inside the circle show how each element controls another: water quenches fire, fire melts metal, and so on. (That same relationship carries over to human function.) The arrows of the circle reflect generation: wood produces fire, fire generates earth (ashes), etc. [3]

FIGURE 41

our bodies are over 80 percent water, a deficiency in the Water Element will lead to weakness, reproductive debility, and a tendency of the body to shrivel and dry up. In aging, the Water Element tends to diminish; if not countered, this can manifest as decreasing libido, depression, and memory loss.

The Fire Element brings heat, ardor, and aggression. When excessive or not properly contained in the "boiler room," it can spill out and cause conflagrations: temper tantrums, "angry" rashes, and fevers. On the other hand, when it's inadequate, we feel cold, unenthusiastic and "unable to get fired up about anything." A balanced, steady flame produces the sort of intelligence, creativity, and warmth of personality that everyone feels drawn to. The Fire Element burns food, distributes its energy, and radiates it from the heart.

The more ethereal Elements of the Tantric system—Air and Ether *(Akasha)*—are given a totally different spin by the Chinese. They, too, are brought down to earth. The Air Element becomes Metal, practical and serviceable. Metal has to do with wires and connecting devices, with holding and letting go. It suggests issues of relatedness that you might associate with the heart and with the arms—extending from the chest where the Tantric Element of Air is based. But the Chinese focus is on how the issues and organs relate to worldly concerns, rather than on their connection with the realm of spirit. So the Metal organs are those that take hold of and let go: the lungs, which seize oxygen and release CO_2, and the large intestine, which absorbs water and discharges feces. To see what this has to do with metal, you might picture a large electromagnet, which can pick up and drop scrap metal, or the mechanized arms of a robot of the sort that now works many of our assembly lines and that grasps and releases continually.

The Element of Metal relates to our capacity to end one relationship and begin another.

> *When a friend offered me an acupuncture session for the recurrence of the cough that had precipitated my retirement from the Himalayan Institute, she took my pulse and said, "It seems to be a problem with the interaction between Metal and Fire." At the time I fell ill, I had been overwhelmed by my countless responsibilities and yet ambivalent about letting them go. I felt they were the means of expressing my creative Fire. But there were too many of them—I was smothering.*
>
> *The cough had begun when I returned from a lecture tour in South America. All attempts by well-meaning colleagues to reach a conventional diagnosis failed, and the cough worsened. Soon I could not take more than two breaths without coughing, and the cough also became more violent. Unable to eat, I lost weight and strength. Eventually, after several weeks, the racking cough was too much for my body to sustain. Ribs began to crack. One of the physicians who worked with me, alarmed, taped my chest in an effort to prevent fur-*

ther fractures. But my skin reacted to the tape and it had to be ripped off—leaving a raw, oozing surface. I began to feel like Job.

One night, lying in a semi-stupor, I found myself half-dreaming. I had a very vivid image of myself throwing things out—tossing the burdens of my life up and away. A feeling of lightness followed, and at that moment I realized that I had taken four or five consecutive breaths without coughing! Once the Metal issue of release had been solved, the lungs, the prime organ associated with that Element, were free to work again. The Fire Element would find a new—and more realistic and manageable—outlet for creativity.

If Metal is the Chinese counterpart of the Indian Element of Air, then Wood corresponds to *Akasha* (which is Ether or "space," see Fig. 42). Tapping on a log or looking at a section of it under a microscope will make you aware of what a perfect manifestation wood is of "captured" or structured space. It is emptiness delineated and staked out—within which something has manifested, or might in the future. In Chinese medicine, it is said that the Element of Wood involves the structuring of

FIVE ELEMENT CORRESPONDENCES

INDIAN	EARTH	WATER	FIRE	AIR	ETHER
CHINESE	EARTH	WATER	FIRE	METAL	WOOD
ORGANS (YIN)	SPLEEN	KIDNEY	HEART	LUNG	LIVER
(CHINESE) (YANG)	STOMACH	BLADDER	SM INT	LG INT	GALL-BLD
CHAKRAS (INDIAN)	ROOT	GENITAL	SOLAR PLEXUS	HEART[4]	THROAT
DISORDERS	ANOREXIA	STIFFNESS	ULCERS/ DEPRESSION	ASTHMA	ADDICTIONS
STRENGTHS	STABILITY/ GROUNDEDNESS	FLEXIBILITY	INTELLIGENCE/ TRANSFORM'N	COMPASSION[5]	WILL/GRACE
ISSUES	PRIMAL FEAR	SENSUAL DESIRE	POWER	ATTACHMENT	EGO

FIGURE 42

potential into experience—what has been called "the Plan," your program for your life. Wood also relates to the liver and gallbladder; the liver
bears the brunt of our "worry"—obsessing over the Plan and the countless ways it might miscarry (see Fig. 41).

The Chinese version of the Five Elements is more "user friendly" for
the westerner since it relates to practical issues like the organs and how
they interact with the world. Though it is holistic and inclusive of the
subtle, it takes its point of view more from the outside. The Indian
approach to the Elements, on the other hand, is more "otherworldly"
with its references to the realm of Spirit. Nevertheless, it connects more
directly to our own inner experience.

ELEMENTS AND CHAKRAS

The Tantric tradition, probably the most intensely personal and
introspective of the various Indian schools, connects each of the Elements
with a *chakra,* which is a focused field of internal, experiential awareness.
Each of these foci is a point where the different levels of your being connect, a node of interaction between your physical body, the energetic level
of your being, and your mind. If you could *see* subtle energy, that point of
interchange among the different levels would look like a swirl or a
whirling wheel; in fact, *chakra* is Sanskrit for "wheel." Each of the first
five of these chakras, or energy centers, has a theme or set of issues associated with it that relate to the part of the body where it is located and, at
the same time, to one of the Elements.

The first chakra, situated at the base of the spine, is the foundation of
this energy system, and involves the Element of Earth. It might be sensed,
for example, as tension there when your feelings of security are undermined by threats of being expelled from your "tribe" for having violated
group taboos.[6] Or you might get a sense of it standing on a cliff overlooking a steep drop-off—moving toward the edge, you may feel a sinking sensation in the anal region. Attention, energy, and physiologic
activity gravitate there when you regard a situation as threatening to your
survival (see Fig. 43).

It's the presence of the Earth Element, and the grounding in life it
represents, that disintegrates when the gravest miasmatic disorders disengage the vital force from animating your physical vehicle. The result is
the erosion seen in Hahnemann's syphilitic miasm—where the structures
that maintain life crumble.

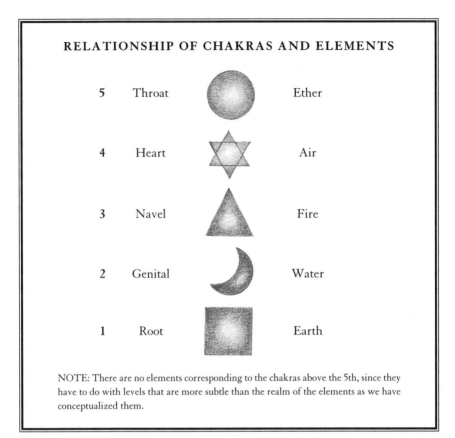

RELATIONSHIP OF CHAKRAS AND ELEMENTS

5	Throat		Ether
4	Heart		Air
3	Navel		Fire
2	Genital		Water
1	Root		Earth

NOTE: There are no elements corresponding to the chakras above the 5th, since they have to do with levels that are more subtle than the realm of the elements as we have conceptualized them.

FIGURE 43

Functions associated with the Water Element are concentrated at the second center or chakra, and relate to the *flow* of life from one generation to the next.[7] This is where endocrine, energetic, and psychological operations that relate to the genitals and sexuality are focused. The connection with the Element of Water here might be most concisely captured by the word "sensual": water has to do with the urogenital system and the fluids of sexual expression, but it also has to do with the delight you experience in savoring your food—taste buds will only register that which is in solution, dissolved in water. Efforts to extract sensual delight from repetitious experiences (such as sexual ones) that no longer satisfy real needs or open new doors result in the pointless oozing of watery discharges—a prime expression of the homeopath's sycotic miasm.

The Fire Element is especially felt at the solar plexus—your own internal "sun," which constitutes the third chakra. Fire is the transformative Element, converting the material substance of Earth and Water, characteristic of the first two chakras, into the subtler elements (of Air and Ether), which are dominant in the chakras above. Organs powered by this Fire are the small intestine, pancreas, and adrenals. The effectiveness of Fire is undermined when attention wanders from being in the present and being in your body. Pulled out of the solar center, displaced to the skin, Fire can produce the rashes the Ayurvedic physician would call *pittic*. If there's a more ingrained tendency to drift outward, the itching and burning of the skin may begin to look psoric and develop a miasmatic depth.

The Chinese physician sees Fire as extending up to the heart, while his Ayurvedic counterpart will focus on the relationship between the heart and Air—which dominates at the fourth chakra. This next center, which is the heart chakra, is located in the chest, the "hollow," air-filled cavity in your body. This is where the nourishing current of inhalation is received, and this theme of nurturing carries over into structural expression with the breasts.[8]

But breasts are not only involved with suckling; they are also the focus of weaning. Here the nurturing and sustaining theme we saw earlier with the Earth Element is revisited, but with a new layer of development added—the ability to let go of and to separate from the source of that sustenance. The processes of connecting and letting go that are the keynotes of the Chinese Element of Metal are central to the cardiorespiratory organs of this chakra and their process of gas exchange. The heart is constantly taking in and releasing, as are the lungs. On an emotional level, when the releasing phase of the cycle here is difficult, this fourth center also becomes the site of grief. Releasing ties to family and establishing new ones is a Metal issue.[9]

The fifth chakra involves the element of Ether, *Akasha* (Chinese = Wood), and relates to sound, vocalization, and creativity. This Element is important for healing in the Tantric scheme, being the medium through which sound moves and through which you reconnect in Akashic space with the point from which the phenomena of the world are felt to emerge. The perspective you gain as you move toward that universality allows increasing degrees of understanding and insight and makes possible the most profound reorganization.

While the Chinese system is not focused on the Infinite, but rather on the challenges of incarnation, its Element of Wood still carries some flavor of spiritual concern. Since its Plan points the direction for your life, disturbances of the Wood Element involve confusion about where you're going and why. Anger about being out of synch with your Plan leads to liver problems—hence the connection between this Element and the liver (even though the liver is not in this location anatomically). The Chinese system doesn't occupy itself with chakras—it's more concerned with the circle of interaction with the practical world.[10] The chakras belong to that more vertical connection with the infinite which is tantric territory. But the Five Element associations that come from the Chinese tradition often complement and enrich our understanding of the chakras.

For example, each Element is associated with one of the five senses, but the two systems, Chinese and Indian, do not always agree on which sense goes with which Element. Hearing is associated with the tantric *Akasha* or Ether, while the Chinese physician thinks of vision as the sense that goes with his corresponding Element, Wood. But the two might best be seen as complementary: the Chinese doctor is looking with the eye down at the unfolding of life's Plan, while the Indian tantrist is listening back with the ear to hear the origin of that life's purpose.

AYURVEDIC TASTE PHARMACOLOGY

This Five Element concept provides a sort of foundation for the Ayurvedic principle of taste testing,[11] an experiential system for assessing foods and herbs to see how they might affect you. It's deceptively simple, but extremely elegant and highly useful. The sweet taste, for example, is an indication that the food or herb carries a strong expression of the Earth and Water Elements. Sweets will strengthen those Elements in those who take them—i.e., lead to more matter. That's clearly no surprise for those who have watched a box of chocolates add inches to their most sensitive measurements.

A sour taste indicates both Earth and Fire, and while its Earth aspect provides nourishing and building, the Fire Element in sour foods stokes the digestive furnace. My grandmother's Victorian dining room always had a cut-glass cruet of vinegar on the table—for those who wished to splash a bit on their greens so they would be more digestible.

Pungent or "hot" foods, like peppers and ginger, invigorate the Fire even more than those that are sour, and are not a good idea for the already overly hot type. That doesn't mean the presence of an excess of Fire always acts as a deterrent to taking in more. Sometimes the fieriest people crave the hottest food. A red-faced man who worked in my father's office when I was a child was famous for his irritability and outbursts of temper. As a little boy who had come to work with my father, I was taken to lunch with my father and him, and watched with fear and fascination as he poured huge quantities of Tabasco on his food. To me he looked like a dragon exhaling fire as he gobbled it down—talking furiously all the while.

Bitter foods and medicinals are said by Ayurvedic physicians to feed the two most intangible Elements—Air and Ether. Too much of them throws one into a spacey, disoriented state. This is especially true of conventional pharmaceuticals, which are almost without exception bitter. The next time you encounter a prescription pill, bite off a tiny piece and taste it. You will find its bitterness unbearable.

The old Ayurvedic doctors who taught me used to laugh and say, "Of course you have to take your 'bitter pills.' That's because you eat only sweet and salty foods. Every now and again you may have something sour or hot, but because you never choose to eat what's bitter, you become imbalanced and then sick. To right yourself, you have to take your awful bitter medicine." Traditional Indian cuisine at its best provides all the tastes—and hence all the Five Elements—in every meal. Indian spices run the taste gamut. And then there are delicacies—like bitter melon— which baffle westerners. Why, we wonder, would they lick their lips over something so atrociously bitter?

To the traditional Asian physician, that which is bitter has something beautiful about it. It is the sobering aspect of human experience—the flooding of consciousness with awareness of the downside, a more realistic appraisal of the situation—an inducement to change and to reorganize.[12] When you avoid what is bitter, you become superficial or phony, limited by denial of the disappointments in life that might rein you in.

Besides adding a hint of bitterness, basic spices like turmeric are also used for their astringent taste. Astringency is not even considered a taste by modern physiologists, since there are no taste buds that correspond to it. In fact, astringency is a sensation registered by the whole mouth, and from the Ayurvedic perspective it reflects one of the fundamental properties of food and medicines—the ability to pull together and close. We have largely chosen to omit this taste, too, from our experience—with the possible exception of certain pickles that are treated with alum, a strongly astringent chemical. By spanning the spectrum of Elements (see Fig. 44), an astringent taste creates a sort of contraction and is valued for its ability to close up hemorrhaging vessels or to "tighten" a "loose" bowel that

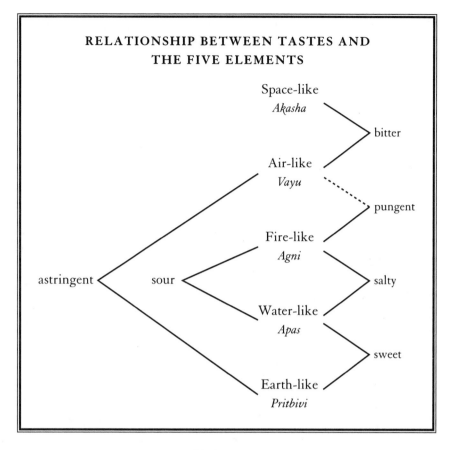

RELATIONSHIP BETWEEN TASTES AND THE FIVE ELEMENTS

FIGURE 44

is in the throes of diarrhea. Blackberries are unusual among fruits, because of their combination of sweet and astringent tastes, and blackberry liqueur is an old remedy for loose bowel movements.

"You have a laboratory in your mouth," my teacher of Ayurveda used to say. When he smiled, I could see the empty space where a tooth was missing; he eschewed dentistry and all its paraphernalia, which might distort his sensitive contact with the world of the natural. "You can test any food or herb to see what its properties are. All you need to do is taste it!"

After years of thinking that medicine had to depend on vast laboratories with high-tech autoanalyzers and spectrometers, and on huge and incomprehensible pharmaceutical factories, I found it exhilarating to think that, equipped with a tongue and palate, a knowledge of the Five Element system, and nature's bounty, I could treat the sick. There was only one more piece, my teacher insisted. I had to have a way of sizing up the situation so I would know exactly what the person in question needed. This is accomplished in Ayurveda not by a Western-style allopathic diagnosis, but by a formulation based on *tridosha,* the basic three-pronged conceptual tool of the Ayurvedic physician—one that is easier to wield than the more complex Five Element system.

Vata/Pitta/Kapha: A Simplified System

Chinese medicine outlines five constitutional types based on the Five Elements. Practitioners of Traditional Chinese Medicine often formulate their understanding of a patient on the basis of an analysis of the interaction of the Five Elements (or Phases, as they are more often termed in this context), and do elegant work on this basis. Though the study of human nature through the lens of the Five Elements is rich and full of insights, I find the concept difficult to use as a clinical tool. The interactions of five factors is a lot to keep up with; I can't seem to keep all the permutations and combinations straight in my head. I suspect that unless you immerse yourself in the system and work with it constantly, you will find it unwieldy.

Fortunately, there is an easier way. In contrast to the Chinese system with its five variables, Ayurveda is simpler, reducing them to three (see Fig. 45).

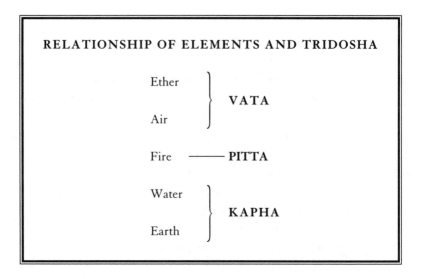

RELATIONSHIP OF ELEMENTS AND TRIDOSHA

Ether
}   **VATA**
Air

Fire ——— **PITTA**

Water
}   **KAPHA**
Earth

FIGURE 45

The two material Elements—those that represent the substance of the body, i.e., Earth and Water—are combined. The amalgam that results—muddy, if you will, in some metaphorical sense—is treated as a unity. This is called *kapha* in Sanskrit. The term comes from the same root as our word "cough," and is used in colloquial Indian languages to indicate mucus—the most common manifestation of excess *kapha*.

The Fire Element remains free-standing—*pitta* is the term that designates it. It holds a central, transformational position, having the ability to convert the matter of Earth/Water *(kapha)* into the subtlety of the remaining Elements, Air and Ether. These two are also treated as one, and it is termed *vata*. As the invisible, intangible aspect of the person, this "spacey" Air/Ether factor, *vata,* is responsible for motion and animation. It is implicated in many, if not most, disease states, since it is the movement of Air/Ether or *vata* that can sweep the fire or *pitta*, for example, out of its home in the solar plexus chakra (where your own internal fire belongs) and carry it afar to manifest as red eruptions or burning pain.

This triune distillation of the Five Element concept has proven most useful. Simple enough for the average person to master, yet profound enough to encompass much of the complexity of human nature, it has equipped Ayurveda to become the traditional medicine of one-fifth of the world's population. Though there are Ayurvedic practitioners in every village and hamlet throughout South Asia, and in colonies of Indians living all over the world, Ayurveda is at least as much a system of self-help as it is a school of medicine designed to be applied by a professional. It is used as an approach for dealing with your own health—how to keep it in balance, and how to right it when it is overturned. Central to that undertaking is understanding which Elements or, in this shorthand Ayurvedic system, which dosha of the three, is customarily strongest and weakest in you. In other words, what is your "constitution"?

THE STOLID OR *KAPHA* TYPE — ELEMENTS OF EARTH AND WATER

Larry was born under the sign of Taurus. The bull is not an inappropriate symbol for his personality. He teaches kung fu, and when attacked, his short but stocky frame seems welded to some concrete foundation. He is immovable. Rarely raising his voice, he has a steady gaze that reminds his students that they need to focus on what he's saying. He always shows up on time and seems inseparable from his rou-

tine. Calm, cool, and complacent, he's a friend that you know will always be there when you need him.

Earth/Water or *kapha* types are the persons who are solidly built, have smooth, thick skin, and lustrous, healthy hair. With an ample endowment of the Elements of Earth and Water, they are "well incarnated," solidly grounded in their earthly existence (see Fig. 46). Their big, moist eyes and mouths, with beautiful, evenly aligned, large white teeth might remind one of the soulful presence of a cow—calm, steady, and complacent. They are good at being nurtured and in giving nurturance. *Kapha* types know how to be content and are not easy to fluster—or easy to change from their customary course. In fact, they may tend to get in a rut and be resistant to change.

Contrary to popular misconceptions about Ayurveda, obesity is not an indication of a *kapha* or Earth/Water constitution. While *kaphic* types are solid, and may tend to get heavy, they are not automatically given to being fat. Their solidity has little to do with actual weight. When Sky, my eldest son, was a child of three, he could walk across the floor upstairs and you could feel it through the whole house. It wasn't how much he weighed, but the firm way that he planted his feet on the floor. My second son, Galen (who's more like his father), at twelve can walk through the room and you don't know it. He's of a more *vatic* nature. Air and Ether predominate, and sometimes, especially when lost in a book, he totally forgets where (and I suspect at times even *who*) he is.

KAPHA

- HEAVY
- SMOOTH, THICK SKIN
- THICK, LUSTROUS (COARSE) HAIR
- LARGE EYES, MOUTH, (EVEN) TEETH
- STEADY, STABLE APPETITES
- AVERSE TO ACTIVITY
- COOL, CALM
- COMPLACENT

FIGURE 46

The *kaphic* type will tend to oversleep, crave sweets, and overeat especially when it comes to dairy products and heavy, sour, *kaphic* foods, like avocados or puddings. Of course, those are exactly the foods that will overbalance him toward ill health, creating coldness, heaviness, swelling, and congestion.

Nevertheless, the *kaphic* constitution is a strong one, and these folks tend to have good health. When they do fall ill, they are prone to disorders of accumulation, with mucus congestion, edema, calcium deposits, and heaviness. They also tend toward lethargy and can get into a sort of blue funk—a kind of bored depression. They are likely to stop moving simply because they are content to stay where they are, and can easily turn into good-natured couch potatoes. At their worst, they can go on to become lazy, greedy, and severely self-indulgent.

THE HOT OR *PITTA* TYPE—ELEMENT OF FIRE

Pittic types have a medium, balanced build. They usually have fine, often reddish hair that is, by their second or third decade, already tending to thin. The men go bald early, and even the women notice an alarming amount of hair loss. Their eyes flash with intensity. They have brisk appetites and good endurance unless they get overheated (see Fig. 47). *Pittic* types have a sort of love/hate relationship with heat.

Here's a typical case:

Anne is a very industrious and quick mother. She has a face that is often flushed with the intensity of her life. She perspires easily, but

---

PITTA

- MEDIUM, BALANCED BUILD
- FINE, STRAIGHT (REDDISH) HAIR (OR BALD)
- FIERY EYES
- BRISK APPETITES
- GOOD ENDURANCE UNLESS OVERHEATED
- ANGRY, FORCEFUL, INCISIVE (CUTTING), IMPATIENT

FIGURE 47

does poorly in hot weather. She hates spicy food, and a trip to the trop-
ics is not her cup of tea; skiing in Vermont is much more appealing.
Yet, after a day on the slopes, she loves nothing better than to slip into
a steaming hot bathtub and cook until she is red. Her husband and
children know this is tricky, a bit too hot and she is impossible—she
will bite your head off.

Pittic persons are at home with anger and aggression. Their nature is
to be forceful and incisive. The incisions they inflict, however, may not
only open up the innards of the matter at hand but may also leave
bystanders lacerated and wounded. Quick and intelligent, the *pittic* type
will penetrate to the heart of the matter in a flash. A moment later they
are on to the next thing and are at least mildly irritated by the inability of
the rest of the world to keep up with them. Unfortunately, what they
don't grasp in their rapid-fire analysis may be missed forever. Often that's
left to their more plodding *kaphic* brother or sister who stays around to
ponder the other side of the story—or their *vatic* counterpart who skit-
ters off into realms of infinite possibilities and dizzying turns of thought.

Because they are "on fire," *pittic* people are more prone than other
types to oxidative stress, and should be careful to get enough antioxidants.[13] They are also given to illnesses like hypertension and acid stomachs. The liver can become overheated, and their lives can be distorted by
the difficulty they have controlling anger.

Kala was an Indian woman who was built like a tank—not the
more graceful solidity of the kaphic *frame, but armored for war. She*
dominated her frail husband with an ease that suggested neither of
them had ever considered relating otherwise. She ran their house—as
well as any house she happened to be in. One day she called me and
said that she was having a lot of trouble with acidity in her stomach.
It was, I suppose, what a westerner might have called "heartburn"—
a sort of burning that kept rising into her chest. But when I asked her
what she thought was going on, she answered simply, "I think it's just
pitta." I said, "I think you're right." She had tried adjusting her diet,
decreasing sour, salty, and spicy hot foods, but that wasn't enough.
The process had gone too far and the pittic *overflow had become*
entrenched. It took a course of cell salts—Ferrum phos 6x (for red
inflammations) and Kali mur 6x in combination—to quell the con-
flagration.

The prime characteristics of *pitta* are hot, oily, and sharp. They tend to get hot physically, emotionally, and mentally. They're oily—their bodies tend to produce oily sweat, and there is something about their personality that comes across at times as greasy or "slick" in some metaphorical sense. Oil is not good for them, and they should avoid greasy foods, which will only cause them distress—more acidity and burning in the belly. Their sharpness is like the tongue of a flame that flashes with the slightest provocation. The sparks that fly when they light into something (or someone) can ignite the oil and set off a brushfire that may quickly get out of hand.

THE SPACEY OR *VATA* TYPE—ELEMENTS OF AIR AND ETHER

The third constitution, the spacey type, is dominated by a preponderance of the Elements of Air and Ether. In Ayurvedic terminology, this is the *vata* constitution. This person tends to be thin—often tall and "rangy," though sometimes, paradoxically, abnormally small. Irregularity is a keynote here (see Fig. 48). Irregularly tall or short, with limbs that seem (even when they're not) ill-proportioned. There's a sort of tentative awkwardness about the *vata* type that is missing from his stolid *kapha* sister or his assertive, muscular *pitta* brother. *Vata* often looks as though he doesn't quite know what to do with his body. Arms and legs akimbo, he blunders

---

VATA

- TALL, RANGY
- LEAN, DRY HAIR & SKIN
- SMALL EYES, IRREG. TEETH
- VARIABLE APPETITE
- POOR STAMINA
- LIGHT SLEEPER
- FEARFUL, ANXIOUS
- SPACEY
- CHANGEABLE

FIGURE 48

through life avoiding embarrassment by simply spacing out. The obvious natural flow of life that the *kapha* and *pitta* types immerse themselves in is not obvious at all to *vata*. He often looks a bit baffled and confused and quite uncertain about who he is or, indeed, what this whole world is about.

> *I was long intrigued by John. He regularly paced the streets near my home in Chicago, looking around at the trees and houses each time as though he'd never seen them before. He was a sight to behold. I fantasized that someone had created a perfect prototype of the* vata *constitution—and it was he. His hair was coarse and dry and stuck out randomly—as if he had, years ago, grabbed a live wire and had, like some cartoon character, been zapped by electricity that sent his hair bristling and thereafter into lifeless disarray. His skin had a gray-ish, wooden quality to it that looked as though he had been indoors for the last decade—though I knew that he was out wandering quite fre-quently.*
>
> *He somehow appeared both taller and more stooped over than he really was, and had a tentative, aimless air about him. There was a sense about his gait that at any moment he could reverse his course or make an abrupt turn to the right or left. I loved him for his archetypal purity, but found myself wondering if there was anyone to take care of him. How did he manage? The habits that maintain most of us must have fallen away like so many dead branches, for he always seemed to be wearing the same faded, stiff-looking clothes. I pictured him sleeping in them—sitting in a chair or on a park bench where he happened to drift off.*

The most unique quality of *vata* is its dryness. Dryness is an inherent aspect of how we age. *Kapha,* the fullness of embodiment, is most exu-berant in childhood, when we are in the honeymoon phase of our romance with material existence. In adulthood, we burn with a desire to leave our mark and accomplish our goals that brings *pitta* strongly into play, and it becomes more visible and predominant through those decades. As we get older, the fire burns lower, finally reduced to a few smoldering coals.

Meanwhile, the *vatic* or subtler forces gather strength, and our invest-ment in this earthly, physical life is gradually withdrawn until the body begins to wither and our minds become progressively spacey and absent and finally we leave. The last scene in *Godfather III* offers a beautiful depiction of this last stage of our life cycle: The Don has become old. He is sitting in his patio, a blanket wrapped around his legs. It is fall, and the wind is loosening the leaves from the trees overhead and carrying them across the yard. Finally, you know that life has left him as though he might also crumple and fall from the chair, like one more dry leaf blowing away.

Just as different *doshas* dominate through the cycle of the seasons of life they also do so through the seasons of the year:

> *Katherine complains that every spring she comes down with a cold. There is a great outpouring of mucus. She doesn't want to simply treat it when it starts, but to understand what's going on so that she can prevent it next year. "How do you come at this from an Ayurvedic point of view?" she asks. "In winter the body wraps itself in a coat of kapha," I explain. "It's both a method of storage and a kind of insulation. In the spring, this is thrown off. If we help the process along— do a few days of juices and some washes—we don't have to suffer through a cleansing crisis."*

James may discover that his ulcer really flares up in the heat of the summer when the *pittic* predominance becomes powerful, owing to the intensity of the sun. And when autumn comes and the leaves shrivel and the wind blows, that's when Linda gets her arthritis. The *vatic* or spacey Element is strong, and joints begin to dry out and crack and ache. Or bronchi spasm and lungs wheeze—asthmatic flare-ups in the fall are also typical.

Similar to this seasonal cycle, there is even a minor but perceptible shift in the dominance of the *doshas* through the course of a day. Obviously midday—from about 10:00 A.M. to 2:00 P.M.—is when *pitta* is at its peak. But there's a corresponding burst during those same hours at night. That may be why some folks get another surge of energy—a "second wind"—around 10:00 P.M. that gets them fired up again and can carry them on a frenzy of activity well past midnight. *Vata* and the spacey Elements come into play during the transitional times—at dawn and dusk, when one phase of the day is giving way to another (see Fig. 49). At that point the changeability of *vata* predominates and one has the urge to sit quietly and drift off into other realms. Those are the hours when people are most likely to die, as there is a natural inclination during this time to shift, to let go and move on.

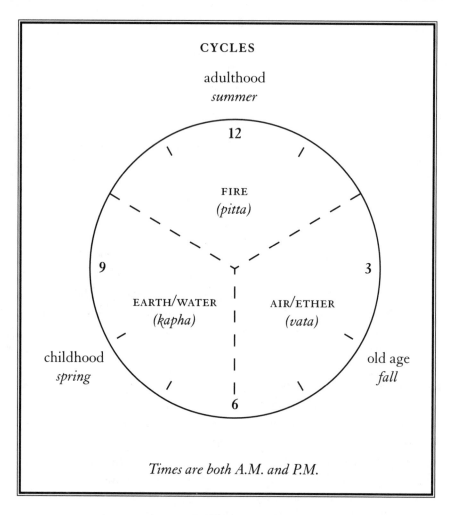

FIGURE 49

The time between six and ten o'clock, morning and evening, is when the dew falls. This is when there is a moisturizing, nurturing process going on that reflects the restorative and strengthening effect of an influx of *kapha*.

Your Constitutional Diagnosis

Knowing your constitutional type can be of obvious use. A *kaphic* type may not want to take a nap during the day—especially at dusk—or he might wake up congested and on the verge of a cold. The *pittic* type will want to avoid the midday sun—or he's asking for trouble. Pure *vatic* or *kaphic* types, by contrast, may find that the sun brings them to life. There are mixed types, too. Not everyone is going to fall into one of these three extreme categories. The *vata-pitta* type will find the heat helpful, but has to be careful or he can get overheated.

A simple way to peg your type is to look for the unique characteristics of each (see Fig. 50). *Pitta* is hot, while both *vata* and *kapha* are cold. So heat is the distinguishing characteristic of *pitta*. If that's a strong aspect of your makeup, it's a sure bet that your constitution is, at least in part, *pittic*. *Kapha* is the only one of the three that has solidity and heaviness—as the other two are light. If your personality and body reflect a complacent, substantial, slow-to-change tone, chances are you're *kapha*, or a combination of *kapha* and one of the other two *doshas*. *Vata*'s dryness is distinctive. If you are plagued by dry skin, dry lips, and dry eyes, chances are that there is a strong *vatic* Element in your makeup.

Or try checking your pulse again. This time just get a sense of the general quality of it. The spacey, *vatic* type of person will have a pulse with a thready, zigzag, irregular feeling. We're not trying to do anything very complex here. This is not the focused, organ-specific investigation of the Chinese pulse diagnostician, or that of the traditional Ayurvedic expert.

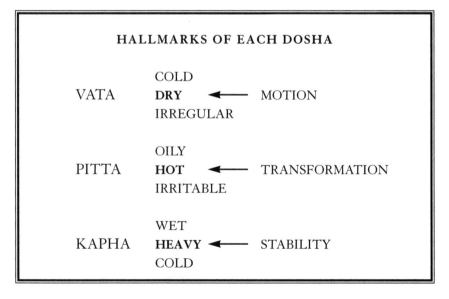

HALLMARKS OF EACH DOSHA

VATA	COLD **DRY** ⟵	MOTION	
	IRREGULAR		
PITTA	OILY **HOT** ⟵	TRANSFORMATION	
	IRRITABLE		
KAPHA	WET **HEAVY** ⟵	STABILITY	
	COLD		

FIGURE 50

This is simply a bird's-eye view of the overall tone of the person. The pulse of the *pittic* type will tend to be bounding and taut—the *vaidyas* say it moves like a frog, with a regular, distinct hop, hop, hop—while the spacey type's pulse moves in a more wriggly manner, like a snake. They compare the Earth/Water *(kapha)* pulse to a pigeon, which you might have noticed waddling across a sidewalk in its deliberate, heavy fashion.

You can also go back to the tongue. Now we can look at it in light of the three *doshas—vata, pitta,* and *kapha* (see Fig. 51). The *vatic* tongue will be thin, often dry, and tend to tremble. The *pittic* tongue, of course, will likely be red and hot-looking—though if there's lots of accumulated matter in the body, it may have a coating that will be yellowish. This may at least partly obscure its red color. The *kaphic* tongue is wide and thick and will often have a white or creamy coating.

ASSETS AND LIABILITIES

The list of "markers" in Fig. 52 may also be of some help in discovering your constitutional type. If you use it, imagine you're looking at yourself with your eyes not fully focused, as you would in sketching the

---

TONGUE DIAGNOSIS II

	VATA	PITTA	KAPHA
GENERAL	thin, small, trembling	medium-sized maybe pointed	large, round, thick
COLOR	pale, dull	red, yellow, green	pale, white
COATING	brown or black	yellow	white mucus
MOISTURE	dry	moist or red and dry	wet

FIGURE 51

CONSTITUTION MARKERS

	Earth/Water (K)	Fire (P)	Air/Ether (V)
Body type	solid, sturdy	medium, muscular	extremes (tall, short, thin)
Hair	thick, lustrous	fine, thinning	coarse, dry, wild, unruly
Hands	wide, strong, cool	medium, red, warm	dry, cold, pallid
Response to temperature	cold, damp, mucusy	hot and greasy	cold and dry
Activity	prefer to relax	assertive and to the point	fits of excitation followed by fatigue
Mind	slow, but good memory	quick, certain	drifts off
Temperament	calm, difficult to ruffle	easily irritable	changeable, erratic
Common symptoms	heaviness, congestion	irritability, acidity	nervousness, exhaustion, jumpiness, and gas

To use for self-assessment, circle the markers that apply to you, then go back and write in each circle a number: 1 if it's mildly true, 2 if markedly accurate or 3 if *extremely* descriptive of you. Then add the numbers for each vertical column. If two of the columns have high numbers that are close, you're a mixed type.

FIGURE 52

outline of a figure. Don't get caught up in concerns about whether you are the "most desirable" type. This is not a system for ranking health. *Kapha* is not "healthier" than *Vata*. There is no value judgment implied in these constitutional labels. Each has its peculiar liabilities and assets. *Vata,* for example, because of its connection with air and gas, is particularly susceptible to problems of the colon and lungs. Its changeability and restlessness affect the nervous system and can lead to such disorders as tremors, numbness, confusion, and dizziness.

Vata's lack of Fire, Earth, and Water may also mean poor digestion, and a tendency to weight loss, exhaustion, and debility. But this is just the downside. These spacey individuals will also often have a marvelous imagination—with minds that can go wonderful places. Though they may need help turning that into productivity, and may need to remember to ground themselves so they can do something creative with their mental pirouettes, they are remarkably adaptable, can be home almost anywhere, and are often able to sample a breadth of life that most would covet.

The Fire type, the *pittic* constitution, has its pros and cons, too. As a veritable locomotive, its energy can accomplish amazing things. *Pitta*'s quickness and sharp intelligence is the envy of all who know him. But his irritability, temper, and sharp tongue are often not much fun to be around, and the excess fire in the solar plexus can cause acid indigestion, fevers, heat, burning pains, and angry red eruptions over the surface of the body. *Kapha*'s steady consistency and affability is her strength, but she is prone to stubbornness, indifference, lack of motivation, and diseases that result from the accumulation of too much matter.

Certainly there are other ways of formulating your constitution besides this traditional Asian system. One of them is the choice of a homeopathic remedy of the constitutional sort. This is a much different proposition: there are scores of choices possible, though only a handful of types that are very common. Though constitutional prescribing is a powerful and, to me, indispensable approach to reorganizing the subtler realms of functioning and prompting personal evolution, its use doesn't eliminate the need for, or undercut the value of, Ayurvedic typing. Though you can choose the homeopathic remedy without pinning down an Asian constitutional diagnosis, there are other areas of your life where it is indispensable: in deciding which foods are optimal for yourself, or which of the dozen herbs recommended for this condition would be best to take, or what kinds of thought processes you tend to get caught up in and had best watch out for. These are all places where knowing your constitutional type can really make a difference in managing your life skillfully.

There are other versions of this, too. Latin American traditional medicine focuses primarily on the distinction between the hot and cold tendencies of people and of the foods and medicinals they might use. This is a very fundamental point, and one that is emphasized in both the Ayurvedic and Chinese systems. Chinese medicine, too, is very rich and complex, but, as we have seen, probably better suited to the practitioner than to the layperson. The threefold system of *tridosha* seems a happy medium, offering a clear distinction, for example, between the hot tendencies of *pitta* and the two variations on the cold: *kapha,* which is heavy and congested, and *Vata,* which tends to be dry and depleted.

I have chosen to organize much of this book around the triune concept of *tridosha,* because I feel that, rooted in the experiential traditions of yoga and Tantra, it is optimally conducive to cultivating self-awareness. Learning these basic concepts, you can immediately begin your own experimentation. Sitting on cold concrete steps outdoors on an early spring evening without long sleeves, sipping iced tea and bypassing the offer of a walk to help digest a heavy dinner, will allow you to watch in living color as *kapha* increases and begins to show itself in the form of mucus, heavy-headedness, and lethargy. Or we can observe, especially those of us who have some *vatic* tendency, that a walk in the dry fall wind can throw us into a tailspin of dizziness, confusion, and indecision.

Worry and fear also disorganize the *vatic* type, as does staying up late or overexerting. Sexual excesses are particularly draining for the airy type. He doesn't have so much substance present that it can be expended without feeling drained and depleted. The Indian doctors say that riding along a bumpy road in a rickshaw is disruptive to *vata,* but I can vouch for the fact that a ride in a New York taxi can also be murder.

INDIVIDUALIZING ACCORDING TO CONSTITUTIONAL TYPE

Equipped with the tools of the Ayurvedic trade—*tridosha,* taste pharmacology, and your own self-scrutiny—you can begin a great adventure of self-discovery. The more you learn about yourself and your unique characteristics, the more skillfully you can negotiate the rough waters of life on this rather polluted and chaotic planet. You will be able to take a trip and stay well, while others succumb to the stresses of different climates and strange foods. You will be able to pick up a book off the current best-seller rack and, instead of wondering, "Can this also be the answer to what I should eat, or how I should exercise, or what would improve *my* sex life?" you can flip through it and quickly conclude whether it's for you or not. A sproutarian diet might be just the ticket to lighten up a *kaphic* man, but if his *vatic* spouse tries to join him on it, she may end up full of gas and too weak to function. *Tridosha* is invaluable for individualizing.

To take another example: massage is great for everyone, but different techniques are good for different people. *Vatic* people need massage more than anyone else, because they need the sense of touch and connection to ground them—they're so close to simply floating away—but they also need a gentle and nurturing kind of touch. They're sensitive and easily rattled. They benefit most from using warming oils like sesame, almond, and mustard and slow, rhythmic strokes. *Vatic* folks should have a massage regularly—at least once a month.

Fire types like variety in massage, to try all sorts of things because it keeps their active minds busy. But they need a soothing kind of *cooling* touch, and the best oils to use are olive oil, cocoa butter, or coconut oil, since these will calm their fire a bit. The earthier *kaphic* type requires a firm, vigorous massage. They need stimulation to wake up a sluggish body and get their circulation moving. They really do best without oil—skin to skin—or with cornstarch as a medium for the massage. If oil is going to be used, then they would do best with a lighter variety, like mustard or sunflower seed oil (see Fig. 53).

The three factors, Earth/Water *(kapha)*, Fire *(pitta)*, and Air/Ether *(vata),* might be thought of as three fundamental forces or vectors that act within us to prompt us to function or move in one direction or another. The first grounds and nurtures us, the second warms us and burns our fuel, and the third throws us into motion and helps us soar to the clouds. In traditional Ayurveda, they are not only seen in the constitutional makeup of each person, but also as acting from moment to moment to shift the dynamic balance within us. You might think of it as a two-layer affair. The deeper layer, the constitution, is the enduring ground on which the more transient, changing events occur. So a *kaphic* person who eats too many hot peppers and is out on the beach all day playing volleyball can also come down with a bad case of burning stomach pain—

MASSAGE FOR DIFFERENT TYPES

	Technique	Oil
V	gentle, rhythmic strokes	sesame almond mustard
	regular frequency	castor (but all are good)
P	soothing, cooling touch	olive cocoa butter coconut
	variety	(but less is best)
K	brisk, vigorous motions	sunflower safflower mustard
	stimulation	(but none are good)

FIGURE 53

though he won't be as susceptible to it as his redheaded, balding, hyper-active friend.

In other words, *tridosha* can be used to make acute diagnoses as well as to understand and conceptualize your basic nature or tendencies. In the chapters that follow, you will have a chance to use this understanding to individualize your own tailor-made diet and exercise programs.

Concluding Thoughts on

Assessment/Diagnosis

As a result of what we've done in this section of the book, you should be able to free yourself from some of the diagnostic conditioning you've absorbed previously in your life, and to get a new fix on how to evaluate yourself. With the tools of Asian medicine, you can begin to discern hints as to your constitutional makeup. This gives you a fresh angle on how to choose what is right for you: If you have clear *vatic* tendencies, you may decide to forgo that walk out in the wind, or that last frantic activity that would stretch you far beyond your comfortable capacity and leave you drained. If you're more *pittic,* you will think again about the ginger tea recommended for your digestion, and look for something more cooling.

There's no counterpart to this in Western medicine. "What do you use for a cough?" is not a question that makes sense to an Asian doctor. What *kind* of cough? A cough in *whom?* A *kaphic* cough will bring up thick, white mucus and there will usually be coldness and congestion. The *vatic* cough is most often dry and painful with perhaps a headache and wheezing as well as anxiety or insomnia. The drying agents that will help the *kaphic* cough will make a *vatic* one worse. *Vata* needs demulcent herbs such as slippery elm and marshmallow, herbs that would magnify *kapha*'s congestion.

In homeopathy, there are literally scores of cough remedies, each with its characteristic pattern that details a specific cough picture. So what could it possibly mean to a holistic practitioner to ask, "What do you have for a cough?" Yet conventional medicine answers readily, "Oh, this is the latest cough medicine. It's very effective." My teacher used to shake his head in disbelief. "They try to drive all cows with the same stick," he would mutter with a sigh.

Overlooking the obvious differences between people is a shortcoming that has plagued Western medical traditions. Even the naturopathic schools have labored under the handicap of lacking of a constitutional typology or even, for that matter, any systematic approach to diagnostics. Meanwhile, as we've seen, the diagnostic approach of conventional medicine has focused on detailing physiologic and psychological patterns of structural deterioration and creating fearful disease entities, rather than on exploring the individual characteristics of people so that healing could be tailored to each person's needs.

There is, however, one promising development in conventional medical assessment, and that's the identification of habit patterns that can lead to dysfunction and suffering. Your doctor will now tell you that smoking or a high-fat diet is a "risk factor" for heart disease. The massive amount of data accumulated on disease is finally making it impossible to ignore these connections. A few short decades ago, the person who insisted that vitamins or exercise kept his arthritis at bay was dismissed as a health nut. Now doctors are beginning to prescribe more green vegetables or a course of supplements to reduce risk. But the change is awkward. A medical system that focuses on reductionistic pinpointing of cellular pathology, and whose thinking is trapped in military metaphors of war on disease, is ill equipped to plumb the depths of the habit-ridden person and reach a resolution of the issues that push him toward self-destructive behavior.

Some years ago we were visited at the Himalayan Institute by Ernst Wynder, one of the country's primary researchers in preventive medicine and the editor of the journal by that name. He had been asked to create an educational program for the public on smoking. It was, by some measures, immensely successful. After it had been in place for some time, random polls showed that the public was much better informed about the dangers of smoking. But when the man on the street was then asked if he had stopped smoking as a result of what he now knew, the answer was most often "No." Dr. Wender was baffled and disappointed.

Knowing that something is harmful often fails to deter you from doing it—there are irrational underpinnings to your self-destructive habits. Hidden beneath those habits that lead to suffering and disease are mental and emotional knots, and unraveling them can lead you toward personal and even spiritual evolution, toward a fuller expression of your creative potential, and to the fulfillment of your agenda for this life. What you need to accomplish this are ways of working that don't simply condemn habits and order them to stop, but that inspire you to explore their role in your life, to use your strengths to find the opportunity for growth buried in the habit and ride it into further unfoldment and self-realization. This will be your challenge as you move into the next section of this book.

FOUNDATION STONES

Wait! Don't skip this section. It's not what you might think, judging by the chapter titles: "Diet, exercise, cleansing. Oh my God! All the stuff I *ought* to do." Wrong. This is not about prescriptions or the mechanical compliance with tiresome routines of ought-to's. But such fears would not be unreasonable. That's what this section of a book on health usually is. That just doesn't work—at least not for long. No one wants to face the drudgery of repetitive workouts and designated diets. If you're fearful of disease, you might do it for a while, but eventually the fear wanes, and so does the routine.

The intent of this section is different. It is to explore what your habits of eating and of movement tell you about who you are— how your actions are a key to your inner self. That self is always there to see, but most of the time you may be too busy to see it. You eat with friends, you walk from your office to your car— busy with the distractions of life. In this section you'll look with full attention at *how* you move and *how* you eat. An exercise session, for example, will become a time to focus on how you move spontaneously, not a time to go on automatic pilot, looking forward to the end of the session. You'll learn to immerse yourself fully in the experience, feeling the emotions or the memories that connect to using different parts of your body, acknowledging the attitudes and impulses that arise with a certain posture or movement.

When patients say, "I won't follow a diet," I congratulate them. I won't, either. Diet is not something to be conformed to slavishly; it is an opportunity for constant experimentation, a laboratory into which you are pushed several times a day by your appetite. It can be great fun—or it can deteriorate into rote compliance or disobedience, guilt, and self-condemnation. What you eat *is* important, but if you examine the meaning behind your impulses, you'll end up with both a better diet and some understanding of yourself. That's why diet and exercise are "foundation stones."

Watching yourself and tuning into your body, its cues and its promptings, will provide important skills in self-observation and self-regulation. These skills will become a solid foundation for further work you will do toward healing yourself or others. They will be applied to working with the subtler aspects of yourself— observing energy and consciousness and fostering their reorganization. Of course, the better food and freer movement toward which you inevitably gravitate will also keep your body functioning well, and thereby offer a foundation in a more obvious way.

By now we all know a lot about nutrition and exercise—we've tried low-fat, high-protein, and meat-free diets, we've done aerobics and we've jogged and maybe we've even had a go at yoga— so our discussions of these subjects can move beyond the prescriptive. But the topic of cleansing is different; it's unknown territory for most modern folks. Maybe you've tried a brief fast, but chances are you've not delved into the intricacies of liver and colon physiology and skin and kidney action. The second chapter of this section does just that. It's basic training in the mysteries of detoxification.

Though self-discovery remains the keynote in our approach to each of these three areas of your life—nutrition, exercise, and cleansing—it will be useful to feel your way toward cultivating regular times for them. This is not to revert to mindless repetition. Awareness and curiosity are crucial, but it is also important to cultivate and strengthen strong, constructive rhythms in your life. The regular pulsation of rhythmic nourishing, cleansing, and movement are the heartbeat of a healthy life. By choosing and creating patterns that work for you, you can ride on the momentum of satisfying habits, and free yourself from having to re-resolve and re-initiate, day after day.

Most important, a predictable framework of life routines creates a lab where changes will stand out. A regular tempo of meals, exercise sessions, and cleansing techniques, when approached in the spirit of experimentation and curiosity, provide a setting in which the discovery and resolution that make healing possible are likely to occur.

To work successfully with these tools, however, you must start where you are. First, let's look at the reality of your current diet and what's going on in the everyday world with food and nutrition. You must deal with promptings and influences, day in and day out, and the reflexes you have absorbed from your surroundings. We will see how you can step out of those social ruts into a more playful and enjoyable encounter with your food—and one that will contribute powerfully to your health and healing.

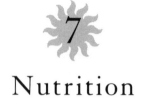

7

Nutrition

*S*andra and Julie, aged four and six, had been diagnosed with a fatal blood disease, the name of which I'd never heard before. The pediatric hematologist had told Mary, their mother, that fewer than a dozen cases were reported in the literature. This was the first time the disease had been seen in two children in the same family. The prognosis was poor. No one had survived more than a few years. Mary was, of course, devastated, but had come to me in the hope that I had some alternative treatments. "Can you help?" she asked, with a tearful, terrified expression.

I squirmed. I'd never worked with something like this. "I'm happy to do my best," I started, then hesitated. After a moment's reflection I realized all I could do was what I always did: give the indicated remedies, for example, and work on their diet, which consisted of hot dogs, Twinkies, and PBJ's. Diet would have to be a priority. She was willing to do anything, she said, relieved, I think, that I was even willing to try.

But when she came back the next time, I didn't see much evidence of progress. And though I emphasized the importance of diet again, and though she agreed again, on the third visit, the diet record looked very much the same. At that point I was not very experienced with giving dietary advice, and felt frustrated and helpless. "Do you work outside the home?" I asked, with an edge to my voice. "No," she answered nervously, shrinking back a bit. "You devote your life to taking care of your children," I asked with a staged tone of disbelief, "and this is the best you can do with their diets?"

She began to cry, and I immediately regretted my harshness. "I don't know what you want," she said through her tears. "I buy all-beef franks and the best brand of peanut butter!"

Suddenly I understood. She had no inkling of what a good diet was. She had grown up on hot dogs and PBJ's herself. We had to start from scratch. "You know the part of the supermarket where they have the fresh vegetables and fruits?" She hesitated. "I know what you're talking about . . . I never get stuff there, I use the frozen ones." It was a hurdle. She was willing to cross it, to buy fresh produce, but confessed she had no idea what to do with it in the kitchen.

Fortunately she was a willing student, and it didn't take her long to learn. As their diet improved and they took the homeopathic remedies I prescribed, the girls perked up. Color came into their faces, and they had more energy. Eighteen months later the hematologist seemed puzzled. All evidence of the syndrome was gone. I last heard of them many years later, when both were on the girls' basketball team at their high school.

It's hard to witness something like that without wondering how many of the odd diseases that we see are related to the diets that we have fallen into. This chapter will only deal briefly with current information on molecular nutrition, and often a simple approach to supplements. Though there's a lot to be said about supplements, I have kept this passage concise. I have previously written two books on nutrition that deal with the subject from a holistic perspective. All the detail you might want is available there.[1] Here I want to focus primarily on a system for dealing with food choices in a way that is creative, fun, and contributes to healing. It's a five-step program, and each step brings up a series of key issues in holistic nutrition. Like any other aspect of human structure or function—e.g., the palm, the face, how you move—your dietary patterns will tell you much about yourself, and working with them can provide powerful leverage for healing. But first let's try to get a bird's-eye view of the strange food habits we modern folk have fallen into.

We're Eating *What?*

In the Ayurvedic tradition it is said: "If you have a good diet, of what use is a doctor? And, if you *don't* have a good diet, of what use is a doctor?" Felicity and I seemed to fall into the latter category. She had a bad diet, and I seemed to be of little use. I'd been pushing her for months to clean up her food habits. Her joints swelled and hurt, and she'd been told she had rheumatoid arthritis, but she'd reached her limit with this business of dietary change.

"I've tried the diet you suggested," she began, "but it's hard to find the kind of stuff you told me to eat." Then she looked straight at me and said, with a mixture of irritation and exasperation, "I just want to eat *normal food!*"

It wasn't the first time I'd heard that. It's very difficult to limit yourself to healthy foods and still function in the world today. I was sympathetic, but how was she going to recover her health on the white bread, meat and grease, and frozen-vegetable diet that her record revealed? *I* wanted to ask *her,* "How can you consider what you eat *normal* food?"

It's difficult to disentangle ourselves from our habits, to get any real perspective on what's become familiar. I try to imagine an anthropologist five hundred years from now, looking back at this era with amused detachment: "You know they almost made themselves extinct. They were taken with the notion of creating fake flavors and appearances that would be more appealing than natural foods. They set up outlets along every street and road with stuff geared to those tastes that had fallen into a sort of addictive craving—heavy on the sugar, salt, and grease. After a couple of generations they actually began to consider this pseudo-food they had created for the marketplace normal, as if it were the real thing. They convinced themselves it could be used as regular fare. They had to reach a crisis point of immune collapse before they began to realize what they were doing. . . ."

A careful analysis of nutritional physiology shows that the gulf between sane eating habits and what has become the norm has widened increasingly. Less and less do we provide ourselves with the simple foods we need.

Change in diet is far and away the most common first step taken by those who are searching for a more natural approach to managing their health. Health-food stores often serve as a point of entry—a sort of shimmering borderland where one reality shades off into another. Crossing that boundary may be difficult. It often requires courage and determination. Changing your eating habits can be like walking away from what is comfortable and familiar—like leaving home.

So much of our identity and group affinities are tied up with how we eat. I explained to Antonio, a patient with gallstones who didn't want surgery, that gallstones are simply crystallized cholesterol. "Cut the fat out of your diet and they can dissolve," I told him. I was also thinking that for a New York businessman in his mid-forties, cutting down on fat and lowering cholesterol wasn't a bad idea anyway. I was happy to see that he took the advice to heart and began to make major changes.

But when he went home to celebrate the holidays with his large Italian family, his new dietary practices were not greeted with enthusiasm. When the sausage was passed, he declined. Ditto the prosciutto. There was an uncomfortable silence. His mother, keeper of the tribal bonds, looked at him askance and asked, with an edge to her voice that belied her forced smile, "What's the matter, Tonio, you not *Italian* anymore?" He could feel the deep threat of being cast out of the family circle tugging at the pit of his gut.

Stepping out of your dietary patterns is a radical move. Often, in the secret recesses of your inner world, it's just plain scary. You may be giving up that sense of warmth and nurturance that you associate with a big slice of buttered white bread, or that feeling of "being good" when you swallow the same sugary treat you were rewarded with as a child. Making these changes is, in a quiet and inconspicuous way, revolutionary. It breaks the momentum of habit and releases the mind from patterns of repetition. It opens the door to examining other aspects of the way you live. It's radical—shift the diet, and other life changes follow.

When I gave up meat, my headaches went away. So did lots of my friends. As I moved more toward vegetarianism, I became a problem. "Where are we going to have dinner? Last time he ate nothing but lettuce because everything on the menu had meat in it. And we can't stay at home, because he won't eat anything *I* know how to cook."

Besides, they were worried. A good friend warned me (this was 1970) that my vegetarian diet was dangerous. "Look," he said, "I know what I'm talking about." He was, in fact, enrolled in a graduate program in nutrition. "You can't keep it up. I asked one of my professors. Without some meat, you can't survive." That set me back a bit. I'd been feeling better and better as I cut out first red meat and then chicken, but I wasn't willing to depart this life to hold onto the diet. I decided I'd better do some reading.

TOO MUCH INFORMATION, NOT ENOUGH NUTRIENTS

Nearly three decades of study later, having written two books on nutrition, I still often feel like a novice. There seems to be an endless amount to learn. When I wrote the introduction to *Diet and Nutrition* twenty years ago, I quoted Clive McKay, a pioneer in the field, who had said, forty years before *that,* that in order to keep up with the volume of research being published on the subject, he would have had to read an article every three minutes, seven days a week. In the sixty years since then, the volume of information available on nutrition has increased exponentially. At this point there is no way that even a team of experts can keep abreast of it. And most of it is biochemical.

Biochemical nutrition is the study of the molecular components of food and of the metabolic machinery of the body. It's the best medical science has been able to do—this cataloging of molecular nutrients, counting how many are present and measuring how much they have dwindled. But, as a basic approach, it seems myopic. It's a little like having the bride fail to show up for the wedding and making a list of body parts that are missing.

Yet even the data that have come out of this mechanistic approach are sobering. The most recent U.S. Department of Agriculture survey, done in 1996, showed widespread dietary deficiencies (see Fig. 54). Less than half of the adult population gets adequate amounts of calcium, magnesium, or vitamins A, B_6, and E. And the diet of nearly three-quarters is deficient in zinc. And this study looks at only a limited number of familiar nutrients. The trace minerals, for which there is voluminous data showing even more alarming deficiency, are not represented at all.

What has struck me is that the vitamin bottles on the shelves of health-food stores and pharmacies have proliferated as the presence of vitamins and minerals in our food has dwindled. Mineral depletion of the soil has come about through poor soil management. The use of chemical fertilizers as a substitute for composted organic matter has left soils vulnerable to erosion and to the loss of minerals. Plants grown on those soils are not as healthy and vibrant nor as rich in nutritional value. A study some years ago showed, for example, that the corn grown in the traditional Navajo fashion had fourteen times the mineral content of that grown on current farmlands.[2]

Already having lost much of their minerals to erosion, our grains are further fragmented by "refining." Wheat, for example, already much poorer in vitamins and minerals than it was a half-century ago, is milled, removing much of what might have remained in nutritional value. Meanwhile, as the nutrients have disappeared from our foods, entire industries have arisen to fill the vacuum. Supplement producers offer

PERCENTAGE OF INDIVIDUALS IN USA TAKING IN RDA*
(Recommended Daily Allowance)

Nutrient	Percent of Population
Calcium	35%
Iron	62%
Magnesium	38%
Vitamin A	44%
Pyridoxine (B$_6$)	47%
Folic Acid	67%
Vitamin C	62%
Vitamin E	30%
Zinc	26%

*Source: *Results from USDA's 1996 Continuing Survey of Food Intakes by Individuals,* Food Surveys Research Group, Beltsville Human Nutrition Research Center, Agricultural Research Service, U.S. Department of Agriculture, Riverdale, Maryland, 1998. Figures are for adults over twenty years old, and do not take into account vitamin or mineral supplements.

FIGURE 54

nutrients, and the food processors add flavors and colors in an effort to re-create the appeal of natural food.

I often find I'm faced with an impossible task—to reassemble from supplements and available foodstuffs some semblance of what our bodies are designed to use. Doing detailed nutritional work with patients, looking at formulas and calculating doses, I sometimes feel as if I need a computer with space-age software to deal with the increasing complexity of it all. And even if I were to succeed, the patient's needs might well change from one day to the next.

At a certain point we have to abandon that reductionistic approach, commit ourselves to using fresh, wholesome produce, and put together a diet of simple food that is satisfying and nurturing. But first the supplement questions: To what extent does it make sense to turn to pills to supply what is missing from your food—and how do you ever decide *which ones?*

A SANE APPROACH TO SUPPLEMENTS

Supplements have proliferated and invaded pharmacies and grocery stores. They are lined up now by vitamin. All the Vitamin A's, different strengths and brands, then the various B vitamins—so many of them they may occupy a whole section of shelves. Usually there's a wall of vitamins and minerals—sometimes an entire storeful! For the consumer, it can be overwhelming. A few simple guidelines might serve to make the subject more manageable. These are practical measures that will tide you over until your diet falls into place and is strong enough to sustain you by itself.

The first point is that more supplements are needed in the city than in the country. More accurately, more nutrients are needed for a hectic, chaotic life than for one that's quieter. I first figured that out when I was alternating one week in New York City and one week in rural Pennsylvannia. The weeks I was in New York, if I didn't take vitamins, I would drag. During the periods in Pennsylvannia, especially if they extended longer, I felt less and less of a need to take the supplements, and I would begin to find myself echoing the words of friends and patients who lived there full-time: "I find these pills unpleasant—like some foreign stuff in my system that I don't need."

So make your own adjustments. If you're running around madly, increase your doses. If you're relaxed and quiet, give your system a vacation and a chance to clean out excesses that might have built up when you were pouring in the pills. Note that it's not always the obvious stresses that increase needs. Your environment may be quiet, but if you're going through lots of emotional upheaval, you're probably going to burn more B vitamins. Folks dealing with acute schizophrenic states, or a highly amped-up emotional crisis, often use enormous quantities of one or more of B_6, niacin, and/or vitamin C. If you're not in the sunlight, take more D. If there's a flu going around, up your C.

Read about supplements, but don't get crazy about them. There *is* a point of diminishing returns. If you don't draw a line somewhere, you'll end up needing extra B vitamins just because you're so frantic about which vitamins to take! A homeopathic remedy, chosen according to your present symptoms or tailored to your constitution, might reorganize how your system operates and decrease, or even eliminate, your tendency to use more than your share of a vitamin or mineral. So might insights that come through meditation or by working with a therapist. But in the meantime, using a supplement to supply your special needs for that nutrient is a reasonable temporary measure.

The second point is, take a summer break. Stop your supplements for a while. Even if you live a hectic life and are an adrenaline addict, your body needs an occasional breather. Summer is a great time to do this, because generally you'll get more fresh fruits and vegetables, sunshine, and fresh air then, and as a result you'll need less supplementation. And since you don't wear a computerized intravenous dispenser, you are doomed to dose yourself in a way that is not precise. The stuff you take in that isn't needed must be gotten rid of. Give your body a chance to flush it all out.

Third, make peace with the fact that you've probably had multiple minor deficiences for years. Even the good diet you're going to get won't be able—at least not for a long time—to replenish those depleted inventories. So take a multivitamin for a while. Once your diet's in place, stop. You have some idea of how long to do this because you know how bad your diet has been, and for how long! (A little honesty with yourself here is helpful.) Even after you've stopped, keep a supply handy and resume at times when you feel the need—for example, when subject to extra stress or during seasons that are harsh—or just during those periods when you feel "run down."

My grandmother, who remained alert and "fit as a fiddle and fine as silk" (in her words) until she died peacefully at one hundred, once asked me, as she was turning eighty, to help her get some vitamins. "What is it that you need?" I asked, having little interest in supplements myself back then. She told me the name of the proprietary formula, and I looked it up. It contained megadoses of vitamins E and D. I was alarmed. I could see the utility of the E, since I had just begun to hear of the use of vitamin E to slow aging. But the huge doses of D concerned me. "How long have you been taking this?" I asked. "For many years," she said. Then, apparently noticing my serious tone, she added, "Well, I don't take it all the time." I was puzzled. Still in medical school, all I knew was prescribed doses. "So when do you take it?" I asked. "I take it when I need it," she answered, as though that shouldn't need explaining. "And for how long?" I asked, a bit scandalized by her cavalier attitude toward such a potent preparation. "Until I've had enough," she answered with a finality that made it clear to me that the discussion was over.

The use of supplements provides an excellent opportunity to begin to learn how to watch our internal signals and see what we need and when.

My grandmother, I later found out, had some vague sense of heaviness in her back and legs that the supplement corrected. When it was better, she stopped. She didn't need any literature on the use of vitamins E and D, or any warnings about potential toxicity. She took her walks until the last year of her long life, and never concerned herself with fractures or bone disease.

And that's the essence of the fourth point: If you have chronic symptoms, use them as cues that you are lacking a nutrient. Pimples and pustules might be telling you that you need zinc, as would a chronic or recurrent sore throat. Anxiety and fatigue can signal thiamine (B_1) deficiency. Puffiness in the hands or ankles could be an indication of low B_6. Carpal tunnel syndrome may be another "request" for that nutrient.

> When we were in the midst of building our house, with subcontractors lined up to come in on a tight schedule, our head carpenter suddenly announced he would be gone "for a few weeks." This would leave our plan in shambles. "Why?" I asked, pained. "I'm going to have surgery," he explained. "I've been numb and weak in my right hand, what they call carpal tunnel syndrome. I won't be able to use a hammer for several weeks after they operate." I thought for a moment. "Do you really want to have this operation?" I asked. "If you are willing to wait a couple of weeks, here's something you could try." I suggested he take 100 mg of B_6 twice a day. A few weeks later, I asked him about his hand. "Oh, it's back to normal now." He smiled. "I canceled the surgery. And you know what? I used to be tired in the morning. Now when I wake up I feel pretty frisky!"

The B_6 wasn't simply a treatment for carpal tunnel symptoms; it was something our carpenter was low in, and the numbness in his hands was merely a warning light. When he took the vitamin, his whole system could function more optimally. Similarly, broken capillaries can be asking for bioflavonoids, while mitral valve prolapse can be a sign that magnesium levels are low. Muscle cramps often suggest a need for both calcium and magnesium. If you have two or more symptoms of a deficiency of a vitamin or mineral, that's pretty sound evidence that you are running low in it.

Bleeding gums might call for vitamin C. So would easy bruising, slow wound healing, or a tendency to respiratory infections. Blood sugar problems can be based in part on chromium deficiency. There are scores of such simple signs of vitamin or mineral needs, some of which are in Fig. 55, others of which you will find in the Self-Help Index in Section V of this book. The need for a nutrient is probably not the only message such symptoms are trying to convey to you. But the request for the vitamin or mineral is a start. If you can learn to hear that and address it, you'll be better prepared to deal with what's there on other levels, too.

NUTRIENTS AND INDICATORS OF DEFICIENCY

Symptom	Nutrient
slow wound healing	Zinc
sunburn	vitamin E
shingles	vitamin B_{12}
prostate enlargement	zinc
gum disease	coenzyme Q-10
neuritis	vitamin B_1
Ménière's disease	manganese
wheezing in kids	B_{12}
diabetes/hypoglycemia	chromium
eyes slow to adapt to darkness	vitamin A

Note:
1. This is not about using megadoses as medicine, but about correcting deficiencies.
2. These are the easy ones—one symptom indicating a need for one nutrient. With so many deficiencies prevalent today, we more commonly see multiple defiencies. For more help dealing with those, see the Self-Help Index at the back of the book.

FIGURE 55

SUPPLEMENTS MADE EASY

**1. How much you need depends on
how much you use up.**
(Live sanely, use less.)

2. Take a break from time to time—
summer is perfect.
(Let your system clean out.)

**3. Replenish your stores until
your diet is solid** (with
supplements e.g., a multivitamin).

**4. Let your symptoms tell you
what you're low in.**
(Use a simple reference.)

5. If you're still confused, then
see a nutritionist (to help
you learn to do it yourself).

FIGURE 56

After all this (see Fig. 56), if you're still hopelessly confused, see a nutritionist. But try asking her or him to help you make the approach outlined here work; don't just hand over total responsibility for deciding what you need. Chances are, with a little expert guidance, you will be able to replenish your stores of vitamins and minerals, discover the nutrients that you are characteristically liable to use and need most, and get established on a diet that will sustain you with only limited and/or intermittent supplementation.

Nutrients in pill form are, after all, only adjuncts to a diet. They are supplements, not substitutes. There is no way that fragmented nutrients can replace whole foods—despite sci-fi fantasies or industry hype to the contrary. The whole food bears some complex and intimate relation to the digestive tract and human physiology and resonates on subtler levels in ways that are also nurturing. Whatever you do with supplements as a temporary or ongoing compensation for defects in your food supply or inability to assimilate and use nutrients, a good diet remains of major importance.

What is a "good diet"? Interestingly enough, we may be among the first people to ask. Until recently, everyone *knew* what to eat, which was what their mothers or grandmothers had fed them. In this era of commercialized food, nothing is so clear. We are increasingly suspicious of the food products we are offered—and usually appropriately so.

Though loss of ethnic traditions and the advent of commercial foods have created a sense of confusion and uncertainty, the good news is that there's an unprecedented openness to rethinking what we eat and why. Increasingly liberated from tribal strictures on our eating habits, we become free to explore how we relate to food in a way that can be enlightening and healing. How you deal with your food speaks volumes about your inner struggles, and as you learn to hear what it reveals, you will make empowering discoveries that have an impact on your health and your personal evolution.

What follows are five basic principles for working with your diet. Taken together, they provide a simple yet profoundly comprehensive approach to what otherwise may often appear to be an impossibly overwhelming subject.

Dietary Principle Number 1. Back to Eden: Whole Foods and Wholesome Impulses

The first principle is to create a context within which food choices can be free and spontaneous. This means putting oneself in a space where the options are all relatively wholesome and natural. Though this may seem like a big order, when approached gradually, it is quite possible. The following exchange with one of my patients is typical:

> *I realized that I was stuck in the middle of another struggle over diet. Victoria sat across from me with her lips set grimly. Though I could see how much her eating habits were setting a limit on her progress, we weren't getting anywhere. Her symptoms were many. Some doctors had called her condition "fibromyalgia" (literally, pain in the muscles and fibrous tissues, which she certainly had). Others said it was chronic fatigue syndrome (it was true, without a doubt,*

WORKING WITH DIET

1.

Limit yourself to natural foods
to set up a playground.

2.

Stay away from oils/fats, salt, and sugar
to avoid addictions.

3.

Evaluate what's left with your constitution in mind
to clean and attune your instrument
of gut-level assessment so you
can trust your impulses.

4.

Analyze
what you eat in terms of
its effects on consciousness
so you can "get high"
from your food!

5.

Play with your "mistakes."
they are creative dramas
with a story to tell!

FIGURE 57

that she was also chronically fatigued). Other diagnoses ranged from candidiasis to irritable bowel syndrome. Each seemed to capture the truth of some facet of her suffering. I knew there were as many angles on her treatment as there were on her diagnosis, but diet was a big one.

I also knew she was struggling, as was I, to prevent our interaction from degenerating into a power struggle. "Well, I guess it's true that whatever tastes good is bound to be bad for you and whatever is good for you is bound to taste bad!" she commented, attempting a smile. As much as I wanted to support her effort to lighten up a bit, I couldn't go along with this. I shook my head.

"It doesn't have to be that way," I began hesitantly. "What I want for you is to reach a point where you can look at food and say, 'Um, that looks good!' and know that if it's appealing, then it has to be just what you need." She shot me a look of disdain.

Nevertheless, I plunged ahead. "Your taste buds weren't put there to trick you into eating something that will hurt you," I argued. "It's only reasonable to assume that they were designed to lead you to what you need. Like poorly schooled students, however, they can be confused and mistrained. What they need is retraining. They only need the experience of reconnecting with what makes you feel nurtured and energized—then they will catch on pretty quickly. You just need to offer them a range of choices that is more natural, foods that they were designed to encounter and evaluate—not chemicalized, altered stuff that they can't deal with." I could see her face darken again as she saw Restriction and Deprivation lurking ahead. To reassure her, I explained, "You have to start with a range of choices that your taste buds are familiar with and enjoy. You don't say, 'I'll only eat sprouts and raw greens.' You won't get far like that.

"You want to continue to enjoy your food—otherwise it won't do you any good." She relaxed a little. "The body won't digest or assimilate what you find repulsive." Now she smiled. "The goal here is to offer yourself a selection of fresh, wholesome fruits and vegetables, grains and fish—and even meat, if you are accustomed to it—that is vibrant and delicious. You want your tongue to become more discriminating and selective, to find higher levels of enjoyment. This will lead you to more pleasure in your eating, and energy and aliveness in your body."

I think I had her then. I was only slightly glossing over some of the less attractive aspects of this path. I didn't mention that at first some of these foods would seem tasteless because her palate had to recover from being blasted by huge quantities of sugar, salt, and artificial flavors before it regained its sensitivity to the subtler flavors of fresh, natural foods.

In my experience, this process of dietary change is best undertaken gently and gradually. Forcing yourself to eat what you don't want doesn't work. The diet plan taped to the refrigerator door has an average life span of about two weeks. It's crucial to preserve a sense of playful exploration of new flavors, and to study the effect that these foods have on your sense of well-being—your energy, spirits, and clarity of consciousness. You will naturally learn to love that which makes you alert, clear-headed, and exhilarated. A major part of nutritional work is creating a situation in which such learning can occur. The other part is to identify what is interfering when it doesn't—what underlies the tendency to eat blindly, even when doing so creates discomfort and disrupts your sense of well-being.

When the Himalayan Institute first moved its headquarters from a small building in suburban Chicago to a former Catholic seminary in the Pocono Mountains of northeast Pennsylvania in 1977, we had, for the first time, a large institutional kitchen and enthusiastically turned out regular meals for the whole group as well as for visitors. With so much energy going into the food, we thought it was sure to be good. But something was wrong. People were complaining of painful gas and distended bellies. Why would there be *more* problems with better food?

I decided maybe I should spend some time in the kitchen. What I found might have been predicted. The zealous crew was going overboard in the whole-foods direction. Fruits and vegetables were not peeled, so that nothing would be lost nutritionally; stems and roots were to be tossed in, too, since they were "an integral part of the plant." Other crusaders had decreed white rice off limits, and used only brown. Meanwhile, the bread crew had its own campaign going, it was using only full-grain whole wheat flour, and was adding generous quantities of extra bran to the bread dough. It all added up to enough fiber to start a paper mill.

The higher content of fiber in a primarily vegetarian diet is the basis of many of its advantages: its ability to collect and pull toxic substances out of the body, for example. I am horrified by the nearly total absence of fiber in the standard American diet, which is largely meat, white flour, milk products, eggs, sugar, fats, and oils—all of which are fiberless. The occasional addition of potatoes or green salad, which do contain a bit of fiber, comes nowhere close to remedying the situation. But we culinary adventurers at the Himalayan Institute had gone too far to the other extreme—especially for the digestive systems of people who had grown up on the typical American fiber-free diet. The result was an explosion of gas from intestinal bacteria as they broke down the large quantities of fiber in the food. When we took the extra bran out of the bread, peeled the vegetables, composted the stems and roots, and alternated lightly

---

DIETARY PRINCIPLE NO. 1

Limit yourself to natural foods.

Eat fresh, unprocessed, preferably organic,
largely vegetarian foods,
emphasizing whole grains, legumes,
fresh-cooked vegetables, fruits, salads,
and dairy or fish.

FIGURE 58

milled basmati rice with the coarser brown, stomachs began to deflate and abdominal distress diminished.

Had we all chosen what felt right to our bellies, what was appealing and satisfying, rather than what some new dietary doctrine dictated, we might have made a smoother transition to healthy eating. Our hyper-austere approach was revealing—though not particularly surprising in a group of would-be yogis who often made the common mistake of thinking you could torture yourself into enlightenment. It was a valuable lesson. Had I been a bit more open to that insight, I might have saved myself the affliction of further years of inattention to my own inner voice.

So the first principle of healthy eating is to surround yourself with choices that are natural, fresh, unprocessed, and preferably organic, emphasizing whole grains, legumes, fresh-cooked vegetables, fruits, salads, and dairy or fish.

THE QUESTION OF VEGETARIANISM

There are many reasons for moving toward a vegetarian diet. Economically and ecologically, it's almost an imperative. It takes 2,500 gallons of water to produce a pound of hamburger—more than you would save in a year by switching to a water-conserving toilet or putting low-volume showerheads in the bath. We read daily of the thousands of acres of rain forest cleared to create grazing land for beef cattle. Obviously we cannot afford to give up oxygen and water for meat.[3]

Medically the data is equally compelling: your intake of toxic chemicals drops dramatically as you decrease animal foods. Heart attacks are seven times more frequent in meat-eaters than in vegetarians who are matched so that other aspects of their lifestyles are the same. Cancer, arthritis, and osteoporosis are also much less likely to appear in those who don't eat meat.[4] With the world's population growing and the cost of medical care soaring, the move toward vegetarianism seems inevitable. This may be perfectly apparent to our minds, but what do we do when the body resists?

> *"It just doesn't agree with me," Julian, a man in his fifties, said flatly. "I tried being a vegetarian, and it didn't work. The grains gave me headaches and I started getting weak. I felt confused and couldn't function." I couldn't tell whether his exasperation came from feeling pressured by his wife and friends who were mostly not meat-eaters, or from his own frustration at being unable to join them. "When I started back eating meat, I regained my energy and stamina. My body just isn't meant to function on a vegetarian diet." He sat back in his chair and crossed his arms in a posture reminiscent of a defiant adolescent.*

Many factors are thought to militate against adjustment to a vegetarian diet. The kind of work you do, for example, might affect your desire for meat. Some of my patients believe surviving in a world of aggression and competition may be easier with the "edge" that meat provides. In classic Vedic times in India, architects of the caste system harnessed the aggressive energy they saw meat providing, and prescribed meat-eating for the Kshatriya or warrior caste. The Brahmins, who were the spiritual teachers and priests, were, by contrast, forbidden to partake.

The climate you live in could also have a bearing on the ease with which a vegetarian diet might be accepted. Even Buddhists eat meat in the mountains of Tibet, where the cold is harsh and vegetables are unavailable for most of the year. When I was a child in the American South, we ate little meat in the summer—not only because the garden was overflowing with tasty produce, but because meat seemed too heavy to digest in the hot weather.

Race has something to do with it, too. If you are from ancestry with a long history of vegetarianism, it's probably easier for you to thrive on an all-plant diet than for someone from a line of meat-eaters. The dietary patterns of your childhood are formative as well. My children, raised totally vegetarian, have absolutely no desire for, or interest in, fish or poultry, not to mention red meat. But I was not raised vegetarian, and after twenty years as a lactovegetarian and then five years as a vegan (no dairy, either), I found I needed a bit of seafood or even an occasional small portion of organic[5] chicken to replace milk products if I was to remain strong and energetic.

Your constitutional type is also key. Earth/Water or *kaphic* types can do very well on a vegan diet, while at the other end of the spectrum, the airy, spacey, *vatic* person may need some animal food to ground him or her. Dairy might suffice, but if it's not tolerated well, fish is a reasonable second choice. Meanwhile, the fiery *pittic* soul is spurred to problematic levels of aggression by eating red meat. As a *vata/pitta* combined type, I would probably have trouble with meat, but the watery nature of fish is helpful for me. Some nutritionists feel that blood type can be a clue to what will suit you best, adding another possible piece to the puzzle.[6]

On one level, the obstacles to adjusting to a meatless diet represent specific physiologic responses and even what appear to be characteristics of the "hardware" of the system, such as enzyme deficiencies. That leads us to see the problem as "permanent," unalterable, irreversible: "I can't be vegetarian, my body doesn't work that way. I have to eat meat." When we think that way, we are reasserting the primacy of the physical. But even when rooted physically, such a characteristic may not be so immutable that it can't change. A shift on the level of consciousness, if thorough enough, will redirect and reshape the physiologic responses.

From one perspective, physical functioning is a simple fact, but from another perspective it is only the material, outward manifestation of something internal—of our belief systems and our deeply ingrained patterns of emotion and thought. These belief systems are far from insignificant; they are the warp and woof of the prevailing planetary mindsets that have us trapped in self-defeating habits of relating and thinking. The lifestyles that result from these attitudes and mindsets often perpetuate the problems—medical, social, and ecological—that cause our suffering and limit our individual and collective evolution.

Julian, who complained that he required meat, turned out to feel that giving up meat undercut his male power. His wife, well-meaning in her way, seemed to him an adversary in this struggle. His case fit the characterization of the meat-eater's identification with a warriorlike image of masculinity and domination that still prevails on the planet.

I once had a conversation with a reporter for an Indian newspaper as we drove into New York together. We fell into a discussion of the pros and cons of a meat-based diet. "I'm not vegetarian and wasn't really raised to be," he explained, "but as a concept it was very alive in my upbringing." Though he seemed curious about the whole issue, he didn't seem to be defending a position. "I guess I grew up accepting the traditional idea that meat-eating promoted aggression. I'm not sure it's true, but I am reminded of it sometimes. A few weeks ago, for example, I was invited, along with a group of friends, for dinner. Before we ate, the conversation was quite pleasant. After dinner, which was heavy on the red meat, the atmosphere seemed to shift. Everyone seemed sharper, and a couple of nasty arguments broke out. I was struck by the difference."

Even if it is true that violent and destructive energies emerge in the course of meat-eating, this doesn't necessarily mean that meat should be stopped to avoid them. Instead, we might take a different tack. We might say, "These dark energies are within us and are part of the intricate network of impulses that grip our world. Better to deal with them consciously and not banish them to the unconscious." Such work was accomplished in the Tantric tradition by the ritual consumption of meat. Repression was not tolerated on that radical spiritual path.[7]

Whether you address this issue by grappling with meat-eating and the impulses it arouses ("warrior"), or whether you explore the challenges of living in the light ("priest"), a gradual, progressive clearing of consciousness is what will lead us past a dependence on meat. As a collective goal, this may become crucial, since producing enough healthful meat to feed a burgeoning world population is likely to be impossible.

If you, personally, feel weak and confused from the dietary changes you make, however, that's counterproductive. Back up. Increase the quality and freshness of your food—including the animal products. Adopt an attitude of reverence for the lives—both plant and animal—that were surrendered for your sustenance. Affirm your intention of using the nurturance you derive from those life forms to heal and transform yourself and the world.

As your physical body, your energy/emotions, and your consciousness feel stronger, experiment gradually and gently with decreasing and eventually phasing out red meat. Next, try to remove the poultry from your diet. Once you have finished with reducing it as far as you feel comfortable, don't force the issue further. Next, ask yourself whether you need fish or dairy products.[8] Determine whether the reluctance or resistance you feel is the residue of upbringing, racially determined physiologic reactions, or metabolic traits. Your impulses and resistances are opportunities for healing, and they are your piece of social transformation.

Dietary Principle No. 2.
Watch Out for Sugar, Salt, and Grease

Once you have narrowed your choices to these wholesome foods, you should be able to experiment freely and eat what you want. But there are three saboteurs lurking in the shadows, waiting to spoil your diet. They are sugar, salt, and grease. Even "healthy" foods such as those that come from health-food stores or veggie restaurants can harbor dangerous quantities of these three culprits, the most malicious of which is sugar.

The blood level of sugar controls our sense of when we need to eat. Physiologists like to talk about the "appestat"—the feedback mechanism that controls appetite. When blood glucose levels go down, we feel hungry. Eating sugar is like mainlining appetite satisfaction. We have an immediate sense of having gotten what we needed, a sort of "high." I first became aware of the intensity of this reaction when I took a group of ten- and eleven-year-olds to a movie as part of my son's birthday celebration:

> *On the way there, they were polite and calm. When we arrived at the theater, I rushed ahead to the concession stand, having rehearsed in my mind how I would buy everyone lemonade and popcorn to limit their consumption of chemicalized sugar. But I hadn't figured on their determination. Each produced his own money, stepped around me, and purchased his own personal supply of candy—a couple of boxes per child—which they had devoured by the end of the film. I was amazed.*
>
> *I knew it tended to speed them up, but I was not prepared for the ride home. They were literally bouncing off the walls of the large Chevy Suburban, throwing each other over the seats and breaking into fights that required vigorous intervention. Nothing I said had a lasting effect, and with their glazed eyes they were clearly in an altered state. For most of them a sugar high was their first "drug experience." I wondered how much it would prompt, a few years hence, the search for other "highs" and a reliance on more serious drugs to create excitement and energy.*

Sugar's potential for "abuse" seems to be related to the central role it plays in the energy economy of the system. "It's the energy food," advertisers like to say. More accurately, it's the energy *extracted* from the food.

Though the sugar is the energy-providing aspect of food, in nature it is packaged with the ancillary nutrients needed to burn the sugar efficiently. Natural sources come with an appropriate complement of vitamins and minerals—and even the protein needed for structural maintenance. Taking the sugar alone is cheating, like trying to extract the pleasurable aspects of life—bypassing the rich, complex mixture of other feelings and experiences. Just as the addict must eventually come to terms with this lack and go back and recover the piece of his past that can teach him wisdom, so must the sugar junkie retrace his steps and restore the missing nutrients—as well as subtler nurturance that comes from relating to a whole plant with its complex patterns of energy and information.

Though glucose (also known as dextrose) is the form in which sugar is tranported in the bloodstream, sucrose (table sugar) seems to have the most potential for abuse. In my clinical and personal experience, as well as in my experience as a father, sucrose arouses the strongest craving and seems to produce the most dramatic behavioral changes. Simple glucose, produced by the splitting of the double molecule of sucrose, is a close second and fructose, the other half of the sucrose molecule, a slow third. Fructose, or fruit sugar, seems best tolerated of the three, perhaps because it does not require insulin to cross from the blood into the cell.

In a whole-foods diet, most of the blood glucose comes from the breakdown of starch, which is simply a chain of glucose molecules. When we cheat and take in the energy essence of the food without the rest, a whole sequence of consequences begins to unfold. First we miss the accompanying nutrients, so our food is of "low nutrient density"—a situation we can partially remedy by taking supplements. Second, we disrupt the normal gradual flow of energy—which would result from a piecemeal release of glucose during the stepwise breakdown of the complex carbohydrate of starch. Simple carbohydrate, or sugar, blasts the bloodstream with glucose, and the pancreas must release a corresponding burst of insulin to deal with it. Repeated episodes can exhaust the insulin-secreting cells and lead to difficulty in regulating blood sugar, usually first hypoglycemia and later, perhaps, diabetes.

The adrenals respond to the energy crisis that results from erratic blood sugar levels, and this stresses them in a way that can lead to adrenal exhaustion. A similar process goes on in the liver, which shares the responsibility for maintaining a constant blood glucose. A roller coaster effect in the blood sugar plays havoc with our ability to remain calm, to focus, and to concentrate. Kids become hyperactive and have trouble

```
┌─────────────────────────────────────────┐
│                                         │
│      RESULTS OF "SUGAR ABUSE"           │
│                                         │
│   • Low nutrient density                │
│                                         │
│   • Disruption of stable energy         │
│     Pancreatic stress                   │
│     Adrenal stress                      │
│     Liver stress                        │
│                                         │
│   • Cultivation of yeast overgrowth     │
│                                         │
│   • Undermining of immune competence    │
│                                         │
└─────────────────────────────────────────┘
```

FIGURE 59

learning, and adults may suffer from anxiety and depression as they try to control unstable emotions. The man who murdered San Francisco mayor George Moscone in 1978 pleaded not guilty by virtue of insanity, which his counsel attributed to his having eaten sugar-laden junk food; this became known as the "Twinkie defense."

Though the human system has remarkable resilience and can comfortably accommodate occasional disruptions in blood sugar levels, this capacity is crippled when the adrenals and the liver are already disabled by constant stress, anger, and emotional upheaval. If regular sugar intake is piled on top of that, the result can be a breakdown in the system's adaptive mechanisms. There are further consequences, too.

When sugar intake consistently exceeds the body's ability to handle it, the excess sugar in the intestinal tract begins to encourage an overgrowth of yeast. The yeast ferments the sugar, producing gas, bloating, and alcohol. It's my clinical impression that the alcohol can reach levels where it affects consciousness, produces hangovers, and contributes to the craving for more sugar.

If this sounds exaggerated, remember that the average person eats nearly his body weight in sugar each year. This is a startling change in a relatively brief period of time. As recently as a century or two ago, sugar was an expensive luxury. As production became automated, cutting its cost, and as the storage and preservation of food became a major challenge in the distribution system, the imperishable table sugar became a cheap substitute for more natural whole foods. Now practically every processed and packaged foodstuff has sugar added, from breakfast cereals to canned beef stew. And now economic pressures *favor* the consumption of sugar, and the ghettos of our indigent are populated increasingly by obese people rather than the emaciated and undernourished. The undereducated and ill-informed, swayed by the constant bombardment of television advertising, load their grocery carts with gallon containers of colored sugar water, and struggle helplessly with emotional instability, learning disabilities, and physical diseases stemming in part from their nutrient-deficient, high-sugar diet. Marie Antoinette's "Let them eat cake" has become "Let them drink Coke."

But sugar addiction is not limited to those who are mired in its most severe versions. Many of us are suffering from its milder forms. Leslie, my health-conscious but sugar-addicted editor, asked me, "How do you break the habit?" It's not an easy question to answer. Once the body has been sensitized to sugar and has become accustomed to functioning in an addicted mode, it has trouble handling even small amounts comfortably. A large percentage of my patients and I have had to think of ourselves as "recovering sugar addicts" for some time. Even a little bit seems to set the whole downward spiral in motion again. So totally eliminating the sugar from one's diet is the first step to finding a new way of relating to food.

Maybe the answer to the question of breaking the sugar habit is to learn to look for and enjoy the subtle flavors of organic, full-flavored fruits and vegetables, salads with nasturtiums and marigold petals. Next to them, sugar seems crass and intense—in an almost abusive way. It loses its appeal. But if the food in front of you is tasteless, dull, and of low vitality—frozen, canned, processed—sugar becomes the only source of energy and "oomph" to which you have access, and you will begin to crave it again. During lecture tours when I am forced to eat in hotels where the food is dead and lifeless, I am amazed at the sharp desire I feel for sugary desserts—for the sort of sweets in which I normally have little or no interest.

MARCH TO THE SEA

It's tempting to wonder whether the principles of sugar addiction might carry over to salt. If sugar levels in the blood are the body's index of the need for fuel, then it could be that salt is the body's marker or index of a need for minerals. Just as our food supply is often lacking in energy or vitality, it's also often low in trace minerals. Salt as a marker would

BREAKING THE SUGAR HABIT

- No SUCROSE
  includes molasses, brown sugar, maple syrup.

- DON'T add sweeteners like honey to tea or food.

- AVOID the super-sweet fruits—grapes, pineapple,
  very sweet apples, oranges.

- HANG ON—you may have a brief period of withdrawal
  and detox, when you feel very bad and are sure
  you NEED sugar!

- Use tea sweetened with STEVIA—you can also cook with it
  (plus small amounts of malt syrup or fructose).

- MINIMIZE very contractive foods like meat and salt,
  which will call for sweets for balance.

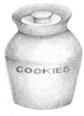

- REWARD yourself with luscious organic fruits and veggies,
  and *remember,* they will taste sweeter and sweeter
  the longer you're OFF THE SUGAR!

FIGURE 60

make sense, since our primal contact with salt was seawater, and it not only contains sodium chloride, which is table salt, but also has a full complement of other minerals—including the trace minerals. What's more, they are present there in exactly the same proportions as they are found in the bloodstream. Crude sea salt will contain this spectrum of minerals, but unfortunately it's rarely available since, in its unrefined form, it's gray and lumpy and draws moisture.

As with sugar, eating the refined substance, the table salt, might be "fooling" the body—so the original clever biochemical mechanism, the use of sodium chloride as the marker for a concentrated source of minerals, would miscarry. Dr. Ehrenfried Pfeiffer, author of the book *Mental and Elemental Nutrients,* had a clever solution to the trace-mineral shortage. Living in New Jersey, near the coast, he went regularly to the beach and collected seawater, which he brought home and boiled down until the sodium chloride crystallized. Then he poured off the liquid remaining, put it in a bottle, and kept it on the table to season his food. Mildly salty, it was also very rich in the trace elements that are now so disastrously absent from our food supply.

While I never made the pilgrimage to the sea, I have used a similar liquid trace-mineral preparation that is from prehistoric salt deposits. Its advocates say that it's less likely to be contaminated than present-day seawater. Other researchers in the field contend that trace minerals are best given to the body in forms that are complexed with organic food molecules—such as what is found in fruits and vegetables grown on mineral-rich soil. Unfortunately, such ideal produce is still in limited supply. So I cook with the Great Salt Lake mineral product and bank on the possibility that its minerals will complex with the food while it simmers.

Meanwhile, I am convinced that the effort to limit our salt intake is worthwhile, at least for some of us. Pure *vata* types may benefit from a limited amount, but it's especially contraindicated for *pitta* and *kapha*. Even mixed *vata/pitta* types like me don't do well with salt. If I eat heavily salted food, what I see in the mirror the next morning is alarming. My face looks puffy, swollen, and angry. What would I look like if I did that regularly, I wonder, and what would that tell me about my internal state?

There are also logical biochemical reasons why sodium chloride should be limited. Potassium is the major positively charged ion inside the cell. Sodium is its extracellular counterpart. When sodium collects, it holds excess water in our tissues—in that space between cells. But if it reaches high enough concentrations, especially when potassium levels are low (as is the case when there are few fruits and vegetables in the diet, or when they have been packaged with salt), sodium can begin to invade the cell and replace the potassium. This undermines normal functions such as the conduction of nerve impulses. Metabolism shifts toward more primitive patterns in the presence of excess salt, those typical of the malignant cell being favored, for example. High-salt diets are especially unfortunate in the case of children, where they are known to predispose to high blood pressure later in life.[9]

FAT OF THE LAND

Our third temptress is the goddess of grease. She slips into our salad dressings, butters our bread, and sizzles our fries. Soon we find that ungreased food tends to stick in our throats. We're hooked. But where does this hankering for fats and oils come from? Are they, like sugar and salt, a marker for something? Doubtless another primal craving is involved here. Just as we speak of "the salt of the earth," we also talk about "the fat of the land," "the cream of the crop," or even the "crème de la crème."

Our language reveals the premium we place on the salty, the "rich" oily foods, and the sweets. We call those we love "honey" or "sugar." Another testimony to the primacy of these hankerings is the persistence with which we pursue them. Friends and patients tell me, "Oh, I don't use salt. I use *sea* salt or tamari." Or, "No sugar for me. I sweeten with molasses and honey." Though slightly toned down, these substitutes are still salt and sugar. Such urges, it would appear, insist on gratification.

If butter's not okay, then we have margarine. If I shouldn't use corn oil, then the market is ready with Canola—the latest "it must be healthy" head on the hydra of fat cravings. But often, such efforts only get us deeper in trouble. In fact, there's evidence that margarine is *less* healthy than butter,[10] that canola oil is *more* of a problem than olive oil.[11] The search for a "healthy alternative" may not be the point here. The real issue is the craving itself. Where does it come from?

Like sugar, fats and oils are pure energy. They are fuels lifted out of their normal context and accompaniments. They are calories without the nutrients needed to burn them—"empty calories," we sometimes say. In fact, fats and oils are an especially condensed storage form of energy. A gram of fat contains more than twice as much energy as a gram of carbohydrate. Just as you take the energy of your work and store it as money, plants and animals store their accumulated wealth as fats and oils. So, in a metaphorical sense, extracting fats and oils is raiding the treasure troves of the natural world. In the same way that eating the purified energy of sugar is "cheating" because you don't do the digestive work of opening the whole-food package and assimilating its vitamins, minerals, protein, and fiber, so eating oils is a similar shortcut, in this case a sort of theft.

And like money you didn't earn, money you wrangle from others, fats corrupt. Saturated fats clog arteries and tissues. The unsaturated oils produce free radicals, which damage cells and tissues and lead to premature aging and predispose us to malignancies. Here our cultural icons are telling. The primitive ideal was a slightly rotund body, bolstered by a comfortable layer of fat. But eating whole food and storing some of its surfeit as fat is a very different process from taking the extracted fat from whole foods and discarding the remainder of the plant or animal. Perhaps this principle gets silent recognition in our "affluent" society—one that uses a disproportionate percentage of the world's natural resources and tends to obesity—through our worship of the skinny model, the anorexic cover girl.

So far there is no evidence that we require more fats and oils than are present in a spectrum of whole foods: grains, beans, vegetables, and fruits. In fact, there is ample evidence that added fats and oils contribute to the diseases common in our society. So one of the challenges of reaching a peaceful, loving relationship with your food is to eliminate from your spectrum of choices the greasy, the fried, the fat-and-oil-added. This also includes large amounts of high-fat whole foods like nuts, cheeses, and most red meat. But, like giving up sugar and salt, this can be a wrenching shift.

> When I was thirty-five, perhaps because I had a strong family history of heart diesease, Swami Rama recommended that I go on a fat-free diet. Already vegetarian, I was to cook without ghee (which I usually used because of its superiority over other fats and oils[12]), eliminate the butter I put on my bread, and put only lemon juice and herbs on my salads. I also was to use skim milk instead of 2% and avoid muffins and baked goods made with butter or oil. I thought this would be easy. It wasn't.
>
> At first everything tasted like paper. The very feel of the food in my mouth was repulsive and it was hard to swallow. I ate less, because my digestion couldn't accommodate the usual amount. I began to realize how much I relied on the oily component of the foods to stimulate my digestive fire. Like salt, fat activates Pitta. Without it, the sedentary person can't digest as much. I needed to exercise more to make up for the lack of oily food.
>
> By the end of a month I had begun to adjust to the new way of eating. By the end of the second month, I had discovered a depth of fla-

vor and enjoyment in food that I had never experienced. After the third month, since I was traveling more and having great difficulty finding food that I could eat, I decided to go off the program. I thought this would be a relief. Wrong again.

Going back to "regular food" was even more difficult than my original adjustment to the fat-free diet had been. Everything seemed disgustingly greasy. I found myself furtively blotting Indian pakoras and Chinese spring rolls in paper napkins, and scanning menus for steamed vegetables, which, though unnecessarily bland, were at least grease-free, and wouldn't slide off the plate in a puddle of oil. I longed for the luxury of my own kitchen where I could prepare well-seasoned, tasty meals without a coating of fat or oil.

A small amount of good-quality oil can be useful. Limit yourself to two tablespoons of total added fat per day. I am not convinced that any of the vegetable oils are desirable—with the possible exception of olive oil, and perhaps sesame. Neither are polyunsaturated and therefore less liable to trigger free-radical formation. On the other hand, there is ample research that butterfat is beneficial. Butyric acid, its unique constituent, has been found to incease natural interferon production, decrease viral growth, and provide some anti-aging benefits for the brain.[13]

Though the prevalance of junk foods in the current diet makes it hard to know what substance creates which effect, it's my impression, after many years of observation, that the sugar, salt, and oils are responsible for many of the obvious negative effects of poor eating.

DIETARY PRINCIPLE NO. 2

Stay away from oils/fats, salt, and sugar.

Even "healthy" foods
—such as those that come from
health-food stores or veggie restaurants—
need to be looked at carefully
with this in mind.

FIGURE 61

A KINDER DIET, A CLEARER FACE

During my midday break from seeing patients in Manhattan, I sit in a lunch bar that serves mostly soups and sandwiches. Watching the people crowd in and rush out, I imagine that each one is on a no-white-flour, no-sugar, low-salt, and low-fat diet. As I look at them, in my mind's eye I see paunches disappear, faces become leaner, younger, steps lighten, and smiles deepen. Diet does affect how you look. After so many years of working with people who are changing their way of eating, I can almost visualize the transformations that the face can go through—moving back into puffiness, bags under the eyes, the purplish swelling of stagnation and overindulgence—or moving forward, losing bulges and distortions, looking calmer, more serene.

Once I had an opportunity to defend this thesis when I agreed to present a half-day program on vegetarianism to the high school students where my daughter, Rebecca, went to school. I had not reckoned with their fierce indifference, the wall they put up when confronted with an adult authority telling them what they ought to do.

They sat before me closed and distracted, one sharp dresser front row center with sunglasses hiding his eyes. I wanted to break through that barrier. I wanted them to see how much they were affected by how they ate, how much choice they have, how much control they can exert over how they feel and think and look, how much the irrationality of our food habits is destroying their environment and producing disease. I wanted them to know that they did not have to repeat the stupid mistakes of their elders, that they didn't have to respond reflexively to the promptings of advertising, that they could be free agents. I flashed a slide on the screen showing the many effects that diet has: physical, mental, emotional, and economic.

I began with appearance. Teenagers care about how they look and don't want acne or scaly, greasy skin. They long to have healthy, well-proportioned bodies. Eager to drive my point home, I said, "Diet does affect the way you look. After twenty years of working with patients, I can look at someone and tell what they eat!"

A young lady in the back raised her hand and asked with a toss of her head, "What do I eat?" I stopped. The kids sat up. My daughter covered her face. The guy in the front took off his sunglasses. I had been appropriately challenged. Could *I tell?*

I did believe *that what you ate showed on your face, and that I could usually see it. So I looked closely at the girl. What I saw were clear features, healthy skin. What I visualized was healthy food.* "You eat a good diet—grains and beans and fresh vegetables," *I heard myself say.*

Immediately I had second thoughts. Exactly what are the chances of a teenager eating that sort of diet? But I had seen what I had seen.

"You're right," she replied. "There's a hyperlipidemia in my family, and we were all put on a diet of beans and rice, fresh fruits, and vegetables years ago."

Rebecca heaved a sigh of relief. I relaxed. The class sat forward in their chairs. I had an attentive audience the rest of the day.

Whole foods without sugar, salt, and grease create a "safe space" nutritionally—a space where you can eat with confidence, satisfaction, and delight. This is a place to experiment freely, reeducate your taste buds, and restore a trusting relationship with your body's natural, spontaneous impulses. It's a culinary Garden of Eden that we can all enter at will. Life inside offers new levels of energy, alertness, and a wellspring of creativity.

Dietary Principle No. 3. Individualize — "You Know in Your Gut"

So far, what we've outlined applies across the board. Everyone needs to limit his or her choices to whole and wholesome foods and to avoid sugar, salt, and grease. Now we shift gears and look at each person's unique requirements. This means finding what meshes with your needs, what resonates with your system. It is the challenge of individualizing.

There's more than one way to individualize. You can use a system, such as *tridosha*, and, on the basis of which type you are—*vata, pitta,* or *kapha*—decide what you need. You can also be guided by your inner sense of what feels right—your gut-level impulse. One way is using your head, the other is listening to your body. By working with both and comparing what you come up with using each of them, you can learn a lot about yourself and transform the way you relate to food.

For example, according to the Ayurvedic teachings, Earth/Water or *kapha* types need to avoid foods with a predominance of Earth and Water

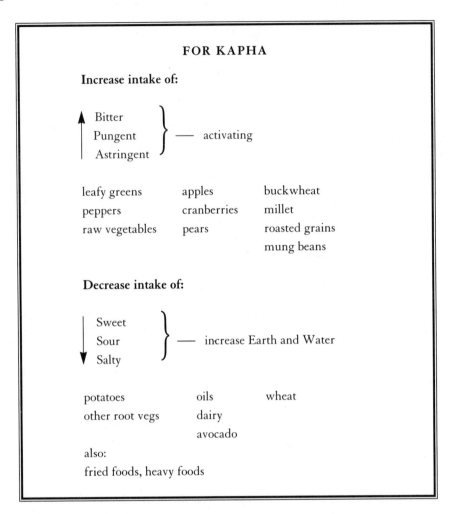

FOR KAPHA

Increase intake of:

Bitter
Pungent   } — activating
Astringent

leafy greens	apples	buckwheat
peppers	cranberries	millet
raw vegetables	pears	roasted grains
		mung beans

Decrease intake of:

Sweet
Sour   } — increase Earth and Water
Salty

potatoes	oils	wheat
other root vegs	dairy	
	avocado	

also:
fried foods, heavy foods

FIGURE 62

Elements. (See the Five Element/taste chart in Chapter 6, page 193.) Too much of such foods will leave them heavy and congested. This is a useful hint for the *kaphic* person, but this is also where experimentation begins. The *kapha* type will find two conflicting urges within himself. Because of his constitution, he will feel a certain affinity for *kaphic* foods—they will provide a sense of comfort and coziness. Ample amounts of *kaphic* grains, such as wheat, or vegetables such as potatoes will wrap him in familiarity and security. But that's a regressive tug. He will note a sense of retreat when he gives into such *kaphic* indulgences.

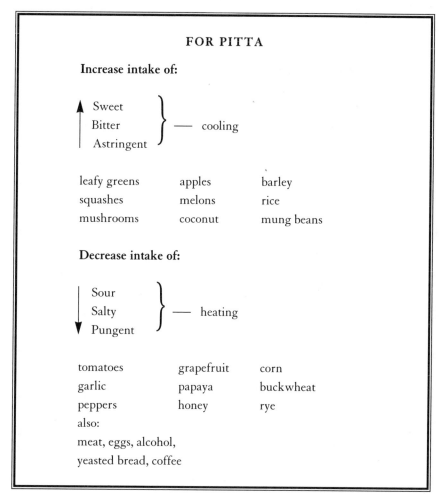

FIGURE 63

Foods with more Fire or with Air and Ether elements will, by contrast, offer him stimulation, the exhilaration of stepping into the unknown. That has a certain appeal, too, but this is a totally different kind of pull. Playing with the different sense of attraction that each of these offers can be an extremely valuable game. Much of your skill in moving through your own process of healing will depend on how successfully you can learn to distinguish between the two impulses.

Fire or *pitta* types will be faced with a similar choice. Fiery foods will ignite their hotheaded impetuousness, blasting them off into fits of

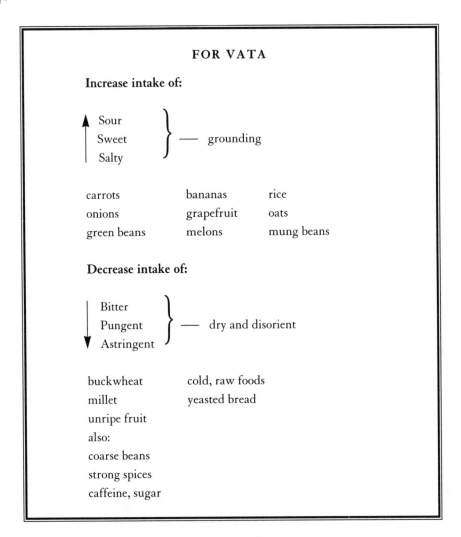

FOR VATA

Increase intake of:

Sour
Sweet   } — grounding
Salty

carrots	bananas	rice
onions	grapefruit	oats
green beans	melons	mung beans

Decrease intake of:

Bitter
Pungent   } — dry and disorient
Astringent

buckwheat	cold, raw foods
millet	yeasted bread
unripe fruit	

also:
coarse beans
strong spices
caffeine, sugar

FIGURE 64

aggression or anger. This is their familiar territory. So they will have a certain tendency to move in this direction. But it's the cooling effect of the more *kaphic* and *vatic* foods that will balance them out and offer them a sense of adventuring into more tranquil realms.

If the spacy *vata* type eats too much raw food, coarse beans, or yeasted bread she will bloat, filling with the gassy Air Element that predominates in those foods and in her system. Yeasted bread is bloated—puffed up by the fermentation of yeast. "Sweet" foods such as rice and onions are nurturing for *vata*. But sugar in the digestive tract of the *vata* person ferments like the yeast in bread, producing more gas and encouraging the growth of yeast in the gut. These events occur most dramatically in the colon; hence the large intestine is considered the "home" of *vata,* just as the duodenum, the center of digestive juice production is the home (or, in Sanskrit, the *kosht*) of *pitta.* This is where the digestive fire is focused. The home base of *kapha* is the stomach—where a major production of mucus occurs and where mucus often collects.

Thus each of the three, *vata, pitta,* and *kapha,* is housed in its own specific location within the gastrointestinal tract. From the Ayurvedic perspective, the intestinal tract is at the center of the organizational plan that governs human function. It is the crux of the matter. This notion is echoed in other traditions, too. The digestive organs are represented along the center of the tongue in Chinese diagnosis (see the tongue map in Chapter 5). The iridologist sees the markings closest to the pupil, the central circle in his map of the iris, as depicting the state of the gastrointestinal tract. There seems to be a sort of consensus that it is here where health is rooted and where disease originates.

Certainly, connecting and relating to food is the essence of how your subtler nature takes on form in the physical world. This relationship with your food can be seen as an elaborate metaphor for other aspects of your life. If the ego, or sense of "I am," has difficulty in wooing and merging with its beloved, the food, disorders of nutrition and physical disability will present themselves as well as analogous problems in relating to other people.[14] The digestive tract is also where the Ayurvedic physician sees the disturbed dosha build up and begin to overflow into other parts of the body to create disease. *Vata,* for example, when sufficiently aggravated and overstimulated, will spill over to produce trembling, shaking, coldness, and irregularity throughout the body and even as far as its surface, as dry, cracked skin or deformed nails.

In traditional Asian medicine, good nutrition and the sound health that follows are based on a resonance of the food with your individual system. Just as you resonate with the organizational pattern of an herbal remedy when you need it, so does your body resonate in some more general way with the subtle energy of a food when you need it. This congruence of your nature and the food can be felt first and foremost in the intestinal tract. When you attend to it, there is a "gut level" sense of what is right for you and what is not.

From your constitutional type or acute imbalances and from which *dosha* needs balancing, you can decide which taste or tastes you need to supply yourself at this time. After taking foods with that taste, your inner signals will confirm or reject your hypothesis. Flipping back and forth between what makes sense Ayurvedically, and how this gut-level "bio-foodback" compares, you can refine your diet to a high degree. This should help you to eat exactly what you need and even, as a result, to begin to use your food as a kind of medicine. But when instead you neglect to attend to the subtleties of what meshes with your uniqueness, trouble begins to brew in the belly.

MICRO- AND MACRO-ECOLOGIES

Your intestinal tract is the interface between you and the external world—at least that part of the external world you have chosen to ingest. The simplest diagramming of an animal shows it as two not-quite-concentric circles. The outer circle depicts the outer surface of the animal, and the inner circle the digestive tract. The space between the two is the body itself. Our least complex brethren, such as the earthworms, follow this plan with little elaboration, and, crawling through the soil, "surround" a certain portion of it, which passes through them and is converted into "castings" in the process. Something has been extracted from that soil, and something added to it. We interact basically in the same fashion with that part of the outer environment that we have brought inside of us. The part we extract from ingested matter we integrate into the tissues of our being. The rest we get rid of. So that space inside the digestive tract is a sort of way station—temporary housing for building blocks we may or may not end up incorporating into the body.

For that reason, what's inside the gut is a part of you and yet not quite a part of you. It reflects your nature, but it also reflects the larger nature outside you. Like that world outside, it has its own ecological balance of life forms, being populated with a complex assortment of microbes—bacteria, fungi, single-celled animals, and even viruses. These microbes exist in complex relationships that carry over from their lives outside. For example, fungi and bacteria are old rivals; they have been feuding over territory since long before humans showed up on the scene. The fungi, whose numbers include the molds, yeasts, and even mushrooms, long ago learned to secrete a sort of toxin that will kill bacteria or keep them at bay.

We learned to use those fungal toxins, such as penicillin, to eradicate bacteria that had begun to proliferate in the body, but the bacteria are not about to go down without a fight. They have their own tricks. They learned to counter the toxins, becoming "resistant" strains. They even discovered, somewhere along the course of their evolution, to communicate this ability to resist antibiotic toxins to fellow bacterial strains—setting up their own information "underground." The battle between bacteria and fungi continues—among other places in your intestinal tract. Here the fallout from their war can have serious consequences for your health.

We have begun to realize that the web of life on the surface of the planet is intricate and interdependent, and that the removal of one species can disrupt the whole, even resulting in substantial changes in the earth itself, such as erosion, desertification, and major shifts in climate. The same principle applies to the intestinal ecology. Encouraging an overgrowth of fungal forms will displace and disrupt bacterial growth. But bacteria are not merely innocuous bystanders; they are essential to the healthy functioning of the lining of the intestinal tract. Without them, normal processes of digestion and assimilation are crippled. Losing them amounts to losing a component of the lining itself, and the result is irritation and inflammation.

The current assaults on the integrity of our intestinal ecology are many. First, the ideal bacteria for colonizing the gut may be missing in the outside world, having faded away during shifts in bacterial populations caused by toxic environmental chemicals. Their absence already makes the intestinal tract a bit "weak"—often from birth. The replacement of breast milk with infant formulas probably further complicates the process of establishing an optimal population of bacteria.[15]

As we saw earlier, a diet high in sugar encourages an overgrowth of yeast, and the addition of oral antibiotics, sweeping intermittently through the gut, must be like a series of nuclear attacks, devastating populations of bacteria that were trying to maintain themselves there. It's certainly been my clinical impression that the combination of sugar and antibiotics functions as a powerful and destructive juggernaut, blasting through the intestinal tracts of a large percentage of people today and creating havoc.

When the intestine is in such a state of extreme disorder, nothing you eat feels very good. You lose your sense of what "sits right" and what "disagrees." How can you "know in your gut" when your very instrument of knowing is disordered? Making poor choices leads to more disorder, which in turn makes choices even more difficult.

THE LEAKY GUT AND FOOD ALLERGIES

The usual outcome of a disordered intestinal ecology, what many holistic physicians call *dysbiosis,* is an intestinal lining that doesn't work well. It's less able to serve both its main functions—bringing things in that are needed and keeping things out that are not. First, its capacity for absorption and assimilation is decreased. This means you're less able to get from the food the nutrients it contains. Second, its ability to serve as a barrier is lost. A raw, inflamed lining is like a fence with holes in it. Protein molecules that have not been fully digested pass through. Normally, proteins are broken down into their constituent amino acids before they are absorbed. Those components are reassembled to create the structural proteins we need for maintenance and repair in the body.

Intact proteins should be allowed in only when they are "invited," absorbed actively for a purpose.[16] Other proteins that slip through holes in the lining of a leaky gut are targeted as "foreign" and the immune system makes antibodies against them. When that happens with a food protein, it's as if you've been vaccinated against that food. When you eat it, your immune system reacts with a "food allergy"—an immune response. Some of these reactions are to high-protein foods like milk or eggs. Others are to the protein components of grains, vegetables, or fruits.[17] A sensitivity to gluten, the protein of wheat, is very common—probably because we eat so much of it.

Some of these reactions are immediate, like common allergies to shellfish or nuts. Others are more delayed. They may come on as late as a day or two after the food is eaten, and may not manifest as classic allergies with redness, swelling, or rashes, but may show up as stomachaches, fatigue, confusion, or even emotional instability. These delayed reactions involve a different set of antibodies—those based on IGG (immune globulin G) rather than the classic IGE—and have therefore been largely ignored by conventional allergists. In my clinical work, a substantial portion of what is called "chronic fatigue" appears to be related to unrecognized food reactions of this delayed type.

In fact, milder versions of this may be more common than we are accustomed to thinking. I was first struck by the prevalence of food reactions during a dinner meeting of the medical staff at a psychiatric hospital where I was a consultant. We were served a less-than-inspiring institutional-style standard banquet menu, with white bread no doubt "kept fresh" by preservatives and offered with a dish of margarine pats.

The salad was iceberg lettuce accompanied by little foil envelopes of chemicalized oil dressing. The main course was chicken with frozen peas and carrots, followed by a little dessert bowl, in which was a chunk of oily pie crust floating in a sugary syrup and hiding a few pieces of some no-longer-identifiable fruit.

None of this was new to me. I had long bemoaned the quality of the food at this facility. However, what I saw on this night that I had never noticed before was how the physicians and psychologists were reacting to the food. Before we had gotten well into the main course, a number of them were wiping their eyes and blowing their noses. By the time dessert came, you would have thought there was a sudden epidemic of hay fever. "Doesn't anyone see this?" I wanted to yell. "This stuff is killing us!" Of course, it wasn't so much the toxicity of the food additives or even the nutritional deficiencies that had developed from eating so many meals like this that were the immediate causes of the symptoms. It was the intestinal disruption that had allowed us to become sensitized to not only the additives, but even to some of the otherwise useful nutrients remaining in our highly processed food.

Is your sinusitis really a food reaction? Your fatigue? They may well be, but that doesn't mean they are not also related to psychological and emotional factors. Russell Jaffee, a physician whom I came to know in the early seventies when we were both beginning to venture into the uncharted territories of holistic medicine, devised a very reliable test for food sensitivities called the ELISA/ACT.[18] What he stumbled across during his research led him to suspect that the reaction of the immune system to foods may be entangled with memories and associations.

When Russell was establishing normal values for his test results, he grabbed everyone in sight to test. One of his subjects was his secretary, a young woman in good health with no complaints. Yet her test came back with some strongly positive results. Moreover, Russ was struck by the foods ticked off on the report: wheat, bananas, peanuts, and honey. Suddenly it made sense. "Did you ever eat peanut butter and banana sandwiches?" he asked her. She let out a shriek. He shrank back. "What did I say?" he asked apologetically.

"Nothing, nothing." She laughed. "That just made me remember my grandmother. My *grandmother!* Oh God, she was such a *pain.* I had to go live with her for a year when I was eight, and she sent me off to school with peanut butter and banana sandwiches every day! I *hated* them. I still can't face a banana or a peanut butter sandwich."

Food reactions result, I think, from a complex interaction of physiological and psychological triggering experiences. What emerges from all this is a sort of "fingerprint" of sensitivities, intolerances, and cravings that can reveal traces of our history. My own experience certainly confirms this.

By the time I was approaching the twelfth year of my marriage, I was in grim shape. I had developed a constant severe pain in my right neck and shoulder, and my joints were aching and swelling. I was stiff, and without regular and intense hatha yoga, I would lose mobility. I was entering some sort of arthritic state. Along about this time I had a food sensitivity test done. What came back shocked me. Spinach, rice, milk, ginger, these were the staples of my diet—the foods I ate regularly, whether I wanted them or not, because they were "good for you." I had to set an example for the children. And I had to follow my own dietary recommendations that I prescribed in lectures and books. It simply wasn't possible that such foods could be bad for me!

But I looked down at my hand. The joints were swollen and painful, and my fingers held a cup of "tilk"—tea made with milk instead of water and spiced with ginger. Suddenly I realized the potion I sipped constantly was making me sick—and I became aware of a revulsion for it that I must have been sitting on for months or years. I threw it out, knowing I had to stop milk, though it was the backbone of our lactovegetarian diet. My wife was furious.

I had taught her to cook—healthy food, modified Indian-style, lightly spiced, with lots of legumes and plenty of milk—milk added to the cooking vegetables, fresh cheese (paneer), whipped and served on fruit salad, and milk and spinach blended with onion to make a luscious "green soup" that, served with piping hot whole wheat buttermilk biscuits, was our standard supper. It was a wholesome, hearty, and delicious diet. And it was unthinkable without milk.

"It's not a problem," I reassured her. "We can do the soups and breads with soy milk, and I can pass on the paneer." But she wanted no part of it. Running a household with four kids and trying to figure out a different diet for a finicky husband was pushing her beyond her limits. We entered a phase of kitchen warfare. "Here!" she would say angrily, throwing in front of me the special dinner she had struggled to make dairy-free. I would look at it wondering whether to respond to the love it took to try, or the irritability and anger that resulted.

One thing I was clear about. Off the dairy, my joints quit hurting and returned to normal size, my neck pain disappeared, my mind cleared and my energy returned. Back on the dairy—and I tried several times—I collapsed into a painful, lethargic heap.

What was ultimately the most fascinating part of the whole experience was the emerging connection between milk and nurturance. As I dug into the past, I remembered that my mother had not only not nursed me, but, following the fashion of the day, had put me on a cow's-milk formula. Researchers now say that anything a child is given before four months of age—other than mother's milk—he is likely to become sensitized to. The lining of the gut has not matured by that time; it is still "leaky." But my issues with milk went beyond that. I had thrown up the cow's-milk formula, and my mother had had to boil the milk and skim off the top before I could keep it down.

Lurking beneath these apparent conflicts with wife and mother were deeply rooted reservations about accepting nurturance from anyone. Psychologists would term it a problem with trust. Spiritual teachers might see it as holding out for the Infinite. After many years, I found peace when I discovered that in some sense the earth is my real mother and from her I can accept nurturance. In the meantime, getting off the milk and rice and spinach and other "dutiful foods" gave me the energy and clarity to begin to deal with my life differently and to untangle the threads of my deeper feelings and aspirations.

A LOW-TECH APPROACH TO FOOD ALLERGIES

Blood tests and restricted diets are only one mechanical and usually temporary approach to dealing with food intolerances. If you can't shell out hundreds of dollars for the lab work, there are other ways of tackling such a problem. One way to do it is to avoid repeating foods—especially wheat, dairy, and soy—that are common allergens. The typical recommendation is to wait at least four days after eating each food before you have it again. This is called a "four-day rotation diet." Though the principle is sound, I find it can be applied less mechanically and with even better results if you modify the routine according to what you observe.

Still better is to go a step further and engage in what could be called "dietary meditation," in which you regulate what you eat by sharpening your sense of what is right for you. The point is to pay close attention to what your body is asking for. I first understood the power of this technique many years ago when I discovered a tiny book called *One Bowl*. Its author, Don Gerrard, had overcome a serious weight problem by breaking all the rules of dieting.

He simply ate whatever he wanted. In his one little bowl, he would place a small amount of whatever struck his fancy—choosing from a spectrum of healthy options. Arriving at that choice is a process he called "hunting": You tune in carefully to what your inner cues are saying, then sharpen your perceptions until you can see the precise food that will satisfy your inner need. Finding it, you eat it mindfully until you have satisfied that urge. Once you've had enough, you stop. If you're still hungry, you go through the procedure again: *"Now* what do I want?"

Gerrard's approach attains the height of refinement and elegance when he finds the color and aroma of a kidney bean to be exactly what his appetite calls for, eats one of them slowly, with utter delight, and discovers after he finishes, to his amazement, that he is completely fulfilled by that single bean, and really wants no more.

Such an approach turned out to have profound effects for Gerrard, and may be a crucial key for many folks who are struggling with excess weight. Research on obesity shows that people who tend to be overweight respond to external cues—the clock ("It's time to eat!") or the presence of

---

THE "ONE BOWL" APPROACH

1. Get a bowl.

2. Think of what you want.

3. Put a small amount of it in the bowl.

4. Eat very slowly, with full attention and enjoyment.

5. **STOP** when there's an inner satisfaction.

6. Repeat until you're content.

FIGURE 65

DIETARY PRINCIPLE NO. 3

Individualize.

Evaluate in terms of your constitution
(e.g., *vata, pitta, kapha*),
check your gut-level impression, and eat
only what
you really want and
only as much
as you really want.

FIGURE 66

food—but attend poorly to the internal cues that would suggest exactly what and how much they really want. Once you establish for yourself a healthy range of food choices, you can bring into play your inner sense of what appeals to you and what you need. Without that consciousness, even the best food can be counterproductive, and you miss the potential that diet holds for sharpening your awareness of how to live creatively and joyfully.

The second point in our psychotherapeutic approach to food allergies is to "be in your power." Fulfilling activity intensifies the fire at the third chakra, and a strong and focused solar plexus fire burns the food thoroughly, leaving little undigested residue to cause trouble. A vigorous digestion supports a healthy intestinal lining, one that is not "leaky." Not having found the way to express one's inner drive and purpose is at the heart of many if not most of the cases I've seen of food allergy and the intestinal disorder that leads to it. The result is commonly a Gordian knot of hypoglycemia, yeast overgrowth, leaky gut, and food sensitivities. Stella is a good example:

She doesn't seem fifty years old, so hesitant and childlike is her manner. Her face is lacking the lines and battle scars that usually bear witness to a half-century of struggling with this world. Her present concern is a lingering earache. It seems worse from certain foods, and she fits the typical profile of a "food reactor." But then again, it was fine after she went out to dinner with friends, forgot her diet, and ate a number of things that she "shouldn't have." And the night after she went dancing—it felt great!

We agree that she's dealing with a general weakening of her immune system. "There are three basic angles to work from to strengthen the immune system," I explain. "The first is to decrease the burden of immune drains—in your case, clearing the chronic vaginal infections, and the yeast growing in your intestine. The surface of your intestinal lining, because of all the villi and microvilli, if it were to be flattened out completely, would be as large as a football field. Your immune system is faced with producing enough antibodies to keep in check the overgrowth of abnormal microbes across this vast space.

"The second angle is to support immune function with supplements, herbs, and other natural remedies. Let's add Astragalus, *and you may repeat the* Pulsatilla 200C."

The third angle, and probably the most important, was for her to do something spontaneous and self-expressive that could bring her to life. While eating what she shouldn't—probably sugar—was an act of emancipation in some limited way, it would most likely rebound after the physiological effects kicked in. What she really needed was not an adolescent defiance of the good dietary habits she had developed, but an unleashing of her true self on some more fundamental level.

As a chiropractor, she worked long hours and gave all the energy she could muster to her patients. Like many caregivers, she had become so mired down in a routine of dutiful giving she had lost sight of her own needs, her inner spark of creativity. Maybe she needed to go to Hawaii and study traditional Huna medicine, or meditate in the mountains for six months! Or maybe she needed to take dance classes and combine movement with chiropractic—who knows? "Only you can figure out what your direction needs to be, by tuning into your heart or feeling it in your gut—that sense of which way to move next. When you are on your path—doing what you need to do in this life, living through the experiences you came to live through—then you feel a certain joy, a sense of being engagé, *which activates the solar plexus and strengthens the flame there."*

This also affects the immune system. "We might imagine the directors of your immune system saying, 'Okay, we can defend this! Now that you know what you want and you are throwing all your energy into it, we're happy to protect and maintain the integrity of the physical instrument of your intention.' And they might add, by way of explaining past lapses in managing your resistance to disease, 'But don't ask us to defend this body when you're not using it for what's meaningful to you. Our standing orders are: when the will disconnects from the body, recycling microbes should be allowed to dismantle it, break down its components, and return them to the general pool of biological material for other uses.'"

Dietary Principle No. 4. Eat for Clarity

Narrowing your choices to whole, high-quality foods with little sugar, salt, or grease, and tailoring your intake to suit your digestive capacity and constitutional type will create a diet precisely geared to your needs. But even more fine-tuning is possible. We can choose what we eat according to how it affects consciousness. This has little or nothing to do with "nutrients" of the sort that we call vitamins and minerals. Though applying this fourth principle may take into consideration your digestive response, it is not focused on that, either. Rather it is based on judging how the subtle effects of various foods lead to either a clouding or a clearing of your awareness.

Western nutritionists have not explored how food affects one's sense of clarity and balance, though Eastern dietary systems have done so in great depth. In Chinese medicine and nutrition, for example, foods may be classified by their expression of one or more of the Five Elements, here often termed the "Five Phases."[19] Balancing a meal on this basis is almost an art form. For example, a plate with yams (Earth), mustard greens (Fire), seaweed (Water), lentils (Wood), and rice (Metal) would have a balanced effect on consciousness. Adjustments are made for season and weather, as well as for the makeup of the person being fed. But, as we've seen before, keeping five different categories of foods straight in your mind is something of a challenge, so those who follow the philosophies of the Far East have tended to deal with diet most often in the simpler terms of yin and yang, the dichotomy which is a basic organizing concept in Chinese medicine. It is echoed in the Indian Tantric teachings by the left and right breaths, qualities of receptivity and activity, and their relationship to femininity and masculinity. The Chinese, however, have applied this dualistic concept most thoroughly to the matter of what we eat and how it affects us.

When it comes to understanding how food affects consciousness, it's often useful to differentiate between those foods that have a contractive effect and those that are expansive by nature. Contractive foods pull you tighter and make you more compact physically and mentally. Expansive foods do the opposite. Salt, which is contractive, will give you, when taken in excess, a headache that feels like it's pressing inward to a painful point of implosion. Too much sugar, on the other hand, can produce a headache of overexpansion in which the sensation is one of pushing outward in all directions, feeling scattered and confused.

We acknowlege this distinction in a semiconscious way by offering ourselves both sweet and salty snacks—providing the opportunity to select what will maintain balance. Too much fruit and raw food (expansive) leaves you feeling uncentered and produces physical symptoms of bloating and gas. Too much cheese or animal-based food will tend to do the opposite and interfere with your capacity to explore new inner spaces or play with different identities and senses of who you are.

The expansive/contractive differentiation helps us understand one basic aspect of how food affects consciousness. These qualities are often considered yin or yang, but unfortunately different schools of Eastern thought use those terms in exactly opposite ways when referring to the expansive and contractive qualities. Traditional Chinese medicine considers contractivity a yin quality, while macrobiotics, a Japanese Zen school, sees it as yang. With writers on diet coming from both of these schools, the confusion can get pretty thick. I tend to follow the lead of my

---

DIETARY PRINCIPLE NO. 4

**Analyze what you eat in terms of
its effects on consciousness,**
using
tridosha
Five Elements
expansive/contractive
or, best, whether it leaves you feeling
restless/hyper (*tamasic*),
dull/lethargic (*rajasic*), or
energetic/serene
(*sattvic*).

FIGURE 67

friend Annemarie Colbin,[20] who helped me untangle all this, and simply use the terms *expansive* and *contractive* when referring to those qualities, and save the yin and yang for other contexts.

While the expansive or contractive quality of foods, their Five Element attributes, or their tendency to affect *tridosha* are all useful and reflect some of the effects that food has on consciousness, there is an approach more explicitly geared to deal with the subtleties of how consciousness responds to diet. This is a system from the classic philosophic traditions of India. It is based on three categories and is somewhat reminiscent of the *tridosha* system of *vata, pitta,* and *kapha,* though the two are different.[21]

UPPERS AND DOWNERS

Foods and, for that matter, other environmental influences are classified as creating one of two extremes of disturbance—either hyperactivity or lethargy—or as supporting a third and totally distinct state, one of serenity and clarity. The hyperactivating foods act like "uppers," exerting a "speedy" effect, with rapid thoughts and restlessness, much as you might expect from amphetamines or caffeine. In fact, coffee and tea, along with hot, spicy foods and red meat, are the classic items in this category. In the Vedic tradition they were termed *rajasic*—the *raja* was the ruler, the king or prince whose restless preoccupation with the world of objects and ownership led him to conquest and power over it. Such food, though "fit for a king," may be a bit too rich, too seasoned, salted, and sweetened to leave your senses unclouded. It seduces you into overindulgence and leaves you relentlessly seeking more. It's the sort of delicacy of which you might say, "Get this stuff away from me. It's *too* good."

Though meat was one of the foods permitted the *raja,* you can't always expect its effects to be purely *rajasic.* Much of our meat supply is frozen, canned, preserved, or even purposely "cured" to alter its flavor. This means it has undergone some deterioration. Overcooked and over-processed foods, along with those that are fermented or partially spoiled, are the typical lethargy-producing ones. In this schema they are known as *tamasic,* a term that also connotes ignorance and darkness—caught in the heaviness of the material without the lightening effect of awareness. Alcohol fits here, as do the long leftover remains of meals gone by.

This is a principle that I rediscover periodically. Recently pressed for time, I searched through the freezer compartment of my fridge and

FOOD AND CONSCIOUSNESS

	Food	Mind
SERENE/ENERGIZED *(sattvic)*	fresh veggies fresh fruit grains beans dairy(?)	serene aware calm joyful peaceful
RESTLESS/HYPER *(rajasic)*	strong spices coffee/tea red meat raw onions/garlic salt	aggressive contentious controlling worldly workaholic
DULL/LETHARGIC *(tamasic)*	old leftovers fermented preserved, canned, or rancid foods	fatigued confused ignorant abusive addicted

FIGURE 68

fished out a veggie burger of considerable vintage. The only bread I found—good, but again of unknown age—was frozen, too. I made a meal of it, with condiments and unsalted chips, but forgot all about the compromises in quality involved until later in the day when I found myself obsessed with taking a nap. "I don't usually nap during the day," some routine censor in my head commented. "But then again, I don't usually feel so heavy and drained." It was only then that I remembered the mummified burger and the boardlike bread. My mind was in a *tamasic* funk, and it took a twenty-minute snooze to recover my energy and enthusiasm. If you have any doubts about the validity of this principle, I highly recommend you do this experiment for yourself. (I hope I won't need to do so again anytime soon.)

Food that gave up its life long ago has also lost its vibrancy, the subtle energetic quality that nourishes you on a nonphysical level. Since the transfer of the physical components of the tissues of plants and animals to our own has been the exclusive focus of nutritionists and biochemists, how we might be taking up their energy has been largely overlooked. We are only beginning to develop technology that will allow us to tap into this level of what's going on. Perhaps the study of the energetics of food will be the nutritional science of the next millennium.

If so, it will once again confirm and reconnect us with the wisdom of the past. Ancient Asian physicians and spiritual teachers thought of Earth, Water, Fire, Air, and Ether as the Elements from which the life forms of the planet were composed. You might think of your assimilation of food as a process of sifting through it, gleaning the subtler Elements to "nourish" and sustain the higher vibration of your consciousness, using some portion of the grosser Elements to bolster your physical existence, and, finally, discarding the excess of these grosser Elements, as feces, urine, etc.[22] That denser part is "sacrificed" in order for you to be able to amass the quantitiy of subtle energy necessary to create and sustain human consciousness.

But what happens when what you take in are predominately the grosser Elements—when the subtler Elements have already dissipated? The obvious answer would be that you feel "heavy," lethargic, *tamasic*. Frozen food (especially when frozen a long time ago), canned food, packaged cookies and cakes—these will lose their vibrancy. Even with sugar and stimulants added—like salt or spices or caffeine—you will not feel the enlivening effect you might get from fresh, vibrant foods. And your consciousness is affected accordingly.

HOW TO BE ENERGETIC *AND* CALM

The third category of food and the consciousness that corresponds to it embody this quality of vibrancy and subtle aliveness. What's unique about this concept is that it is not based on a simple polarity. You can't put the hyperactivating foods and beverages on one side, the lethargy-producing ones on the other, and attain this third state by mixing equal quantities of the two. For example, you can't get there by eating frozen, dead food and following it with a cup of coffee. You may be able in that way to produce a certain moderate level of activity, but you won't create the clarity of consciousness and the serenity that are the hallmarks of this third state and that are supported by simple, fresh, live foods.

If your attention is fixed solely on how active you can be, having a heavy, *tamasic* meal and following it with a stimulant drink may look like it's working just fine. You may also use tranquilizers or sedatives or alcohol as the downer, rather than a deadening food. Uppers can include substances that range from from coffee to cocaine. You may think all you need to do is find the right proportions of the two, but what you lose in the equation is clarity of consciousness. Without it, you may not see what's going on clearly enough to notice that you're missing it! Then you get stuck in a repetitious cycle of hyperactivity and fatigue that you keep trying to manage by juggling the balance of uppers and downers in your life.

The masters of meditation who developed this system[23] were focused on charting the inner world, learning to move freely there, and staking out new realms of consciousness. They were less interested in the ability to be active in the outside world, valuing clarity and equanimity over either *tamasic* escape or *rajasic* conquest—no matter how attractive or successful they might look on the surface. The foods that supported their inner search, that were most likely to encourage calm clarity and a relaxed but super-alert state, were called *sattvic*—the root *sat* referring to truth or wisdom. We're interested in the *sattvic* state because it facilitates the discoveries and insights necessary for healing.

The foods considered *sattvic* were fresh fruits, vegetables, rice, beans, nuts, and seeds—and milk from healthy, contented animals. Whether such foods lead to a clear, alert, *sattvic* state of consciousness will depend on whether you select and take them in the proper proportion for your current needs. Even the most ideal foodstuffs must be put through the filter of your constitutional type and requirements of the moment. When that's done, and the food meshes perfectly with the state of your being, an electrifying resonance occurs that energizes and awakens. This resonance is similar to that which occurs between the informational pattern of an herbal remedy and the organizational structure of the person who needs it. When the congruence or resonance between the two is corrective, we think of the substance as medicinal, and call it a remedy. When it's supportive and sustaining, we think of it as nutritional, and call it a food.

Many of the substances we ingest don't fall solely into one category. They may be primarily nourishing and have a minor remedial effect, or vice versa. Either way, cooking with natural foods is therapeutic. There's an old Chinese saying: "I don't need a doctor, I just need a good cook." In the Ayurvedic school where I studied, I was given a list of one hundred plants that were both food and medicine. Food preparation takes on new significance in light of the principle that food is medicine. Preparing food can no longer be considered a menial chore or even merely an act of love.

It is a method for cultivating and shaping the consciousness of the people you feed. Food preparation is art, medicine, and science all rolled into one.

It may be helpful to stop for a moment and notice how far we have come from talking about the chemistry of protein, vitamins, and fiber. You are now engaged in an approach to diet that enlists input from all aspects of your being—your intellect, your intuition, and your gut-level responses. Calculating grams of protein and structuring meals to support the biochemistry of the brain may be one useful angle on this complex thing we call nutrition, and it may be one step toward lifting you to a "zone" of clarity and energy, but it cannot be more than one small part of the puzzle. If you get some mileage out of it, great, but explore other perspectives, too.

Dietary Principle No. 5. Listen to the Poetry

Limit your selection of foods to those that are whole and wholesome; pass up salt, sugar, and grease. Learn what your constitutional type might be, and listen to what your gut tells you when you attempt to satisfy your type's needs. Finally, learn to watch which foods contribute to a clarity of mind and a sense of equanimity. If you observe these principles, even a bit, then your food choices will most often be just what you need. When they're not, you will have sharpened your awareness so much that you will be able to learn something useful from any lapses that occur.

And this is where the fun begins. The accurate application of the first four principles will give you energy, alertness, and a sense of well-being in your body. The times when you fail will give you glimpses of the other side of yourself—the part that needs to be uncovered, accepted, and outgrown. With the strength that comes from even partial success in refining your eating habits, you can tackle this other self. "Slips" and "mistakes" will eloquently reveal that less evolved you. In fact, they will portray it with a poetic flair that can be quite entertaining. All you have to do is listen to the poetry. Here's an example:

I was going to make a scrumptious meal. Usually I set about such work more tentatively, asking my body what it wants and choosing from what is available with deliberate slowness. But this was different—I already had a clear picture of it. In fact, I had eaten it a few days before—it was a vegetable stew with kabocha squash, onions,

DIETARY PRINCIPLE NO. 5

Celebrate your "errors."

Departures from the sensible
are grist for the mill—
"food language" expressions of issues
to be addressed/resolved.
Allow inner promptings to manifest
and
listen to the poetry!

FIGURE 69

celery, and carrot. I had invented it as I went, prepared it fresh, eaten it immediately, and was so energized from it that I felt almost stoned. I'd gone into the living room, stretched out, and simply luxuriated in the vibrancy I was experiencing. And I couldn't wait to repeat the performance! I wanted to feel that way again.

Recalling what I had done, I re-created the original masterpiece with reasonable accuracy. But somehow it didn't look quite as exciting. Nevertheless, I ate it with anticipation, waiting for the surge of vitality I was sure would follow. But it didn't. In fact, all I got was a slightly upset stomach. Then it hit me: I'd tried to recapture what was wonderful in the past, rather than creating what was right for the present.

How many times had I watched myself take a second serving of that delicious whatever, only to be utterly astonished that it didn't taste as good as the first (when it had been just what my body needed), and stubbornly push on to have a *third,* sure that I could re-create the pleasure of that initial plateful. Of course, I'm not the only person to make this common human error. We do the same thing with relationships, with work, and on pretty much every front of our lives—we try to recapture the fulfillment of the past, and in the process we miss out on the possibilities of the present. When the games I play with my kids are repetitions of those we've done before, there's something dead about them. When the way I touch my lover is routine instead of exploratory, some sense of aliveness evaporates.

Seeing this principle expressed in how my food tasted and how it felt inside me in *this moment* was a living allegory for a theme of my life that I needed to grasp more clearly. Eating habits are one of the most obvious places where "core issues" are displayed. Several times a day we enact our inner conflicts on this stage. Just as different features of the tongue express physical health, aspects of eating behavior reflect character. Of course, our core issues are also evident in other areas of our lives, such as relationships and intimacy. If my sexuality makes my emotional issues too painfully obvious, however, I can always shut it down. But chances are I will eat regularly and pretty much without fail.

Attending to the poetry that your food behavior expresses will tell you many things about yourself—how you nourish yourself on other levels besides the physical, for starters. If you find yourself constantly reaching for trashy snacks, do you also obsessively gobble up televised "junk food for the mind"? If you've struggled to curb erratic, random eating, watch to see if the tendency shifts to expression on the mental level, as careless consumption of whatever's close at hand: an article in a supermarket tabloid as you stand at the checkout counter, a television soap opera you don't bother to turn off during lunch, or pop music with trash lyrics on the car radio.

If you gravitate toward *vatic* food—dry chips and cold salads that make you spin out into intestinal storms and twitchy limbs—do you also seek out the cacophonous "high" of heavy-metal rock and strobe lights? Or do you counter your *vatic* tendency by deliberately nurturing yourself with calming, grounding thoughts? And how do you nourish yourself energetically? Do you soak up the angry vibrations of the argument going on in the hallway at the office, or have you become conscious enough of what you take in to say "No thank you," when that particular platter is passed? Do you feed yourself energetically on a regular basis with intentional hugs and random acts of kindness? Or do you neglect to "eat" on that level, and suffer energetic exhaustion and emotional emaciation?

A major step on the journey of healing is to become conscious of how you accept and use the nurturing bounty that nature and the web of life extends to you. If you open yourself to that wellspring of sustenance, joyfully and yet with discrimination, you will thrive, mentally, emotionally, and physically. If you close yourself off or indulge carelessly in what doesn't feed your body and soul, you will fall ill.

Perhaps the ultimate payoff in studying the subject of nutrition comes when we begin to hear the poetic message proclaimed by each of the ways

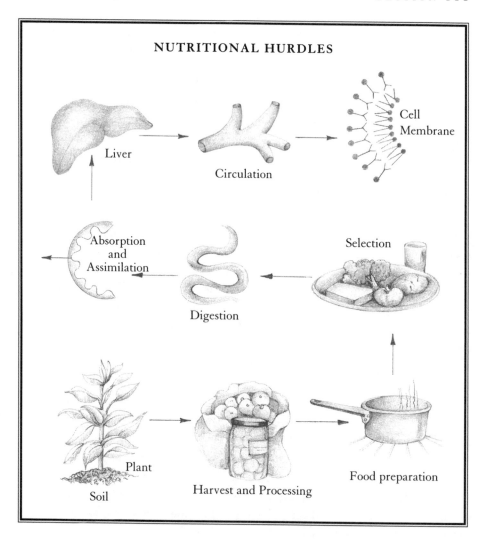

NUTRITIONAL HURDLES

FIGURE 70

we use to cut ourselves off from the abundance of the earth. (See Fig. 70.) Our commercial exploitation of farmlands—using chemical fertilizers and leaving depleted, eroded soils—expresses our parallel exploitation of the nurturing intent of the feminine principle. Our disdain for the loving art of cooking betrays our loss of a sense of what a joy it is to cultivate the unfoldment of another being. Our selection in the cafeteria line of the greasy, the sugary, and the fake reveals our inattention to how we choose the experiences we want from life. Our weakness of digestion shows our lack of empowerment, our waning sense of being able to harness inner strength to transform what we incorporate from the world in order to ful-fill our creative mission. Our inability to take into the cell what we did manage to bring to the bloodstream bespeaks our crippling belief that we do not deserve to be free, radiant, powerful beings.

The subject of nutrition is full of potential for those who wish to study it from a truly holistic point of view and to plumb the depths of its complexity and of its eloquent symbolism. Working with diet goes far beyond merely counting milligrams of vitamins or grams of protein, beyond maintaining physical health or healing disease. It can be a trans-formative practice. But even when you nourish yourself in the most enlightened way, you will make mistakes. There will be times—in fact, there *need* to be times—when you choose to take in something you can't—or don't really want to—incorporate into your being. That *stuff,* be it physical, energetic, or mental, must be got rid of, yet our under-standing of how to do so is sadly deficient. In the next chapter we will look at the matter of cleansing from a holistic perspective, and see how releasing the residues of your past so that you can move freely into a new way of being is another foundation stone in the work of healing.

8

Detox:
A Lighter and Clearer You

"*I can't eat grains,*" *Sharon says.* "*One bowl of granola and I'm out. People think I'm crazy. 'Granola! That's health-food stuff—you can't be serious.' But it's true. It just messes me up. One bagel and my intestinal tract is off for three or four days. I just can't do it.*"

I was grasping yet again how crucially important it is to listen to your body and respect its unique needs. Sharon managed to see this clearly when most of us just keep on refusing to believe it possible that a single bagel or something as wholesome as a bowl of granola could cause a problem—certainly not a serious one. Yet she listened to the signals and stopped. I wondered why.

Then I remembered that ten years ago Sharon had been in a wheelchair with multiple sclerosis. Determined not to fulfill the grim prognoses offered her by her medical doctors, she took matters in her own hands, watched carefully everything that affected her, and decided to stop eating anything that made her feel heavy and numb. Initially this meant eating nothing at all—and gradually feeling her way toward what she could handle. Now here she was, nearly forty, strikingly attractive, looking vibrantly healthy and frequently being mistaken for someone half her age! "Why?" I wondered again, this time out loud.

"*Because I had that experience,*" *she said,* "*of fasting and feeling so wonderful—so clear and so alert and energized! I know what it does. When I'm clean inside, I feel wonderful. I can look twenty years old on those days.*"

I was reminded of a spring day when I had stopped by the motor pool at the Himalayan Institute. The maintenance man, a feisty old exprospector, was arranging his fleet of lawn equipment in neat rows, ready for the summer mowing. I marveled at how old some of the machines were. He turned his well-wrinkled but lively face toward me and gave me an amused smile. "Machinery doesn't break down because it's old," he said. "It breaks down because of dirt that collects inside. That's what wears out the moving parts and ruins it. If you keep it clean, it will last almost *forever!*"

Indeed, my training in Ayurvedic rejuvenation had always stressed the central role of cleansing techniques. When Swami Rama would return from one of his intermittent retreats, during which he fasted and cleared his mind with long periods of meditation, close students would whisper that much of the gray had gone from his hair and that his face was that of a man several years younger. If cleansing is really the secret to vibrant health and turning back the clock, then it deserves more than passing attention. You need to know what you must clean out, and where it comes from. Then you need to know the details of how to do the cleaning.

As it turns out, there are two major sources of "stuff" that obstructs—one from outside us and one from inside. In this chapter you'll get some perspective on the ones from outside, called environmental pollutants, and the immediate threat they pose to your health. You'll also come to understand more about the ones from inside, for which we have no name yet. Then you'll see exactly how these various accumulations give rise to disease, and finally learn some of the many time-honored techniques for clearing them out. You may be surprised by what a powerful tool this can be for reversing and preventing disease, or for simply rejuvenating and revitalizing yourself.

Environmental Pollution

"How do you spell that?" the patient asked, frowning. I had just informed him that his blood test showed a strong immune reaction to *phthalates.* These are a family of chemicals used in products ranging from cosmetics and construction materials to plastic food packaging. Their use is not restricted, even though it was found that "shock lung," a condition that killed many soldiers in Vietnam, was caused by the phthalates in blood storage bags. More than a billion pounds a year are produced in the United States and poured into our environment.

If that sounds like a lot and you suspect it's an exaggeration, think again. It is, in fact, only a tiny portion of the chemicals produced in the

United States. In 1992 the total amount of carbon-based chemicals made in this country was in excess of 435 billion pounds. That's 1,600 pounds per person. And the problem is not limited to highly industrialized countries. There are now approximately 100,000 synthetic chemicals on the market worldwide, and each year another thousand *new* ones are introduced. Safety data exists for only a handful of these.[1]

Thirty-five percent of food tested in the United States has been found to have detectable pesticide residues, and tests pick up only about one-third of the roughly six hundred pesticides in use here. Contamination in less industrialized countries is even higher, since laws there are less restrictive. In 1991, the United States exported more than 4 million pounds of pesticides that are no longer used here, including nearly 200,000 pounds of the long-banned DDT. Though a great deal of ballyhoo has accompanied the removal from production of a few high-profile chemicals, thousands more such chemicals continue to be produced at ever-increasing rates.

Our food and water are also contaminated by heavy metals such as cadmium, lead, and mercury. These metals, formerly buried in the depths of the earth, continue to be mined and dispersed in the biosphere, where their concentrations build up. Despite more than a century of denial by dentists, the mercury in dental amalgam is a matter of growing concern, and several progressive countries have banned its use. Although elemental mercury, the "quicksilver" of thermometers used in dental fillings, is relatively inert and nontoxic, bacteria can convert this simple mercury to highly toxic compounds such as methyl mercury.[2] We discovered the toxicity of mercury compounds a century ago, when workers using them to block hats became agitated and confused—a picture caricatured by the Mad Hatter of Alice's Wonderland.

Though the human system is very resilient and can tolerate a great deal of environmental stress, it has limits. Running parallel to this disruption of the environment with man-made chemicals and unearthed toxic metals is the loss of natural elements from the soil and the food supply. The result is double trouble. For example, the complex system of enzymes, which nudges metabolic reactions along so that they move fast enough to sustain life, is disabled. Enzyme molecules are dealt a one-two punch to their vital center by a combination of trace-element deficiencies and heavy-metal contamination. Each enzyme depends on an atom of some specific mineral to provide its "spark plug." This is installed at the active site of the enzyme megamolecule, where the compounds it acts on are formed or decoupled. If the trace elements are in short supply, this critical site may not be filled. What's more, an atom of a toxic metal can fill this position, displacing the needed mineral, and yet not fulfilling its function.[3]

Though our general understanding of such mechanisms is growing, little headway has been made in studying the intricacies of how these principles apply to the actions of specific chemicals in specific diseases. Nevertheless, it is interesting to note that toxicologists describe the earliest symptoms of chronic poisoning as follows:

- recurrent fatigue and general lack of energy
- digestive complaints
- muscle weakness
- inability to concentrate

To most practitioners, this list will sound quite familiar. These are among the most common complaints of the majority of patients I see. What role environmental toxins are playing in the problems from which we suffer today remains a gnawing question. Untangling this biochemical/pollution knot could occupy a whole generation of medical scientists unless some thorough and immediate solution is found for the problem of our widespread toxic disruption of the environment. I do not mean to imply that this solution has to be purely political or social. I often find it necessary to remind myself and my patients that although each of us may have relatively little leverage as far as the environment in general goes, we do have some control over what we expose ourselves to. A famous photo of banner-bearing demonstrators in the sixties says it best: their message reads "Stop Air Pollution," and the leader of the group has a cigarette dangling from his lips.

The one disease where chemical pollutants have received lots of attention is cancer. Here the links between exposure to toxic substances and the development of the disease have become increasingly clear. Now many researchers are saying that two-thirds of the causative factors in breast cancer are environmental, most of those factors being toxic pollution. In fact, cancer has become our "index" for serious levels of chemical toxins. In places where dangerous industrial wastes have been dumped, such as the infamous Love Canal, near Niagara Falls, it was the growing incidence of malignant conditions, especially leukemia, that flagged the areas of highest contamination. Tests for the safety of a food additive often focus on whether it is carcinogenic, or cancer-causing. In fact, we have come to operate from an unspoken assumption that if it doesn't cause cancer, it's safe.

ENDOCRINE DISRUPTORS

We may be wrong, according to a burst of new research. It indicates that chemicals, including many that we have heretofore considered relatively harmless, can cause serious disorders at concentrations far below what is necessary to cause cancer. In other words, the amount of pollution we can tolerate is a lot less than we thought. A recent book, carefully researched and highly acclaimed, *Our Stolen Future,* by Theo Colborn, Dianne Dumanoski, and John Peterson Myers, redefines the subject of toxic pollution. While they may not cause cancer, toxins at levels we thought insignificant can play havoc with our hormones. As a result, they may assume a causal role in a wide variety of disorders from ADD to sterility. Endocrine systems disabled during fetal development, for example, are seriously undermining fertility rates and may actually threaten our future capacity to reproduce.

Carcinogenic chemicals tend to do their dirty work at concentrations in the range of parts per million, though some of the most potent ones might cause disease in the parts-per-billion range. But the endocrine system functions on the basis of much less. Hormones are active at levels of parts per *trillion.* That's an incredibly minuscule amount. The authors of *Our Stolen Future* explain it this way: if you put "a drop of gin in a train of tank cars full of tonic, one drop in 660 tank cars would be one part in a trillion; such a train would be six miles long." Such a tiny amount would seem inconsequential. Yet chemicals that find their way into your body at concentrations this low can displace your hormones and disrupt their normal actions.

Researchers have identified more than fifty synthetic chemicals and *families* of chemicals, many of them widely dispersed in the environment, that disrupt the endocrine system in one way or another. A number of these mimic estrogen. This includes persistent residues of DDT and chemicals like dioxin and PCBs. It also apparently includes tiny amounts of compounds that leach from plastic containers into our food and water. If such chemicals can act as estrogen in our bodies, they can not only change how our metabolism works, but also affect our emotions and behavior.

When I first learned of this, I had not seen this data and I was skeptical. I had come with my eldest son and his mother to talk about his school problems with Dr. John Diamond. John, a brilliant maverick and innovator in the field of holistic psychiatry, felt that the crux of Sky's problem was the conflict between his mother and me—the same difficulties that had caused our marriage to founder.

Chief among those difficulties had been an unfortunate combination of my depression and her irritability. He explained that this is a common problem, one he saw as rooted in the impact that estrogen-mimicking pollutants are having on our endocrine systems. To demonstrate his point, he put a drop of progesterone oil under each of our tongues. In the female, progesterone counters excess estrogenic substances and brings a sense of relaxation and tranquility. In the male it is converted to testosterone. I was busily discounting his theories when he asked me to notice how the quality of my voice had changed, becoming stronger, and how the coloring in my face had brightened. He was right.

HORMONE REPLACEMENT TO COUNTER CHEMICAL TOXINS

Our response to hormones is very rapid—especially when they are taken sublingually. I have no trouble remembering to take my tiny drop of progesterone oil daily, for if I don't, I begin to "wilt." Minutes after I put it in my mouth, I have a remarkable increase in energy and stamina. John maintained that pollutants with estrogenlike activity have affected both men and women in ways that make relationships between them more difficult. Women become more irritable and angry, while in men the estrogen-mimicking chemicals undercut testosterone's action and cause weakness and depression.

Among the hormone-disrupting pollutants, the estrogenic chemicals have been most intensely studied because of concern about the growing incidence of sterility in males—sperm counts have been dropping at an average rate of approximately 1 percent per year over the last five decades.[4] They are now half what they were in the mid-1940s. If this trend continues, only a small number of men will be able to father children twenty years from now. But this may be only the tip of the iceberg. There is evidence that there are also pollutants that disrupt thyroid hormones. Holistic practitioners have been insisting for decades that there is an epidemic of thyroid weakness. Broda Barnes, M.D., whose followers continue to pursue his work, wrote in 1976 that the high incidence of heart attacks was related to hypothyroidism.

In my clinical work I monitor metabolic rate—what I consider the best index of thyroid status—by using Dr. Barnes's simple, low-tech test: Each morning before you get up, take your temperature. Dr. Barnes preferred doing it under the arm, but an oral temperature will do. If it runs more than a degree below normal (98.6 orally or 97.6 axillary), then you probably have a functional hypothyroidism. Blood tests are not, I think, very accurate, because they often show normal levels while patients complain of the fatigue, hair loss, and raspy voice that are classical symptoms of low thyroid function. I puzzled over this for years, and now suspect that it may be because, even though the thyroid is producing enough of the hormone to bring blood levels up to normal, chemical disrupters are interfering with the proper use of it. Though iodine seems to help some, and many people find taking small doses of thyroid glandular extracts[5] helpful, avoiding the pollutants responsible and clearing the body of those which have accumulated may well turn out to be the most useful approach.

How much we will find that toxic chemicals disrupt and disable other hormonal systems remains to be seen. I can't help wondering if that's what's behind "hot items" like DHEA. Dehydroepiandrosterone, or DHEA, is a steroid hormone secreted by the adrenal gland. Present in concentrations a thousand times that of other hormones in the same family such as estrogen, testosterone, and cortisone, it seems to act as a sort of pool from which they can be produced. But it's not merely a precursor or intermediate in their production. It appears to have many of its own effects, too.

Though research on DHEA is relatively recent, it's thought to increase fat metabolism, decrease stress, enhance immune function, and prevent osteoporosis by improving calcium absorption. Its anti-aging effects remain controversial, but it is known that DHEA levels often drop with age, especially in those persons who show the most deterioration with the advancing years. It's my guess that slowing DHEA production is a way of expressing our conviction that aging is due, and that sinking levels are often an expression of a waning desire to participate in life.

If that's true, then taking the hormone would be contradicting what your autonomic nervous system has instructed your hormones to do. In that case, our struggle with aging would be another example of how we fight ourselves: We hate to grow old, yet our belief systems are so organized around the assumption that debility and deterioration are inevitable that we implement them on a level that never reaches the point of being a conscious decision.

Another possibility is that chemical interference cripples the action of DHEA in the same way it has been shown to overwhelm progesterone/testosterone and displace thyroid hormone. If that's true, taking DHEA would be a logical step.

Even if falling levels of DHEA are caused more by psychological factors than by pollution, and even if the supplement is undoing what you are unconsciously doing to yourself, it could still be a useful way to "buy time"—time to unravel some of the self-defeating belief systems that might have prompted you to program yourself to age. The time you buy for deeper work in this way is less "expensive" than what is bought with drugs like antibiotics and chemicals that are foreign to your metabolism. Here you are only bolstering a normal internal secretion. While purists may object—and often with good reason—to hormone replacement therapy of this sort, its use may be practical at times.

I personally found that my body and mind functioned better on a very small dose of DHEA—5 mg, five days a week. More seemed to overstimulate me in a way that I found irritating, and less left me with skin that was losing its resilience and a memory that wasn't quite as sharp as I needed to write and teach. So I have, with trepidation, entered the world of the "hormone enhanced." Should you? That remains, I think, a very personal question. The safest approach to DHEA is to have levels measured, and if they are low, take gradually increasing doses until they normalize. At this point, however, there is no evidence that small amounts are harmful, so if you are feeling a loss of vitality and symptoms of premature aging, you might try it and see how it works for you.

MELATONIN AND SLEEP

By the time I had decided to experiment personally with DHEA, I had already become a melatonin devotee. I noticed, as I approached my mid-fifties, that my sleep was not as sound or as refreshing as it had been in the past. So I tried a small amount of melatonin. It worked. On 2.5 mg—half a tablet of the lowest sublingual dosage I could find—I slept better. What's more, my memory improved noticeably, as did my digestion. There was only one problem: it wore off at about 3:00 A.M., and I sat up, wide awake. This little snag yielded to the "sustained release" version,

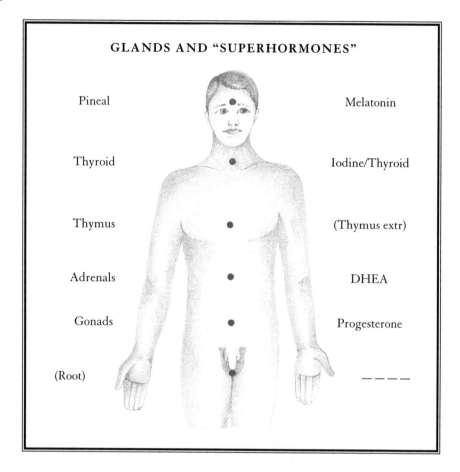

GLANDS AND "SUPERHORMONES"

Pineal	Melatonin
Thyroid	Iodine/Thyroid
Thymus	(Thymus extr)
Adrenals	DHEA
Gonads	Progesterone
(Root)	————

FIGURE 71

and I now take 2 mg of that preparation nightly. Even my kids borrow one occasionally to combat jet lag, or to restore their sleep patterns when they need to get back on schedule after having slept till noon over the weekend or during vacation.

By now we have set up a nearly complete program for endocrine support that covers the whole spectrum of hormonal functions. Since each of the glands is the physiologic aspect of a chakra, we might conceptualize the use of the supplements accordingly (see Fig. 71). That points up the psychological effects that follow from their physiologic action. Progesterone tones the gonads and helps deal with the energies of the sexual sphere at the second chakra. DHEA relates to the adrenals at the third chakra, with its issues of mastery and assertion. Iodine or thyroid glandular preparations enable the fifth chakra's challenges, which have to do

---

MINIMIZING HORMONE DISRUPTION

- Avoid animal fats.

- Use organic foods when possible.

- Minimize contact between plastic and food.

- Don't use pesticides in home or garden.

- Keep foods and beverages covered to avoid dust.

- If unsure about your water, consider investing in a home distiller.

FIGURE 72

with creativity and expression, to be met, and melatonin, which is a pineal hormone, gives aid in the area of our relation to the "unseen"—the sphere of sleep and of connection with other dimensions of our existence. This is the aspect of consciousness that spiritual traditions associate with the "third eye"—the point between the eyebrows, or sixth chakra.[6]

All we missed in our endocrine/chakra sweep was the fourth or heart center. The closest gland to this is the thymus. Its intricate network of hormonelike activators and inhibitors serves to coordinate the complex and far-flung components of the immune system. In view of the pattern that has been emerging here with other glands, we would be justified in wondering whether chemical disrupters might be hampering the function of the thymus, too. That might be another piece in the puzzle of immune weakness which plays such an important role in so many of the diseases confronting us currently.

And Then There's "The Stuff from Inside"

In my work, I found a strategy that yielded fascinating results—one that many other workers in the field of holistic medicine have also discovered. It consists of searching out a principle or a technique from the traditional teachings of an ancient and successful culture, working with the technique personally to experience what it does, and then going to the scientific research literature to find the theory and research that corresponds to it—that will back it up from a more modern, reductionistic point of view. Finally, when fully convinced and comfortable with what I've learned, I begin to prescribe it for my patients. Most of the concepts and approaches presented in this book took shape in that way. Once I've validated the effectiveness of a given technique experientially, the correspondences and confirmations almost always turn up.

But what we're going to talk about now has been an exception. For years I've been exploring traditional teachings on the buildup of matter in the body and cleansing. I've been doing the nasal wash, swallowing cloths to clean my stomach lining, seeing amazing results in myself and even venturing to offer some of the approaches to patients. But I have found very little corroborating work in the medical world. There seems to be a huge void in the literature where I should find mention of the accumulation of waste in the body. The closest thing I ever found was a thread of disdainful references to "the now discounted notion of auto-intoxication."

In the late 1970s, when I was researching intestinal physiology for my book *Diet and Nutrition,* I came across writings from a half-century before on how drastically a stagnant colon could affect one's health. Semitoxic by-products of the microbes growing in "putrifying" wastes were identified, and the idea that they could enter the bloodstream so that you "intoxicated yourself" led to a wave of dismay that swept through a concerned public. "Health reformers," as they were called in those days, seized on this alarm to push programs of better diet, exercise, and bowel cleansing.

It all made sense to me, even if it seemed a bit blown out of perspective. But where had it gone? The idea and its followers had disappeared from the conventional medical literature, almost without a trace. Curious, I began to phone medical school professors, experts on intestinal physiology and gastroenterology, to inquire. "Oh, that!" I heard. "That was discredited a long time ago." "How so?" I asked. I could tell by the vagueness of the answers I got to this question that my respondents hadn't given the matter much thought. It was an idea that had been dismissed in their training as absurd, so they had stepped around it, unwilling to take it seriously and run the risk of jeopardizing their own credibility.

On further probing, I discovered that the idea had been dropped after the publication of an experiment that involved stuffing the lower bowel with an inert material or inflating it with a balloon. Each produced a feeling of discomfort much like that of constipation. This was quoted thereafter as evidence that auto-intoxication was a myth. Though this simple experiment did not even address the question of whether toxic by-products from abnormal microbes might poison the body, it seemed to have served as a convenient pretext for brushing off the whole issue.

The fact is that we have a cultural bias against poking around too much inside ourselves. It's the surface of our bodies that we hold to high standards of cleanliness. What's "in there," we often seem to feel, is better left alone. When I taught a session on yogic cleansing in India, the class consisted of both American and Indian students. Standing in a row, early one morning, we were drinking salt water and throwing it up. This "stomach wash" is designed to remove the excess *kapha* that collects there during the night, so there was lots of stringy mucus coming up from some folks' tummies.

Though my Indian participants were sanguine about the whole thing, the Americans were repulsed. "Yuk!" one lady said with a grimace. "That is *disgusting!* I don't think I'll ever do *that* again!" "Why," wondered her Indian counterpart out loud, "would you want to keep it inside if it's so awful?" Perhaps it's because of our Westerm aversion to this inner mess that our modern scientific research paradigm is not designed to look at the question of what's there that shouldn't be, and how it affects us.

Our microscopes and chemical assays are geared to focus on and measure a chosen target substance. We go in to look for something, and when we find it, we quantify it. We're not well equipped to simply see what's there. You hear, "They sent the drink to the lab for analysis," and think, "Aha, now they will find out whether it was poisoned." In a play or a movie they might, but in real life it's not that easy. If a lab technician is told to look for a specific poisonous substance, he can test for its presence, and state-of-the-art equipment may be able to test for scores of different substances. But it's a limitation of our focused, reductionistic approach that we have no way to look without preconceptions, to explore in an open-ended, curious way.

This allows us to miss what we don't want to see. One of the things we don't want to see is the physiologic clutter that has resulted from our common tendency to overeat and to undereliminate. I suspect there are many times when we blame a sluggish metabolism on an absence of essential nutrients, when that's not what's wrong at all. We take more vitamins or minerals, thinking they'll help, but they don't. The real problem is not what's missing, but what's there that *shouldn't* be—the obstruction of the cellular environment with accumulated molecules that serve no purpose, and which overburdened systems of elimination have been unable to throw off.

AAMA

Though this accumulation of molecular clutter in the tissues is a situation our medical science has overlooked, it did not escape the notice of Ayurvedic physicians, who were closely attuned to the presence of burdensome excesses in the body. Perhaps that's because they were operating in the context of a culture that put a high premium on simplicity and on freeing oneself from attachment to the material things of the world; or perhaps it was because the method used by the developers of Ayurvedic medicine was to look inside themselves, opening up a different realm of information.

When I was a postgraduate fellow at an Ayurvedic medical college in north India, my preceptor, who was also the president of the college, paid me a compliment. "You are learning Ayurveda in the way it's supposed to be learned," he commented. "You are making your body a laboratory. I wish I could get my faculty to do that." He looked wistful. He was a student of meditation, and lived the introspective approach—thinking of Ayurvedic research as based on the use of a highly refined and sharpened sensitivity to what was going on in one's own mind and body. His professors didn't share this enthusiasm for the traditional "sister sciences" of Ayurveda such as yoga and meditation; they were more interested in making their field appear "scientific" in the modern, Western sense of the word.

The introspective methodology may miss some of the things the "looking from the outside" instruments of technological science manage to pick up, but it also may catch much of what those instruments don't. Of course the two approaches are not mutually exclusive. As my teacher knew, they can be quite complementary, the introspection providing us with valuable hypotheses and the scientific methodology of the laboratory giving us a place to confirm them.

In any event, Ayurveda does have a term for the stuff that clogs us: it calls this *aama*.[7] (The first vowel is long, as in *a*rm—the second, barely vocalized, as in *across*.) It's internal gunk, most often the residue of incompletely assimilated food. Sometimes it's spoken of as *aamdosh,* a sort of stepchild fourth *dosha* after *vata, pitta,* and *kapha,* since if it's present to a sufficient degree, it may play a role in the development of disease that is on a par with the other three. Overprocessed or partially deteriorated food, such as that which has sat too long—that which we have called *tamasic*—contributes to the formation of this gunk or *aama.* A great deal of such food is not usable, its nutritional value lost as the molecules are altered during its processing or degradation. What can't be used often remains in the body, however, and can "gum up the works." That leaves you feeling dull and tired, with bad breath, indigestion, and a coated tongue. Much of Ayurveda is organized around how to recognize when *aama* is there, and how to remove it when it's found.

Aama is produced in two ways: the first is by taking in what is of poor quality, such as *tamasic* food; the second is by incomplete digestion of that which is of good quality and potentially healthful, but which your system fails to assimilate properly. If, in the early stages of the process of incorporating the food into your being, the developing merger breaks down, the food becomes *aama.* This incompletely digested food may be treated as an antigen—a foreign substance—and targeted by your immune system.[8] If so, antibodies are built to attack it, and the merging of the antigen molecules with the large antibodies attacking them swells the mass of substance that can lodge in tissues and obstruct normal functioning. The symptoms of the diseases we consider autoimmune are based mostly on the accumulation of such antigen/antibody complexes, produced when the immune system attacks body tissues.[9] From an Ayurvedic point of view, it's *aama* that collects in the joints and makes them stiff and painful in arthritis.

Why we would attack our own tissues, or food that is potentially useful, is a question that may be answerable only by looking at what is going on at a level other than the physical. As in the case of Dr. Jaffee's secretary (whose bad memories of Grandma and her sandwiches showed up in an immune reaction to peanut butter, bananas, and bread), to find where such responses originate, we must sometimes probe the mind, and often the part of it that operates outside our usual awareness. But here we fall into another circular dilemma like that which we encountered in talking about diet. If your diet is deficient, you may not be able to think clearly enough to see what the problem is. If your system is clogged with *aama,* its circuits don't fire as well, and consciousness is clouded. So you're back to needing a "jump start"—which is what cleansing techniques, such as those in Ayurveda, can offer.

There are other mind-body links here, too. The *aama* we see on the physical level will often have its mental counterparts. When I'm lecturing and extraneous thoughts come up, I often stall to refocus. What I hear my mouth say at those moments is, "Aam ... uh ..." as though I'm naming the mental clutter that sidetracked me. What is taken in through the eyes and ears that you are unable to assimilate creates a sort of mental *aama*. A friend who's writing a book on how to stay healthy in New York asked me for a brief statement she could use on what I found most important. "Be careful when you walk down the street about what you take in and what you don't," I found myself saying. "Be selective." The mad chaos of the mega-city offers countless wonderful morsels of nutritious input, but even more poor quality stuff that you will find dissonant and troubling.

The homeopath might say that the accumulation of matter in the body is a result of a miasmatic tendency—the overdoing of *sycosis*. Ignoring inner signals and taking in what your gut doesn't cue you to take disrupts intestinal health and produces a leaky gut with all the complications that follow. Years of overdoing, disregarding the feedback signals that would help you to eat exactly what you need and the right amount of it, lead to the accumulation of *aama*. The same overdoing on a psychological level leads to a mental *aama* that will also need cleaning out.

The beauty of working with these "foundation stones" is that what you do with the physical is like a basic training for dealing with subtler levels. Applying the strategy to your body is concrete, straightforward, and relatively easy to grasp. Carrying out a similar strategy in the arena of thoughts can be more slippery. But when you've already developed the

From outside the body
    environmental pollutants
    (xenobiotics)
 	
Inside "gunk" or *aama*
    by-products of metabolism
	TOTAL BURDEN OF ACCUMULATED "DROSS"

FIGURE 73

skill by working with your body, the reflexes required are in place, and you can more easily get through those difficult moments when you might otherwise lose your bearings.

A Heavier Load, A Compromised Outlet

While the Ayurvedic wizard of a millennium ago might have been keenly aware of the matter of *aama* and how it obstructs healthy functioning, he certainly had not developed the concepts necessary to deal with the load of environmental toxins that we face today. These two sources, the external and the internal, combine to produce our total burden of "stuff." I am again at a loss for a term to apply here. *Aama* won't quite do, since it is more correctly used to refer to that coming from the inside.

Researchers today have begun to call environmental toxins that enter the body *xenobiotics*—literally biologically active foreign substances (as in *xenophobia,* fear of foreigners). But that label does not include *aama,* since it's generated internally and/or is the result of improperly processed food.[10] What we need is a generic term that would encompass both. I often find myself falling back on the word "dross." From a good four-letter Anglo-Saxon word, *dros* (meaning "dregs"), it encompasses both waste *and* foreign matter.

The systemic burden or total dross is normally gotten rid of through four prime channels: lungs, colon, bladder, and skin (see Fig. 74). Each is important and plays a unique role in dispensing with a specific kind of waste. The colon and bladder are what we normally think of when we say "elimination"—feces being the solid waste and urine that which is water-soluble. But the skin is an ancillary route of exit for wastes in solution.

Naturopathic physicians sometimes speak of the skin as "the third kidney." As a matter of fact, when the kidneys are damaged, the sweat glands have been observed to grow in size, taking over some part of the load that the urinary system usually handles. Patients with kidney failure, when not on dialysis, can develop a "uremic frost" from the copious water-soluble wastes that exit with perspiration and remain as salts when it dries. Yogis who train their bodies to amplify the action of the sweat glands through intense breathing techniques ("pranic bath") reportedly experience the same dusting with crystals over their bodies and must brush them off.

NORMAL ROUTES OF EXCRETION

Organ	Product
colon	feces
kidney/bladder	urine
skin	perspiration
lungs	exhaled air

Overflow

mucous membranes	mucus
uterus	menses

FIGURE 74

Exhalation is also a more important route of excretion than you might have thought. This is the preferred route of elimination of volatile wastes—those that easily vaporize and leave the bloodstream as gases. Of course, the bulk of the gaseous waste from the lungs is carbon dioxide, but there is often an admixture of the breakdown products of fats and oils, as well as medicinally active substances. Garlic, if added to an enema, is absorbed, enters the blood, and its odor can be detected on the breath in a matter of seconds. Many of the by-products of bacterial degradation of fecal matter in the stagnant bowel are volatile, and their presence in the exhaled air is a common cause of bad breath in constipated persons. This "constipation breath" is often a tipoff to me that someone needs bowel cleansing. I learned this in an amusing way.

When I first came back from India, I began to practice kappal-bhati, *a breathing exercise that exaggerates the throwing off of wastes during exhalation. It's done in a sitting position by sharply contracting the abdomen to create a forceful outbreath. The inhalation is more relaxed. This is done in rapid repetition, and is said to cleanse the blood and leave the forehead radiant. (The name* kappalbhati *means "shining skull.") During my travels, I had not always found clean or healthful food, and had ended up with a mild chronic dysentery. To try to recover some of the weight I had lost, I was eating more than I really wanted, which further burdened my digestive system. It's probably safe to say that my gut was a disaster area.*

I was working more or less as an itinerant physician for the moment, staying with a friend. He gave me his study to use as my bedroom. Sitting there doing kappalbhati *one evening, I became aware of an unpleasant odor. It occurred to me that since this was a new apartment building, perhaps something was wrong with the plumbing. I thought that the bathroom of the apartment next door must be adjacent to the room I was using, and that somehow I was smelling the sewer line. But as I slept there that night, there was no odor, or the next day—at least not until I started doing* kappalbhati *again. It took me several days to finally accept the fact that the bad smell was coming from* me.

If we were dealing with a moderate level of wastes and pollutants— of physiologic dross—the four main routes of exit should comfortably handle all necessary elimination. Unfortunately, as we saw above, the influx of foreign substances such as synthetic chemicals and heavy metals currently swamping our bodies is far beyond what must have been present in the environment during the evolution of human physiology. Moreover, the internal production of wastes, the *aama* in the system, is probably at a level unknown in the past—largely owing to the prevalence of food that is highly processed and preserved, and to leaky guts that have developed from repeated antibiotics and excess sugar.

In addition to this increased burden of wastes, the four main elimination systems are frequently not up to par. The colon, the mainstay of elimination, is frequently sluggish. A low-fiber diet and suboptimal water intake, along with lack of aerobic exercise, are probably major reasons that disabled bowels have become the norm, and why we have become laxative addicts. Many folks think that a bowel movement every other day or so is just fine, and the idea of more than one in twenty-four hours seems strange to them. By contrast, yogis who delved into what was needed for alertness and longevity advised that the residue of one meal should be eliminated before the next meal is taken. Even if we fall short of that rigorous ideal, having at least one regular bowel movement a day should be a priority.

To understand fully why the colon functions so poorly, we may have to look not only at physical factors but also explore its mental and emotional significance. The movement of the bowels is a physical expression of our willingness to let go the residue of the past. Constipation often reveals a tendency to hold on to the old—relationships, possessions, or thoughts and memories. Sometimes cleansing the bowel can catalyze a more global process of release—mental, emotional, and physical.

The colon is not the only excretory channel that is compromised in its free flow. The lungs are often blocked, too. They are dependent for their cleansing action on the efficiency of your breathing habits. Unfortunately, our manner of breathing expresses our emotions as much as it does our physiologic needs. We sigh with disappointment. We gasp in amazement. We sputter with rage. Many if not most of us do not breathe in a way that will energize us, but rather in a way that expresses our fears and inhibitions.

ARE YOU DEHYDRATED?

The last two of the four main excretory routes, the urinary tract and the skin, have their problems, too. The full use of them for elimination depends on adequate water intake—as does, to a great extent, the optimal function of the colon. That makes water the key to much of your detoxifying and cleansing efforts. But busy people often complain that they don't have time to drink water or, for that matter, to urinate. "Drinking more water just keeps me running to the bathroom," patients explain to me. Yet it is precisely that—a free flow of water through the body—which is needed to wash out the molecular clutter that interferes with normal healthy functioning. This is especially important as we get older, since, as we saw earlier, it is the nature of the body to become more *vatic* with age, and the keynote of *vata* is dryness.

In the *vatic* body, water is difficult to absorb. It may seem as though it "runs right through." In that case it is important to take fluids with a *low surface tension*. The surface tension of water is what causes it to pull together into drops, or to form a meniscus at the edge of its surface. But this property also makes it more difficult for the water to disperse through the membranes of the intestinal lining and the capillaries, or to move freely through the extracellular spaces, enter the cells, and wash away molecular debris.

The surface tension of fresh juices is low; that of carrot juice one of the lowest known, which may be why it is highly regarded as a cleanser and nourisher. In recent years, a number of workers have experimented with natural preparations that can be added to water to reduce its surface tension.[11] These work by rearranging the water molecules so they are not random, but patterned in some fashion. Attention to this reflects, I believe, the beginning of a significant advance in biological science. It is evidence of a dawning realization that water, which makes up more than 80 percent of the body, is *not* merely an inert medium in which active compounds float. It is also alive, its molecules complex, changing, and charged with information. The more we learn about water, the more obvious it will become that a good quantity and quality of water is a cornerstone of sound health.

Optimal water intake is about eight ounces (roughly 250 ml) per twenty pounds of body weight—about two quarts a day for the average adult. If the surface tension of the water is high (as in the case of "hard water"), one will need to take more. The *vatic* person will also need a bit more than this. Everyone will need more when the climate is very dry and/or hot and large amounts of moisture are lost by perspiration. So tailor your exact intake to your specifics (see Fig. 75). There's room for some flexibility here—listen to what your body tells you. But many of us are so out of touch with our water status that we may find a glass of water repulsive, even when we are clearly dehydrated. Our need for water is something that has to be brought back into consciousness. I have my own little running struggle with this.

At least once a week I go through the following scenario, or something very similar: I am developing a slight headache. I notice a cer-

		WATER NEEDED		
	Weight	Normal daily requirement	Quarts	Dry, hot and/or windy conditions
Child	60 lbs.	four 6-oz. glasses	¾	1–1½ qts.
Adult	120 lbs.	six 8-oz. glasses	1½	2–2½ qts.
Adult	180 lbs.	nine 8-oz. glasses	2¼	2¾–3½ qts.

FIGURE 75

tain tension in my jaw, and I begin to feel restless and a bit irritable.
I am having trouble concentrating on my work. My breath is getting
short and tight. When I finally register, with full consciousness, that
"something is wrong with me," and run a sort of internal scan, I
notice the dryness in my mouth. Suddenly I see very clearly a sublim-
inal thirst that I've been denying and, connected to that, a feeling of
physiologic urgency bordering on panic that is a response to the emer-
gency situation resulting from too little water in my body. I stop what
I'm doing, go to the kitchen, draw a glass of distilled water and add a
trace mineral/surface tension reducer, and drink it. I immediately feel
all the symptoms melt away. Relaxed, serene, and tranquil, I resume
my work.

"Emergency" and "panic" may sound like overstatements, but research suggests that if water intake falls far below the optimal levels, and the body begins to experience a relative dehydration, a person's entire physiology goes "on alert." According to biologists, the evolutionary shift from life in water to life on land was a difficult and challenging one. Getting enough water to sustain a system whose original design was water-based has remained, after air, the top priority of your body. When you fail to do so, your internal system may shift into an emergency mode and shuts down all sources of water loss.

Dr. Batmanghelidj, author of *Your Body's Many Cries for Water*, carefully studied the research on the physiology of water and concluded that when the water content of tissues falls to a certain point, the bilayer membranes that surround cells contract in thickness. This forms a barrier that prevents further dehydration (see Fig. 76). But it also obstructs the free movement of molecules, so that metabolism and elimination are limited. Essentially, the cell moves into a survival mode of operation. A wide variety of symptoms can flare up at such times, such as allergic reactions. That's why upping your water intake will not only facilitate the effective elimination of the systemic dross you need to get rid of, but may also improve chronic problems you wouldn't have connected with water needs at all.

What seems to work best is to set a time for drinking water. For me, it is on arising and at about 4:00 P.M. An hour before lunch is also good. Two or three glasses at each of those times will satisfy the bulk of my requirements for the day. Even more ideal is to drink small amounts continually. About four ounces an hour is suitable for most people. This

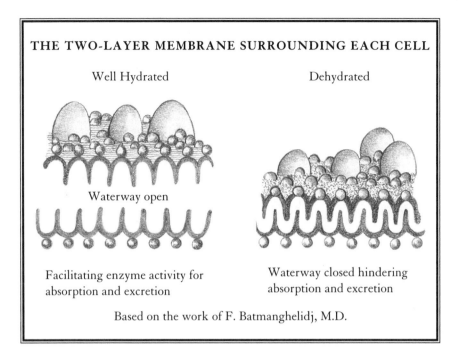

THE TWO-LAYER MEMBRANE SURROUNDING EACH CELL

Well Hydrated   Dehydrated

Waterway open

Facilitating enzyme activity for   Waterway closed hindering
absorption and excretion   absorption and excretion

Based on the work of F. Batmanghelidj, M.D.

FIGURE 76

works especially well for those who have already developed some degree of dehydration. It takes persistance and patience to rehydrate, and the body may accept only small amounts of water at a time.

Even when you drink enough water, the skin may not do its part in the waste-removal effort. That's because we thwart it. Perspiration has developed a bad image. I'm not sure why, but I suspect that it's due in part to the fact that we have so much internal pollution. When we do perspire, what comes out is foul and smelly. In any event, we've developed clever devices to foil the sweat glands. Called deodorants, they are usually strongly astringent aluminum compounds that constrict the pores so that they don't work, primarily under the arms. One can only wonder about the advisability of blocking the removal of toxins and water from this area, since here are the lymph nodes that drain the breasts, where cancer so frequently occurs.

Some of the obstacles to excretion by the skin might also be psychological. Deodorant commercials reinforce the cool, aloof ideal, and a desire to keep yourself separate might be expressed by shutting down your skin.

ACCESSORY OUTLETS

When the colon, lungs, bladder, and skin can't do their jobs well, then the body resorts to accessory outlets (see Fig. 77). There are two of these: the secretions of the mucous membranes and the menses. Though mucus is, in conventional medical terms, a *secretion* rather than an *excretion*—i.e., it is produced to moisten and protect, rather than as a form of waste—it can, according to most traditions, serve both functions. When

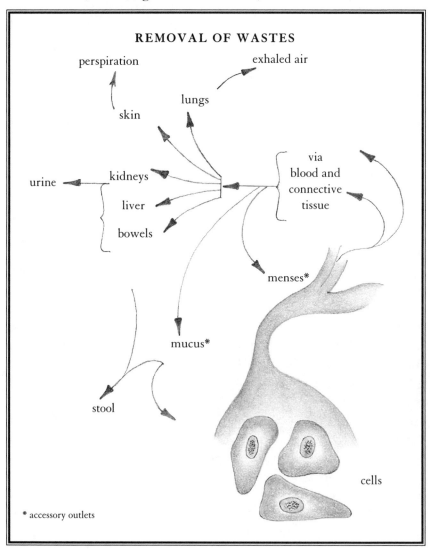

FIGURE 77

it's strictly a secretion, it will be present in small amounts—only what is required to lubricate the lining membranes of body parts such as the eyes, nose, mouth, vagina, and rectum. But when the four principal elimination channels are blocked for some reason, or when their capacity is exceeded, then the mucous membranes provide an outlet for the overflow.

You might have experienced a mild version of this as a spring cold. Spring is the time when your body mobilizes the substance, the *kapha,* that kept you insulated through the winter. When this happens, it can overwhelm your body's exit routes. A light diet at this time, or even a brief fast, can head off the crisis and allow your spring cleaning to proceed without tipping you into respiratory troubles. More dramatic crises can occur when a high-potency homeopathic remedy triggers a thorough reorganization and "everything has to go."

A few days after I took the dose of *Calcarea mur* described in Chapter 2, I had to lecture at the first Himalayan Institute Congress. It wasn't easy. The remedy had loosened a flood of yellow mucus that was practically gushing from my nose and throat. I was embarrassed to climb up to the podium, and had to stop frequently to blow my nose or clear my throat. I asked Swami Rama if I could take *Calcarea sulph* 6x. I was grasping for something to stem the tide enough that I could function more comfortably. But he advised against it. "Don't interfere," he said. "Let it come out."

While men must rely on mucus as an accessory route of elimination, women have a second choice: the menstrual flow. A Victorian gentleman may have openly hacked into a brass spittoon but his lady friend discreetly excused herself to attend to her monthly menses. In this day and time, however, a woman's monthly discharge may be problematic. I find that it is those women who have accumulated a considerable burden of toxins who are most likely to struggle with a crescendo of symptoms leading up to the menstrual period. Then, once the period is underway, there's dramatic relief.

The psychological/emotional facet of this distress is implicit in the function of the uterus as container and creator of life. The pain has, I think, to do with the frustration of being caught in a female role in a world where the feminine principles of nurturance and love are not honored. For a woman, to reproduce means to condemn herself to some degree of complicity with the dominant order, to raise her children within it and see them (to her horror) express it. Forced to be the container of so many destructive values and emotions, not to mention a heavy

burden of chemical toxins—the physical evidence of a patriarchal society's failings—the body rebels. Holding all this becomes agonizing.
Finally throwing it off provides some measure of relief, if only temporarily. Dietary improvement and a good detox program have been
found to be effective in reducing the symptoms of PMS.[12]

The four basic routes of elimination and these two ancillary ones
depend on an underlying network of internal cleansing (see Fig. 77). This
includes the lymph, liver, and kidneys. The lymphatic system drains the
spaces between cells where wastes collect as they are pushed through the
cell membrane. The liver catches toxic chemicals and "bundles" them into
a form that won't cause damage until they can be excreted through one of
the exit organs. The kidneys filter chemical and metabolic dross out of the
blood and send it down the urinary tract. As we've noted before, the liver
and kidneys are often overstressed and undernourished and not up to the
huge demands that are being placed on them.[13] But it's at the initial stage
of lymphatic drainage, just outside the cells, where trouble first begins.

Overburdened and Backing Up:
From Congestion to Disease

When the cumulative load of environmental toxins and metabolic wastes
exceeds the body's capacity to throw it off, it has to go somewhere. The
first place it is likely to build up is in the spaces between the cells. This
space is another example of the sort of blind spot in medical research that
we discussed before. The general tendency in conventional medicine is to
focus on specific, circumscribed components of the body. What gets overlooked is the background—the field, so to speak. What is the context
within which these specifics operate? In the case of the cells, it is the
extracellular space or "ground substance."

Wastes pushed out of the cell (and toxins not allowed in) may accumulate in this space. It constitutes an extensive drainage system that takes
up what's given off by the cells and sends it away through the lymph
tracts—or, when that's not possible, holds it in temporary storage.
Systemic waste can come to load the fluids in this extracellular space and
saturate the connective tissue that runs through it. There are mechanisms
that condense the molecules of this extraneous matter into more compact
forms so they take up less room and are less disruptive to the processes
around them.[14] Even so, the extracellular connective tissue space has lim-

ited storage capacity. As it becomes overburdened, one may begin to
experience stiffness caused by the deposits in it, and pain throughout the
body as a result of irritation from them—symptoms that sound very
much like what is currently called "fibromyalgia" or what was known as
"rheumatism" a century ago. Perhaps the pain is there to remind us that
the buildup of substances in this extracellular space must be limited. It
cannot be allowed to become a sort of cesspool, for it has its own functions
to carry out.

Though it has been largely ignored by the cellular- and later the
molecular-oriented medical scientists of the last two centuries, this space
between the cells is quite important. It is, in a sense, a living matrix—a
place where many systems intersect and are coordinated (see Fig. 78).
Here active substances, on their way in or out of the cells or the capillaries, interact with sympathetic and parasympathetic nerve endings. What's
more, according to current German scientists, this "ground substance"
conducts its own electrical impulses. This is not a new idea. Schuessler,

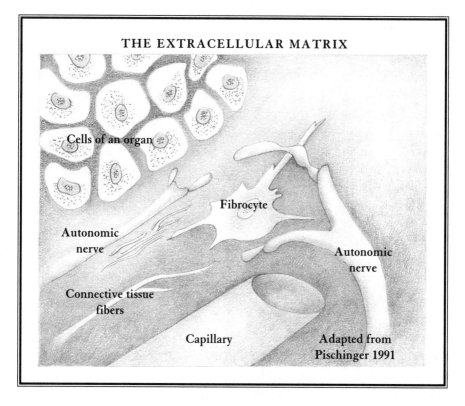

THE EXTRACELLULAR MATRIX

Cells of an organ

Fibrocyte

Autonomic
nerve

Autonomic
nerve

Connective tissue
fibers

Capillary

Adapted from
Pischinger 1991

FIGURE 78

who developed the cell salts long before electrical impulses could be measured, seemed to sense this and called the connective tissue "the matrix through which the most secret currents pass."

Recent research suggests[15] that subtle electrical currents and molecular and ionic shifts in this pervasive ground substance create an intricate communications network operating alongside of, and interacting with, the nervous and endocrine systems. If the nerves are your cable TV and the hormones your mail, the ground matrix might be thought of as your Internet. It was discovered that tiny bundles of nerve fibers and capillaries emerge from this ground substance to penetrate the skin surface at certain points. Where they do, they bring a microscopic cylinder of the extracellular matrix with them. This point is a "window" onto the ground system, and when it is punctured by a fine needle, shifts reverberate throughout. As you might have already guessed, these little points correspond to those marked on the acupuncturist's chart.

If the extracellular connective tissue matrix is overburdened with toxic substances, the communications it normally conducts are blocked. Its "energy channels" are obstructed, and as a result, you don't feel up to par. To diagnose exactly where the obstruction is most severe, the electroacupuncturist will run a low-level current through each meridian. Where resistance is altered, he knows that the sphere of functions the channel serves are likely to be "off." But when widespread excesses of general dross clog the ground matrix, symptoms are likely to be more global. The Ayurvedist lists signs and symptoms such as as tiredness, bad breath, and dullness of the mind and senses as indications of an *aama*-burdened system (see Fig. 79).

Though the extracellular space is a first stop-off for all sorts of metabolic dross, it is the favored site for long-term deposition of protein substances. Other types of waste have their final destinations of choice, too. Fat-soluble toxic chemicals will tend to end up in the adipose tissue, cholesterol in the arterial walls and as stones in the gallbladder. Minerals are usually deposited in the joint spaces, or become kidney or bladder stones. Glycoproteins—part carbohydrate and part protein—are thought by some naturopaths to form "mucoid" deposits in the connective tissue space, and it is probably there where many of the *aama*-like deposits end up.[16]

Bulky collections of deposition in the connective tissues can produce visible distortions of the normal body shape. Some naturopaths of the last century liked to refer to these lumps and thicknesses as "encumbrances." Much of what we consider aging has less to do with age than with the progressive accumulation of such matter (see Fig. 80). You can examine a

---

SIGNS AND SYMPTOMS OF *AAMA*

- Heaviness/tiredness

- Lack of strength

- Turbid urine with foul odor

- Indigestion and/or constipation

- Undigested food in feces

- Offensive odor of feces

- Bad breath

- Tongue coated:
  vata—brown
  pitta—yellow
  kapha—white

FIGURE 79

face for its encumbrances, then compare what you find to the face maps in Chapter 5 to come up with some hypotheses about which organs are likely to be most affected—and even which psychological and emotional baggage might correspond to the physical burden.

CLOGGED CORNERS AND FOCI OF DISEASE

When you've accumulated more environmental and internally generated waste than the connective tissue space can hold, the surplus may be disposed of by "sticking it in a corner." Just as a lazy housekeeper will stuff cabinets and drawers with useless junk he doesn't know what else to do with, *aama* and environmental toxins may be shoved into less critical structures such as joint spaces or nasal sinuses in order to protect vital organs and to preserve some degree of normal functioning in the extracellular matrix. These spots then become like stagnant pools that encourage the growth of microbes.

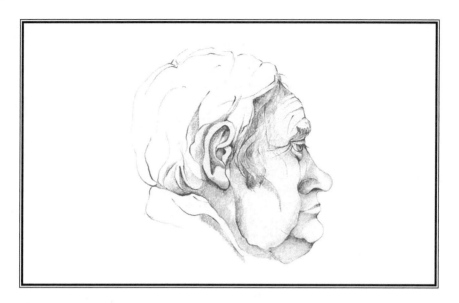

FIGURE 80

Practitioners of Functional Medicine, a German holistic school, refer to such pockets of inflammation as *focal diseases*. Foci probably develop for a number of reasons, only one of which is the need for a "dump site." Psychological and emotional factors doubtless play a role, putting a strain on organs or structures that bear some relation to those issues, so that they become vulnerable and give way to the pressures of built-up dross. For example, chronic congestion and infection in the middle ear in children is often related to not wanting to hear the domestic squabbling going on around them.

Another example is periodontal disease. The gums are what support our teeth, and problems with them can be an expression of a difficulty in backing up our "bite"—the decisive stances we adopt. Periodontal problems would suggest, then, a wishy-washy approach to implementing what we believe is right and know we should do. Gum infection is extremely common. This is not only because there is a huge gulf between our ethical values and how we conduct ourselves in the world, but also because oral hygiene is commonly poor. Here in America, cleaning the mouth after eating is not a cultural norm. We tend to brush only in the morning or at night.

When I first went to India, I met a young man on a neighborhood square in Old Delhi. We were eager to exchange information and

observations about the two backgrounds we came from. He asked me,
with charming innocence, "Is it true that in America, people's teeth
fall out?" "Of course not," I said, laughing. Then I stopped. The
smiles of the elderly sitting around me revealed teeth that were their
own. I thought about our bridges and crowns and other high-tech
restorations. Few here could afford that. Without the elaborate inter-
ventions of our dentists, the truth of his query would be more appar-
ent. "Well," I began to correct myself, "in a way it is true. . . ."

I came to learn that people there were as horrified by Americans
walking away from the table with food between their teeth as we were
horrified by the use of the side of the street as a latrine. I remember
squeamishly negotiating such a filthy road one day when I caught sight
of a beautiful woman in a sari, obviously poor, emerging from her simple
lean-to shelter. Having finished her meal, she walked gracefully through
the squalor with a cup of water and began to clean her mouth. While our
cultural ideal of purity is represented by dry underarms and manicured
lawns, theirs is symbolized by the lotus, rooted in the muck, but rising
above it, radiant and lovely.

Perhaps as a result of such values, clever techniques for cleansing are
found in the Eastern traditions. Gandhi made the world aware of the use
of a branch from the *neem* tree to clean the teeth. The end of the stick,
chewed and frayed, is the traditional toothbrush of the Indian peasant.
Neem has medicinal qualities thought to tighten the gums and discour-
age infection. Periodontists today have developed a modern equivalent: a
soft "blotting" brush that, used without toothpaste or water, can, through
its capillary action, "vacuum" the spaces between the gum and tooth
where food collects, remove plaque, and stimulate circulation.[17] This,
coupled with the traditional Indian practice of rinsing and massaging the
gums after eating, can eliminate them as a locus of chronic infection.

When such foci are allowed to remain, they become a major drain on
the immune system, which must constantly struggle to keep the growth
of microbes in the area under control. The nasal sinuses are a prime
example. Sinusitis is so widespread that it probably affects most of the
population at one time or another. Dusty, polluted air may be one of the
main reasons for this, but again, the mentality that produces such a polluted world must also play a role in most cases. Tension in the area of the
sinuses is usually a by-product of our "effortful" approach to life, and the
postnasal drip that develops is a sort of internal weeping that results from

Common Foci of Disease	Techniques for Rx/Prevention
Gums	Blotting brush, gum massage
Sinuses	Nasal wash
Intestinal tract	High-fiber diet, water
Tonsils	Nasal wash
Gallbladder	Low-fat, high-fiber diet
Middle ear	Nasal wash

FIGURE 81

our sadness at being cut off from those spiritual forces that might guide and nurture us if we let go our stubborn effort to control. When we refuse to do so, life becomes a headache.

> One of the first patients I treated for headaches had come to me after going the rounds of specialists and headache clinics. I was doubtful that I could help, but Swami Rama assured me I could, and suggested that I teach the patient the nasal wash. This simple cleansing technique, developed by the yogis, involves nothing more that pouring warm salt water through your nose. Using a special little pot with a spout that fits into the nostril, you let the water fill one side of the nasal cavity, course behind the nasal septum into the other, and run out the opposite nostril. Then you tilt your head the other way and do the opposite.
>
> I taught the patient this and sent her home. A few days later I received a frantic phone call. "Something horrible has happened!" she exclaimed. I was frightened. What had I done? I should have known better than to prescribe things I hadn't been taught in medical school. "What is it?" I asked, my voice cracking. "This is terrible," she went on. "I did this nose-pot thing you told me to, and"—she stopped as though she couldn't bring herself to say it—"and a bone fell out of my head!" "A what?" I asked incredulously. "A bone fell out of my head," she repeated.

What had fallen out of her head, or her nose to be more precise, appeared to be a large piece of hardened mucus that must have been accumulating there for years. Exactly how the irritation it produced had set off her headaches, I never knew, but after her little incident, they disappeared once and for all.

The nasal wash prevents and often corrects the congestion and focus of infection that develops in the sinuses. Other sites in the body that are likely to become foci of disease are the appendix, the uterus, and the gall-bladder, each of which can come to harbor a little cauldron of brewing inflammation and infection (see Fig. 82).[18] We can't really consider the intestinal tract an isolated "focus" like these others, since it belongs at the center of the picture. But like the foci we have discussed, it can (and often does) function as a reservoir of undesirable microbial growth, and as a major drain on immune reserves.

The perspective that is emerging here is that of a system that is over-burdened and backing up. When our organizational integrity, our ability to coordinate, clean up and restructure, is weak, then, as the Ayurvedist says, "alien identities begin to flourish in the muck of *aama*."[19] One example of this is what we call "infection"—the growth of undesirable microbes.

LITTLE ENEMIES AND BIG PARANOIA

The sages who developed Ayurveda sensed the presence of microbes. The Sanskrit term for them was *krimi*. They did not, however, attribute

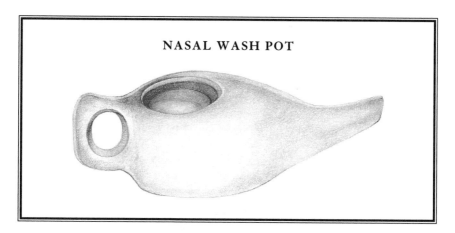

NASAL WASH POT

FIGURE 82

to them a primary causal role in disease. When I was studying in India, I sometimes found the self-assured attitude of the old *vaidya*s irritating. I knew I had lots to learn—that was why I was there. But I had had a lengthy medical education and I thought it deserved some acknowledgment. "Don't ignore what Western medicine has accomplished!" I finally said one day, tight-lipped. "Yes?" came the amused response. "Like what?" "Well, like the conquest of infectious disease with antibiotics," I declared defiantly. "Oh, you mean killing the *krimi*s with mold?" They chuckled. "Actually, we've been doing that in Ayurveda for thousands of years. But it doesn't work all that well, you'll find." I had no comeback. I walked away, feeling irritated and defensive. But the exchange had knocked another little chink out of my wall of resistance to seeing the world from a more holistic perspective.

Actually, in the West there is a long line of research going back over a hundred years that questions conventional ideas about microbes and infection. In the late 1800s, even as Pasteur was framing theories of "infection" that would hold sway for more than a century, a distinguished contemporary of his, Antoine Béchamps, was developing a different perspective. He observed tiny particles in the blood that he said permeated all living systems. These *microzymas,* as he called them, were, he felt, the basic building blocks of life. From them, he claimed, bacteria arose as well as the cellular components of our own bodies. Though Pasteur's name went down in history as the "discoverer" of the germ theory, it is said that on his deathbed, he recanted, admitting that the microbe was incidental, and that *"le terrain est tout"*—the condition of the body is what determines whether the microorganisms will flourish or not.

Adventurous microbiologists ever since, usually with no apparent awareness of Béchamps' work, and often with no knowledge of each other, have taken issue with the accepted Pasteurian ideas that bacteria and other microbes must be introduced into a system and can only reproduce themselves in a tight, unchanging lineage.[20] They have described a variety of intermediate "cell wall deficient" bacteria and surprising shifts from one species to the other.

Gunther Enderlein, working in Germany during the first half of the twentieth century, pulled together a spectrum of such ideas and observations. Through decades of careful study, he and his associates charted the course of the development of organisms from the tiny particles Béchamps had described through a sort of life cycle that included the metamorphosis to intermediate forms and finally into microbes associated with disease.[21] This concept has been echoed, though in a somewhat different form, in the more recent work of Gaston Naessens, a Frenchman working in Canada. His life cycle of the microbial forms in the human includes bacterial versions as well as yeast and fungi (see Fig. 83).

In both cases, the ideas are revolutionary. Conventional microbiologists are indignant at the suggestion that they might have overlooked something so fundamental. But that possibility is not as outlandish as they might assume. As we have seen, current research often misses the connecting observations, the threads that tie the whole picture together. Moreover, conventional blood work and even high-power electron microscopes require that the blood smear or tissue being examined be killed and "fixed" with chemical agents and dyes. The work done by such

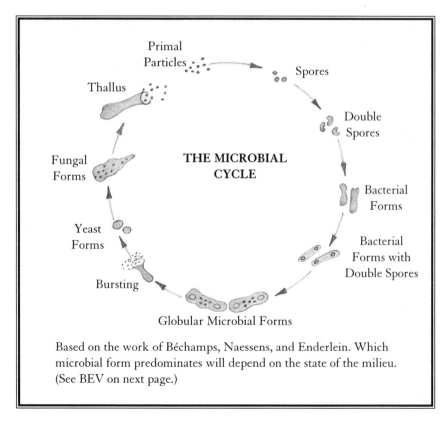

THE MICROBIAL CYCLE

Primal Particles

Spores

Double Spores

Thallus

Fungal Forms

Yeast Forms

Bursting

Bacterial Forms

Bacterial Forms with Double Spores

Globular Microbial Forms

Based on the work of Béchamps, Naessens, and Enderlein. Which microbial form predominates will depend on the state of the milieu. (See BEV on next page.)

FIGURE 83

researchers as Enderlein and Naessens was based on the use of specially designed microscopes which produce a high degree of magnification and employ a darkfield technique which makes it possible to study the blood while it is still alive.

The common denominator in all such work is a conviction that the condition of the body is the main determinant of whether microbes will grow there and, if so, what kind. BEV, a German high-tech, multidimensional measurement of pH, resistance, and redox potential done on urine, blood, and saliva, locates the condition of the tissues in one of four physicochemical quadrants (see Fig. 84).[22] In one of these, disease-causing bacteria proliferate, in another yeasts and fungal forms will grow, and in a third, viruses are likely to take over. This last is the state that tends toward malignancy, and when conditions are such as to push the graph far into the outside corner of this quadrant, cancer virtually always appears. Areas near the center of the graph correspond to optimal conditions where more normal and more desirable microbes flourish.[23]

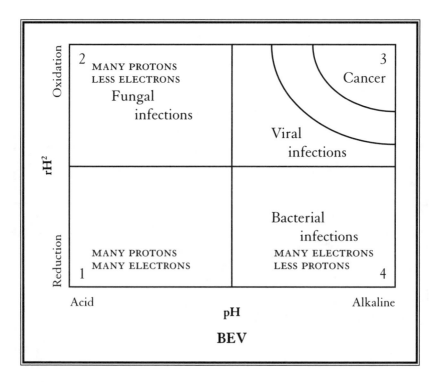

FIGURE 84

Techniques for Freeing Ourselves

"There are two ways to clean a dirty water glass," my teacher observed, with the studied deliberation that told me he was going to say something simple but with vast implications. "The first is to turn it upside down and wash it out." He paused for me to digest what he'd said. "The second is to let fresh water run into it, fill it, and overflow—continuously running in and out over a long period of time." Then he asked, "Which do you think works best?" I hesitated, suspecting it was a setup. Before I could venture a reply, he volunteered, "You think it's the first, the emptying and the washing, but it's not. The gradual approach is more thorough in the long run."

There are basically two approaches to cleansing—to releasing the residue of the past—in order to free ourselves to move on. The first, more gradual approach is simply to bolster the normal routes of elimination so that they can do their work better. These are the "big four" we discussed earlier: the colon, lungs, urinary tract, and skin. If they are working well, they will provide a constant cleansing effect. The second is what we would call "heroic" cleansing—in which more-drastic measures are brought to bear, and you are "turned upside down and washed out," so to speak. Such techniques as fasting, colonic irrigation, and Ayurvedic *panchakarma* fall into this second category. Though they are more exciting and dramatic, they have their drawbacks. Unless used judiciously, they can weaken your digestive system, deplete your energy, and complicate existing problems. Before you resort to such methods, first strengthen and support your body's ability to do the necessary cleaning out in a more comfortable and routine way. Besides, the regular routes of cleansing should be put in top working order before heroic measures are undertaken anyway. And after any intense program of elimination you will need to switch back to a maintenance mode again so that normal routes can continue to keep you clear.

Some of what supports the normal outlets so they operate more thoroughly, you've already heard about. The colon requires plenty of water, a high-fiber diet, and regular aerobic exercise. Once those habits are in place, if you are not having at least one full, satisfying bowel movement a day, then you can go to the first step of gentle intervention: take a pint of hot water with lemon, a bit of honey, and a pinch of salt on arising in the morning. A simple exercise of squatting and moving alternate knees toward the floor with your hands, helps move the hot liquid through the intestinal tract to stimulate the bowels to move. If your colon needs extra help beyond that, substitute *trifala* for the lemon drink for a while. This Ayurvedic formula cleanses the bowel without exerting the kind of laxative effect that might weaken digestion or create dependency (see Fig. 85).

If you tend to puffiness beneath the eyes, pay particular attention to the kidneys. A pint of plain lemon water at room temperature on arising is helpful. When it's hot, it tends to run through the gut quickly. Cooler, it is absorbed and leaves via the kidneys. An intake of too little water results in a concentrated urine that is irritating to the delicate membranes of the renal apparatus. A high-fat diet produces a milky lipemic blood plasma that is difficult for the filtration system of the kidney to process. High-salt and high-protein diets also leave strong, concentrated residues that stress the kidneys. Watch to see what swells or shrinks the bags under your eyes.

After the continued presence of highly concentrated urine in the collection system of the kidney over a long period, crystals may have formed. When you begin to drink more water and to drop some of the oil, salt, and excess protein from your diet, your urine will become more dilute and flow more rapidly, and these crystals will begin to dissolve. Stones that had been lodged because of their size may then wash down the ureter. Occasionally one will get stuck at this point, and you may wonder whether your cleansing efforts are backfiring. That's exactly what happened to Elena.

HOW TO USE *TRIFALA**

Though tablets and capsules are now available, the traditional and most effective way of taking *trifala* is to put a teaspoon of the powder in a cup, pour boiling water over it, let it stand overnight, and in the morning strain and drink it. It may take you a while to adjust to it—it's bitter, sour, pungent, astringent, and, at the end, thankfully, slightly sweet. But it's worth getting past the taste. Based on *amla,* the Ayurvedic miracle fruit, it has a tonic and rejuvenating affect as well as cleansing the intestine.

*Trifala means "three fruits": *haritaki* rejuvenates *vata, amla* rejuvenates *pitta, bibhitaki* restores *kapha*.

FIGURE 85

We'd been successfully clearing up a series of physical problems that Elena had: Kali mur 6x *was "terrific" in dealing with flare-ups of her recurrent bronchitis,* Magnesium *had helped her mitral valve prolapse and, along with vitamin* B_6, *had taken care of her carpal tunnel symptoms. It was also, I thought, addressing her tendency to kidney stones. But kidney stones are often considered little lumps of unresolved anger, and we had just begun to deal with the buried feelings she carried from childhood for her abusive father.*

She called me as she was preparing to leave for an international conference. The little bursts of pain in the small of her back that flashed on and off from time to time had returned with a vengeance. She was panicked. "What should I do?" I suggested Berberis vulgaris *tincture,[24] which will usually relax the passageway and allow a kidney or gallstone to pass. After a couple of doses, the pain subsided and she attended the meeting with no trouble. I have, on a number of occasions, dispatched little bottles of* Berberis *to patients scheduled for surgery to remove such stones, and so far all of them have escaped the knife.*

The skin needs you to exercise vigorously if it is to work at its maximum capacity, and thorough sweating is one of the major benefits of aerobic exercise. Breathing and visualization can magnify this: Extend your exhalation twice as many counts as your inhalation, and imagine that your whole body is a sponge that is being squeezed as you exhale. (In fact, it is—it is full of water, which, when extruded through the skin as perspiration, carries wastes out—just as dirty water is expelled from the sponge.) Brushing the skin with a natural-bristle brush may also help open the pores and is thought by some naturopaths to stimulate the breakdown and removal of material that is deposited in the connective tissue spaces.[25]

The last of the four major routes of cleansing is exhalation. You can increase elimination through the lungs by breathing more fully and by strengthening the diaphragm. The diaphragm will get stronger if you use a sandbag on the midriff as you do diaphragmatic breathing (see Chapter 10). Full use of the lungs involves three phases, diaphragmatic, thoracic, and clavicular. To do this "complete breath," simply imagine yourself as an empty tube of toothpaste that is returning to its filled state. Your mouth is the opening, and on inhalation you start from the bottom. The lowest part, that near the diaphragm, fills first, then the thorax or chest proper, and last, if your inhalation is the fullest possible, you feel a slight lift in your clavicles, or collarbones.

Bolstering the "big four" normal elimination routes is of limited value unless we also tend to the internal systems that package and relay wastes to them. These include the liver, kidneys, and lymphatic system. Initiating a large-scale cleaning-out when these organs can't handle the extra burden won't work. There are simple techniques for helping these, too. Movement of the lymph can be stimulated by the mechanical pressure of massage and through the effects of gravity using a mini-trampoline or "rebounder." This also ensures the good kidney function we just discussed. But the most important supporting role, played by the liver, requires a bit more thought.

The liver is the center of metabolic activities for the body. It contains more enzyme systems than most of the other organs of the body com-

---

ATTENTION TO MAJOR CLEANSING CHANNELS

	Maintenance	Extra Help
Colon	exercise	lemon/honey/salt
	high-fiber diet	drink
	water	*trifala*
Urinary tract	water	whey
	diet low in fat, salt,	cell salts: *Natrum sulph* 6x and
	protein	*Kali mur* 6x
Skin	water	brushing
	aerobics	exhalation twice as long as
		inhalation*
Lungs	complete breath	diaphragm breathing with
		sandbag*

*See Chapter 10.

FIGURE 86

bined, and is responsible for the bulk of detox processes. If overburdened, it can't convert mobilized toxins into forms that can be excreted, and they will build up and make you feel worse.

The liver is commonly overworked, because of nutritional deficiencies that weaken its capacity and the heavy demands placed on it by a polluted external environment and a disturbed internal one: everything coming from the intestinal surface, the inner ecology, goes first to the liver. If the lining of the intestine is irritated by a disturbance of the normal microbes there—causing a "leaky gut"—the liver will have an extra onslaught of debris to deal with. A stagnant colon adds the metabolic by-products of bacterial degradation.

Incoming drugs also stress the liver, since you must rely on it to take them up and convert them into an inactive form for excretion. This responsibility is not limited to pharmaceuticals, but includes caffeine, alcohol, and nicotine—as well as many of the medicinal compounds in herbs or even those in fruits and vegetables. In fact, everything that has been absorbed goes directly to the liver. It is a stopover point where not only are toxins pulled out, but nutrients are sorted and essentials stored for later use. You also use your liver to filter out and package for excretion all the chemical pollutants you take in with food, water, or air. If you continually overwhelm your liver with an intake of toxic substances, it is not free to work on cleaning out old accumulations.

Psychological and emotional issues also affect the way you use your liver. Anger, frustration, and worry are intricately bound up with liver function. The Plan, which is there (or not) to guide your life, is the mental/spiritual expression of liver energy in Traditional Chinese Medicine. The spiritual alienation of modern man often leaves him feeling trapped in a job or life situation that he hates, and frustrated and angry at the way his ego-oriented Plan isolates him—so he's not a happy "liver" of his life!

In fact, if we were to design a lifestyle that maximally stressed the liver, it would look very much like the urban life of the late-twentieth-century man with his deficient diet, high intake of toxins, and angry frustration. It's not surprising, then, that so many of us are suffering from overburdened livers that are sluggish and struggling. To return them to efficient capacity so that they can keep up with detoxing what is coming in—as well as be available to clean out what's stored—we will need to follow a reasonable diet, eliminate the bulk of toxic substances, and bring our stress level down a few notches. There are medicinal supports that can help, too, such as the herbal remedies chelidonium, milk thistle (silymarin), and traditional Chinese formulas containing bupleurum (see Chapter 1). Supplements, as we will see soon, can also be used to supply the liver with the nutrients it needs to deal with an extra load of toxins.

If your diet has been "normally" excessive in fats, protein, and sheer quantity of food for numbers of years, your liver could be clogged with sludge and stones. Naturopaths stimulate the liver to throw off this accumulation, which is called a "liver flush." I tried it, drinking a combination of olive oil and lemon juice. My book said hundreds of stones would be passed. But despite the most careful scrutiny, I found not even one. Apparently, several decades on a low-fat, vegetarian diet will not yield a bumper crop of liver stones. But if you think you need a liver flush, do it with supervision, or at least with careful reading and preparation. Other techniques we have discussed so far are totally safe, but the more aggressive cleansing techniques we are about to consider will also require a bit of caution (see Fig. 87).

Heroic Measures for Major Housecleaning

Bob and Maureen live in a small house in rural Illinois—temporarily, they say, though they have been there now for four years. The Christian community that they lived in for twelve years went through some organizational upheaval, and they found themselves moving out with the accumulated belongings of those years. Their bedroom is crowded with boxes. So is the hallway. The bathroom counter holds more cartons of toiletries, towels, and medicines. Underneath the counter are other things: a vaporizer that can be used for coughs, a Water Pik that needs some repair, and a large box of bandaging material that had been bought for a scout trip, but wasn't needed. In the living room there are aisles between more boxes that barely allow the normal routines of family life to continue. There's more, too—part in a storage room they rent, and part in a friend's barn.

Maureen is reluctant to get rid of too much. She reasons that without a clear direction and without a new, well-paying job, they may need any number of the things they have stored. Indeed, they may be unable to buy replacements if they were to let them go. As mother of two children, she feels a responsibility not to be foolish and throw away what might prove necessary. On the other hand, she sometimes spends hours looking for things—despite an intricate system for cataloging the contents of the boxes. So much energy goes into managing

---

MAINTENANCE CLEANSING

1. Keep the "big four" working well.
2. Keep the liver in good shape and
       lymph flowing.
3. Keep potential foci clean
       and flushed regularly.
4. Minimize input—i.e., environmental
       toxins and *aama* production.

MAJOR CLEANUP FOR A BACKLOG
"Heroic measures"

Panchakarma
Colonics
IV chelation
Liver flush
Oral enzyme Rx
(Sauna/steam)

FIGURE 87

*the bulk of their possessions that it seems difficult for Bob and
Maureen to see their way clear to move into the future.*

In a situation like this, it's not enough to establish a regular recycling
routine, to make sure that someone is responsible for taking out the
garbage and to take the clothes the kids outgrew this year to a local
garage sale. There's a serious backlog here and we're talking major remedial work! It's time for some heroic cleaning efforts.

FASTING—IS IT RIGHT FOR YOU?

Perhaps the most universal of the all-out cleansing techniques is fasting. Its efficacy is probably based on fundamental body rhythms. You are
designed to alternate nourishing and cleansing. Like inhalation and
exhalation, they work in tandem. When you are taking in and processing
nutrients, you are not geared to pulling out and discarding wastes. You
don't bring out the vacuum cleaner and start the laundry when guests
ring the doorbell. But when the input of nutrition is stopped for a while,

then a flurry of cleaning starts up. The rugs are lifted and the dirty dishes are brought out of the cabinet where they were stashed. Cleaning begins in earnest.

There's only one problem with fasting. Cleaning takes work. The physiologic effort involved in mobilizing stored wastes and eliminating them is not negligible. Not only is fuel burned, but vitamins and minerals are used up in the process. If you supply no energy whatsoever—that is, if you do a water fast—the body may be forced to dig into its existing resources to make do. Then it will raid structural protein and steal vitamins and minerals from the least vital tissues. If this continues, the cells robbed become unable to function and die. Like a freezing man in a blizzard, stranded in a cabin with no firewood—who strips boards off the walls to burn—you begin to cannibalize your own tissues. Though such a scenario may be called "water fasting," it's not. It is more correctly termed *starvation*.

The destruction of starvation and the cleansing and repair that happen in a well-managed fast are polar opposites (see Fig. 88). Unfortunately today, when the average person is overburdened with wastes and environmental toxins, and when reserves of essential nutrients are low because of the ubiquity of "empty calorie" foods, what is intended as a fast may well end up as starvation. Your best insurance against such a catastrophe is to do a juice fast. Juices can eliminate much of the trauma of fasting—as the following story demonstrates:

> Mr. M. was an influential member of Parliament in India. He was in Washington to meet with the Secretary of State. But the day of the meeting, he found that he was unable to walk across his hotel room to the door. Carrying a weight of more than three hundred pounds, he had a heart that was on the verge of giving up. His wife and a friend helped him to the car, and soon he realized they were heading out of the city. By the time he arrived at the Himalayan Institute, he was resigned to "being captive," as he joked, but he wasn't prepared for the treatment prescribed. After examination by several physicians, including two cardiologists, he was handed a slip of paper with his regimen boiled down to two words. I saw him gasp. I walked over and glanced at the paper he'd dropped. It read, "NO FOOD."
>
> This was no small change for him. He had been, he said, "a meat-and-potatoes man." That was more than a figure of speech. The religious background he came from in India was not vegetarian, and generally for breakfast he would have "a large platter of meat and

---

FASTING

- Cleansing
- Energizing
- Exhilarating

Brings:
- Rejuvenation
- Cellular repair

STARVATION

- Draining
- Depleting
- Exhausting

Brings:
- Premature aging
- Cellular damage

FIGURE 88

potatoes." But he would often, he explained, "skip lunch—I'm trying to lose weight, you know." By dinnertime he was famished, and would arrive home to a late but ample dinner of—what else?—meat and potatoes. With next to nothing in the way of fruits and vegetables, and an excess of fat and protein, he was in difficult straits—sick enough to acquiesce to a fast. After three days of juices, I was asked by one of the staff, "What happened to Mr. M.? I saw him running up the stairs to his room!" Running might have been a slight exaggeration, but the change was remarkable. With that improvement, we couldn't hold him down any longer. He was off to his meetings. But before he left, he expressed his heartfelt thanks. Then he shook his head in disbelief. "Nearly three days without food! And what was really amazing—I was never hungry, not even once!"

What his body needed most was a rest from the onslaught of rich food it could no longer accommodate, a generous supply of the nutrients he was missing, and the energetic vitality of fruits and vegetables. The juices supplied all that, so he was satisfied and comfortable. Though his diet changed little afterwards, he remembered what had worked for him and bought a juicer, and when his symptoms recurred, he would stop and do a few days of juices.

Freshly squeezed and extracted fruit and vegetable juices contain a wealth of vitamins and organically complexed minerals. They will also supply the four hundred calories or so that is your minimal fuel requirement. Without that, your body begins to break down protein structures to get it. What's more, fresh juices have a cleansing effect of their own and, as an added bonus, if they are taken immediately after being made, they are energizing and exhilarating. A balanced regimen of juices should be made from a spectrum of fruits and vegetables—those in the evening taken hot if the fast is done in a cold season (see Fig. 89).

Fasting sets off a cleansing reflex. Do it when you can relax and let your energy go into repair and renewal. *Don't* do it when you are rushing madly about, under a lot of stress. During a fast you may discover a slightly altered consciousness that is quite pleasant. That may not be true the first time, however. Fasting more than a day or two can mobilize fat deposits, and, as a result, some of the fat-soluble chemical pollutants stored there will be released. As they enter your bloodstream, you may feel toxic—at least until you can get rid of them. Taking extra water along with the juices helps flush all this out, and first attempts at fasting are generally best limited to twenty-four hours. Even after that, more than three days is not a good idea unless you are in a situation designed to support intense detox with appropriate herbs and nutrients and with expert supervision. Otherwise, stick with a day once a month—maybe two or three days spring and fall.

A gentler way to accomplish what a fast does—and, in the long run, a better way—is a cleansing diet. This is basically a low-fat, high-fiber vegetarian diet that exerts a continuous cleansing effect without the stress of a fast (see Fig. 90). This is the diet that has been successful—along with regular yoga and group support—in cleaning out the coronary arteries so that bypass surgery is not necessary. This diet can be continued until the system is cleared of dross and until weight normalizes; how long that takes will depend on the condition of your body. It should then be expanded to include more nourishing and building foods. If the cleansing diet is continued too long, you will end up so cleansed that you feel washed out and depleted.

It's tough to be objective and rational here. I have noticed for decades that those who come up to me after a lecture on nutrition with questions

---

JUICE FAST

6–10 oz. each,
depending on body weight:

6:00 A.M.	Lemon (honey/salt) water
8:00 A.M.	Grapefruit/orange juice (fresh!) (3:1)
10:00 A.M.	Carrot/apple juice (3:1)
12:00 noon	Grapefruit/cucumber/lettuce juice (5:3:1)
2:00 P.M.	Carrot/apple/celery juice (3:2:1)
4:00 P.M.	Green juice (e.g., carrot/spinach)
6:00 P.M.	"V6 or V8" carrot, zucchini, celery, tomato, green pepper, onion, etc. (heated—not boiled—if weather cool)
8:00 P.M.	Hot herbal tea according to indications (your constitution, condition, season, etc.)

Note: Best to use organic fruits and vegetables to drink immediately after extraction, and to sip slowly. Once you get a sense of the above recipes, try coming up with your own.

FIGURE 89

about how to do a fast are those who are already as thin as a rail and teetering on the brink of a *vatic* crisis. Their more rotund friends have already quietly slipped out of the room. This led me to formulate the First Law of Fasting: "Those who need to don't want to; those who want to don't need to." Exceptions definitely exist, but when you study your own attitudes toward fasting, keep this little principle in mind.

Though many traditions have used cleansing techniques like sweat baths and fasts, the two most developed schools of cleansing therapy have evolved in Europe and India. Perhaps this is because each has had its turn

---

CLEANSING DIET

Breakfast
Low-sugar fruit, e.g., one grapefruit with outer peel
removed, eaten whole

One Hour Before Lunch
Water

Lunch
Steamed Vegetables
(Grain—e.g., brown rice—and possibly legume or tofu*)

One Hour Before Supper
Fresh vegetable juice

Supper
Soup or salad

*Grains soften the cleansing effect a bit; adding the legume or tofu does so even more.

FIGURE 90

at being the center of affluence for the world of commerce and trade. Affluence leads to experiments with overeating, overproduction, congestion, and pollution. It also provides a class of people who can afford the luxury of professional help to clean themselves out. In Europe the tradition of spas, offering the wealthy a place to slim down, "take the waters," and recover their tranquillity, is closely interwoven with the development of the school of Naturopathy. The cleansing centers that developed in Germany in the early nineteenth century were where Father Kneipp perfected his water therapies—a mainstay of the natural approach that moved from there into America.

PANCHAKARMA

In India, Ayurveda's *panchakarma* stands as perhaps the most sophisticated and coherent formulation of heroic cleansing therapeutics. It explains how the disease process can be reversed by cleansing. The *dosha*—*vata, pitta,* or *kapha*—is brought back from the area where it is causing distress to its point of origin—its home base—and then eliminated. *Panchakarma,* because it's grounded in the principle of *tridosha,* allows you to tailor the cleansing process to your unique constitution and your current condition. By contrast, without a way of individualizing, the few Western cleansing approaches available are liable to be misapplied and to cause untoward side effects. Though *panchakarma* techniques are not immune to misuse, the theory behind them, if understood and followed knowledgeably, will protect you from that danger.

The literal meaning of the term *panchakarma* is "five actions." This refers to five basic cleansing techniques, though currently only three are commonly used. They are the enema, the purgative (laxative), and the emetic.[26] My stint in an Ayurvedic hospital included a rotation on the panchakarma ward, supervised by a physician from South India, where this discipline has been most highly developed. (Because the southern parts of India do not have access to the same spectrum of herbs and medicinal preparations as does the North with its greater climatic variations, attention has focused more intensely on the development of the cleansing techniques.) During my time on the ward, we were working on a research project, treating asthma with *vamankarm* (emesis or vomiting therapy). Sticking a finger down the throat of a wheezing child to make it throw up is an old folk remedy, used when no other help is to be had. The Ayurvedic version uses an herbal preparation to provoke vomiting, and we saw impressive results with the approach.

Ayurvedic researchers had found that most asthmatics tended toward low gastric acidity, which improved with vomiting therapy, and suggested that it worked by strengthening the solar plexus fire. In the midst of our series, I evaluated a patient who was, unlike the others, muscular, fiery, and clearly a *pittic* type. I thought he seemed a poor candidate for the treatment. Since he was already enrolled in the study, however, my rather hesitant reservations were ignored. As it turned out, the *vamankarm* only made his asthma worse. When I was commended by my preceptor for having predicted that, my growing confidence in the sound logic of Ayurveda was strengthened.

Vamankarm is designed to remove the mucus from the stomach and, at the same time, from the bronchi (see Fig. 91). In Ayurvedic terms, this is emptying *kapha* that has collected in its home place or *kosht*. What yogis call the stomach wash is a gentler equivalent. It uses no medicine to pro-

---

STOMACH WASH
(to remove *kapha*)

Best Done in A.M., Early, Before Eating.

- While squatting, drink 1 quart plus of salt water (to taste like sea water).

- Stand, bend over, and empty stomach (tickle back of throat with finger).

- Best to empty stomach thoroughly.

- NOT ADVISABLE for strongly *vatic* types, or weak, emaciated, anorexic, or aged persons.

- Best done in late spring.

- Good for asthma, bronchitis, swollen glands, diabetes, obesity, sinusitis, and migraines.

FIGURE 91

voke vomiting, but relies instead on warm salt water, the tickling of the back of the throat with the finger, and some degree of conscious, voluntary effort to throw up. I've taught it to many patients with bronchitis and "gastric catarrh," with good results. But conquering your aversion to vomiting can be a major obstacle.

Ellen was a lawyer who had to speak before juries on a regular basis. But she was often embarrassed by a cough that came from a sort of mucusy rattle in her chest. She called it, not so fondly, her "guggle." We had tried everything to get rid of it: herbs, homeopathics, tissue salts, Vitamin C. I kept coming back to the possibility of learning the stomach wash. She consistently refused, considering the whole idea unspeakably repulsive. But finally, out of desperation, she agreed. I arranged for someone to meet her early one morning before she had breakfast, to teach her the technique. It's not complicated, but it's helpful to have someone with you who has done it before, to provide encouragement and support.

After a few days, the "guggle" began to clear up. She was overjoyed. "Why didn't you make me do this before?" she demanded. I threw up my hands. She laughed. But she was hooked. She continued the practice for years. Some time later she called me in a dither. She was to have dental work, and had been told that afterward she should avoid vomiting. "Do I have to stop the stomach wash?" she asked. I told her that in any event it should be left off from time to time. Though initially it stimulates a positive gastric response, constant repetition could weaken the digestion.

ENEMAS AND COLONICS VERSUS LAXATIVES

Just as the stomach wash and its Ayurvedic equivalent, *vamankarm*, are designed to remove excess *kapha* from its home base, you can remove excess *vata* from the colon with an enema.[27] Adding herbs that calm *vata* is a helpful adjunct (see Fig. 92). Otherwise your enema, while removing the buildup of feces and gas, may also have an irritating effect on your colon and stir up *vata* more. You may also wish to add oil, which soothes the bowel, to the mixture, and if your constitution is strongly *vatic,* you would be wise to follow the wash with an oil-retention enema: Simply instill an ounce or two of sesame oil and/or ghee into the rectum with a small bulb syringe, and leave it there to be absorbed.

But don't do the cleansing enema until *vata* has reached its *kosht,* or "home base," as indicated by specific symptoms such as increasing flatulence and constipation (see Fig. 93). At that point the *vatic* tendencies—the gassiness and the tightness in the first chakra that represents the *vatic* effort to hold on and not drift away with the winds—are now concentrated in, and specifically localized to, the colon. You are capitalizing on the body-mind principle that thoughts and emotions are expressed in the body. Here you draw them into physiologic expression, bring them to a focus, and expel them.

My preceptor of Ayurveda authored a book on the treatment of mental illness by *panchakarma*—primarily the skillful use of this technique, called *vasti.* When I mentioned this to a fellow psychiatrist, he was amused. "Enemas for schizophrenia, that's quaint." Simply giving an enema is not, of course, what we're talking about here. Skillful preparation and careful timing are necessary to return the vatic complex to the

---

ENEMA
(to remove *vata*)

**A Mild Therapy, Frequently Useful
(Contraindicated Only in Severe Debility):**

- One quart of a weak, *vata*-pacifying tea (e.g., fennel), with a teaspoon of salt and ⅓ cup sesame oil makes an ideal enema.

- Without oil and/or soothing herbs such as licorice slippery elm, the enema may be too drying or depleting, especially for *vata* types.

- Lie on your back and insert the nozzle, keeping the bag 2 feet above your body. Hold liquid 5–10 minutes before sitting to release.

- Best to follow with an oil-retention enema (sesame oil and/or ghee)—especially for *vata* types.

- Best done in summer or early fall.

- Good for chronic constipation, arthritis, anxiety, insomnia, sciatica, low back pain, and other vata disorders.

FIGURE 92

physiologic point where it can be eliminated. If that hasn't been done, merely washing out the colon can, instead of curing *vata,* aggravate it. Ayurvedic teachers despair of colon therapists who ignore this principle and end up with dizzy, shaky, disoriented clients who give up—deciding colonics "aren't for them." Timing is crucial, especially for *vatic* patients. A crisis with increasing bloatedness, constipation, and sleeplessness probably suggests it is time to empty the *kosht,* and an oil-retention enema after each colonic is a safety measure.

The process of moving the *dosha* back to its home base so it can be eliminated with *panchakarma* is facilitated by steam baths, which "open up the passages," both physical and energetic, through which the *dosha*

SYMPTOMS WHEN DOSHA IS AT "HOME BASE"*
(kosht)

Kapha:	↓ appetite
	fatigue
	mucus
Pitta:	fever
	irritability
	excess acid
Vata:	gas
	constipation
	insomnia

*But not yet removed.

FIGURE 93

moves (see Fig. 94). Oiling before the sweat bath is helpful, especially if you tend toward the *vatic*. A sauna can be used instead of steam when *kapha* or *pitta* are dominant—but it's too dry for the *vatic* person. After this preparation, cleaning the colon can be effective in cases we might diagnose as arthritis, anxiety, insomnia, sciatica, and of course, chronic constipation.

Laxatives, by contrast, are *not* necessarily the best treatment for constipation. According to the principles of *panchakarma,* you use a laxative or purgative (called *virechana*) to empty an accumulation of *pitta* from the small intestine. In the process, what is removed sweeps through the colon, carrying any retained feces along. But problems arise if you use laxatives repeatedly for a *vatic* constipation. *Vata* is cold. Since the laxative removes *pitta,* you will end up depleting an already weak digestive fire. Unfortunately, that's often exactly what is done by older people. In later years, the body dries up as *vata* increases, and the *pitta* of earlier years is reaching a low ebb, the elderly come to rely on laxatives as a convenient substitute for exercise, water, and a high-fiber diet—all of which require time, effort, and exertion.

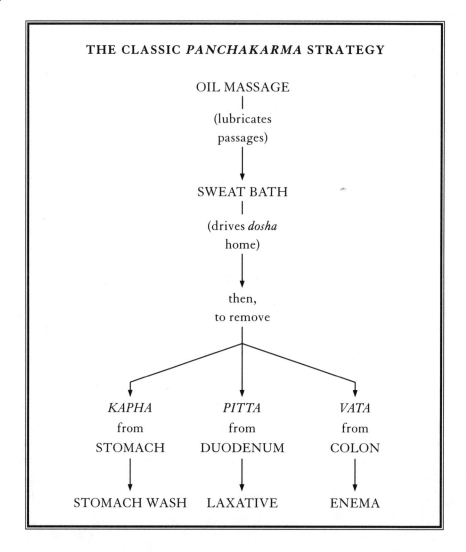

FIGURE 94

FIGURE 94

Strictly speaking, laxatives are appropriate only when there are signs that *pitta* has collected in the solar plexus area. Key indications are feverishness, irritability, and excess acid (see Fig. 95). Here's a personal *panchakarma* story from my own notes:

> *June 14: I've had a cough. I did the stomach cleanse and it helped some with the congestion, but that's not what's wrong now. There's an intense discomfort in the solar plexus. Not quite a burning, but an irritated sort of focus.*

LAXATIVE
(to remove *pitta*)

DO NOT USE in extreme *vata* types, very young or old persons, the weak, debilitated, emaciated, pregnant, or during diarrhea or menstruation

CASTOR OIL (1–2 teaspoons in warm milk with ½ tsp. powdered ginger) is especially good when there is much *aama*.

Other laxatives—rhubarb root, aloe powder, cascara sagrada, senna—are bitter and powerful. Use with fennel and/or ginger to prevent cramps.

Best given in the evening.

Three to five bowel movements should occur next day.

Best done in late spring or summer.

Good to empty excess *pitta* that heats liver and causes excess bile, chronic low-grade fevers, boils, and acid indigestion.

FIGURE 95

June 15: It finally occurred to me that since we had an unusually cool spring, only now has it warmed up enough so that I'm feeling the heat—sweating, in fact. Maybe this is a pittic *thing that has moved back to its* kosht. *That suggests a purgative, but I know, being* vata/pitta, *I have to be careful with the laxatives. They could deplete my digestive reserves. Guess I'll try a gentle version.*

June 16: So last night I took a teaspoon and a half of castor oil in rice milk. I almost immediately felt better—as though something were shifting around energetically. This morning, after a clear and decisive bowel movement, I feel free for the first time in weeks of the cough, the irritation in the stomach, everything! Now I remember my grandfather was known for insisting that everyone needed a major purgative at this change of seasons—as a "spring cleaning."

HIGH-TECH CLEANSING

Drastic cleansing feats are not the exclusive domain of holistic medicine. Conventional therapeutics has its aggressive methods, too. The surgical removal of a kidney stone or a "bone spur" might be considered a cleansing approach—as might renal dialysis. An endarterectomy, the "reaming out" of the arteries (most often the carotid, which helps supply the brain), is another way of removing accumulated excess.

But these are rather crude and intrusive. Chelation therapy, the intravenous input of a compound that can dissolve calcified deposits, is a high-tech but less invasive way of removing arterial plaque.[28] There are a number of other nonpharmaceutical agents that can be used for cleansing. Digestive enzymes, especially when combined with antioxidant enzymes, have been reported to dissolve and promote the removal of the antigen/antibody complexes that deposit in the tissues in such diseases as rheumatoid arthritis and lupus.[29]

But what all these methods have in common is that they are not correcting the underlying problem, nor are they stimulating the patient's system to respond with its own cleansing efforts. They are mechanical or at best mechanistic, done to a passive recipient. This is not to imply that they are not useful. Sometimes, when the condition is far advanced, one of them may offer the only viable option.

TRADITIONAL HERBS FOR CLEANSING

Plant	Heating/Cooling*	Cleanses
Burdock	C	blood/lymph
Cayenne	H	colon
Red clover	C	blood
Myrrh	H	mucous membranes
Trifala	—	bowels
Gugulu	H	blood vessels/ joints

*Heating herbs are best for *vata* and *kapha*, cooling ones for *pitta*.

FIGURE 96

PHASE I AND II DETOX IN FASTING

PHASE I   PHASE II
STORAGE - - - - - - - - - - - - - - ➤ TOXIC - - - - - - - - - - - - - - ➤ EXCRETION
in fatty tissues *(activated by fasting)* intermediates *(assisted by nutrients)* from body
in body*

*Avoiding total fasts (use juices) and providing liver support for Phase II will eliminate the buildup of toxic intermediates in the body.

FIGURE 97

By contrast, techniques that we have discussed from the traditions of Ayurveda, yoga, and naturopathy are designed to provoke or engage an innate urge to throw off the residue of past actions. Natural medicinals such as herbs can be used to prompt this process and, by virtue of their "informational message," may help organize the system's cleansing efforts. They are sometimes divided into heating and cooling categories (see Fig. 96). Burdock cleanses the blood and lymphatic system and, because it's cooling, is good for *pitta* but can aggravate *vatic* tendencies. (You will surmise as much once you taste its bitterness.) Red clover is another traditional cooling "blood cleanser." Heating cleansers like cayenne and myrrh can be used for *vata* or *kapha* types.

Biochemically, detoxification involves two steps or "phases." The first mobilizes toxic substances from their storage sites. Since many toxic environmental chemicals are fat-soluble, when absorbed they gravitate to the fatty tissues of the body, where they may remain for a long time. Phase I reactions convert these substances to water-soluble forms that can be released (see Fig. 97).

Unfortunately, the mobilized forms of the compounds are sometimes more toxic than the stored versions—and they are circulating freely as well. It's important to move them through the second phase rapidly, so the damage they might do is minimized. Phase II hooks these reactive molecules to a biochemical "carrier" so that they can be safely escorted from the body. This step should be accomplished by the liver. But if the liver is unable to keep up, toxic intermediates can accumulate in sufficient quantities to make you feel sick.[30]

If you are carrying a considerable load of chemical toxins when you begin to break down fat deposits, you may find their release agonizing. As a result, you may experience a restless compulsion to eat, even when you're not hungry. Eating shifts the tide back toward deposition and stops the mobilization. While this temporarily relieves the discomfort, it adds another increment of fat. The use of liver-support herbs and supplements may smooth the way, so you can continue the detox.

Vitamin C is a sort of biochemical lubricant for the many metabolic processes going on in the liver, and, along with silymarin (milk thistle), it preserves levels of glutathione, an important biochemical ingredient in the phase-two detoxification processes the liver carries out. Other nutrients that support clearing of toxic substances are pantothenic acid, the various antioxidants, and several amino acids.[31] A combination of tissue salts—*Natrum sulph* 6x, *Kali mur* 6x, and *Ferrum phos* 6x—will be helpful if the excessive demands you've placed on the liver have edged it over into a state of chronic ailment.

Plant extracts rich in the antioxidants called proanthocyanidins[32] may constitute a kind of intermediate between herbal remedy and nutrient. Pine bark and grapeseed extracts of this sort seem to have a potent detoxifying effect—sometimes pulling out such a quantity of toxic substances that the kidneys are overwhelmed. When I tried a dose of 60 mg of a high-potency preparation three times a day, I woke the next morning with a highly sensitive point in the center of the ball of my foot that made it difficult to walk. When I cut back, it went away, but every time I upped the dosage again, it returned. That point on the sole is a major kidney acupuncture point. Despite the power of high-tech tricks to accelerate detoxification, the slow and gradual way is still the best.

Besides, medicinals and supplements don't play a dominant role in the realm of cleansing, merely a supporting one. To expect "taking something" to cleanse you reflects a basic misunderstanding. Medicinals can stimulate and support the cleansing process, but the fundamental and paramount principle is *not* to take in so much for a while, and to provide air and water and *time*. Simply dumping "cleansing herbs," for example, into a clogged, congested system may only add to the clutter. It's much more important to support the natural spontaneous inclination to cast off the old. If that is thwarted for a time, a backlog builds. Be careful—a push at that point can result in an avalanche of emptying out that may reach alarming proportions.

Cleansing Crisis/Healing Crisis

The earliest known writings on medicine in the West, the Hippocratic treatises, speak of a "healing crisis." The Ayurvedic treatment of the subject dates back even further. Thousands of years later, today's naturopaths say, quoting Hippocrates, "Give me a fever and I can cure anything." The notion of a healing crisis is fundamental to natural medicine.

The Greeks thought of the heat or fire of the body as "cooking" the disordered humor—which was, like the Ayurvedic *dosha,* not a purely physical concept, but encompassed the various levels of functioning.[33] This cooking, or "coction" as it was called, was the fiery process going on underneath fever and inflammation as a disease reached its climax.[34] The outcome would be favorable or not, depending on the success with which the inner fire could effect the transformation needed. According to some current German writers, inflammation is an effort to clean out connective tissue, to remove deposits stored there. Bacteria growing in such an inflamed area are serving to create acidity and produce enzymes, both of which dissolve the ground matrix and release substances stored there for elimination.[35]

Western medicine of the last two centuries has had trouble with such concepts. The notion of sickness as a means of feeling your way toward a new mode of being is so foreign to conventional medical thinking that it can only seem bizarre or superstitious from that perspective. But if I can strive to design a computer or build a spaceship, why would my urge to reconstitute myself internally—so as to experience life in a new way—be unthinkable? Holistic schools such as homeopathy, naturopathy, or Ayurveda[36] are organized around the idea of nurturing and guiding such an inner drive to healing and evolution, and clearly recognize that it responds to their nudges—sometimes even in a violent way.

Shifts occurring during the healing process are often personal, evolutionary quantum leaps, fundamental and sometimes "earth-shaking." Reorganization on subtler levels sets the grosser aspects of the person into turmoil. When the Earth's magnetic fields shift, tectonic plates move. When you reconfigure yourself mentally and emotionally during healing, the physical body has to change to conform to a new way of being. Part of that change is throwing off the matter (dross) from your body which reflects held memories and repetitive patterns of functioning.

The dross stored in connective tissue is the physical manifestation of the memories that body workers say are "held in the tissues of the body."

Our bodies have become repositories of the accumulated matter from countless past experiences that were, in and of themselves, not really related to where we wanted to go. It should be relatively easy to move simply and efficiently through the world and the course of your life, toward the experiences that you came here to live through, to reorganize at each step and to blossom as a result of this evolutionary process. But when you are encumbered by physical traces of the past, you are prevented from moving freely into new behavioral patterns.

The matter stored in your tissues is like an incrustation, creating a sort of shell that contains and reinforces the disordered pattern of organization you need to outgrow. In such a situation, even a correctly chosen remedy may not succeed in breaking through and you may well begin to feel frustrated, thwarted, and stymied. Such feelings underlie the suffering that prompts you to open yourself to the possibility of a new way of being, a new internal organization. When your deeper intent brings you through the resistance, and you allow the change to begin despite the physical constraints, then the matter that held you will be discharged in a "healing crisis."

I once saw a patient in Chicago who came in for a minor complaint. He was sold on homeopathy because of an experience twenty years earlier when he'd had lymphatic cancer. He'd seen Dr. Grimmer, an eccentric but masterful old physician, who had given him *Silica* 1M. It was a daring and deep-acting prescription. Soon after he took it, the swollen lymph nodes all over the patient's body opened and began to drain. A copious discharge came out. It was a horrible, disgusting sight that went on for months. When it stopped, the openings healed and the patient had remained in excellent health ever since.

Not everyone is willing to go through that sort of purging. "I have to function in the world," patients tell me when the chips are down and it's a decision between riding out the crisis or resorting to suppressive medications such as cortisone. "Besides, how do I know whether this is a 'healing crisis' or whether I'm just getting worse?" That's an important question, and one that deserves a careful answer.

HERRING'S LAW

Constantine Herring, one of the founders of the homeopathic movement, formulated a rule to guide you in deciding whether what is happening to you is a constructive crisis of needed reorganization or a further deterioration of your health. If healing is under way, he said, it will proceed in an orderly and predictable fashion. The "line of skirmish," that is, the area where the struggle is going on and where symptoms are experienced, will move from within *out*. For example, a patient with asthma may find that as his lungs clear, his skin breaks out. Physicians of the old school liked to call asthma "eczema on the inside." I have seen many patients in whom this progression occurred. The reason it's a move in the direction of cure is that the lungs are more vital than the skin. As we get stronger, we tend to push the disorder out toward the surface. This is the opposite of suppression. I like to call it *expression*. We *express* the disorder the way dirty water is expressed from a sponge. This gets it out where we can see it, as well as freeing our inner world so that we can have the clarity needed to understand and resolve the issues involved.

This expressive move from within out is often undoing some past process of suppression. Many if not most people with asthma have a past history of eczema, though they may be unaware of it. Close questioning usually turns this up. One patient of mine denied any such illness, and when I kept pushing, he became irritated. "I *never* had eczema," he insisted emphatically. I must still have looked skeptical, because he added, "Listen, my mother is coming to visit this week. I'll ask her."

At our next visit, he was shaking his head. "I couldn't believe it," he said quietly. "She said I had severe eczema from *birth*. She spent the first year and a half dragging me from doctor to doctor. It finally cleared up with cortisone creme, and a few months later the asthma began."

Herring's Law of Cure, as it is called, also stipulates that as you move toward better health, old symptoms will return in the reverse order of their original appearance (see Fig. 98). When the asthma goes away, the eczema returns. Herring's Law also offers one more little tip. As your health gets stronger, the symptoms will move from above downward. Early on in my career as a homeopath, I saw a young lady whose complaints illustrated this nicely:

> Sheila had noticed a sort of circular lesion—ringworm is the old-fashioned term—on her ankle. Not wanting to make a big production of it, she bought an over-the-counter steroid ointment and rubbed it on. The ring disappeared, only to reappear promptly on her calf. With another application of the ointment, the same sequence repeated itself—this time the circular eruption popped up on her inner thigh.
>
> At that point she had second thoughts about pushing it any further, spooked, we might guess, like someone who feels a bug creeping up her leg. When she told me the story, I gave her Bacillinum 200C.

HERRING'S LAW OF CURE

The Curative Process Moves:

- from within outward

- from the more important to the less important organs

- in the reverse order of the onset of the symptoms

- from above downward

FIGURE 98

After the first dose the eruption returned to her calf, and after the second, to her ankle. With the third, it left for good.

Herring's Law allows us to navigate seas of symptoms that wax and wane, ebb and flow, and that can sometimes become turbulent and confusing. But what's both fascinating and distressing about this perspective is that the mind is "inside." Symptoms suppressed vigorously enough, the homeopaths maintain, will finally cease to express in the body and cause serious disorder in the psyche.

I remember the first time I heard this notion clearly articulated. I had just begun to study homeopathy, and the principles were beginning to make some sense to me. I was driving back from a lecture with a young physician, and he presented what was, for me, a psychiatrist, a shocking perspective on *my* field: "We have become incredibly skilled at subduing physical problems," he explained. "Our ability to do so has probably never been equaled. We have an impressive armamentarium of drugs that will make the symptoms of disease evaporate. If that fails, we can surgically remove the part that's sick." Then he stopped. "But could that be why we have such a growing epidemic of emotional and psychological problems? Are we just pushing the disorder deeper and deeper until we produce a mental illness?" When he let me out at my house, my head was reeling. Could we have done that? It was a frightening thought.

In the following years, many of the patients I saw provided support for this hypothesis. One of the first was a friend's roommate who was on heavy tranquilizers. His story was sobering:

He had begun with a persistent rash. When it refused to clear up, he was treated with heavy doses of cortisone. The skin returned to normal, but he became hyperactive and began to lose weight. This time the diagnosis was hyperthyroidism. Treatment with radioactive iodine eliminated enough thyroid tissue to return his hormone levels to normal, but after that he developed mental symptoms that were diagnosed as schizophrenic. The powerful medications he was on now controlled the bizarre and frightening thoughts, but at this point, he confided, he felt dead at his core, as though his life were devoid of meaning. "I started with physical diseases, then I had a mental disease. Now," he finished sadly, "I feel like I have a spiritual disease."

Though that picture is pretty depressing, there is one bright light in the darkness. Not everything that is pushed up into the mental sphere has to come back down through the body to be eliminated. Cleansing can take place through mental discharge, too. In fact, that is something we are all familiar with. If you've done your years in psychotherapy, as have so many of us, you know that reliving and reexperiencing old hurts can free you from their effects, at least to some extent. Much of the work of talking therapy revolves around this process of mobilizing and releasing memories of past emotional traumas.

If suppression of physical symptoms has forced the disorder to express in the mind and emotions—then the healing process can be undertaken there. When medicine proper lost its genuinely healing tools, such as herbs, homeopathy, and energy manipulation, and when suppression became the rule, healing work shifted to a new terrain: the mind. Psychotherapy arose to replace the lost art of healing the body. This does not mean, however, that physical measures, such as cleansing, have become obsolete.

You might be tempted to conclude, "If the mind reorganizes, then the body will follow. No need to bother with the tedium of working on the physical level." While it's true that from a holistic perspective the mind is more powerful than the body, and that focusing your healing efforts on the mind is good strategy, it's also true that the physical residues of the past can act as an effective brake. Like a heavy flywheel, or a ball and chain shackled to your ankle, they can prevent you from moving. Removing the physical matter can accelerate movement on other, subtler levels. Otherwise the physical deposit may act as a constraint to the mind's freedom. So our holistic perspective reveals that its best to work on both levels, physical *and* mental.

THE SWEAT LODGE

The nature and significance of the healing crisis was captured and has been passed on to us in the tradition of the Native American sweat lodge. The Santee Dakota tribe tells this story of the origin of the lodge:

> The First Man to be created lived long ago with his younger brother, close to the Great Water. One day, as First Man's brother walked by the shore, the monsters of the depths seized him, dragged him in, and devoured him. All that was left were his bones at the bottom of the Great Water.
>
> First Man went into the water, fought with the monsters, and retrieved the remains of his dead brother. On the shore, he bent together willow poles to make a lodge and built a fire to heat stones.[37] In the lodge he put the bones of his brother, and when the stones were very hot, he brought them in and doused them with water. As steam rose within the darkness, there was a motion. First Man sang and sprinkled more water on the stones. The third time the steam rose, he heard the sound of his brother's breath and a soft voice singing with him. After he sprinkled water the fourth time, his brother stood and walked out.[38]

As is true in many parts of the world, the Native American sweat lodge is regarded as a place of healing—where the older and wiser parts of yourself are guided to bring your inner "younger brother" into new life. This is the reorganization that brings you to a new and unprecedented way of being. The sweat lodge is also a place of testing. There are moments when you feel that you cannot stand it any longer and that you have to get out. Your fears can intensify your discomfort, and confronting those fears is said to be facing your greatest enemy. As you see, contain, embrace, and grow larger than those fears, transformation is under way. Many tales tell of the challenge of passing the test of the sweat lodge. Other stories describe the round lodge as a womb, and equate the experience of leaving the lodge with being reborn.

Sweat was recognized as physically cleansing and health-giving, but it was more than that. Like the alchemist's retort, the sweat lodge was a place where a transformative "cooking" occurred, fusing deep conflicts to forge a new way of being. In one story the Great Spirit takes on the physical shape of a sweat lodge and *becomes* one. "When humans need guidance, they can use me. . . . My ribs will arch over the people and I will hear whatever they say. I will help them when they are troubled and when they are sick."

The sweat lodge is a tangible expression of the intricate mingling of being tested, of being reduced to the mere bones of your life before being guided into a rebirth—a re-creation of yourself—through the ordeal of the cleansing crisis. It demonstrates in a humble, yet eloquent way the connection between physical healing and the realm of the spirit. What is released in the experience of the sweat lodge is the confining consciousness of a limited, fearful ego, and the physical encrustations that hold your body in a form that can only express such a constricted consciousness. Then you are free. The shaman used the sweat lodge to move beyond the limited consciousness of the ego to a place where he could seek guidance for those who were suffering, to transport himself to other dimensions of reality where he could retrieve the spirits of those who were lost, or even to call forth a vision of the future.

To sum up, the subject of cleansing is of crucial importance, but is widely ignored. Though it is almost universally stressed in the major schools of natural medicine around the world, and even emphasized in the great spiritual traditions, it has been dismissed by current conventional medicine. As a result, drugs are pushed to extremes to try to cope with physiological conditions that cry for cleansing. But flooding a polluted body with antibiotics to keep down the growth of microbes is like spraying a dirty kitchen with insecticides to get rid of roaches. Neither works very well, and in both cases you wind up poisoned.

You may find yourself avoiding the issue of cleansing altogether, out of a feeling of helplessness. Currently, environmental pollution looms so large that your personal efforts can seem trivial. But it's important to remember that what you do for yourself is a contribution to solving the larger problem. The definitive solution to the ecological crisis is not merely "cleaning up the environment," but addressing and altering the mindset that has led to the clutter. The current tide of pollution on our planet corresponds to our collective consciousness: it, too, is cluttered. It is jammed with mental garbage that is unrelated to the integrity of our lives—littered and polluted, for example, with random images motivated by the self-defeating greed of countless advertisers.

In the same way that the accumulation of physical dross in the body forces us to deal with what's underneath, what has led to it, so the accumulation of pollution on the planet must bring us to terms with the values and beliefs that underlie our way of life. To change the planetary mentality that has produced our ecological disaster will require seeing within ourselves the microcosmic version of the macrocosmic or planetary consciousness that is causal. The trick here is that because it *is* planetary, it's essentially *normal*—defined into normality by its prevalence. Hence the need for each of us to undertake an intentionally radical course of healing. This, and only this, can get at the root or *radix* of the dilemma. Radical Healing will require digging into the innermost parts of yourself to uproot the deepest causes.

But the Radical Healing this book outlines is not grand and abstract. It is based on the constructive use of every "minor" ailment that presents itself, offering you another opportunity to heal, bit by bit and from the ground up. Your efforts at implementing the techniques in this chapter are not trivial. The shifts you experience in consciousness will be gradual but significant. Study yourself, and try the cleansing tips in the charts and tables when you think they are indicated. When you develop an identifiable condition, look in Section V at the Self-Help Index, which may suggest specific measures for the problem you have.

Like nourishing, cleansing is a basic tool. Besides those two, there is also the art of movement. As cleansing proceeds—as you let go of the residues of the past—you will find yourself free to experiment with how to step into the future, into a new way of being. The time you set aside for "exercise" is your opportunity to play with that possibility—to explore ways of moving forward that are authentic, satisfying, and exhilarating.

Movement
and Exercise

I come home on a Tuesday night. I've seen patients all day and gone shopping afterwards, so I'm tired. But not tired enough to account for the way I feel: disoriented, headachey (though with no real headache), and ill at ease. Maybe I'm coming down with a cold or something. But no, the symptoms aren't really of that sort. I collapse into a chair and think, "Let me get a handle on this." I have a vague sense of déjà vu. Why? Then it hits me: I've done no hatha yoga for four days. That's about my limit. After that, something begins to happen in my body that is uncomfortable. An undercurrent of tension, a sense of being thwarted, stuck—it's hard to articulate. But I know what I need to do.

With no further hesitation, I put a blanket on the carpet and lie supine, my arms together on the floor above my head. After relaxing into this position for a couple of minutes, I sit up slowly into the posterior stretch, reaching for my toes. It doesn't feel good. The tightness in the backs of my legs is at the edge of pain as I lean forward. I am caught between my pride, which says I should be able to stretch farther, and my legs, which are saying "Enough!" I breathe consciously, on each exhalation asking the tension in my hamstrings to release. Bit by bit, I ease down into the posture. This is followed by a Cobra, a Plow, a head-to-knee, and a spinal twist. Twenty minutes of this and I am a changed person. I feel "high"—serene, almost euphoric, and aware that being in my body is now deliciously enjoyable.

I am baffled. Why do I put off doing something that is so wonderfully pleasurable? The answer must be that I am avoiding the initial discomfort and the necessity of facing a backlog of tension and neglect. The more regularly I exercise, the less of an obstacle there is to overcome. Yet every so often it slips down my list of priorities and disappears, and I find myself in the uncomfortable situation described.

So how do we motivate ourselves to exercise? Here's what works for me (most of the time), for my patients, and might just help you: First, maximize the "feel good" quality of your exercise, so it's appealing. Second, cultivate a sense of curiosity about your body and its movement, and develop a habit of approaching them in the spirit of adventure and discovery. To make this possible, it will help to understand more about how your body moves, and what impact that movement has on your emotions and mind. Once that's clear, you will be able to design an exercise regimen that is suited to your unique needs and that you also will look forward to and enjoy.

Life Is Movement

Life flows when you move; it is movement that connects intent and action. The sedentary life is one in which the two become split, disconnected. When you sit for long periods doing mental work, you develop the habit of following a train of thought without expressing what is in your mind through action. This is useful to an extent—it allows for reflection and discrimination before you take action. But it has its drawbacks. Physical immobility risks breaking the link of spontaneity that makes the shift from thought to action a natural, flowing one. Then it becomes difficult to engage joyfully in the process of moving toward your goals and ambitions.

In the early phases of my training in yoga, Swami Rama would often bark at me, "Get up, do it now! What are you waiting for?" After so many years of school and desk work, I tended to stay curled up comfortably somewhere in the recesses of my mind, and found it increasingly difficult to initiate physical action. The spiritual/philosophic tradition[1] that provided the context for my training in yoga, Ayurveda, and holistic medicine put a lot of emphasis on the concept of *spanda* (pronounced "spahnduh.") This term comes from the same root as the Latin *sponte,* which gives rise to our word *spontaneous.* The ancient teachings described *spanda* as a sort of energy of the psyche, a throb or vibration felt in your body that is expressed by your action or, if you haven't acted yet, by your feeling of determination to carry out an action. When you are able to connect with it, you are spontaneous and feel authentic and genuine. When you are disconnected, you feel as if you are "trapped in your head" and cut off from your bodily source of action and joy.[2]

Such a disconnection from your inner spark of intent is at the root of a lot of what we call depression. A chasm separates thought and action. Fears and apprehensions clutter up the space between impulse and expression. It becomes progressively difficult to find your way through all those obstacles to action, and almost impossible to escape a growing sense of uncertainty and frustration. Kierkegaard wrote that depression is what occurs when Spirit wants to move you, and you resist.

What we call exercise, the regular and deliberate movement of the physical body, offers the possibility of cracking the shell of inertia that has developed around us. This initiates a process of restoring spontaneity, of reforging the natural linkage between what feels right to us and its expression in free and creative activity. This can have revolutionary effects on our lives and can occasionally provide the strategic wedge that will pry open a stubborn disease.

> *Francine was a psychiatric nurse from Chicago. She was from a family that had multiple neurological degenerative diseases. Her mother suffered from a condition that had been variously diagnosed as Parkinson's disease and muscular dystrophy. She had an uncle who had died of amyotrophic lateral sclerosis. She herself had been told she had muscular dystrophy. Indeed, her arms showed some muscle atrophy; she couldn't lift them over her head three times in a row, and she had been losing strength and stamina. It was difficult for her to walk more than fifty feet without her legs giving way. Intelligent and analytical, she wavered between feeling empowered by the perspectives of holistic medicine and a lethargic resignation to what seemed at moments like genetic destiny.*
>
> *Though I had seen her regularly for years at the clinic in suburban Chicago, her decision to come to the residential treatment program in Pennsylvania signaled a new level of determination to emerge from this chronic disease. I was happy to see her there, but I didn't have much time. Commuting among four clinics, I had to leave the next day. So I laid it on the line: "You're no novice. You know the ropes, you have only two weeks, so get to work." She was ready.*
>
> *But when I returned she was feeling frustrated. "I can't sit in the classes," she complained. There were several lectures a day designed to*

help patients understand how to manage nutrition, cleansing, exer-
cise. "What do you mean?" I asked, genuinely puzzled. "I just can't
sit still that long," she explained. "I feel like I have to jump up and
run out of the room." This gave me pause. Not that I didn't under-
stand what she said. I remembered stumbling over the desks and legs
of fellow students in a crowded med school physiology lab when I sud-
denly decided I couldn't stay in that room one more minute. I had to
get out of there. But this was different. Here was a woman who
couldn't move, and yet she was complaining that she couldn't sit still!

"So what should I do?" I heard her asking. I had an answer.
"When you feel like you can't sit there, when you feel you have to
jump up and run, then jump up and run!" *I said emphatically. She*
smiled. "But isn't that a bit rude?" she asked, obviously enchanted
with the idea. "It's a prescription!" I said over my shoulder, already off
to another clinic. I was intrigued with the possibility of connecting
this energy for movement with the weakened limbs. It was a hunch
that paid off. When I returned, she had succeeded in harnessing her
restless fire. "I climbed half a mile to the top of the hill!" she informed
me, "And I was hardly tired!"

Though a great deal of attention has been focused on the biochemistry of exercise, I find that what is going on at the molecular level offers
less insight into the essential nature of exercise than what is transpiring
on the level of consciousness and energy. Exercising to generate a dose of
euphoria-inducing endorphins is less appealing to me than exercising to
recover my capacity for free and spontaneous self-expression. Besides, the
world of molecular events is confusing. Even with the sharpest intellect
and the highest level of knowledge of its intricacies, you can get lost down
there. Take a tip from the yogis and climb up to where you can get a better perspective on things. By looking at the situation from the level of
energy or of the mind, the physical aspects of exercise make more sense.

For example, doing exercise is a challenge. There is a barrier to
break through, and though it's primarily psychological it has often
become physical and molecular as well. When you begin to move, you're
likely to run up against stiffness. A great deal of that, especially the stubborn kind that doesn't yield to stretching, may be a result of the accumulation of environmental toxins in the connective tissue. On the
molecular level, antioxidants can be helpful to scavenge free radicals that
cause irritation and damage connective tissue by creating cross-linkages.

Such structural changes in the collagen decrease the elasticity of the ligaments and the fascia.

The accumulation of *aama,* or internally generated wastes, probably also contributes to the stiffness we feel. Stretching might release some of this; more of it can be removed by cleansing techniques. The two work together well. I suspect that moving into an unaccustomed posture stretches ligaments and fascia where toxins have been accumulating, mobilizing them so that they can be removed.

Letting go of the old allows us to move on to the new. The last chapter was about letting go; this chapter is about *moving on.* But again, the letting go and the moving are more than physical. They are mental and emotional, too, and both aspects find a point of interplay in that same connective-tissue matrix we examined in the last chapter, whose passageways conduct subtle currents and store wastes. Now we will see how the deposits it contains, the strictures and stiffness it develops, create an overall shape that constrains and defines your movement in a way that holds you steady but can also, depending on your habitual manner of moving, become uncomfortably confining.

The Fascial Straitjacket

If I ask you how your friends recognize you, you might answer, "They know my face, of course." But they can recognize you from four blocks away—or even on a dark night, when they only catch a glimpse of your silhouette against a wall. Somehow your personality, your character, is reflected in your body shape. Your posture and way of moving are uniquely yours. Let's see how this comes to be.

The story begins with muscle tone. Tone is what gives your arm firmness. Without tone, it would be flaccid and flabby. Tone results from a small number of muscle fibers undergoing contraction. If you are feeling alert and energetic, your body will show an overall tone in the musculature. If you're anxious, some muscles may tighten up more. If you say, "My right shoulder is really tense," I'll wonder what's going on in your mind. From the point of view of mind/body interaction, tension reflects *in*tention. The tight muscle expresses intent, whether you are consciously aware of it at the moment or not.

Let's say you are reading this on a cold day, and somewhere in the back of your mind you picture yourself getting up to go put on a sweater.

But you want to finish this section, so you push the thought aside. You go on with your reading, but you feel the cold, and the intent to get up from your chair has not gone away. It has simply been banished from your immediate consciousness. Meanwhile the muscles that have to do with getting up have developed some increased tone. If the room is cold enough, the heightened tone becomes frank tension. If you sit there long enough, you may begin to feel discomfort in those tight muscles.

Such momentary episodes come and go, and may leave no lasting imprint on our bodies. Those that are habitual, however, may. For example, perhaps your boss criticizes you a lot. Not openly, but in subtle ways. He reminds you of your father. When your father yelled at you, you reflexively shrank, pulling your head down and lifting your shoulders—as though to protect yourself from what felt like a verbal blow to your head. As a teenager, you stopped doing that because it could make you look weak and frightened. Your shoulders didn't move anymore, but they still tensed up.

Now, every time your boss aims another barb in your direction, those same muscles tighten a bit. Not enough to move perceptibly, but a little bit nevertheless. And over the years your shoulders have crept up, shortening your neck and creating a characteristic hint of defensiveness in your posture. You look in the mirror and say to yourself, "Relax!" and let your shoulders drop a bit. But a few minutes later they have crept back up, as though pulled by some invisible force, or snapped back in place by a hidden rubber band. The fact is, that's exactly what has happened.

There are mind-body mechanisms that restore your customary shape. Two forces act to bring your body back into its characteristic posture. The first is the mental—in this case it would be defensive thoughts running like a subterranean stream through the events of your day. That could be changed through insight and the resolution of emotional issues. But even if it were, and if you managed to get past the fear and defensiveness, your shoulders would still tend, for some time at least, to gravitate back to their accustomed position. The rubber band that pulls your shoulders back up is the complex of connective tissue sheaths that surround and encase the muscles. The anatomical term for these sheaths is *fascia*. Unfortunately, re-creating the body configuration that corresponds to the fearful thoughts prompts them to return—just as opening your arms wide nudges you toward feeling openhearted and generous, or straightening your spine bolsters your courage. By popping you back into old positions, the fascial elastic perpetuates mind-body habits.

All the muscles of the body exist in fascial envelopes. In fact, each muscle, however small, has its own little fascial container. All these envelopes are interconnected, one with another. You might imagine a sort of honeycomb of sheaths, with muscle tissue where the honey would be. Because the connective tissue of the fascial envelopes is made of fibrocytes and elastin, they are flexible and can be stretched. But they can only be stretched to a certain point. Then they begin to pull back into their original shape. Elastic, they have a dual purpose: they allow movement, and they provide stability by returning you to your customary position.

The fascial planes of the connective tissue network and the ligaments and tendons that are extensions of it establish themselves around your customary posture and arrangement of body parts. This is their resting point—zero on their scale of movement. You can depart from this so many degrees, but the farther you go, the more they tug you back toward their resting point. If you try to go beyond the range of motion they are designed to permit, you may begin to tear some part of the system. You then experience pain, so you stop.

We might say this network of fascial planes provides a second superstructure or "skeleton" for your body—one that is flexible to a degree but that also holds you close to your habitual posture and way of moving. Because it sustains your habits of movement, it acts, on a physical level, to stabilize your mind and emotions—by only allowing you to enter those positions that will support mental and emotional states that are familiar. So you have a permissible range of motion—physically, emotionally, mentally—and if you begin to depart from it too much, you are pulled back, returned to where you were, like a child lifted by the strong arm of a parent back into his seat.

I often wonder how much imitating the posture of others—especially by children as they're growing up—contributes to creating the uniformity of thought and emotion that are the commonality of a culture. Even more important, how much does incorporating those physical constraints to mind and feeling sustain and enforce the belief systems that give civilization its coherence, but also hold it to a course that may be, on occasion, self-destructive and may contribute to the development of disease?

Sustaining postural habits is a means whereby the unconscious mind contains and restricts your range of choices. The mind has established its arena, beyond which you are not allowed to move. A certain pattern of habits is permitted. If you attempt to step out of that pattern, you are restrained by the fascial network. It prevents you from "going wild." It is, in effect, a sort of connective-tissue straitjacket. Unconsciously you create this internal fascial straitjacket to preserve the security of the familiar—to ensure that you don't do anything out of character.

Many of us have very rigid containers. We are "stiff," we say—an interesting choice of words, since it's also slang for a dead body. In such cases the range of choices open to us is so restricted that the quality of life suffers. A few people are the opposite—so flexible they are amorphous. I once treated a woman who was known for her ability to twist her body into the most difficult yoga positions. But mentally and emotionally she was distressingly unstable. She would weep uncontrollably, and afterward find herself at a loss to explain why. She couldn't set a course for her life, or define herself.

The specifics of your fascial limitations will tell you much about your "forbidden zones"—the areas of feeling and consciousness that are off limits for you. If there are sexual fears, motion of the hips and pelvis will not be free. A collapsed, closed chest protects the heart from being hurt, but shuts off communication and compassionate interchange. With time the bones, which are also dynamic and continually re-forming themselves, will reshape around the position we have established. In healing work, it is preferable to start when the constraints are still largely limited to the fascial network. Bodywork is especially useful here. Rolfing or "structural reintegration" was developed explicitly to rework fascial strictures. At least one Rolfer has devised a system of self-therapy—body positions you can put yourself in to stretch and reshape the fascial envelopes, an accomplishment tantamount to rein-venting (and updating) hatha yoga.[3] Yoga remains, however, a thorough and elegant approach to freeing yourself from your self-created fascial trap.

If you are a do-it-yourselfer, by all means take a yoga class. If you already have, dust off that manual and get down on the floor. Yoga works slowly but gently. By gradually moving a little farther each time into the position, you stretch the fascial planes and bit by bit expand the repertoire of physical positions you can enter. You find yourself walking differently, moving more freely. This implies that you have also expanded the range of mental and emotional spaces you can enter.

Hatha yoga was developed as a preparation for, and an adjunct to, meditation. It's generally assumed that that means loosening up the body so you can sit cross-legged on the floor. Western meditators say, "Not necessary. Just sit in a chair." Sitting in a chair is fine, but that misses the point. To be able to sit for meditation means to be able to have the flexibility to move your *mind* into new places—into those parts of the field of consciousness where you have previously not been able to enter—the areas blocked out, repressed, hidden, shoved into the unconscious. Where the body can't go, the mind can't either—at least not easily.

Consistent use of a few basic postures will go far to loosen your physical constraints and open new possibilities of mental and emotional experience (see Fig. 99). A condensed routine would include one forward bend, one backward bend, and one twist. Lie quietly and observe the effects of each posture after you've done it. Problem areas will need special attention. The rule of thumb is this: the positions that are the most difficult will provide the biggest payoff, because the tightest constraints are hiding the most. Where you feel you are up against a wall, get the help of an expert. Besides Rolfers, there are Phoenix Rising Yoga therapists, and a growing spectrum of other ingenious approaches.[4]

Meanwhile remember that the essence of exercise is twofold: (1) it can spring you from your confines, opening new experiences, and (2) it can reconnect you to your spark of spontaneity and aliveness. The more you use your exercise sessions as a time for exploring yourself, the more of both of these effects you will experience. To encourage this to happen, you need only to be attentive to body, breath, and mind. Most of the rest of this chapter will be devoted to explaining how to do this and what to look for in each of these areas.

Watching Your Body, Part 1. Where You Move *To*

If loosening your constraints so you can move into new spaces is what yoga is for, actually moving into those spaces, actively and exuberantly, is what aerobic exercise is all about. Both are important. The yoga opens you up and the aerobics gives you a chance to move in the world with this new openness. To approach your aerobic exercise with a spirit of curiosity and discovery, you will need a context within which to examine it. That context is the physical space within which you move. We interpret motion in the world on the basis of what it does—where it takes us, and toward what. One simple framework for looking at movement can be derived from the game of tennis. Whether you play or not, the layout of the court provides a perfect grid for charting the meaning of your movements in almost any situation.

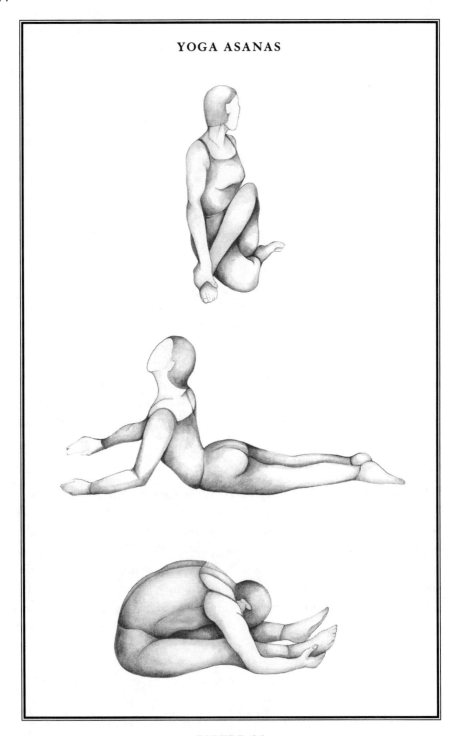

YOGA ASANAS

FIGURE 99

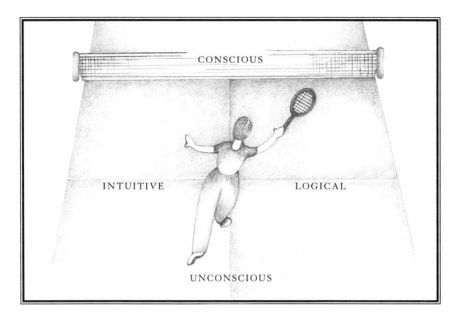

FIGURE 100

Tennis was known as "the game of kings." As the royal player, you are faced with constant decisions and make repeated moves within the context of your "court." When I was learning and exploring tennis, I worked with a friend who held a Ph.D. in linguistics. Ricardo Melo analyzed body language in terms of what he called the "syntax of the court." The net represents the "other" to whom you must respond. The space surrounding you is divided into front and back. That part behind you corresponds to your unconscious; you reach back into it for the depth of feeling that impels you forward. Players who make short stabs at the ball, without a deep backstroke, fail to dip into this well of inspiration. The space before you is your conscious mind and world.

I played tennis once with a young meditation teacher from India. Sincere and guileless, he stood squarely facing the net. He could not remember to put his left shoulder forward so that his right arm could reach deeply into the backcourt. That would have allowed him to extend the racquet back into the realm of the unconscious, where his personal power was hidden, and bring some of that out to propel the ball forward.

There's also a right/left division of the court. The right side is dealt with logically and linearly, while the left, where the backhand takes place for most people, is a reflection of your intuition. When you reach into the space on the left with your backhand stroke, you are showing how you use your intuitive faculties. The very hard-nosed, super-rational businessman will often have a lot of trouble with his backhand. Unusually artistic and intuitive types may find it easier, and may instead have a weak forehand. In contrast to these ground strokes, which demonstrate your ability to *respond,* the serve is about *initiating* an action or interchange with another person.

> *Though my ground strokes were pretty good, my serve was a disaster. So I wouldn't have to deal with it, I avoided real games where I would have to serve. Instead I found a friend who would rally with me endlessly. This sort of block didn't surprise me—it wasn't limited to the tennis court. If I were asked to write an article, I would stumble along through one false start after another. When I finally had a rough draft in front of me, no matter how rudimentary, I could alter, rewrite, modify, and in short order end up with something quite good. My lectures were the same. "I didn't know what you were talking about for the first fifteen minutes," friends would say, "but then you got going and it was great!" Initiating anything was hard for me.*
>
> *Though I was convinced the tennis court was the place to work out this problem, I'd not made much headway. Experts had broken the serve down into its component movements for me, and I had practiced each separately. But it simply wouldn't come together. I felt like a machine trying to go in three directions at once. Then I had a lesson with Terri, a tennis pro in Florida. Sturdy, good-natured, and down-to-earth, she was just perfect for me. "Well, you jes' get so wound up in this servin' business, don't you!" she drawled, laughing. "Try this." She tossed the ball up and executed a simple serve. "Just throw it up an' hit it!" So I did. I was thrilled. I tried the same thing with my writing. I just sat down at the computer and started hitting keys. It worked.*

I learned lots more from tennis, too. My reluctance to bend my knees told me I was too aloof. I didn't get down to other people's level. On the basis of this insight, I took the flower essence Water Violet, which is for aloofness and condescension, and gradually my stiff knees softened. I started listening more to the viewpoints of those who were doing the practical work, and my effectiveness as a leader improved. I am convinced that this sort of work is preventive medicine and that without it I might well have ended up with seriously disabled, arthritic knees. I still take notice when I feel a twinge of pain in my knees, and search out the place where I am reverting to haughty disregard for others.

I also got insights into friends with whom I played that helped me understand the roots of their medical problems when they came to me for help. Measured against the ideal stroke and the optimal position, how much your movements tend to deviate will tell you much about yourself. Each day on the court brings another series of lessons.

Of course, not everyone can—or wants to—play tennis. But these principles for analyzing the spatial grammar of movement are easily extended to other forms of exercise. You might apply them to aerobic dance, for example. Into which quadrants of your surrounding space do you tend to move your body? Do your shoulders and arms actively move into the space behind you—that part that represents the unconscious, from where you might access feeling and inspiration? If not, try reaching back, extending your movement into that space. Are your feet planted wide, do you bend your knees? And what about your hips—do *they* reach back and up, or do they maintain a sanitized stillness—keeping the territory of unconscious, instinctual energy off limits?

If there is a segment of "your space" that you avoid during your movement, that represents a piece of yourself that you are cutting off from your consciousness. In Africa, where the instinctual life has been more accepted and integrated, dancing is freer. The European legacy of stiff-torsoed minuets and a consciousness dominated by the intellect provides a fascinating contrast, and is still strongly with many of us. Free-form and African, Haitian, or Brazilian dancing are especially great for reconnecting with abandoned "spaces." Working with this, you may run up on problem spots that are hard to move into.

After a lecture I gave, a woman from the audience who was attuned to auras shared with me what she had seen. "I saw you surrounded by a bright blue light with no dark spots in it. When I watch speakers, I often notice that they stand with their heads tilted to one side. Usually I'll see a dark spot in that area—as if they're holding themselves away from it— to avoid it." If character is reflected by our posture, then deformities of that posture must reveal those areas we haven't integrated.

Exercise time is your opportunity to begin to playfully approach these avoided and unintegrated areas of consciousness. Let yourself get into the forbidden space and explore it with your body and movement. Experience the feeling tones and/or thoughts or memories or images that are associated with it. "Push the envelope"—the connective-tissue one *and* the mental/emotional one!

Watching Your Body, Part 2. What Part Moves?

If at this point you're thinking, "My God! Do I have to analyze every little movement I make?" Relax. Of course you don't. You may decide that this is the perfect time to simply enjoy the movement of your body or the feel of the water as you swim. That's great! That is full participation in your exercise by all levels of your being—mental, emotional, and physical. But when you find yourself thinking, "Okay, I know I have to exercise. I want to lose weight and I don't want a heart attack like my brother-in-law. But this is such a drag. It's so *boring*," that's when the approach we're sketching out here is priceless. When you begin to get bored, open your eyes to the eloquent language of what your body is expressing.

Besides the space you move *into,* and the way you position your body to do that, there is also the matter of what parts of your body you chose to move. If your chest remains stiff and overinflated when you move, it may reflect an effort to armor yourself and hide your feelings. If your midriff is rigid, you may have issues around control. If your neck is shortened, you are probably feeling defensive.

These regional significances are conveniently decoded in terms of the chakra system. The lowest or first center, related to the element of Earth, has to do with primordial fear—the fear of being annihilated. This could be annihilation physically, by death, or socially, by being cast out of your primary group. We might think of this center as involved with survival—the squirrel or rabbit twitching its tail, looking around to pick up any signs of an imminent attack from behind, illustrates the feeling tone that is prevalent when this center is the focus of our consciousness. The muscles associated with the first chakra are the hamstrings, and tightness there is usually an indication of preoccupation with fear of this sort.

Kevin was admitted to our treatment program with weight loss and fatigue. The yoga instructor who worked with him remarked that he had great difficulty with the posterior stretch. In fact, he had the tightest hamstrings she'd ever seen. Though young and lean, he could barely touch his knees. As he settled in to the program, I discovered that he was terrified. He had AIDS, and was coming to terms with his impending death. When this center is tight, all the yoga postures that involve stretching the back of the thigh will be problematic. In aerobic exercise, the butt may be held tucked in and closed.

The second chakra, the one we have connected to the Element of Water, is related to the reproductive organs and expresses issues around sensuality and your use of sexuality. It has more to do with the muscles of the front of the thigh, the quadriceps, rather than the back side. Tightness in these muscles will tend to pull the knees toward the belly, closing the pelvis in the front—as if you are hiding your genitals. (The bravado of overcompensation in one who is fearful but can't admit it may show up as an exaggeration of the opposite.)

It's when fear for survival and fear of sexuality coexist—which is not rare—that your pelvis can become pretty well "frozen," without much mobility in either direction. Hatha yoga is a systematic therapy for this, as are body techniques like Rolfing, especially if done by someone who is attuned to encouraging you to identify and reintegrate the feelings released by the forceful opening. As we shall see in the next section of this book, work in this area—to gently free up the huge amount of energy trapped by the repression of sexuality—is often critical for any thorough healing to take place.

Stiffness in the midriff is an indication of issues around mastery and control and the Element of Fire. In Tantric symbology, the third (solar plexus) chakra was related to the god Rudra, literally, "he who makes one cry." This center is a focus of aggressive energy—it's the point from which you attack. Attack may be destructive aggression, but it may also be an effort to strip and burn away what is confusing and deluding for you. A lack of flexibility in the solar plexus region is, however, an indication of stubbornness and of using aggression to avoid truth and to exert rigid control. The art of belly dancing requires a profound mastery of the energies here, and its beauty suggests the ability to use one's fire seductively, skillfully, and playfully.

If your chest is collapsed and your shoulders are pulled forward, your back may begin to become hunched. This doesn't mean you have no capacity for the expression of feelings from your fourth chakra, or heart center; it may simply indicate that you are an especially sensitive person and have been hurt before when you opened your heart to someone. Swimming provides an opportunity for opening the chest and concentrating on breathing fully while immersed in the safety of a nurturing medium. Yoga postures such as the Cobra and the Bow also offer you a chance to explore the feelings and thoughts that emerge when you open and loosen up your chest.

The chest can also be overexpanded. The barrel-chested person doesn't exhale fully, but creates a tight, inflated wall of protection around the heart. There is usually a fear here of softening and letting down one's guard. Such folks tend to have a determined pride about them, along with logical, though rigid, standards of how people should act, and they usually place a strong emphasis on performance and success. Therapeutic work with movement and breathing will bring out their desire to be free, and their rigid defenses may crumble into sobs. Recalling the connection of the Metal Element with the lungs and with issues of taking up and releasing, it makes sense that the overexpanded chest reflects an inability to let go easily, while the collapsed chest suggests difficulty taking in emotional vitality.[5]

Creativity is the keynote of the fifth chakra, located in the region of the throat and neck. Defensiveness raises the shoulders, shortens the neck, and stifles creativity. When we're not living up to our creative potential, we become narrow-minded, "bullheaded," and stiff-necked, and refuse to see things from other perspectives. I suspect this stance is what most often leads to arthritic degeneration of the cervical spine. I've found rotation exercises to be very helpful for people with compression problems in this area. It's crucial, however, for the rotations to be done while *extending* the neck. To do this, stand or sit and imagine that you are lifting your head as you rotate it, trying to reach the ceiling and trace a circle on it with each rotation.

Similar rotation *with lengthening* has been a great help with other joint problems.[6] Your joints represent how you connect one part with another to move and switch directions. Scrunched-up joints bespeak a recoiling from forward motion. Lengthening the joints reasserts your willingness to reach into the future toward your goals.

Watching Your Body, Part 3. Where You Move *From*

We've looked at how you move into the space around you, and we've looked at what parts of your body you use to move. But there's another aspect of movement we haven't touched upon, and in a way, it's the most important. That's where you move *from*. From what point inside yourself does the movement begin? When it comes to the process of healing, this is critical. As before, the physical is a reflection of how you are functioning on other levels. The way you come up with the movement of your body corresponds to the way you come up with how to move in your life. Much of the work of the holistic practitioner is organized around getting you in touch with that internal source from which your "gut level" decisions, as well as your bodily movements, originate. But this is a tricky thing to talk about. To get some clarity on this issue, we'll need to explore a couple of basic points about how the body is organized. It has a dual set of structures, one oriented to the outside and one to the inside.

First, imagine an armored fish. This is not some sci-fi creature from the arcane world of video games and Magic cards. This is a real animal that paleozoologists tell us was one of our ancestors. It was largely covered by massive bony plates that protected it from predators. That's known as an exoskeleton—an external bony system that stands in contrast to the internal one. In the fish, the endoskeleton, the central version, consists mostly of the spine. It has little to do with protection, but it has everything to do with the undulating movements that propel the fish through the water. You might wiggle your own spine in a somewhat similar way when you are feeling good, or simply luxuriating in the delight of being in your body.

As the fishes evolved, it is thought, most of the armoring plates were dropped, but several were retained and modified to become side fins or flippers. These were the structures that grew in complexity and detail, giving rise to our arms. In fact, the whole of your shoulder girdle and arms is said to be derived in part from such external protective elements. This is easiest to see in the case of the shoulder blades, where the internalization of armoring plates is more obvious.[7] In other words, your upper extremities originated in structures that were designed to deal defensively with the outer world.

Meanwhile your spine (including the ribs which developed by extending little side protrusions off the vertebrae) originated for a different purpose. It provided the central structure or axis of the body, around which everything else revolved. You might say that this axial skeleton is for orienting you in relation to yourself, while the appendicular skeleton is for moving in relation to the world.

Each of these two skeletal subsystems has its own set of attached and related muscles. Ida Rolf called the external ones "bandaging" muscles— they wrap us and hold us together—and the internal ones "scaffolding" muscles—they hold us upright. I prefer the terms "surface and core" or "extrinsic and intrinsic." During meditation, it is helpful to relax the surface muscles and keep the core ones well toned. Doing this tends to draw the attention inside, where it can explore the inner spaces of the mind and consciousness. If the meditator uses muscles related to his appendicular skeleton to hold himself up, the activation of these surface muscles will tend to bring into play thoughts of the external world and his possible responses to it. For example, using the shoulders and arms to brace creates tension there. That activates the intent to use the arms and, by implication, the hands, which reach out, seize opportunities, possess things, or touch others.

Anatomically, hands are probably the most characteristic feature of human beings. They express our enchantment with manipulating our environment. Imagine what the mind of a dolphin must be like—with no hands or feet, and none of the busy detail of thought they imply. The dolphin must be a paragon of inner awareness—mostly axial muscles, traveling by flexing them and energizing the core of his being! It's intriguing to take note here of reports that some autistic children, who refuse to interact with our world, have been transformed by contact with dolphins—strengthened and reoriented, perhaps, in their inner world by these gentle preceptors, so they can deal more successfully with what humans have created.[8]

Since tension in the extrinsic muscles activates thoughts of the outer world, it breaks the flow of consciousness toward an inner focus. Surface muscles also tend to call into play their antagonists. A tense arm reflects both an intention to move and an inhibition of that movement. This is the physical corollary of thoughts that bounce back and forth between "yes" and "no." The simultaneous push and pull tightens the bandaging effect or, perhaps more aptly, cinches up the straitjacket. Without being anchored in or initiated from your center, your actions are *uncertain*— undecided, ambivalent. Hence they are thwarted by antagonistic muscles. Movement from the center reveals a clear and coherent intent, and the straitjacket begins to fall away.

Yoga postures, originated as a preparation for meditation, are designed to strengthen preferentially the core muscles, those related to the spine. The trick is to do the posture through the use of these inner scaffolding muscles rather than by relying on the externally oriented ones. If you are doing the spinal twist, for example, it is possible to use your arms to push your shoulders around so that you turn at the waist and move into the posture. Much preferable, however, is relaxing your arms and using the intrinsic muscles that run up and down the vertebral column to rotate it. If you regularly do a balanced series of postures in this fashion, you will systematically strengthen these core muscles and create an intensity of awareness along the center of the spine that establishes a firm base for self-awareness.

Strengthening, toning, and balancing the intrinsic muscles will also begin to set them up as "primary movers." That is to say, if your customary upright posture is based on the action of this set of muscles rather than on your body being propped up by the surface ones, then when you move, your body will tend to move *from* this center. This creates a very different feeling from what you will experience when you move yourself with the outer muscles. A sense of operating from this inner point also prompts you to look at the world from your own perspective, rather than relying on the opinions and suggestions of those around you.

Years ago, when I was a medical student, there was a lot of excitement over a line of research done by Dr. John Lacey. He and his wife devised a test that would determine whether you were "field dependent," i.e., whether you relied on cues around you to orient yourself, or whether you took your cues from inside yourself. Sitting in a dark room, you saw, illuminated, a rod inside a frame. As you watched, the objects would disappear, then reappear in a new position. It was your task to determine whether the rod was vertical or not. But it wasn't only the rod that moved; the frame did, too, and there was no guarantee that it would be aligned with the true vertical and horizontal. Sometimes the rod was "vertical" in relation to the frame, but not in relation to the gravitational field—in other words, not *really* vertical.

Some people took their cues from the frame, while others ignored the misleading position of the frame and made their calls on the basis of their own sense of gravity, i.e., their own internal body cues. What was exciting about this work was that those who were field-dependent— influenced by the frame—were the people most influenced by others in social situations. They were hard put to act on their own feeling of what was right. Though as far as I know the hypothesis was never put to a test, I would bet their surface muscles were more developed than their core ones. My work with patients certainly tends to support that conclusion. Here's an example:

> *Toni is a vivacious, talented woman in her forties, who has had scoliosis since age ten. She remembers that she had to stand in ways*

that felt odd to her "in order to be straight." At fourteen she had surgery, after which she had to remain immobile in bed for six months. She attended classes by use of an intercom—a novelty in those days. It was, as she put it, "a disembodied experience."

Toni is also plagued with fears—of cancer or some other disease. "It doesn't feel safe to be in my body—I fear it will turn on me." A talented artist, she couldn't seem to get her energy into her art, and had worked at jobs she hated for the last several years. "Fear runs my life," she observed. "If only I could stand straight and be fearless."

I felt the problem with her spine was her most eloquent articulation of her impasse in life, and that working with that was most likely to pay off. She agreed that her spine was "like it's dead. Is that why I get panicky—because I can't feel *myself?" I asked her to lie on the floor, put her hands over her head with her palms together, and imagine a line running from a point between her feet to one between her palms, straight through her midline.*

She tried for a week, but couldn't do it. "I can only feel that center line if I have my husband trace it by running his finger along the surface of my body. Then I can begin to get in touch with it." This was especially difficult where the spine was not straight. "That place is like a bump that the energy bounces over when I breathe up my spine." But we persisted. After several sessions, she was beginning to be able to maintain some consciousness of this central fulcrum of her body. As this change occurred, she felt stronger. She was able to get the job she had wanted teaching art. We were rebuilding her axial musculature and establishing a beachhead in the sphere of consciousness that corresponds to it.

Without that anchoring in the axial, you can become, as Toni said of herself, "swept up in the mechanics of life." She knew there were things she should do for herself, but to try to get them into her busy schedule just meant making "another list to be obsessed with." Unable to rely on the inner impulse, she had had to "fool herself" into eating or resting or taking time to be quiet. This became less of a problem as she became more established in her axial self.

Arms and shoulders are barely attached to the central structural system. The shoulder girdle "floats free"—almost. Its only point of bony contact with the axial skeleton is the collarbone, which is easily fractured when the arms are pulled too hard. When you are exercising, see if you can position your arms and spine so that your shoulders float effortlessly around the axis of your body. This does much to relieve neck and shoulder pain. It's a statement of your intention to remain centered and let the matters of the world take their course—not to take in your hands or on your shoulders the responsibility of making sure that things go the way they "should."

The pelvic girdle is another matter.[9] Through it you relate not so much to the busy world of manipulation and possession, but rather through your legs to the earth. The lower extremities provide a resilient interplay between your body and the pull of gravity. If your axial skeleton and core muscles are taking the lead in this response to the gravitational field, then your movements will reflect a constant harmonious melding of the earth influences and the input of your spontaneity. As this fusion of energies then flows outward to the surface muscles, your every movement will be infused with poise and grace. By contrast, if movement is *initiated* by the outer muscles, it will seem mechanical. The difference can be seen in dancers. Some are technically perfect but boring; others give you goose bumps. The same is true of skaters.

I once took my kids to Lake Placid to see champion ice skaters from around the world. Their level of proficiency was amazing, as was the intricacy of their routines. But after a while we tired of it. There were a few skaters, however, who jarred us back to attention. They were especially captivating. Even though they may have been unable to do triple turns, and fell more than once, their moves were like poetry. Watching them took your breath away. There was something about the way they interacted with the surface of the ice that seemed inspired. If you looked closely, it seemed as though their arms moved out from within, like a flower opening. I felt that we had witnessed the essence of gracefulness.

You, too, can play with gravity the way an expert skater does, or the way the dolphin cavorts in the sea. Do it when you run or when you dance. Use the experience to sharpen your awareness of the inner core of your body. This will not only revolutionize your exercise sessions; it will prepare you to become your own healer. A clear focus on inner signals is essential to the process of coordinating what you need.

I remember the family of a friend that returned from a trip to India with its own mini-epidemic of dysentery. My friend, his wife, and his two daughters all saw gastroenterologists and other practitioners of both conventional and holistic persuasions. What followed were days of debate about which kind of treatment was wisest, and whether antibiotics were justified. Indecision ruled while bowels ran. Finally one of the daughters decided to take a stand. She put the antibiotic on a table in front of her and said to herself, "If my body moves toward it, I'll take it; if it moves away, I won't." Her belly seemed to tilt slightly toward the bottle, so she started the medication with no further ado. A few days later her GI tract was back to normal, while the controversy (and the epidemic) raged on in the rest of the family.

I sometimes suspect that the connective tissue straitjacket we create for ourselves is intended to restrain those of us who can't be trusted to act from our center. If it's the surface muscles that are controlling us—tugged by suggestions and pressures from the world, like strings jerking a marionette about—then we need some limit on how far we can go! The fascial constraints at least guarantee that we will remain in a predictable and fairly stable rut. But clearly there's not much room for *spanda*, our inner spark of spontaneity, here. Disconnected from our center, strapped in by physical restraints, it's no surprise that we feel a bit down at times. A combination of yoga and aerobics, done mindfully and with an eye to reharnessing our inner vitality, can help bring us out of such a chronic funk.

Otherwise we are running on a sort of fake alternate system—cerebrum to surface muscles—as opposed to going from gut feeling to core muscles (and *then* to external muscles). Of course, the ideal is actually more complex than that. Perhaps we should say "from body-centered feelings coordinated with higher consciousness, to core muscles, and then outward to surface ones." True spontaneity is a melding of our own unique impulse with Spirit flowing through us. Still, a fundamental step in healing is the reinstatement of an inner sense of the central core of your being and a sharper awareness of *spanda*. Attention to the breath is one of the quickest ways to return to awareness of the axial fulcrum. We will explore the complexities of this in Section IV of this book, but first let's see what simple aspects of breath and energy might be attended to during exercise.

Watching Your Energy

So far we've concentrated on watching what goes on in the physical body: into what space it moves, what part of it does the moving, and where in the body the movement originates. Watching these aspects of yourself when you exercise is guaranteed to transform the experience into something quite different from what you've known before. But there are two more areas to keep an eye on if you want to get the most health and healing from your exercise time. These are the nonphysical levels of your functioning—mind and energy.

Some forms of exercise are really exercising the energy body rather than the physical body. These include the Chinese movement forms of t'ai chi and qigong. Here the expert practitioner is aware of the energy body, and of "putting it through its paces." If you could shift your vision to perceive only energy phenomena, you would see something like the illustration in Fig. 101—swirling currents of energy coalescing to shape a vague semblance of the physical body. Without extensive training, few of us can see that, but the martial arts master, if he is sufficiently adept, is primarily aware of that "body." He is moving it, exercising it, and strengthening the parts of it that are weak by using his mind and breath to amplify the currents moving into those weaker areas.

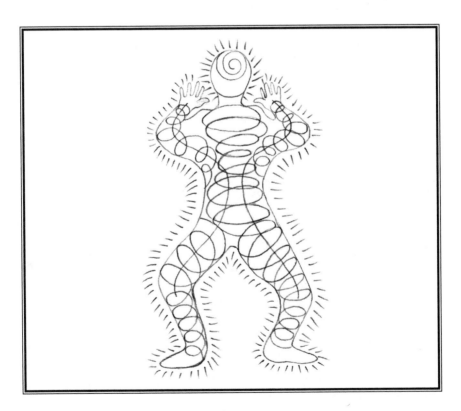

FIGURE 101

That's all pretty advanced stuff. Long before you are ready to do that, there is a series of other more basic points you can monitor with regard to the energy aspects of your exercise. First, just tune into a general sense of your energy status. This is nothing esoteric, it's just a matter of whether you "feel energetic" or not. Do you arrive at your aerobics class tired? Do you feel it's an effort to hold yourself up? If you stopped pushing yourself, would you collapse? These are the initial questions to ask as you begin to assess the general state of your energy. If the state of affairs is critical, you need to bring that up to full awareness.

Unfortunately, you're not unusual if you are in the throes of your own little energy crisis. The tempo of modern urban life is such that many of us run on the rhythm of the crowds around us, rather than on our own awareness of our physical and energetic capacities and resources. Getting back in touch with your center through the use of yoga and other mindful techniques that heighten central tone and sharpen awareness of the inside of your body will set the stage for you to begin to be more attuned to your energy and its current status. Though you don't need to become a qigong master, it is essential to be tuned in enough to your energy to know whether your exercise routine is leaving you energized or depleted. Being pleasantly tired after exercising is fine, but you should also feel an increase in vitality. The juices should be flowing.

If you finish your sessions drained, do something different. Otherwise it's counterproductive. Whether you are replenished energetically or not will hinge, you will find, on several rather simple things. The first is how you enter the session. If you are exhausted when you start, all you will be able to do is exhaust yourself further. This is an especially important point for the *vatic* type—who, in the enthusiasm of the moment, will fail to attend to his shaky stamina. Caught up in his zeal, he will push and push and end up having nothing useful for his efforts. *Vatic* types should take careful inventory of their energy reserves before beginning any strenuous exercise. If they discover that they are exhausted, they should rest a bit before beginning.

The second point is how you pace yourself. A simple run or even a walk can either exhaust you or boost your energy, depending on your speed. Again, this is a matter of most importance for the person with some *vatic* coloration to his or her constitution. *Kapha* types will not be easily exhausted, and need to push themselves a bit to get going. *Pitta* types will have good stamina, too, unless it's hot—or they are. But although the *vatic* person may have to be most careful about energy conservation, this may become an advantage, because she will learn about this energy business and become skilled in managing it. The challenge is to find just the right speed. I learned this on the slopes of the hills overlooking Big Sur.

I had partnered with an aquaintance to climb up the trails that led into the mountains away from the coast. He was an experienced backpacker, and more or less took me on as an informal apprentice. But I felt sure there wasn't much to learn about something so simple as walking along a trail, and soon, in a burst of overconfidence, I struck off, leaving him to poke along at what seemed to me a snail's pace. It was exhilarating to bound up the mountainside, but the fun was short-lived. In less than an hour I had to stop. When my friend caught up, he explained to me how to set a pace that could be sustained indefinitely. Once I did that, climbing felt very solid and satisfying, but I had to watch my friend pull away and gradually leave me behind, promising to find a campsite and wait for me there.

When you walk or run, experiment with the pace. A bit too fast and you will feel progressively tired, a bit too slow and you will not get things cooking. But there is, between those two, a pace that is just perfect for energizing you.

Next, how you breathe is important. Breathing through the mouth is not conducive to clarity of mind or to physical strength and stamina. Aerobic exercise is that which you can do without exceeding your capacity to supply oxygen. A test of whether you are exceeding your oxygen supply is whether you can breathe through your nose and continue to run. If your nose is stuffy, you may need to open your mouth, but if you find yourself panting, you've clearly moved beyond the aerobic range.

Once you get the hang of keeping tabs on your general level of energy and making sure that what you do increases it, you might want to go on to the next step. This is a bit more specific. See if you can notice what *part* of your body is being energized. Though useful in monitoring your aerobic workout, doing yoga is the best way to learn how to do this:

> *Lie down on your back and stretch your arms over your head, letting them relax as far as they will go down toward the floor to align with your body. As you do this, where do you feel the flow of intensity and aliveness? Usually this will be in the head and arms. This is a shift of* ch'i *or* prana *(energy). If you can't get in touch with anything at that moment, continue the posture—in this case the posterior*

stretch—by raising your torso and grasping your ankles (or as far down as you comfortably can). Remain in that position, relaxing any muscles you can locate that are tense.

When this begins to feel uncomfortable, lie back down, leaving your hands at your sides with your palms up. Your feet should be about one foot apart. Your head should be resting on a thick carpet or a thin pillow. Now, breathing gently and regularly, pay attention to what you can feel in your body. Where do you feel any shifting of inner sensation? This way you will begin to identify those subtle currents moving through you that we have been calling "energy."

Notice how the way you breathe affects the shifts of energy. Notice where nothing much is happening—the parts of your body that are blank or "dead" when you are scanning it. Experiment with "breathing into" those parts. Do they "wake up" when you do this? If so, you have discovered how to send healing energy where it's needed. If not, don't despair. As your skill improves, it will work better. In the meantime, you've noted what parts of yourself are cut off from energy nurturance—now you can keep an eye on them so that when they need some special attention you are prepared to give it.

If you've gone this far and want to go further, take a course in qigong or work with a yoga teacher who is attuned to *pranayama* (literally, the control of energy). This and basic pranic currents will be described in the next chapter. Like yoga, many of the martial arts also offer excellent opportunities to work with energy. In fact, the remarkable feats that martial artists are famous for, such as breaking bricks, are accomplished through energy manipulation.[10] Traditionally such knowledge was not shared with students until they had served a long apprenticeship—often many years. Now that seems to be changing, and more teachers are willing to focus attention on the energy work, but insisting that to do it you have to clean up your diet, cleanse your body, and clear your mind. Otherwise the subtle phenomena of the energy body will be drowned out by static and noise.

Athletes talk now about "being in the zone"—reaching a state, after intense training, in which their responses are so finely tuned that they are operating from a sort of altered state of consciousness. Videos show that at such moments a receiver may turn, for example, with no way of having seen the quarterback's position or movements, and reach up to the precise point where the ball is. I shared with my sixteen-year-old son my own experience of running after ten days of intensive meditation and silence. "I could swear that my feet were hardly touching the ground," I confided hesitantly, afraid I would sound absurd. He blushed. "It's happened to me, too," he said, "but I never told anyone." What is the capacity of the human to use the body in ways that are light, delightful, and mind-opening? Though we cannot break the laws of nature, there may be some we've not discovered yet.

Watching Your Thoughts

In addition to watching your body in the various ways we've discussed, and observing your energy and breath, there is a third and last area to be monitored during your exercise. That is the mind. The mind is like a

---

WHAT TO OBSERVE DURING EXERCISE

Looking at ...	to see ...	during (e.g.) ...
1. **Rate** of exercise	whether you overdo or not	jogging
2. **Use** of body parts	how you approach the world	tennis
	whether you use core or surface muscles	yoga
3. **Way** you breathe	how you manage your emotions	swimming
4. **Flow** of energy	where you send your resources	qigong/t'ai chi
5. **Thoughts** and images	how you see yourself	trampoline, yoga

---

FIGURE 102

background television monitor flashing images and information overhead as you do your workout on the gym floor. Check it out every now and then, and see what it adds to your understanding of what's happening. Here are some of the clues you might get from it:

It may tell you that you've forgotten to initiate your movement from your center. If you were tuning into your energy, you might have already picked that up—by the tightness of your breathing or lack of vitality along the spine. What the mind will probably be doing in this less-than-happy situation is regaling you with downer thoughts and images— mostly the usual stuff about what a bore exercise is. What you need to do is bring the point of initiation of your motion back to your center so that you can get back in touch with the joy of movement. It's potentially there; it only needs your attention to take hold and build.

If you don't focus on the good feelings that can flow from the exercise—if you don't cultivate an appreciation of them—then old habits take over. You slip into a negative frame of mind and further lose your center. That increases the likelihood that you'll move in a way that is awkward and *not* enjoyable. Soon you've fallen into a vicious spiral: mechanical movements feed negative thinking, which makes movement more mechanical, etc. Prevention of or cure for this dilemma will depend on cultivating a constant inner awareness.

If you do something that works, something that is increasing your vitality—and that on some level feels *great*—but you don't notice, because you're not attuned to that part of yourself, then you won't feel encouraged to continue. It's of no use to do an experiment if you don't collect any data. Many of our efforts toward good health flop because we are not learning from what we do. You can't learn from what you did if you don't notice its effects on you, and the best information on that is available by tuning in to your inside. Reliable data is collected from what you feel in your body, but watching the train of thoughts is useful, too. It may give you some insights into how moving into previously unoccupied and unexplored spaces affects you. If you play tennis, see what flashes through your mind when you deepen your backstroke, or, if you dance, when you let your hips loosen up a bit more. You don't have to talk about it; some of it may be X-rated. Stretching into a new yoga posture is especially likely to bring up images and memories.

Harry came to the residential program at the Himalayan Institute to work on his emotional instability. He had been diagnosed as manic and was on heavy medication. He learned hatha yoga and discovered that doing the postures intensively had a profound effect on him. "I hold a posture for several minutes. Then I lie in the corpse pose. My mind is suddenly flooded with wave after wave of emotionally charged thoughts and pictures. I breathe through it, keeping my breath steady and constant." He would simply be with the chaos, and when the fireworks dissipated, he would go to the next posture. After each especially intense session, he was able to lower the dosage of his medication a bit.

What appears on the mental screen during movement can be quite instructive. I noticed when doing Nautilus machines that those that required me to pull the weight toward my chest were easier than those involving pushing away—for which I had to change the setting lower. That puzzled me until I suddenly pictured myself pushing patients and projects away, and realized how difficult that was for me. I had no trouble drawing the world to me, but often failed at telling it I needed time for myself.

But that wasn't the whole story; the process went on. I noticed that my bench press wasn't too bad. How did that fit? That was also a "pushing away" motion. As I watched myself, I discovered it was the triceps that was the weakest. The image that popped into my mind was that of sweeping objects to the side with a motion like a swimmer's breaststroke. That's where the triceps is used, and the image brought back a memory of my teacher's voice explaining that you must push aside your attachments to the world in order to move forward. "If you try to swim by pulling the water toward you, you'll drown," he used to say, laughing.

Suddenly I realized that pushing away was not of much use to me if what I was trying to get rid of was still right in front of me. It's the putting aside and leaving behind that will allow me to move on. Then I remembered a healer commenting on some of my physical ailments: "You seem to have trouble letting them go, they keep recurring." It all fell into a pattern. I watched the insights click into place as I observed my movements in the gym and the images they brought into play.

When you watch your mind, you may find that the rapid pace of an aerobics class or the clamor of a gymnasium is not producing the calmness and tranquillity you need. Adjust your routine accordingly. Gardening is a wonderful type of exercise, which, though not for the most part aerobic, has other marvelous effects. It is very grounding and stabilizing. It clears away confusion and brings you back to a sense of the simple verities of life and the basic rhythms your body and mind crave.

When I'm writing I can get overwrought, caught up in the excitement of what I want to convey and the pressure to put it down on paper. When I reach that point, I know it's time to go out and weed or water. It usually takes only about twenty minutes to bring me back to sanity. At first it's a struggle just to be there and do something so apparently mundane. Gradually, I calm down and begin to enjoy it. My guiding rule is to stay in the garden until my indoor work begins to fade in importance, until I no longer feel I need to rush back to it. Then it's okay to go back inside.

Gandhi considered gardening one of the best forms of exercise. He thought of it as exercise for the mind as well as the body. Though he said, "Exercise is as much of a vital necessity for man as air, water and food," he added that "the mind is as much weakened by want of exercise as the body." The life of the farmer, he felt, provided the perfect workout for both. He was not, however, thinking of the farmer who drives heavy equipment, spreads toxic chemicals, and wrestles with profit margins and mortgages.

What he had in mind was the tiller of a small piece of land who lived in close communion with the forces of nature and coordinated his bodily toil with the phases of the moon and the shifting of the seasons: "He knows the state of his immediate surroundings thoroughly well, he can find the directions by looking at the stars in the night." He could tell a great many things from the ways of the animals: "He knows, for instance, that rain is about to fall when a particular class of birds gather together and begin to make noise." He is aware of the subtleties of the soil, and, "Since he lives under the broad open sky, he easily realizes the greatness of God."

Of course, he admitted, we cannot all be farmers. Yet experiencing this coherence, this interconnection of man and nature with its sense of completeness and coordination with the Divine, was too valuable to be regarded as dispensable. "The best thing for ordinary men would be to keep a small garden near the house and work in it for a few hours every day."

Gardening is a priceless metaphor for how to relate to your body and its needs and impulses. My teacher frequently repeated that "animals are governed by nature, man is not." He spent countless hours outdoors, weeding, pruning, planting, and guiding those of us who helped. "I don't try to *conquer* nature," he explained. "Nor do I simply leave it to its own devices. I work *with* it." As I watch my flower beds shift and metamorphose, shaped by a bit of strategic cutting or transplanting, by a choice of what to pull out and what to leave, I feel I am being schooled in the art of working with my own nature, blending the guidance of Spirit with the spark of *spanda*.

Setting Up Your Routine

I know. I know. I promised no "shoulds" or "ought to's." But I did say that routines could be helpful. Think of them as temporary—preparatory. Eventually you won't need them. After doing hatha yoga for some years, I found that when I lay on the mat, the image of the posture my body needed flashed into my mind. When I did it, it eased some deep longing to be stretched and moved. Afterward, when I lay quietly, the next position would come into view in my mind's eye. What you are moving toward is a reconnection with your inner promptings so that at some point you will not have to resort to exercise sessions, but can trust that your impulses to movement will provide what you need when you need it.

This will depend on honoring—not suppressing, denying, or ignoring—what your body is saying to you. We are like a parent who provides feedings on schedule to a child whose communications we don't yet hear. Until we can hear more clearly, we are treading a fine line. We need to try to strike a balance between regularity and spontaneity. I am often asked, "Should I eat on schedule or when I'm hungry?" My answer, never received with much enthusiasm, is simply "Both." With a little finesse you will move increasingly toward listening to your body and organizing your life so that it can eat or move when it wants to. And you will realize with increasing clarity that its inclinations are cyclic. It likes rhythms.

So, with the insights you should have gleaned by now from this chapter on how to make of your exercise something that offers at least moments of fascination and exhilaration, you should be in a position to design a program for yourself that will be both supportive of your physical health and enjoyable enough to look forward to. As you begin to sketch out what this might be, keep in mind that you will need to include both aerobic and stretching exercises. Though they offer different benefits, both are important. The trick is to find some way to make room for both in your life.

For example, your aerobic sessions might alternate between jogging and swimming. Let's say you do each twice a week. Mondays and

Thursdays you jog, and Tuesdays and Saturdays are when you go to the pool. Maybe midweek you take an evening yoga class, but do brief sessions on your own before bed the other nights before a workday (see Fig. 103). This leaves your weekends free—from Friday noon until Sunday evening. Even if you are away or have a lot planned, your schedule won't be disrupted. If the weekend includes physical activities, a skiing trip for example, great; if not, you still have the bases covered.

This is a pretty pared-down plan. It's almost as minimal as it should get—maybe you could reduce the yoga to three or four times a week instead of five. Four aerobic sessions per week is the barest minimum, however. And they're best spread out a bit, rather than done four days in a row. Each should last at least twenty minutes, not including warm-up and cool-down time, and a bit more is preferable. A half-hour session, done five or six days a week instead of four, will probably provide a noticeable extra boost in your energy and sense of well-being. I like to do an additional brief stretching session on waking in the morning.[11]

SAMPLE WEEKLY EXERCISE SCHEDULE

	A.M.	P.M.
Monday	Jog 25 minutes	Bedtime yoga (15–20 mins.)
Tuesday	Swim 40 laps (30 mins.)	Bedtime yoga
Wednesday	——	Yoga class
Thursday	Jog	Bedtime yoga
Friday	Swim	——
Saturday	——	——
Sunday	——	Bedtime yoga

FIGURE 103

Running or jogging is a great choice for aerobics. Swami Rama was a jogging enthusiast. Visitors to the Himalayan Institute were surprised to see the founder in his latest sweatsuit, pumping his arms as he made his way around the grounds of the campus. He offered specific guidelines on jogging,[12] and insisted it was essential (see Fig. 104). The beauty of running and jogging is that they lend themselves to being outdoors—through much of the year, in most climates—and you reap the benefits of natural light[13] and fresh air.

Stretching includes hatha yoga and other techniques that are used as preparation for running or for other types of workout. If you don't do

---

GUIDELINES FOR OPTIMAL JOGGING

- Dress warmly and
  stretch first.
- Run on the bare earth if possible;
  if not, use well-cushioned shoes.
- Set your pace so you can go a long
  time without tiring.
- Nose-breathe (if you can't, slow down);
  exhale twice as long as you inhale.
- Stay on the front half of your foot
  as much as possible.
- Keep shoulders relaxed, head up,
  and fists loose.
- Move arms and shoulders
  with a churning motion.
- Concentrate on what you are doing,
  especially the breathing.
- Move smoothly, rhythmically,
  and with grace.
- Stop if in pain—let it teach you what to
  adjust so running feels good.
- Be gentle with yourself, but firm,
  so you can *enjoy*.

FIGURE 104

regular hatha, then you will need to stretch before and after your aerobic workouts to prevent your muscles from tightening up over time.

The major decision you will face as you design—or refine—your routine is which form of exercise to choose. What you enjoy is a prime factor in this matter, but before you settle on anything, stop for a moment and recall your constitutional type as it emerged in reading Chapter 6. Equipped with that, you will avoid some significant pitfalls. *Pitta* types, for example, will gravitate toward the fiercest of competitive sports, but that's not what they need. *Vata* folks will tend to get carried away with overly ambitious plans, which they follow fanatically for a few days and then drop when they are exhausted and disheartened. The *kaphic* person will, of course, postpone starting, and may never get going without a bit of a nudge. Being aware of which tendency applies to you allows you to avoid getting caught in the usual traps, and can be a vital asset in putting your program into effect.

The different forms of physical exercise can be analyzed in terms of which of the constitutional types they benefit most (see Fig. 108). This doesn't mean that's the type of person who will be drawn to do them, as

---

AEROBIC EXERCISE FOR *VATA* TYPES

- Prone to become exercise addicts and to overdo.

- Exhaustion further aggravates *vata*.

- Tend to have weak joints, therefore should avoid jarring impact sports (substitute rebounder).

- Best is slow, rhythmic motion—swimming is perfect, tennis is good, martial arts, too.

- Sweat baths and hot tubs may be useful to get going when cold and not inclined to exercise.

(*Vata/pitta* types may follow similar guidelines.)

FIGURE 105

AEROBIC EXERCISE FOR *PITTA* TYPES

- Like competition and aggressive sports,
  but they increase *pitta*'s irritability.

- Team sports are best, or activities where
  one competes against oneself.

- Important to avoid getting overheated.

- Swimming, water skiing, and snow skiing
  are all excellent (cooling).

FIGURE 106

we've seen, nor is it necessarily the type that will excel in a given sport. Some of the most famous and successful tennis pros are *pitta* types, but they are also notorious for their outbursts of anger and frustration. Look for an activity that has a balancing effect on your nature. If you're not sure what your constitution is, you can always fall back on the half-dozen forms of exercise that are good for all types. Swimming, jogging, and cross-country skiing are great for everyone, though some adjustments and refinements are best made with your particular needs in mind. The

---

AEROBIC EXERCISE FOR *KAPHA* TYPES

- Need vigorous exercise.

- Tend to avoid intense exertion, but need it badly.

- Difficult to get started, but once going,
  kapha will keep to the routine.

- Activities that push to the limit
  are appropriate for this type only.

FIGURE 107

EXERCISE AND CONSTITUTIONAL TYPE

Exercise	Type Drawn to It	Most Beneficial For	Precautions
Aerobic classes	V *(vata)*	K *(kapha)*	P *(pitta)* can get overheated
Basketball	KV*	K	P starts fights
Cross-country skiing	V, P, K	V, P, K	V will tend to overdo
Biking	K	V, P, K	K needs to speed up, V must set a slow pace
Downhill ski	P, K	P	V gets overchilled
Golf	K, P	V	P loses temper, K excels (but not vigorous enough for K)
Walking/hiking	K	V, (P)	Vata must set a slow, steady pace
Riding (horseback)	K	V, (P)	Not vigorous enough for K
Martial arts	P	V, P, K	Less competitive and aggressive forms for P
Rollerblading	P	V, P, K	Speed and style should be individualized by type
Rowing	P	P, K, (V)	Only in moderation and better on water for V
Running/jogging	P, V	V, P, K	V on softer surfaces
Swimming	V, P, K	V, P, K	Chlorine is hard on V
Tennis	P	V, P, K	V and P do best with doubles

*Mixed type.

FIGURE 108

kapha type will need to make sure he or she picks up the tempo enough to get an aerobic workout while enjoying Nordic skiing.

Tennis, as we have seen, is full of potential and fascination, but *vata* and *pitta* types do best, at least until they are well grounded in careful self-awareness, to stick with doubles in order to avoid getting overwrought. The martial arts provide an incredibly rich experience, but the "harder" forms are meant for the *kaphic* person—not for *pitta* or *vata*. They need a "softer" form, such as aikido or t'ai chi.

With such a spectrum to choose from, you should be able to find just the right thing for yourself, and if you tire of it, to find something to shift to for variation. If for some reason you can't do any of the more aerobic activities, then walk. Walking is great for those who are unable to do more vigorous exercise—for example, during pregnancy. Gandhi called walking the "queen of all exercises." Go out into the fields and forests where you can have a taste of nature, he urges, and a mile or two is not enough. Thoreau, he reports, walked four and five hours a day, and insisted that the writings of those who stayed indoors would be as weak as their bodies.

Gandhi tells the story of a patient who went to the doctor for indigestion and lack of appetite. When he asked for medicine, the physician encouraged him to walk a bit each day instead. But he pleaded that he was too weak to walk at all. Then, the doctor took him for a drive in his carriage. On the way he deliberately dropped his whip, and the sick man, out of courtesy, got down to retrieve it. The doctor, however, drove on without him and the poor man had to trudge along behind. When the doctor was satisfied that the patient had walked long enough, he took him back into the carriage again, and explained that his ruse had been a device adopted to make him walk. By that time the man was so hungry he didn't care that he'd been tricked, and went home to enjoy a hearty meal![14]

So even those who find some obstacle to other forms of exercise can walk, though there are rare exceptions. Some folks can't get up and out. But, as one of my teachers said, if you can't even walk, at least laugh. Laughing burns calories, exercises your respiratory muscles, increases oxygen intake, boosts endorphins, requires no special equipment, and can be done anywhere!

If you're not limited to walking, but find that the jarring of most exercise is difficult for you, try a rebounder. A sort of mini-trampoline, it offers the benefits of gravity opposition without the trauma of impact. Jumping on a rebounder will not only get the lymph flowing, but the tremendous increase in gravitational pull that is experienced should increase bone mineralization and combat osteoporosis. It also exercises muscles that you wouldn't ordinarily use. It seems to be an all around "upper," restoring lift to sagging connective tissue as well as to drooping spirits.

I notice that when I'm feeling a bit down, that twenty minutes of free-style dance on a mini-trampoline with upbeat music (I especially like that of the African Pygmies) will always turn me around. Afterward I feel energized, enthusiastic, and optimistic (see Fig. 109).

From Exercise to Rest

The role of exercise and movement in healing work is central. Exercise takes the body through its paces in a way that is both necessary and enjoyable. The more enjoyable you manage to make it, the more beneficial it will be. Exercise also helps to loosen connective tissue so that deposits are mobilized and can be eliminated. If used properly, exercise can push the connective-tissue envelope within which you exist and stretch it—opening new possibilities for you to move into physical and psychological positions that you have not had access to before. In the process of doing this, you have the opportunity to learn much about yourself—about your

---

"REBOUNDING" ON THE MINI-TRAMPOLINE

- Start slowly (even a few minutes might leave you *sore* the first time).

- Try to hit the trampoline with arms and legs in varying positions.

- Make it a dance and pay attention to moving into all "quadrants."

- Best music is African drums (my favorite is *Spirit of the Forest* by the group Baka Beyond) or Nusrat Fateh Ali Kahn singing Qawwali (Sufi spiritual music).

- Above all, feel the juices flowing and *have fun!*

FIGURE 109

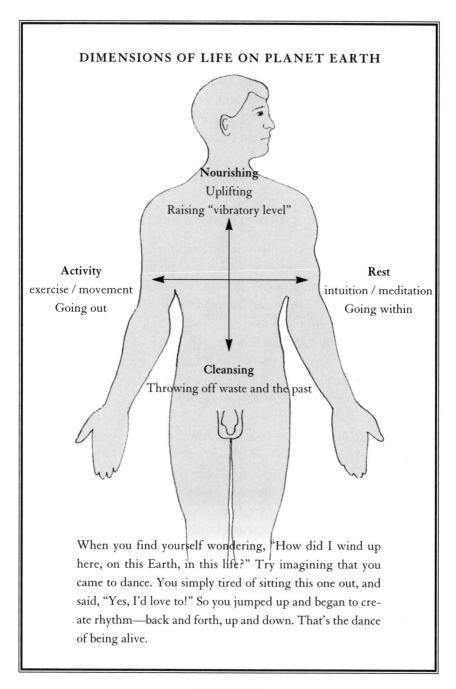

DIMENSIONS OF LIFE ON PLANET EARTH

Nourishing
Uplifting
Raising "vibratory level"

Activity
exercise / movement
Going out

Rest
intuition / meditation
Going within

Cleansing
Throwing off waste and the past

When you find yourself wondering, "How did I wind up here, on this Earth, in this life?" Try imagining that you came to dance. You simply tired of sitting this one out, and said, "Yes, I'd love to!" So you jumped up and began to create rhythm—back and forth, up and down. That's the dance of being alive.

FIGURE 110

fears, your inhibitions, and your potentials. And the techniques and
habits you establish to deal with the movement of your body will serve
you well as you turn your attention to the movement of your mind, or the
movement of your life and the directions it feels best for it to go.

Last and probably most important, exercise can help you get back in
touch with your innate capacity for spontaneity and authenticity. That
spark, *spanda,* in the context of a more encompassing and accepting consciousness, can, as we will see in Section IV, ignite an explosion of healing
changes.

AND THEN THERE IS REST . . .

Just as cleansing is the flip side of nourishing, so is rest that which
alternates with exercise. We might represent the four as seen in Fig. 110.
The bulk of what you do in this life will fall into one of these four categories. The "up" direction on the graph occurs by filling yourself with the
nurturance you take in physically, energetically/emotionally, mentally, or
even spiritually. The "down" direction represents the throwing off, the
getting rid of the negative, the superfluous, the unwanted. Your right
side is active functioning. It's the dimension of asserting your being, of
manifesting—exercise, movement, exertion.

The other side of that dimension, its rhythmic counterpart, is rest. For
every quantum of energy you put into expression, into "doing it," there's
a need for a corresponding pulling back, a time for quiet and for collecting yourself. This is the time when you look inside and reflect, when you
release and relax and go into the inner world. This is the time for rest. The
rhythmic interplay between these four modes of human functioning create a vibratory wave form that sustains life (you might think of the vertical axis of nourishing and cleansing as the amplitude—and the horizontal
periodicity of activity and rest as the frequency—of that wave).

It may seem we've shortchanged the fourth and last dimension—
with chapters on nutrition, detox, and exercise, but none on rest. But
Section IV will explore the inner realm, discuss the importance of reflection, and show how releasing the effortfulness of the external world is at
the heart of healing. But first, let's pull together what we've learned about
foundation principles in Section III.

Concluding Thoughts on Using

Foundation-Stone Principles in Healing

As I hit my mid-forties, I began to have a recurring nightmare: I was a student on the campus of a large university when I suddenly realized that half the semester was gone and somehow, after the first day or two, I had missed going to class. Each day something had come up that diverted my attention and each time I'd think, "Well, I'll go tomorrow." But somehow I never got there. Now I was totally out of touch with the work, with what the assignments had been, and with what had been covered in the courses. Everyone else seemed to know what was going on, but I clearly did not. I looked at my books: I had no grasp of what was inside them. I felt embarrassed, humiliated, and profoundly disappointed. And by this time there was no way to catch up.

I had this dream so many times that I finally made a note and put it on the wall of my study. It said, "DON'T FORGET TO GO TO CLASS!" At first I wasn't quite sure what it meant, but I knew that somehow it was vitally important—that though the years were slipping by, in some sense I wasn't "going to class." Gradually I came to realize that I had not fully engaged in the work with my body. I had not listened to what it was telling me about what to eat, how to move, and what to let go of—either literally or figuratively.

These are the bases of your curriculum here. If you don't deal with these issues on the physical, energetic, mental, *and* spiritual levels, you're not going to class. When you arrived on this planet, you were issued a body. Dealing with it and the challenges presented by providing for its needs ensures that you will deal with the items on your agenda for this lifetime. That's the way the experience is set up: physical plane; physical body. Your body will remind you when you forget what you're here for.

Back in 1975, when we created the Himalayan Institute Combined Therapy Program, the intent of which was to revolutionize the participant's management of his or her health and create a state of high-level "wellness," we set forth a three-point assignment. The enrollee was to spend time every day being aware of each of three areas: (1) how she moved and used her body, (2) how she breathed and circulated energy, and (3) what thought patterns were running in her mind. These are the three levels—body, energy, and mind—on which the four basic functions of nourishing, cleansing, exercise, and rest occur. Here are a few measures that help them along at each level:

	Physical	Energetic	Mental
Exercise	Aerobics	Hatha yoga	Concentration
	Stretching	Qigong	
		T'ai chi	
Nutrition	Food	Inhalation	*Course in Miracles*
	Supplements	Sun/Earth	"Inspirational reading"
		Contact with others	
Cleansing	Urination	Exhalation	"Empty-mind
	Perspiration		meditation"
	Defecation		
	"Washes"		

The term "foundation stones" implies that other treatments—a homeopathic remedy, bodywork, psychotherapy, or whatever—may not work very well without this groundwork. This is the "healee's" part of the contract. While the practitioner brings his skills in homeopathy or acupuncture or bodywork to the healing partnership, you do that foundation work. Even if you are working alone, the principle holds. Don't count on a medicinal to work its magic if you've not provided the foundation. It's in the business-as-usual, daily rhythm of your life where you weave together the approaches that make healing and evolution a way of living—an ongoing process, rather than something that is brought to bear only intermittently when you are pushed by pain and suffering.

Since this is the "warp and woof" of the fabric of your life, both in terms of managing your physical body and in laying a foundation for working on other levels, you might want to assess how you're doing with this and where you need to put your efforts. Here's a checklist for doing that in your own life.

FOUNDATION STONES CHECKLIST

	0	1	2	3	4
Water, 8-ounce glasses per day	0	2	4	6	8
Fresh, cooked, green veggies per week	0	2	4	6	8
Grain/legume combos per week	0	1	2	3	4
Time outdoors each day, average minutes	0	5	15	30	60
Fasting time nightly (hours from last to first meal)	6	8	10	12	14
Aerobic exercise, 30-minute sessions per week	0	1	2	3	4

Total number of
    checks in each column   _____

Number above ×
    number in line immediately at top of column   _____

Sum of numbers in line
    immediately above for total score   _____

Evaluating your score:

        18–24—solid foundation

        12–18—good, but pay attention

        6–12 —need serious work

        0–6 —WAKE UP!

To evaluate your habits: 1) in each line place a check over the number that most accurately applies to you; 2) add the number of check marks in each vertical column and enter on the first line; 3) multiply each of these numbers by the number at the top of the column, entering the results on the second line; 4) add all the numbers on the second line together to get your total score.

Note: This is not intended to be a comprehensive survey—the items were chosen to serve merely as flags—rough indices to help estimate the status of the foundations of your health.

One last point about this concept of foundation stones: Stones, like much of our efforts with diet, cleansing, or exercise, tend to be heavy. You may remember the story of Milarepa, whose teacher required him to lug stone after stone to build a house, only to tear it down and rebuild it again. Though the task was absurd, it finally led him to the realization that busy efforts may have nothing to do with the opening in consciousness that can transform. In other words, he grasped the irrelevance of what he was *doing* and shifted his attention to how he was *being*.

Our work with foundation-stone principles is intended to harness our habit of effortful doing, but in such a way that we move past it, past that overintentional way of operating to a new way of approaching healing— one that is based on *allowing* rather than *doing*. The most powerful healing comes from allowing formative forces to move us into new organizational patterns, new ways of being that we could not have imagined.

In Section III, we have already begun to make this shift in strategy from the effortful to "allowing." With nutrition, you learned to channel your busy mind into organizing supplements and assembling wholesome foods to choose from, so you could then relax, allow yourself to eat what you felt like, and grow in awareness by listening to the poetry of what resulted. In your work with cleansing, you saw how the mechanics of releasing the old and the habits it had perpetuated could allow a new way of being to emerge. In dealing with exercise you devised routines, but only with the intention of using the time they provide to allow the promptings of *spanda* to emerge so you can learn to move with its freedom and truth.

In a word, we are already well along in the process of making a transition from the heaviness of "work" on health to the lightness of *allowing* a healing force to move us into radically new ways of being. Section IV will further illuminate that new and freer world.

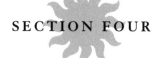

ENERGY AND CONSCIOUSNESS

This is the pay-off in holistic medicine. Playing with energy and exploring new planes of consciousness can lead to new heights of exhilaration and delight. What start off as merely techniques for feeling better become the means to attain high level wellness and ultimately to generate an electric kind of energy that is a ticket to all sorts of creative power. Since sickness holds the clues to your particular blocks to growth, when you deal with illness in the best holistic fashion you "outgrow" it, and find yourself moving into the kind of expanded awareness previously associated only with mystics and spiritual teachers. Holistic medicine is uniquely equipped to use the experience of illness and healing as a training ground to launch into these new realms of living.

Learning how to deal with the flow of energy and the shifting of mental patterns provides perhaps the most important of the therapeutic approaches, the ones with the most leverage for change. But just getting enough distance on our thoughts to see them clearly is not easy—it runs counter to our socialization. And even to talk about "energy" flies in the face of what we have been taught to think of as science. This is not so much due to lack of evidence for its existence as it is due to the different worldview needed to comprehend it. For energy is not a physical, material phenomenon, nor is it easily manipulated by ego-oriented intention.

Working with energy is not based on controlling. It is healed into a pattern of flow that suits you because you are part of a greater whole, a Spirit or Universal intent, that will push for that pattern of flow—if you ally yourself with it. Lacking a worldview that acknowledges this larger Force, the more stubbornly materialistic proponents of conventional science cannot accommodate an understanding of the phenomenon of subtle energy.

Yet, despite the different paradigm required to understand it, familiarity with the nature of energy is spreading. Discussing it seems less strange, and considering it a means of healing no longer bizarre, as reflected by the fact that "energy therapists" are becoming almost commonplace. Such a shift is to be expected, since without tuning into the energetic aspect of your being and making it conscious, it would be difficult to support or sustain the transformation that is the essence of radical healing. For at the heart of that healing transformation, between the opening up to a larger consciousness and the change that occurs in the body, is an energetic shift—a sort of meltdown of an old pattern of energy flow, with the bursting into flower of a new one.

Since energy and consciousness do not lend themselves to the kind of "control" or "management" we may have applied—at least initially—in dealing with the body, the rules of the game will need to change here. As we step into the arenas of energy and thought, it is important to adopt a new attitude, a new tack. Rather than *directing,* we simply learn to remove the obstacles we have unconsciously put up that have stopped energy flow or mental patterns from being reshaped by deeper and larger forces of healing. Because we have long ingrained habits of effort and control, this is not an easy task.

The major blocks to allowing such healing shifts to occur remain the belief systems that deny our potential for change and separate us off in hopeless isolation from the larger forces that both nurture and heal. So in this section our healing work must address the unconscious habits of thought and belief that block access to reorganization, and that create the distortions of function that we have termed *miasmatic*. Such limiting beliefs lose their power over us as awareness becomes more inclusive. The healing force of a more encompassing consciousness is switched on, like a light, when energy is focused at the higher chakras.

The power that turns that light on, and that can energize the most thoroughgoing healing is known in the Tantric tradition as *kundalini shakti*. The energy of this powerful force will need to be disentangled from its unconscious expenditure on issues of security, fear, and sex.

That there is consciousness beyond the ego-dominated field of awareness we generally inhabit is a core principle that links together all the pieces of the holistic puzzle and brings into play the matter of Spirit. By reaching deep enough to catch that essential thread, we can reweave the many into one and complete the reconnection that heals each individual as well as the planet.

10

Energy and Breath

I had long had liver problems—nothing really serious, just nagging aches under my right ribcage. As a result I carried a lot of tension in my right shoulder and my neck. Sandhya had offered me a shiatsu session. As I lay on the floor, I felt her lifting and twisting my shoulder blade. Her pressure was uncomfortable, and I could sense that I was resisting it, but she persisted. Finally I felt something release, and at that moment I could feel a sort of flow of energy gush through the area. "Ah," she said, "at last!" This was my introduction to healing energy.

Your own internal energy system might be compared to a jungle gym. Like a large framework on which you can swing and sit, drop and climb, it provides a sort of subtle structure where your playful explorations can illuminate the connections between thoughts, emotions, energy, and bodily functions. The ancient Vedic description of this system highlights the seven vortices or foci of maximal energy intensity that are the chakras. Most of the great cultures of this planet have described this inner space in nearly identical terms. The Tree of Life in the Kabbalah, as commonly pictured, even looks like a piece of playground equipment! The emphasis on play here is not gratuitous. One must resolve the fear and survival angst that are barriers to a playful attitude in order to be able to access this inner world. Once that begins, however, discovery follows discovery and one soon learns that attending to the flow of energy and allowing it to move more freely can have astonishing effects on consciousness as well as on physical health.

Your Three Primary Channels of Energy Flow

I was on a plane, slumped in the seat. This was my moment of quiet with no telephone ringing, a rare opportunity to check in on my most intransigent patient—me. Running from clinic to clinic and lecture to lecture, wherever I landed there were patients to see, staff to meet with, and audiences that were eager to learn. I was heading to the third in a series of four cities, and I couldn't afford to get sick, so what I was finding now particularly disturbed me: My right nostril was wide open—almost painfully so—and I suddenly realized that on the periphery of my consciousness I'd known it had been that way most of the afternoon. This was not good.

I knew that if one nostril stays open for more than two or three hours, you're bringing yourself to the edge of some kind of difficulty. If it's open for twenty-four hours, forget it—you're coming down with the flu or something. Now my left nostril was totally shut. And the breath in the right one was hot and striking the inside of the nose at an odd angle that was irritating. Moreover, I was beginning to get that feeling of malaise, like "I'm going to be sick soon." I thought, "I can't do this. There's no way I can get through the next three days if I'm sick."

So I shifted in the airplane seat so as to put my weight on the right side. That should have opened the opposite nostril. But nothing happened. I knew I had to get into a more drastic posture. As I twisted into a more extreme contortion, I heard the person sitting next to me clear his throat, communicating, per airline etiquette, that I was overstepping my bounds. This was not going to work. So I retired to the bathroom, thinking, "Now, if I put my left foot higher than my head . . ."

We hit some bumps, and I began to bounce around, upside down, in my little water closet. But I was determined to persist. When I finally unlocked the door ten minutes later and slipped past the waiting line, I breathed a sigh of relief. My left nostril was now open. I sank into my seat, so relaxed that I immediately fell into a deep sleep. When I woke, a half hour later, I was fine. I didn't get sick. I didn't catch cold. But I knew I had been very close.

As we have noted, it's our nature to function in alternating phases: nourishing and cleansing, exercise and rest, inhalation and exhalation. The rhythm of such functions creates the basic vibratory backbone of our existence. These biological rhythms vary in frequency. Some of them are fairly rapid—like the heartbeat or the pulsation of the cerebrospinal fluid. Others extend over weeks—the menstrual cycle, for example. A large number of them cluster around twenty-four-hour ("circadian"— Latin for "about a day") and two-hour ("ultradian") periods of time.

The shorter, two-hour cycles include a number of basic shifts such as alternations between overall activity and rest, and phasic fluctuations in heart rate. There's a similar two-hour shift between right and left hemi-spheric dominance, as indicated by EEG changes (see Fig. 111). The right nostril activates the left brain (and vice versa), and it turns out that all these two-hour cycles move in concert with the breath, as it shifts from from one nostril to the other. And—most intriguing of all—it's the nasal cycle that seems to take the lead.[1] As your breath changes from one side to the other, your mindset shifts from linear to intuitive! (See Fig. 112.)

If you'd like to learn about the relationship between breath and energy, reading about it is not the best way. The field of study is close at hand. Close your eyes for a moment, concentrate on the sensation of air moving through your nostrils, and see if you can tell which of the two is more open. If not, use your fingers to close one and then the other so you can compare. Once you've established which side is more open, turn your attention inside again to see if one side of your body feels more alive, is easier to tune into, experiences more vivid sensations. If so, is that the side with the open nostril? Are you feeling quieter and more reflective, or eager for action?

What psychophysiologists have recently observed about right and left brain functions, yogis had already formulated two thousand years ago. They also specified how it relates to your breathing. The *Shivagama* gives explicit information on how the flow of breath reconfigures energy pat-terns within so that you will know how and when to coordinate your actions with it. The Tantric text says, for example, that "in climbing a high place, in athletic sports or in battle . . . in harsh and hot deeds," the right nostril should be open. This is called the "sun" or active breath, and as it brings into play the left brain,[2] it gears you to act assertively in the world. It also prepares your body to carry out its more active physiologic processes—eating, digesting, or defecating.

Breathing through the left nostril, by contrast, is traditionally associ-ated with the moon (and the right brain), and creates an open and intu-itive state, appropriate when "entering an order of life (monastery), in amassing wealth, in marriage," but also for artistic pursuits, singing, or

BIORHYTHMS IN THE TWO-HOUR RANGE

Right nostril	Left nostril
Logical thinking	Spatial thinking
Left-brain dominant	Right-brain dominant
EEG: minimum alpha waves	EEG: maximum alpha waves
Stomach contractions	Stomach quiet
Salivation maximal	Salivation minimal
Hunger maximal	Hunger minimal
Urine flow minimal	Urine flow maximal
Motor strength maximal	Motor strength minimal
REM sleep	Non-REM sleep

FIGURE III

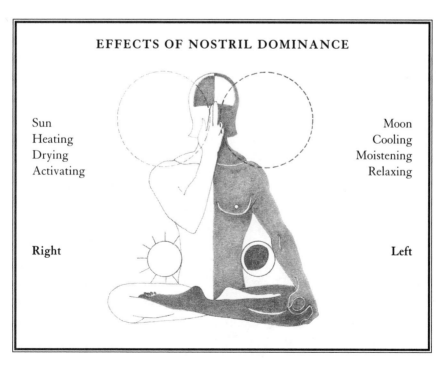

EFFECTS OF NOSTRIL DOMINANCE

Sun
Heating
Drying
Activating

Moon
Cooling
Moistening
Relaxing

Right

Left

FIGURE II2

playing upon instruments. The theme is receptivity; it is best to breathe through the left nostril when "establishing relations with one's people," and even "when the rain is coming."

This concept goes beyond "nonlinear thinking," though it includes that. It's a matter of settling in, receiving and integrating something new. Therefore, the left breath is also best "in disease, sorrow, dejection," when we have to accede to the harder lessons of life. It's during this moon breath that the body processes fluids, when it *flows* with nature, so the left nostril should be open when you drink water or when you urinate.

Touching on so many practical aspects of life, we might be tempted to seize this nasal mechanism and make of it a tool, one that we can apply to control ourselves and give us an edge in our competitive struggles in the world. And to some extent this is possible, but more often it's not. The flow of energies through the nostrils is part of a larger energy configuration that coordinates with solar and lunar cycles. We can, however, bring this complex web of relationships more into awareness, and nudge it back into synchrony when it's amiss, as I did with my airplane water closet gymnastics.

Once you realize that the dominant nostril in use will determine which aspect of your being is engaged, you can move more gracefully through your day. A bird doesn't try to shift the flow of the wind or alter the schedule of seasonal migrations, but it still manages much of the time to soar and dip with freedom and spontaneity. If your breathing gears you to do one thing, but you try to do another, it won't work very well, and you may find yourself baffled by how difficult it seems: "I've done this before, and it was so easy!" Put this notion to the test: Check your nostrils before you eat. If you eat while the right nostril is not open, watch and see what happens. It's a good bet the food won't sit so well.

In fact, even when it's lunchtime, if you have your right nostril closed, you probably are not truly hungry. If, instead, you are breathing fully through your left, chances are you're thirsty. Try drinking water rather than eating. This may surprise you by producing a profound sense of satisfaction and a half hour later you might find yourself genuinely hungry. Now when you check you'll discover that you are breathing fully through your right nostril—and now you'll find that food will taste good and digest well.

I remember telling a couple of friends about this many years ago. We were lounging around a low table after dinner, stretched out on the floor, he lying on his right side, she on her left. They were skeptical about this laterality business—it all sounded pretty strange to them. Then I pointed out that he was in a position that would open the left nostril, and consequently was drifting off—looking drowsy as we talked. His wife was more alert, actively engaged in the conversation. I suggested they each turn to the opposite side. A few minutes later, she was nodding off and he was talking animatedly.

Though normally this nasal cycle is coordinated with daily and monthly cycles in nature, modern life, with its artificial lighting and its insulation from the cues of the natural world, can disrupt that synchrony. The cycle becomes less stable and regular, and may lose its rhythmicity, resulting in problems (see Fig. 113). Fortunately, there are various techniques that can help guide it back into place (see Fig. 114). Change your position, for example, and hang your arm over the back of the chair you're sitting in. In a few moments the nostril on the opposite side will open. As you become more attuned to the flow of breath and energy, you will be able to simply concentrate on the nostril and the sensation of the air moving through it, and it will open more fully.

Yogis, however, do not manhandle the flow of energy according to whim. My teacher once confessed that he often sent students away until later because his breath was flowing in a way that did not equip him to deal with what they needed. When a nostril opens, an energy channel turns on and activates corresponding aspects of body and mind. Being conscious of this mechanism opens the possibility of coordinating your urges and inclinations with the larger patterns of which you are a part. In the co-creative process you share with the forces that shape your currents

---

**PROBLEMS LIKELY TO ARISE WHEN ONE
NOSTRIL IS OVER-DOMINANT**[3]

RIGHT	LEFT
ANGER	DEPRESSION
HYPERACTIVITY	FATIGUE
AGGRESSION	WEAK DIGESTION
ELEVATED BLOOD PRESSURE	SLEEPINESS

FIGURE 113

SHIFTING NOSTRIL DOMINANCE

When you are functioning optimally, the shifting of breath from one nostril to another is synchronized with natural rhythms of the Earth, such as the rising and setting of the sun and the phases of the moon. But since we are often "out of synch" with nature and out of touch with whether it's day or night, artificial forces overshadow such subtleties as moon phases. With the nasal cycle disengaged from natural synchronicity and often erratic, nasal flow can often be shifted deliberately and fairly easily with the following techniques:

LIE on your side with the closed nostril up; after some time, it should open. (How long this takes will depend on *where* in the cycle you already were—if you were about to undergo a shift, it will open quickly; if not, it will take longer.)

SIT with the arm of the open side over the back of a chair, or with the arm and chest pressed against it. The critical factor is pressure in the area of the armpit of the open side. That will tend to open the opposite nostril.

STIMULATE the inside of the closed nostril. This can be done with a tissue, with a nasal wash or in any other way.

CONCENTRATE on the sensation of air against the inside of the closed nostril. Accentuating awareness will bring that side more into play. This requires more mental control, but can be amazingly rapid and effective.

CREATE thoughts characteristic of the opposite side: i.e., think of the hot sun, aggressive actions, and "harsh deeds" to bring the right breath into dominance; cool water, the moon, and quietness and receptivity for the left.

FIGURE 114

of energy, your turn to take the lead is when your right nostril is open. And, like a flexible dance partner, you accede to being led when the left nostril flows.

THE INTEGRATED BREATH

Besides right and left nostril breathing, there is a third option, that brief moment when you breathe through both nostrils equally. As one side is progressively opening and the other closing, they reach a point of equilibrium. At that instant you will tend to space out, to daydream. That's when you're likely to say, "Oh . . . what were you saying? I must have drifted off for a minute." Milton Erickson, a master hypnotist, was found to choose that precise moment, when the nostrils equalized, to step in and induce a trance. Until then he would temporize, making small talk until he sensed this window of opportunity, when the mind was already tending to disengage from the world.

When you're breathing equally through both nostrils, your consciousness is most integrated—it encompasses both sides of you. Tantrists who charted the pathways through which energy flows described three major channels or *nadis* (*nadi* is Sanskrit for "river"). One passes through the left nostril, another through the right. The third is the central channel, and you circulate energy through it when you breathe through both nostrils equally. When you have this central canal open, you should not try to do anything in the outside world. It won't work, it is said. We engage the world around us either by acting assertively or by being receptive. Those are the ways we "plug in"—like the ends of an extension cord that must connect one way or the other. When neither nostril predominates, you're not suited to interact—you'll screw it up, step in front of a car while trying to cross the street, perhaps. But such a time has its own value. It is a moment when you are geared to look inside and understand yourself, to grasp your totality.

This is of such central importance to matters of healing that the oldest symbol of medicine in the West, the caduceus, is based on a depiction of the two lateral channels winding about the central one. They cross at each chakra and end at the sixth—where the two petals that traditionally represent the third eye emphasize the integrated awareness needed to provide a healing insight (see Fig. 115). The crisscrossing reflects how the energy moves away from center as it is drawn into expressing the conflicting impulses of polarization. The convergence at each chakra sug-

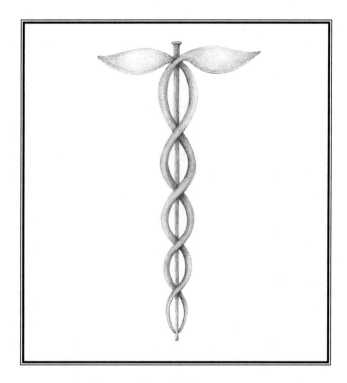

FIGURE 115

gests that it is at these points where there are opportunities for one step after another of resolution and reconnection with a centering sense of the universal.

If your breath seems to you one more thing to deal with, another burdensome responsibility to keep up with, don't feel bad. That's not an unusual initial response. Decades ago, when there was a first flurry of interest in holistic healing, I was invited to appear on national television. After a station break, the director informed us that 14 million people would be watching the show. At that moment the red light came on the camera moving toward me, indicating it was live, and the host, Phil Donahue, sauntered over and asked, "What is this about breath? Do you really expect us to pay attention to how we are breathing all the time?"

My heart pounding, I heard myself answer, "Coordinating your breath shouldn't disrupt your life. You just walked over here, didn't you—perfectly aware of where your legs were, it seems, and managed them nicely. But using your legs didn't distract you from asking me that question. Why can't your breath be a part of your awareness, too?" He smiled, and so did I. His smile was because he made a living challenging guests and liked a snappy response. My smile was because I was watching my breath, riding on its rhythms—and realizing that doing so was what had enabled me to answer his question calmly, instead of being overwhelmed by the anxiety that threatened to engulf me.

THE ANTI-ANXIETY BREATH

The basis of all breath work is diaphragmatic breathing. It is the key to entering the calm, introspective state that will allow you to study effectively the subtler inner world. In over twenty years of teaching classes on breath and energy, however, I find that this subject is usually not understood. Diaphragmatic breathing is done with the middle of the torso— where the diaphragm is. It should be distinguished from belly breathing, where the movement is further down, and chest breathing, where the major motion is up higher.

This is not to say that diaphragmatic breathing is "the right way" to breathe. Just as it would be absurd to ask what is the correct way to move your legs, there is no right or wrong way to breathe. It depends on where you want to go. Each way of breathing has its special energetic effects. In other words, there's a right way to breathe to carry out a certain action or to enter a specific state of consciousness. Diaphragmatic breathing is just one of those ways of breathing, but what makes it special is that it's the breathing pattern that corresponds to a tranquil state of mind.

Moving the most breath with the least effort, diaphragmatic breathing involves a gentle expansion at the midriff that is quieting and calming. How it affects emotions might be understood physiologically if we look at the impact of breath on the autonomic nervous system, which gears you up (sympathetic) or down (parasympathetic). For example, chest breathing creates sympathetic arousal: By design, the chest is drawn strongly into action only when unusually large amounts of air are needed—during exertion, for example, or in emergencies. Breathing primarily with the chest tends to set off a chain of physiologic events that say: "Prepare yourself, something's about to happen!" Belly breathing, with movement at the other extreme of the torso, arouses the energies of the lower chakras, and is therefore a technique that can be very valuable in certain kinds of therapeutic work where you want to bring into play suppressed memories or feelings associated with those centers.

Otto Schmidt, a brilliant biophysicist, once put it this way: "If the autonomic nervous system is the gear box that moves us into one state of readiness or another, breathing is the gearshift, the lever we grasp to shift from

INSTANT TRANQUILLITY:
Correct Diaphragmatic Breathing

The dome of the diaphragm isn't muscle at all, but a sheet of fascia or connective tissue. Picture it like an old-fashioned fringed lampshade—the shade being the dome of the diaphragm and its fringe the muscle fibers that run vertically, lying against the wall of the chest.

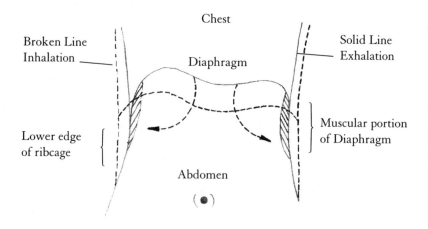

When you inhale, the muscle fibers contract, lowering the whole dome, but changing its shape very little. As the diaphragmatic muscles lower the dome, the abdominal contents are compressed. Since they can't be pushed through the pelvic floor or through the back, which forms a rigid wall to the rear, they may force the belly out as you inhale. This is abdominal or belly breathing, but it's not diaphragmatic.[4]

But if the belly is restrained, then the force is transmitted to the lower edges of the rib cage (arrows) which are pushed outward and, *voila!*—the diaphragm *expands* in diameter as a result of *contracting* its muscle fibers! You can hold the belly in place by contracting your lower abdominals as you inhale or by lying on a firm surface (like the floor) with your forehead resting on your crossed arms. Another technique is to put a sandbag on the belly.

FIGURE 116

one of those states to the next." The pattern of function that diaphragmatic breathing draws into being is one of calmness and tranquillity. Emotional storms, on the other hand, involve dramatic agitation in the autonomic system. This means that if you feel an emotion developing, you can cut through it by deliberately instituting a pattern of diaphragmatic breathing. Here, then, is the leverage needed to be able to explore fearlessly the feelings and conflicts encoded deep in the energetic complexes of the chakras.

From another angle, diaphragmatic breathing is a matter of relaxation and release. It is the least effortful kind of breathing, and by releasing the blocks to it, we reconnect with the larger pool of energy and nurturance that sustains. It is not something to "do" as much as something that happens when you *stop* doing. Over the years, I have taught diaphragmatic breathing to a majority of my patients, convinced that it is a foundation for deep healing work of all kinds.

Because we all have habits of tension that interfere with full diaphragmatic breathing, it is helpful to understand exactly how it works. Unfortunately, the mechanics of correct diaphragmatic breathing are not so obvious as generally assumed. For example, when I ask a class—even those medically trained—whether the diaphragm expands or contracts on inhalation, I get a variety of answers, but usually none that are totally correct. In fact, in a sense—though you might think this impossible—it does both. At the very moment the diaphragm contracts, paradoxically, its diameter increases too. Study Fig. 116 carefully, and you'll see how this can happen. (Without that expansion of the lower rib cage, it's not really diaphragmatic breathing.)

In the lucid, quiet, anxiety-free state induced by correct diaphragmatic breathing, you can explore the energy body much more easily.

BREATH AND ENERGY

The flow of breath is not the same as the flow of energy. There's not a precise one-to-one relationship, but they are roughly congruent—as one moves, the other tends to follow. To get the picture, imagine that your shadow is only loosely connected to your body. When you move, it sometimes catches up with you, but sometimes it lags instead, or slips away.

The yogis like to compare life energy or *prana* to a kite. Your breath is the string you hold that influences its course. But the wind is the natural force pushing it along. If you blend your breathing skillfully with the universe's intent, your energy will dance and soar. If you become over-controlling, it may go where you didn't intend—or even crash to the ground. You can cultivate that delicate congruence between the breath and energy flow by being relaxed and attentive, but by not making an effort to control. Biofeedback therapists call this "passive volition." In fact, training with EMG (muscle) biofeedback is great preparation for breath work. If you try too hard to relax the muscles, they only tense up and the machine beeps louder. Finally, when you say, "Oh, forget it. This isn't working!" then they relax and the biofeedback device lets you know with a slower, quieter signal.

Once you step beyond the physical, you'll find that your greatest power is in allowing, not forcing. The attitude that you cultivate here will carry over and serve you well in many phases of the healing process. Working with the breath brings you back repeatedly to the necessity of letting it flow. Can you focus your attention intensively as you let go of your control totally? That's the challenge here. When you manage to do that—focus, allow, release—your mind starts to move the energy very nicely. What you will discover then is that there are ways of moving energy without using the breath at all—where the mind itself does the work by imagining and allowing.

If you become skilled in shifting the position of the body and the motion of the lungs and also in creating specific images in your mind, and if you align yourself with the universal intent (the level of Spirit), then you can make the energy go anywhere "you" wish—through your hands, for example. This is how Reiki is done, or other forms of energy healing in which the *prana* or *ch'i* is extended outward to heal another.

Words get confusing here because, as we enter the realm of subtleties, the rules change. Forceful control through actions dictated by the ego-dominated mind is possible only on the physical level. As we move into working with energy, effort and force can be counterproductive. We must constantly remind ourselves that here we *allow* rather than manipulate or control. We can remove obstacles to the flow of energy by noting tension and releasing it, and, perhaps more important, by becoming aware of our unfortunate conviction that we are separate from the larger Spirit and its healing intent, and releasing *that*.

PRIMARY PRANIC CURRENTS AND THE BREATH

As a first step to getting acquainted with your energy body, try tuning in to overall shifts—the widely sweeping currents that are easy to

pick up. This isn't something weird, nor is it only the psychically en-
dowed who can perceive it. It's something you already feel; you've just
been trained to shove it to the side and ignore it. But the sensations of
aliveness and of energizing that come and go with the movements of the
breath are always there, on the periphery of your consciousness. We just
want to bring them into sharper focus.

Traditionally, the yogis count five of these currents, which they call
pranas or *vayus* (*vayu* means "flow"[5]; see Figs. 117 and 118). Each might
be noticed as a certain intensity of awareness in a specific area. Most dramatic is the sense of energy swelling upward that you create as you
inhale. This is considered the most important of the five *pranas* and is
therefore, itself, called *prana vayu*.

To become aware of how you are prompting this upsurge of energy
with your inhalation, lie quietly in a relaxed position and follow with
your mind's eye up the spine as you breathe in (see Fig. 119). Don't try to
make something happen. Just be available to notice what is occurring.
When you try to move or direct the energy, your intention creates tension
that blocks free energy flow. (As we learned in the last chapter, the intent
to do something activates the muscles that we would use in our effortful
attempt to act. But that very tension can obstruct the movement of the
current.)

If, on the other hand, you relinquish the goal of making the energy
move, relax, and sweep up the spine with your attention, the movement
along that path will be encouraged and strengthened. But don't make the
mistake of thinking, "Ah! I moved the energy!" or all your "doing in the
world" muscles will immediately tighten up, and the flow will stop. In
some inscrutable way, awareness and flow seem to supersede cause and
effect.

What you may feel as you tune in to the effects of inhalation is a sort
of filling yourself with energy nurturance. You are vitalized and
uplifted—*inspired,* we might say—as the in-breath proceeds. Watch what
happens in the rest of the body at the same time. Most often the energizing effect will spread out to all parts, but it especially moves up. This will
become valuable when you want to support the upward shift of energy to
activate higher chakras, as we will describe in the pages that follow.

The upward tendency is not so much a matter of energy moving up
from below; it's more like you're filling a glass: it's filled first at the bottom and then on up to the top. The air itself moves in a different direction. It comes in your nose and *down* into your lungs, but we're not

MAIN ENERGETIC CURRENTS

Direction of motion	Function served	Ayurvedic name	Associated element
In and up	Nourishing	*Prana vayu**	Air
Down	Throwing off	*Apana vayu*	Earth
At navel	↑ Fire	*Samana vayu*	Fire
Up and out	Expressing	*Udana vayu*	Ether
Centripetal/centrifugal	Cohering	*Vyana vayu*	Water

*This is considered the most important of the five *prana*s and is therefore itself called *prana* and, making matters even more confusing, often *prana vayu*—to distinguish it from the generic use of the term *prana*—but resulting in a sort of redundancy, since the terms *prana* and *vayu* are so close in meaning!

FIGURE 117

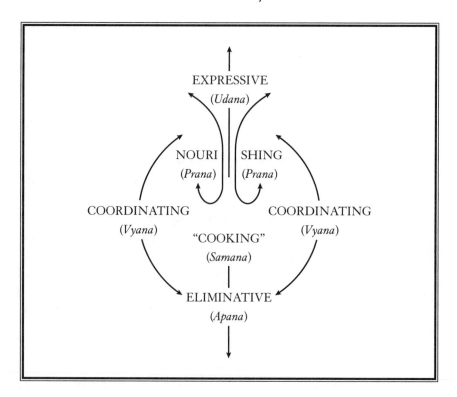

FIGURE 118

talking about the motion of the air. Instead we're looking at the flow of energy that results from that incoming air, and the energizing effect created has an upward lift to it.

When Roy lay on the table, he looked even thinner and tenser than he had sitting up. He was troubled with a tight jaw, and he complained that he didn't assimilate his food well. His breathing was shallow and taut, and attempts to take a full breath were only partially

---

ENERGY AWARENESS
(This is an exercise for tuning in to subtle energy.)

You need to be in a place where you're not distracted by
outside noises and disruptions.

Find a position where you can relax your muscles
—lying on your back on a firm surface,
with your head cushioned, is ideal.

After going through a brief inventory of your body,
releasing tension in those areas that are tight,
begin to focus on the breath.

Extend your exhalation, tapering it so that it becomes finer
and finer but doesn't quite stop until your body
spontaneously initiates an inhalation.

Allow this inhalation to be as full and complete as it wants to be.
Notice any sensation of *filling* and the increase in alertness,
and well-being that accompanies it in the breath.

Allow yourself to enjoy it.

This is an example of what is called *prana* or *ch'i (qi)*.

FIGURE 119

successful. It was as though the effort to breathe itself created tension that limited the opening of his chest. The fullness and nurturing that his breath should offer were not there, though his bony, rigid body seemed to declare that he was starving for it.

"Try this," I suggested. "Focus your control and effort on the exhalation only. Extend it, letting it taper gradually. When your body begins to demand air, let it do the breathing in—however it wants to. Don't involve yourself with the inhalation." He tried it. After a prolonged, slowly diminishing outbreath, his chest swelled spontaneously. His face lit up. "How did that feel?" I asked him. "Wonderful!" he exclaimed. "It was as though I wasn't breathing, I was being *breathed." I laughed. "You were! You let down your guard and opened up freer access to the ambient energy."*

After this primary, nourishing current, the next in intensity—the other one that you may be able to pick up right away—is that which powers elimination. It has a downward push to it, and is operative everytime you exhale. If you are lying quietly, doing diaphragmatic breathing, you may be able to notice a downward sensation that courses through your body all the way to your toes as you breathe out.

This is the cleansing current. While exhalation carries carbon dioxide out of the lungs, energetic wastes are thrown downward and out. Just as physical wastes are returned to the soil, where they are converted to nutrients for plants, negative energy is also absorbed and transmuted by the earth. But tension and tightness in the lower part of the body may obstruct this outlet.

Margot's face was darkened by stress. She had been standing on a subway platform for forty-five minutes waiting for a delayed train amid an impatient rush-hour crowd. I wanted to discuss with her issues she had brought up on her last visit, but I knew it was impossible. There was a barrier between us that preoccupied much of her energy at the moment. "Let's start with a little breathing," I suggested. She lay down, and I took her through a brief relaxation. This decreased the tightness in her face somewhat, but the tension did not totally disappear, and the dark scowl was still very much in evidence.

"Now, as you exhale, do it as though you were exhaling from the crown of your head all the way to the tips of your toes. Follow with your attention down the spine as you do this." After a moment, I went

a step further. "Now imagine that when you exhale, you are exhaling down the spine to the tips of the toes and then right on out. *With every exhalation you are releasing negativity and tension. All your worries and preoccupations are being thrown out below as you release the breath."*

I watched as she continued this for several breaths. With each cycle there was an increment of darkness that dropped away from her face. After a little more than five minutes, she looked calm and peaceful, almost radiant. I helped her slowly emerge from the deep state of relaxation. Now we could talk. She was in a place from which she could look dispassionately and acceptingly at the emotions and thoughts that had been troubling her.

The downward-moving current, what the yogis call *apana,* is active when you urinate or defecate, as well as in childbirth in the female or ejaculation in the male. When it is obstructed, we get disorders like constipation or difficulty with urination. Many of our healing crises develop because this eliminative current is not moving regularly and freely. The psychological correlate of this problem is that of blocked cleansing in general, the inability to release old patterns so that you can move on to new ones. You must release with each breath the attachments and cares of the last moment if you are to embrace the present one fully and joyfully. Sometimes in the morning, when I am having trouble waking up, I find that focusing on the eliminative, downward current moving out my feet brings me back to the world, grounds me, and makes it easier to hop out of bed.

OTHER CURRENTS YOU WILL FEEL

There are three more major currents of energy flow beyond that which nourishes and that which eliminates. They are tied to the breath in less obvious ways than the first two, so they may be a bit trickier to get a handle on. One hovers near the solar plexus and is used to digest food. It's also the energy used to exert, or to dominate, and is related to the third chakra and the Element of Fire. This is the energy that tends to get overly aroused and spill out in the *pittic* crisis. You can also store energy in the region of the navel. It's the original input point for energy uptake—even before you've begun to breathe—through the umbilical cord. Though the physical apparatus for this is severed at birth, energetically it persists and remains an opening through which energy and power are absorbed or extended.

Absorbing energy through the navel center is accomplished consciously through the Chinese technique of qigong. Qigong, of which t'ai chi is one variation, is rich in techniques for collecting and building the vital energy stored at the solar plexus or the *hara*.[6] I visited a hospital in China where I was introduced to several patients who attributed their recovery from cancer to the qigong taught there. When I asked how this worked, an elderly gentleman volunteered to demonstrate.

He walked a short distance across the small room, swinging his arms in rhythm with the breath. At each step, the hand that swung forward rotated so that its palm turned in toward the belly. It was as though his hands were gathering energy from his surroundings and sweeping it toward the abdomen. Then he stopped, looked at me, and smiled, as though to say, "See how simple it is!" Of course, he explained through a translator, he also had to improve his diet and change how he dealt with his family.

But I got the distinct feeling that it was this energy "stoking," collecting and storing *ch'i* with these simple movements, that had been able to give a depleted and sick system the energy required to undertake the other necessary changes. Try it yourself. You can amplify the effect by coordinating your motions with your breathing and letting your hands reach back into the space behind you, pulling in energy from the unconscious realm (see Chapter 9).

A fourth energetic flow is that which moves upward and out, and is called *udana*.[7] Your voice is powered by this energy, which is focused at the fifth or throat chakra. It is most intensely activated during creative vocalization. This current is related to the Element of Ether or space, and is also the energetic force that powers the physiologic act of vomiting. When you begin to think in these energy terms, you may find that problems that had seemed mysterious become simpler to understand.

My teacher of Ayurveda was president of the Ayurvedic medical college in Lucknow. This city also happened to be the home of the premier Western-style medical school in India, and when the mayor's wife fell ill, the most prestigious physicians in town were the professors there, and it was they who were asked to attend her. Unfortunately, her illness did not respond to their ministrations. She had an inflamed gallbladder and was vomiting nonstop. None of the conventional anti-

nausea medications seemed to make much difference. For such an important personage, resignation did not seem a viable option. In desperation, they appealed to Dr. Sharma, my teacher.

*Ignoring the condescension with which he had been treated in the past, he agreed to visit the patient. After careful evaluation, he declared the case to be quite simple. "Yes?" his allopathic colleagues asked skeptically. "Give her an enema," he suggested. "The vomiting will stop immediately." They were indignant. "An enema? Are you mad? The woman has been vomiting for days, and you want to give her an enema?" He was not moved. "Do you have a better idea?" he asked. They didn't. After the enema, the vomiting ceased straightaway. "It was very obvious," he explained. "*Udana vayu *was moving up out of control. All you have to do is bring* apana vayu *into play with an enema, and the flow of energy is pulled back down into balance."*

The last of the five energy currents is in some ways the most difficult to grasp, but is no less important for that. It has to do with the circulation of energy through the whole body and the integration of the gestalt into a coherent system. It's traditionally associated with the Element of Water. Since the bulk of the body is water, this circulating, pulsating coordination force is fundamental to making you feel like an intact, integrated whole. It may be sensed in the periphery of the body as a sort of centripetal/centrifugal reverberation. You might say it's most intense at your outer boundaries, the "surface" of your energy body.

This current provides an undergirding for what psychologists like to call your "body image," and the chakra with which it is most intimately associated is the second or genital one, the focus of your erotic energy. Feeling sexual attraction toward someone may make you more aware of this sphere of energy that surrounds you, and of the biological urge to merge it with that of another. Genital stimulation, or even merely breathing into the second chakra, can intensify your awareness of it. Because of this connection to your sense of yourself, and to your ability to meld with energies beyond yourself, erotic energy can play a key role in healing work. In the next chapter we will explore ways of working with it.

These five energy currents are the functional aspects of *vata.* This makes sense, as *vata* is the subtlest of the three *doshas,* the one that is essentially energy. From an Ayurvedic point of view, derangement of these currents is responsible for the bulk of diseases. In some cases the flow is blocked; in others it becomes locked into a maladaptive repetition. Sometimes this will explain problems that otherwise are baffling. For example, one night my thirteen-year-old son came out of his bedroom squinting and frowning.

"I can't sleep, Dad!" he complained. "What's wrong?" I asked. He lowered his voice. "I keep having to get up to pee . . ." His undercurrent of agitation, along with the disrupted urination, brings up an energetic screen in my mental computer: the downward-moving eliminative current, stuck in a repetitious but incomplete discharge. "Go to the kitchen and get some sesame oil. Rub it into your feet, put on a pair of socks, and go back to bed." He shot me a somewhat skeptical look, but headed downstairs. The next morning I asked him how it had gone. "I went right to sleep and didn't have to get up again!" he replied with a mixture of gratitude and disbelief. The oil soothed the aggravated energy, and allowed a normal rhythm to reestablish itself. Conventional physiological thinking wouldn't have offered much here.

Caring for Your Energy Body

You are constantly—though usually unconsciously—directing the flow of energy through your system by means of breathing patterns that have become habitual without your being aware of it. These are similar to the habits of movement that we cataloged in the previous chapter. They are also related to those habits, since the connective tissues that shape themselves around your repertoire of postures and movements also limit the motion of your lungs.

Once you begin to inhabit your energy body consciously, you will become aware of breathing habits and energetic imbalances that can limit your vitality and creativity. Such energy patterns, if allowed to persist, go on to cause serious diseases. The first step toward remedying them is to remember the foundation principles learned in the preceding chapters.

In other words, the energy body also requires nourishing, cleansing, exercise, and rest. The nourishing comes especially through free and open inhalation, but it also comes from food that is fresh, vibrant, and alive; ideally, food should provide *prana* as well as substance. Sunshine and clean air are also energizing. Energy is drawn from the Earth, too, but the upward pull needed to make it rise seems to depend on the efficiency of the downward-moving eliminative current. When that's not operating freely, the uptake of Earth energy is obstructed. It's as though the channels for lifting it up must be cleared by a thorough release of waste and negativity downward. Effective nourishing depends on effective cleansing.

Like the wastes that accumulate on the physical level, negative energy will build up if it's not released regularly. Then it backs up and moves in reverse. Moving upward, it creates all sorts of disorders, from gas pains and cardiac arrhythmias to nervous and mental derangements. As the negativity moves up, the higher centers can be overwhelmed, the mind becoming preoccupied with thoughts of helplessness, hopelessness, and a distaste for life. Here's one of many such cases I've seen:

Harold looked drawn and uncomfortable. His wife sat anxiously beside him. This was his second family, his wife only slightly older than his children from the first go-round. At sixty he was a successful lawyer, lean, fit, and attractive, but he looked baffled. Headaches, dizziness, and nausea had made it increasingly difficult for him to work, and he felt the need to lie down frequently. He had let go his usual routines of running, tennis, and golf because of lack of energy and waning interest. His sex drive had dwindled to zero. Food didn't go down easily; in fact, it felt more as if it wanted to come up.

"If I could burp for ten minutes straight, I'd feel better," Harold says, moving his hands up his torso in a gesture that showed how the gas was pushing upward.

A gastroenterologist had found Helicobacter pylorii *in his intestine and prescribed antibiotics, which made him feel worse. A few weeks after the medication was completed, however, he began to improve some, and that continued until evaluation of the dizziness turned up nasal polyps, which he had removed under general anesthesia. That set him back significantly.*

"This is a classic case of vatic *disturbance," I began, explaining what the term meant, and that one aspect of* vata, *the downward-moving one,* apana, *was out of whack, and had reversed its direction. "That energy moving upward brings all the negative—physical as well as mental—up toward the upper parts of your body. That's why you feel dizzy, for example, and why you feel like you can't keep food down. Antibiotics only further disrupt the ecology of the intestinal tract, and aggravate the problem. Anesthesia, which is sublethal poisoning—sufficient to cause loss of consciousness, but limited so as not*

to be fatal—is very disruptive to vata. *No wonder you had a setback just as you were improving."*

I explained how to follow a vata-*pacifying diet, and that he needed to get lots of water. Exercise was a must, but he should start slowly. He needed to massage his feet with oil at bedtime to bring down and ground the energy, and take acidophilus to restore normal flora in the gut.* Natrum phos 6x *would help with the gas, while the nasal polyps, along with warts on his left hand, called for a dose of* Thuja 200C.

Three weeks later, Harold was considerably better. He was excited because, with his newfound alertness and enthusiasm, he had come to realize that much of his energy had been sapped by a case he had delayed. This had preyed on his mind constantly, and the longer he had procrastinated, the more serious had been the consequences he imagined. Now that he had identified the problem and talked about it with people at work and at home, it could be resolved. The heavy load of negativity it represented was now being released.

It's helpful to take a moment on a regular basis to focus on the cleansing current of energy (see Fig. 120). This is a powerful technique for freeing yourself of mental and emotional baggage. But again, don't forget the role of the physical. If there's backed-up waste on that level—constipation, for example—then the free flow of downward, eliminative energy will be impeded to a significant extent. Doing the breathing in conjunction with physical cleansing techniques, on the other hand, is a very potent synergistic combination.

Besides attending to the nourishing and cleansing energetic flows, exercising the energy body will involve deliberately bringing the other three currents into play. The upward- and outward-moving one, *udana,* is exercised very effectively by singing. Chants that tune consciousness to the higher centers are a traditional way of doing this that encourages and supports the work of healing. The energy at the solar plexus, *samana vayu,* gets a real workout during aerobics, but it's even more powerfully activated when you're engaged in action in the world that is meaningful and fulfilling for you.

The fifth integrating current *(vyana vayu)* is vigorously brought into play with dance. This is when you celebrate your body and its form. Dance is inseparable from erotic energy (which is why it has been considered revolutionary to incorporate dance into worship). Conscious,

AMPLIFYING THE
CLEANSING CURRENT

Lying on your back in a
relaxed position, inhale from
the toes up to the top of the
head. Then follow with your
attention from the crown to
the feet as you exhale. Don't
force the breath, it should be
relaxed and gentle—it's the
energy flow that you want to
allow to maximize—not the
muscular exertion of the
chest. Imagine that as you
exhale you are throwing out
all your troubling thoughts,
and feelings. As you inhale
you are taking in light, clarity
and serenity.

FIGURE 120

open sexual encounters, where there is trust and a playful attitude, are supreme opportunities for this energy to glow.

That leaves rest. Resting the pranic body doesn't mean turning off your energy any more than resting the physical body means getting rid of it. What energy "rest" does mean is bringing the flow to a state of quiet vitality. This is, in fact, a critically important skill to master. Because the energy body is where emotions manifest, and because they can be experienced as storms there—especially when we have no control over them—it is crucial for the exploratory work of healing to know how to calm emotional turmoil when it threatens to get out of hand.

This does not mean that emotions are bad or even that they are to be avoided. But if we are to be able to explore experiences and relationships playfully, we must be free from the fear of uncontrollable emotions and the harmful actions they might produce. Using the breath to establish the physiologic parameters of equanimity and calm is a clever and effective strategic step in cultivating a healing consciousness.

ENERGY ASSESSMENT

After you learn to take care of the energy body, providing what's needed to keep it in general good order, you are in a position to begin to address its more specific disorders—to let in energy to where it's needed, for example, when it's deficient. The patterns of muscle tension that create your "fascial straitjacket" reflect the resistances you unconsciously put up that block the free flow of energy currents. When you can identify them and release them, you begin to let energy flow *through* you, pulling you back into the overall pattern of the larger energetic gestalt of which you are but one small part.

However unfathomable it is to us—and this is why the modern mind has trouble with the concept of energy—true spontaneity doesn't separate you from the whole, but connects you to it. Your deepest and most individual creative urge, your heart's desire, has a precise and coordinated place within the larger energetic scheme of things. When you are most in touch with your *spanda,* your innermost urge, you are most in synch with the natural rhythms and cycles of energy flow that are trying to move through you.

To see where you are resisting, to find where your muscle tension and emotional conflicts are creating energy blocks, so that you can bring them into consciousness and release them, you'll need to learn to do a detailed assessment of your energy status.

This is accomplished by carrying out an internal inventory of your energy body, systematically moving your attention through a series of inner checkpoints. The routine my teacher used for this involved sixty-one of those points. Using the chart here in Fig. 121, start with number one and let your attention rest for a second or two at each station. This must be done in a state of deep relaxation, with diaphragmatic breathing. You might imagine a bluish light illuminating the vicinity of each point—as though you're a night watchman, shining his flashlight in each nook and cranny to make sure everything is okay. When you find a place where it's hard to get your mind to go, or where the point is difficult to visualize, this is usually an area where something is energetically "off." This is, then, an effective method of energetic self-diagnosis.

But remember, the mind tends to pull the energy along, wherever it goes. So making the rounds inside this way will also, to some extent at

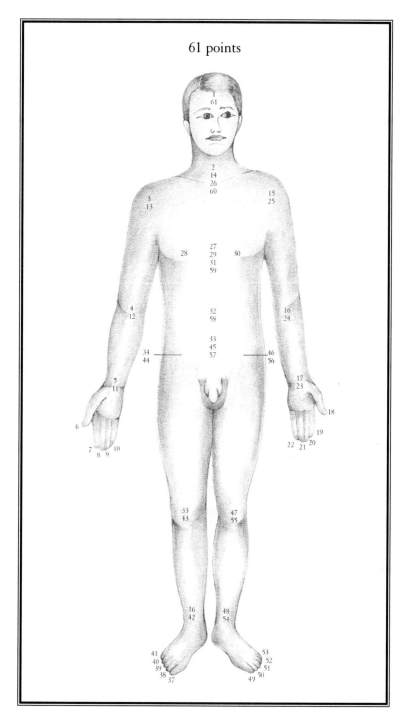

FIGURE 121

least, encourage energy to fill spots that may be lacking. It's like allowing your energy body to reinflate where it was sagging. If you "breathe into" those places, that is, give them permission to expand as you inhale, at the same time you are visualizing them, the effect is amplified.

Incidentally, this internal survey is also a solid foundation for diagnosing others. A basic version of intuitive diagnosis can be accomplished when you sit with another person, resonate with their energy (simply start by synchronizing your breath), and then check the usual points. Any new dim or dark spots you find inside yourself are most likely clues to what is going on in this person you're with.

As you step into this world, you will begin to develop some notion of "energy anatomy." The energy body has its own complex shape and form. You might think of it as a "ghost" or echo of the physical body, hovering about it, occupying much the same "space," only on a different, subtler level. It mimics the physical in some respects, yet is different in others. Unlike the physical body, it is in flux, ever flowing and changing. For this reason, different observers often see it in different ways.

As a result, there are a variety of "maps" of the energy body, and how it's been mapped depends on how it's approached. There are two major viewpoints, one from the outside, the other from the inside. So far we've focused on exploring the body from within, experientially. That leads to a map drawn from the inside, which will tend to be organized around chakras and the streams of energy that lead to and from them, that we've called *nadi*s (see Fig. 122). The other approach, from outside, will discover energy channels nearer the surface of the body; these are the meridians of acupuncture or shiatsu (see Fig. 123).

The system of chakras and *nadi*s corresponds to your experiential center, that inner core from which you feel yourself move when you are truly spontaneous. From there you move out to contact the world. The meridian system, on the other hand, reflects how that energy interfaces with the world around you.

Since the energy body is sandwiched between the mind and the physical body, it is limited to a specific segment of that spectrum of phenomena which run from gross to subtle and constitute our multileveled being (see Fig. 124). But, like a rainbow, it is almost arbitrary where we draw the line between one part and another. Red shades into orange on one side and purple on the other. Similarly, the part of the energy body that is closest to what we would call physical is the part where the meridians are found.[8] This proximity to the material is why this level of energy can be

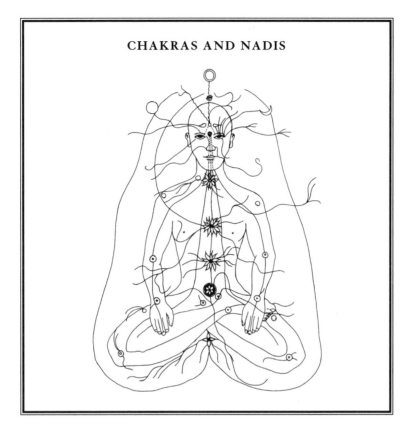

CHAKRAS AND NADIS

FIGURE 122

manipulated through the use of a physical instrument—such as a needle—or with pressure from the hand.[9]

The chakra/*nadi* system, with its energy streams and foci along the axis of your inner world, is located further into the realm of subtle phenomena—closer to the mind and to your larger awareness. Though this has been your reference point in the work we have been doing, and the maps of the energy body based on this approach are those we've used, when you run into a roadblock and need help, you may turn to someone who works from the outside and uses a different set of maps and concepts—those based on meridians, for example, or auras and "energy fields."

Do what you can for yourself. You may use the sixty-one-point check-in, or you may just follow your breath, moving from chakra to chakra, tracing the energy radiating from each center along the pathways it follows—venturing along these channels or *nadis* as an explorer might have followed a river. When you find something amiss, you might find

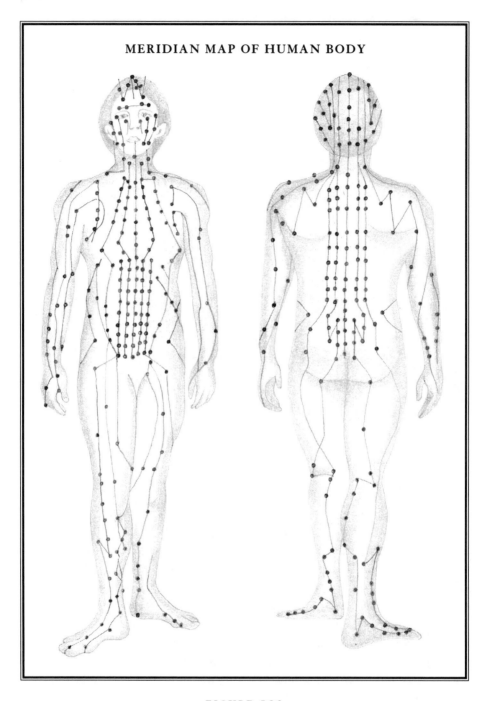

MERIDIAN MAP OF HUMAN BODY

FIGURE 123

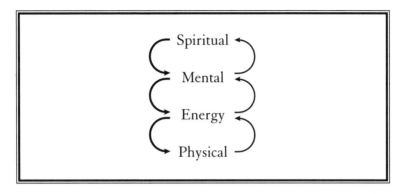

FIGURE 124

you can allow breath into it, or do a yoga posture or qigong exercise to open it up, so it feels okay.

Even if that doesn't work, as long as you're monitoring the energy body, you're in a position to practice preventive medicine at its best— picking up disorders while they're still limited to the subtle. "Early detection" is the buzzword here. When I sensed a vague clunking sound in my car, I insisted on taking it to the shop, even though a friend was sure he heard nothing. "Good thing you brought it in now," the repairman said. "Your steering rod was about to go."

WHEN TO SEE A PROFESSIONAL

I had been in the South. It was spring, and the pollen was a quarter-inch thick on the screened porch of my cabin. By the third day, my eyes were swollen and my nose stuffed. I felt myself yielding to the influences of my natal culture—diet slipping, old fears and images sliding back into place. By the time I left, I felt like a mobile battle-ground. Despite my best efforts with breathing and reenergizing, I was weak and tired and a hint of my old cough was showing through. Though a confirmed "do it yourself" man, I called Lorie and asked for an acupuncture session.

When I arrived, she checked my pulses. "You need more juice," she commented. Then she inserted needles into the major kidney points in the center of the ball of each foot. "Sorry, this may hurt," she warned. It did. I almost jumped off the table. "Opening these points allows you to draw energy from the earth up." Though qigong teachers empha-sized the importance of that, still I was surprised by the results.

Immediately I felt activity in my legs—and up. My face was ener-
gized, almost flushed. "You look different!" Lorie said, smiling.

Though a bit skeptical, there was no doubt I clearly felt tingling
and buzzing sensations streaming up from the still-sensitive points on
the soles of my feet. As I walked away from her office, the contact of
my foot on the earth was a delicious experience. Each sole felt like a
mouth kissing the earth and sucking up nourishment from it. No, it
wasn't just suggestion. I definitely felt calm and quiet—yet more
energetic. The next morning, as I began to jump on my rebounder, the
effect was sensual, especially where my foot touched the trampoline.
Fifteen minutes later, the vibrations moving up my legs were notice-
able. That evening, after a long stint of seeing patients, I was tired,
but not frantic or exhausted as I'd been the week before. Instead it was
a pleasant fatigue. It felt good to let go, as though I were absorbing
renewal through my body as I relaxed.

If you can't fix it, see a professional. There's a growing spectrum of practitioners who specialize in "energy repair" (see Fig. 125). Cranio-sacral osteopaths focus on the movement of energy up and down the spine and how it coordinates with the rhythmic pulsations of the cere-brospinal fluid. They are great for helping restore normal energy flow when the pattern has been distorted by trauma of some sort. Yoga postures, when sustained, can powerfully redirect the movement of prana or energy so that you feel more alive and whole. The problem is, the position you most need to assume is probably the one you avoid most assidu-ously, since it would bring up emotions and memories you've shoved out of sight. A Phoenix Rising yoga therapist will help you find the postures you need to work with, support you through them, and help you process the feelings that emerge.

But use these professionals the same way we discussed using a pro-fessional to assist with your diet in Chapter 7. Just as you don't want to go to a nutritionist and say, "Tell me what to eat," but rather to ask for help in shaping your own diet, you don't want to dump responsibility for your energy management in the lap of another person. Use her or him as a consultant—someone to help you past a block, and to help you learn how to do it yourself more successfully. And whatever you do, don't for-get to watch your breathing. To go to an energy therapist when you're ignoring your breathing is like towing your car to the shop when you're out of gas.

ACCESSING ENERGY MEDICINE

Technique	Directed toward	Useful for
Shiatsu	meridians	muscle tension associated with organ dysfunction
Reflexology	reflex points on feet	general
Craniosacral	energetic rhythms through spinal fluid	especially old traumas held in energy body
Zone therapy	regional energetic zones	general
Homeopathy	overall pattern of energy flow	chronic disorders
Acupuncture	meridians/points	general
Polarity	flow between + and − poles	general
Phoenix Rising yoga therapy	postures to redirect energy	emotional release
Reiki	energy infusion	general
Bioenergetics/ Core energetics	reconnecting to lower-chakra energy	repressed emotions
Breathwork trainings	various: unearthing emotions and/or directing energy	strengthening integrative consciousness and/or dealing with repressed

FIGURE 125

Breathwork will introduce you to your energy body, and that new awareness will enable you to take better care of your energy self. But from the point of view of healing, the real function of breathwork and energy expertise is to activate the higher chakras, which provide the vantage point from which you can delve into the energy knots in the lower centers and allow them to untangle.

Instinctual forces are organized around biological imperatives such as food, sex, and self-preservation. The fulfillment of these requirements for physical survival are hard-wired into the human system to ensure that they are not ignored. The chakras below the diaphragm mediate these drives, while those above bring into play an expanded consciousness that can modulate the fearfulness of a mentality organized around pure survival.

The Chakras: Climbing Jacob's Ladder

The chakras are way stations along the central axis of your being. Each one is a point at which energy can be expressed in a certain set of attitudes, actions, and emotions. When you have "finished" with those experiences and have integrated what you need to learn from them, then the energy stops demanding expression there, and is free to move on up to the next center. The chakra system provides a sort of map of your evolutionary challenges, of your soul's journey—of the road you must move along for healing to happen.

The disorders and diseases from which you suffer point to the region of the body with its governing chakra that expresses the issues where your energy is "stuck." Such a clue can help you identify the issues and the polarities that express them, so that a flower essence or an insight can help you disentangle the energy being expressed there and make it available to activate the chakras higher up, illuminating the inner world even more, and further speeding the healing process.

Energy focused at a specific chakra brings into play a certain consciousness characteristic of that chakra. Mastery of the issues presented at that chakra lays the foundation for the consciousness of the next chakra to emerge. When we are totally invested in the first (the lowest) chakra, and it is not lit by the larger vision of higher centers, it can support only a very frightened, materialistic state of awareness. By contrast, when reworked by activated higher chakras, the lower centers serve to establish our grounding in healthy embodiment.

1. SURVIVAL OF THE INDIVIDUAL
AND THE ROOT CHAKRA

The first center is at the base of the spine near the anus. Here is where the most primal instincts for self-preservation are felt. Energy gravitates here when you regard a situation as threatening to your survival—whether or not it is in fact a threat.

> *Earl stands to tell me his problem. He has hemorrhoids. Not the mild kind that you can treat with over-the-counter ointments, but a horrible swollen mass of angry purple veins that make it almost impossible to go on demo drives of the cars he sells, or to sit at a desk to sign the papers for a sale. But his problems at work started before his hemorrhoids; in fact, he recalls the symptoms really got bad when he was threatened with loss of his job for failing to meet quotas. This job, I discovered, was to him his last chance to succeed in the world, and losing it meant losing his self-respect and his future. Even deeper, I suspected, was a feeling that his very existence hinged on making it work. All his apprehension seemed concentrated in ferocious tension in the anal sphincters and surrounding muscles.*

Fear is the keynote here, but it's not a fear of loss or even a fear of catastrophe—it's an overwhelming, though sometimes unconscious, fear of annihilation. Deep in our biological nature this sort of fear is rooted in attack from the rear—being pursued and hunted. Horror films capitalize on the intensity of this energy, and arouse it to create a sense of excitement. Abject terror, however, can create spasms here of such severity that there is total loss of bowel control.

While blind identification with the physical body is crippling to the human spirit, a solid grounding in this incarnation is necessary for carrying out one's life's intent. Associated with the element of Earth, the first chakra should embody the quality of being rooted in life on this planet. Qigong training provides details on how to direct the grounding force from a larger consciousness, and those who have mastered it are known for baffling the untrained by rooting themselves energetically with such firmness that six or eight strong men cannot move them.

Since we know that the body can be destroyed and that it will, in any case, eventually die, a heavy identification with the physical body leads inevitably to fear, constant agitation of the energy of this chakra, and a

anus   earth
rectum   smell
descending   yellow
  colon   (red)
hamstrings

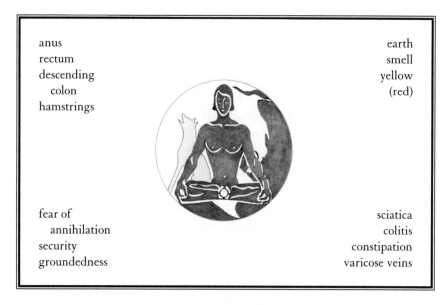

fear of   sciatica
  annihilation   colitis
security   constipation
groundedness   varicose veins

FIGURE 126

disturbance of the healthy functioning of the structures coordinated here, producing local disorders such as sciatica, colitis, constipation, varicose veins, or hemorrhoids. A lack of existential security can also provoke a spectrum of other, more global derangements, from anorexia, weakness, and wasting all the way to schizophrenia. A radical and genuine cure of such problems requires bringing into awareness, at least to some extent, the energy focused here, and reworking the beliefs and attitudes involved.

The degree to which you respond to physical danger with a concentration of energy in the first chakra is a measure of how exclusively you identify with the physical body. If you see yourself as something other than that body, then your survival is not threatened by losing it. Beginning to perceive, explore, and identify with your energy body is a first and crucial step out of being limited to a purely material identity and the terror that provokes. A perfect person to help with first chakra hangups would be a body-oriented psychotherapist.[10] You'll probably find lots of "stuff" about fear of abandonment, constricting family prohibitions, and so on.[11] Looking at all this and coming to see it clearly can result in major changes in your health and consciousness.

Addressing first-chakra issues is a frequently needed foundation for any deep healing work. Fear throws cold water on the process of healing, which can take place only when there is a spirit of play. Survival issues and play don't occupy the same space. As soon as fear and insecurity appear, the exploration and curiosity of play evaporate, you retreat instead to the familiar, and resume repetition of what seems safe.

2. SURVIVAL OF THE SPECIES, AND THE SEXUAL CHAKRA

The genital chakra is the focus of your erotic energy. It should permeate your being and light you up. Remember that the experiential energy current associated with this center is the one that pulls you together into an integrated whole *(vyana vayu)*. If this chakra is not open, your sense of integrity suffers and your image of yourself is fragmented. As we shall see in the next chapter, this is not an uncommon dilemma; much of the energy that should be available here remains tied up in first-chakra self-preservation issues. The energy we do manage to bring here is so colored by those survival fears that sexuality is often used to control and possess another person. This is an effort to provide some small measure of security and buffer ourselves from the death and annihilation we feel constantly breathing down our necks.

The Element of Water at this chakra is the medium of the urogenital system and expresses the inexorable push of nature to perpetuate the generational flow. This is a new twist on the survival concerns of the first chakra. When hormones run fast enough, self-protection measures are

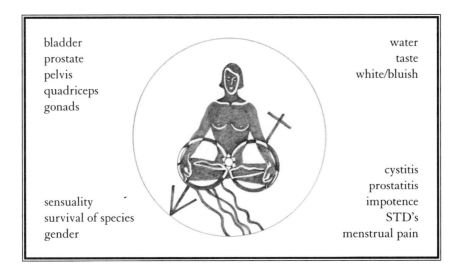

bladder	water
prostate	taste
pelvis	white/bluish
quadriceps	
gonads	
	cystitis
	prostatitis
sensuality	impotence
survival of species	STD's
gender	menstrual pain

FIGURE 127

dropped for total immersion in sexual contact. On a biological level, this is the subordination of the survival of the individual to the survival of the species. On a subtler level, it is an abandonment of fear for the joy of merging with something beyond the limited self. This makes it a first step outside self-preoccupation, an opening into transcendence—a basic model for an evolutionary leap.

Because the energy of this center has to do with the overwhelming urge to meld with another, and because this chakra is a focus for the energy current *(vyana vayu)* that defines your surface and shapes your image, this is where we encounter the issue of commitment. Whether it's commitment to another person or to a goal or project, it's the energy of this chakra that brings the possibility of opening your boundaries and making the object of your commitment part of you. This is how mating, marriage, and gender roles relate energetically to sexuality.

Disorders can develop in the second chakra as a result of a number of different energetic states. Because of preoccupation with first-chakra survival issues, too little energy may be available. Or the frustration of feeling intense energy with a fixation on channeling it into controlling sexual liaisons that are not working may "burn out" organs and structures here. Herpes genitalis seems to be an outburst of this sort of trapped sexual energy. Besides the reproductive organs, the bladder, the muscles of the anterior thigh, and the pelvic structures can also be affected. Menstrual pain, cystitis, infertility, impotence, and prostatitis are problems that commonly arise as a result.

> *Donald was sixty-one. He was short of breath and had to leave the consulting room every few minutes to urinate. The usual diagnosis here would be "enlarged prostate and early emphysema." After three weekly doses of* Thuja 200C, *his breathing had improved a lot, but his bladder symptoms were even more troublesome. Urine dribbled into the urethra so constantly that he continually felt he had to urinate. Meanwhile, his libido had* increased, *and, contrary to his usual lack of interest, he found himself masturbating as often as once or twice a day.*
>
> *It seemed the* Thuja *had cleared his chest and focused the crisis lower. It appeared to have awakened the second chakra, bringing its issues to the fore, where they were now ripe for resolution. Urinary urgency related to genital urgency—irritation that sometimes translated to having to pee and sometimes to wanting to masturbate. I increased the* Thuja *to 1M and repeated it again two weeks later*

when he returned to learn energy-holding exercises. He was experiencing some sexual arousal as we worked with the "root lock," an anal contraction technique, so I told him to lie down and inhale up from the base of the spine in order to move some of that energy up.

Three weeks later, when he returned, he read from his diary: "Got lots of sexual energy going in the exercises—almost like an out-of-body experience. Inhaling up the spine, something opened—it was alarming—it felt like I was floating. Then there was a feeling of being suffused with love."

Meanwhile there had been no shortness of breath since starting the work with breathing. "And now I can hold the urine for three hours—so I can go shopping!" he enthused. I explained that the root lock created a *container*. Before, when unconscious patterns of muscle tension blocked energy from moving up the spine, he had felt compelled to vent it—to pee or to ejaculate.[12] Now that he'd learned to allow that energy to move upward more freely by inhaling up the spine, his urge to urinate was less pressing and he felt less compelled to masturbate. Also his breathing was freer, because he was letting it do what it was meant to do—move energy upward and revitalize him.

3. POWER, MASTERY, AND THE SOLAR PLEXUS CHAKRA

Located in the region of the navel, this chakra is the focus of your Fire. The issue here is the polarity between domination and submission. The wrestler and the business tycoon are playing on this field, as are the S-and-M devotees who do so with whips and leather and the toys of bondage and mock torture. Mastery is the key word. This chakra supports clear thinking, strong vision, and assertive action. This is also the control center for your physical vitality. The nerve center that anatomists call the solar plexus is the largest mass of nervous tissue outside the skull and spinal canal—a sort of abdominal mini-brain.

When the fire is dislodged from its place here, *pittic* problems arise, and are resolved only when it's returned, as the following patient discovered:

Simone is a petite and very attractive woman in her mid-forties who looks twenty-five. Her complaint is tension in her neck and shoulders. "I always carry them up here almost to my ears! I get so tense running around tending to the kids, shopping, and so forth." Her

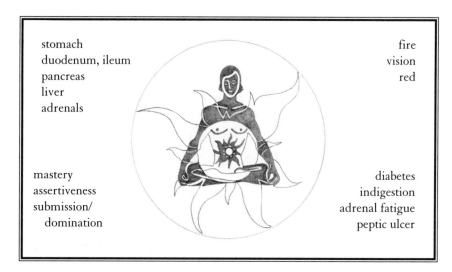

stomach
duodenum, ileum
pancreas
liver
adrenals

fire
vision
red

mastery
assertiveness
submission/
  domination

diabetes
indigestion
adrenal fatigue
peptic ulcer

FIGURE 128

throat is often burning, too. "The doctors did tests and said that it was the acid from my stomach that comes up—'reflux,' I think they called it." She paused. "And my energy is decreasing—I'm running down."

I asked Simone to lie on the table so I could watch her breathe. As I suspected, she was a chest breather. "Let your shoulders drop and let this part increase in diameter as you inhale," I suggested, putting her hands on the lower edge of her rib cage. She did, and it worked. "How does that feel?" I asked. "It's easier!" She answered quickly, flashing me a look of surprise.

Then I suggested Simone sit for three to five minutes for a sort of mini-meditation, which is done as follows: Breathing diaphragmatically, visualize a triangle behind the navel, surrounding the point that seems to correspond experientially to the center of your assertiveness and power. When you've identified the central focus of that dynamic energy, picture a small but intense flame there. Concentrate on that for a few minutes. This simple practice can be a potent support for your solar plexus, stoking and focusing the fire there.

"When you operate from here—when you bring your energy to such a fine point here that it burns like a flame—then you will be able to relax your shoulders," I explained to Simone. This seemed to make sense to her. "Can I make this my center all the time?" she asked. "Yes!" I answered. "That will help you, because what has been happening instead is that you have been pulling that fire up with your

shoulders." I demonstrated, lifting my shoulders and drawing my hand from my solar plexus upward. "So it burns my throat!" she exclaimed. "Exactly," I said.

For the energy of the third chakra to be turned to its proper purposes of mastery and vitality, it must be disentangled from the even more basic survival issues of the first two chakras—safety from annihilation and perpetuation of the species. Simone needed to relax her frantic struggle for survival amid the pressing demands of her life to bring her fire back to a calm, centered focus.

FROM NIGHT TO DAY

Only the diaphragm separates the solar plexus from the next chakra, the heart center. In some Native American traditions, the diaphragm is likened to the horizon. The first three chakras below harbor the instinctual energies (see Fig. 129), moving energy up from the solar plexus to the heart brings your internal sun from the darkness of the centers below to the daylight that shines in those above. It is the dawning of a new way of being, since it lifts you from domination by biological pulls to the possibility of compassion, creativity, and intuition.

This notion of moving energy up is an important aspect of the chakra system of energy dynamics. Without the insight and awareness that comes with the activation of the higher chakras, you will be ruled by instinctual use of your personal energy. If the captain is not steering this ship from the bridge, where he can see clearly and make informed decisions, then it will revert to automatic pilot. The lower chakras are designed to channel energy into biological necessities, and will do so until a switch is flipped for manual override. This is a crucial principle in understanding the process of personal evolution through spiritual practice or psychotherapy, and is basic to any kind of healing work.

The higher centers need to be "turned on" enough to allow you to observe, understand, and learn from your experiments in living. Otherwise you are doomed to repetitive habits governed by biological imperatives. This doesn't mean that the life of the body is inferior. It's your school, your playground—your garden of delights. But without a larger awareness it becomes instead a nightmare of wrenching compulsions, a windstorm of frightening and unpredictable forces, and a struggle for survival ruled by the law of the jungle.

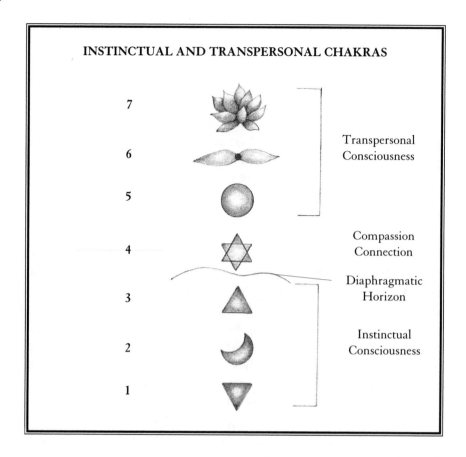

FIGURE 129

4. LOVE, COMPASSION, AND THE HEART CHAKRA

The heart is at the center of your being, hence the significance of the cross and the star of David, symbols traditionally associated with this chakra. This center is the point where the biological issues of the first three chakras are coordinated with the consciousness and vision represented by the three chakras above. It is no accident that this is where our arms extend from, since they enact the Metal Element theme of grasping and releasing. From one angle they represent interaction with the world—holding or pushing away other people, manipulating objects around you. From another angle they suggest letting go of the world of material objects to grasp the clear vision of a higher consciousness.

By this fourth chakra we have crossed the diaphragmatic horizon to enter a new world of light, so now the themes of the lower centers begin to be reworked as seen from a larger, more enlightened perspective (see

CHAKRA	ELEMENT	FUNCTION
7th		Beyond subject/object
6th		Intellect/intuition
5th	Ether	Creative flow
4th	Air	Nurturing, love
3rd	Fire	Assertion, sharp mind
2nd	Water	Generational flow
1st	Earth	Grounding/individual survival

FIGURE 130

Fig. 130). This center leads the way by reframing the Earth issue of grounding. Now security comes from a sense of immersion in a matrix of love, from a sense of inhabiting a transpersonal world of reciprocal nurturance that is reinforced by giving, rather than from the mere fact of receiving the material sustenance and personal support that were the theme of the first chakra. When life is supported by a matrix of love, first chakra fears of annihilation fade.

In the Tantric system, this center is related to the element of Air. It's where the inflow of the nourishing energy current of inhalation, the *prana vayu,* is prompted by the lungs. Here we are nurtured and anchored by connecting with the pool of *prana* that sustains all life. From here we can reframe the question of security, transforming the use of energy in the first chakra by allowing it to be held and used more gently, rather than grasped with a desperation that creates dysfunction and disease. Until that is accomplished, the pressure to ensure survival will distort any expression of energy through the higher chakras, limiting our freedom to express sexuality, twisting the power of the third chakra into compulsive control, and cutting the heart off from genuine openness.

Lee was a dentist and a health fanatic. Like his meticulously perfect dental restorations, his diet was beyond reproach. Low-fat and largely vegetarian, it was exactly what the American Heart Association recommended. But he had just had a serious heart attack, and that baffled him.

As we talked, however, it became apparent that Lee's personal life was as carefully and rigidly arranged as his professional work. A good

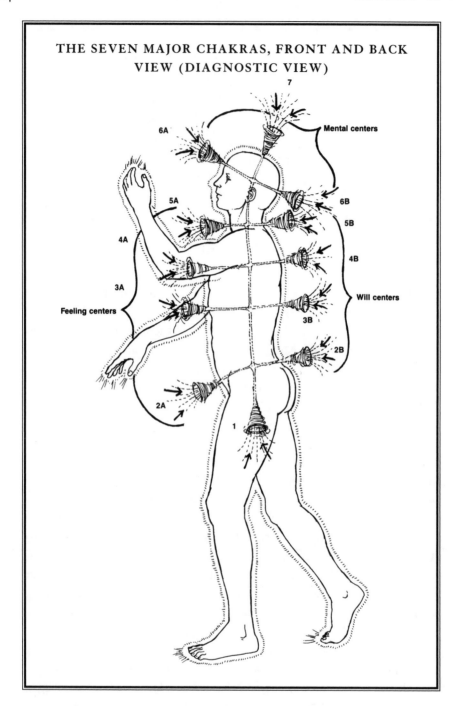

THE SEVEN MAJOR CHAKRAS, FRONT AND BACK
VIEW (DIAGNOSTIC VIEW)

FIGURE 131

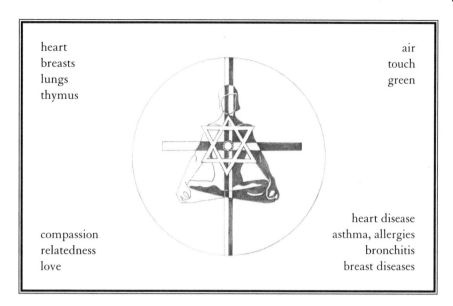

heart
breasts
lungs
thymus

air
touch
green

compassion
relatedness
love

heart disease
asthma, allergies
bronchitis
breast diseases

FIGURE 132

husband and father by all measures, he allotted "quality time" for his kids and for regular times out with his spouse. But there was little room for spontaneity, and even less for sharing the messy feelings that he was keeping a lid on. He had maintained a tidy life by keeping his heart shut down—until it erupted.

Those who work with chakras "from the outside," as therapists, often depict them as opening out to both the front and to the back (see Fig. 131). The front expressions are said to be related to feeling, and the rear to will. Extend your arms and turn in a circle. The figure you've cut is like a top with a steady axis inside a spinning circumference. The vertical axis is your spine. Where the chakras open in your back is where you experience their connection to your core, your source of knowing what is right for you.

The circumference is where you interface with the world as you turn to contact it on every side. It is where you feel the joy and pain of connection and separation, where you taste the infinite variations of the material world, and where scenarios issuing from the chakra take form in your life so they can be experienced, understood, and outgrown. Arranged along the central axis are the hubs of the chakras, where the energetic seeds of such experiences are stored, like magnetic impulses on a whirling disk drive, awaiting their turn to flash on the screen of your life.

Move your shoulder blades together in the back. Then try to pull your shoulders together in the front. Repeat this, alternating the two several times. Now sit quietly with your eyes closed and focus on the heart. As you begin to tune into its motion and the ripples out from it, you will see how its form and function are the most concise expression imaginable of taking in and then emptying out to give—in a constant joyous rhythm.

This little meditation will shift your consciousness to a field above the instinctual, and from there you can more serenely explore the lower centers. By bringing additional energy to the heart center, you begin to see the issues of each of the chakras below from a new vantage point. Since consciousness organizes and guides energy events, this means the energetic dynamics of those lower centers will change, and the scenes they spin out into your world will begin to be different, too. This is the transformative power of moving energy up.

Intoxicated by the possibilities here, some folks decide that such mundane matters as diet and exercise are no longer worthy of notice. They'll just meditate on the upper chakras. But don't make that mistake. Remember that the energetic also interfaces with the physical.[13] The physical can jar and disrupt energy flow. Without the requisite attention to the body you won't be able to perceive energy, or if you can, what you'll find when you look inside will be chaotic. If the energetic level is a confused mess, you can't focus on chakras or make out the obstacles to energy flow that need to be released. Instead of opening to fine adjustments from subtler levels in order to correct physical disorders, you'll be reduced to rushing about blindly from one disaster to the next, taking medicines and fixing body parts as though patching a broken machine with chewing gum and safety pins.

5. CREATIVITY AND THE THROAT CHAKRA

From the throat the upward- and outward-moving current (*udana vayu*) is extended out into the world. This is vocalization—song and poetry—and this center is the focus of your creative energy. Lower-chakra conflicts that interfere with expression here often affect the thyroid, as the following case illustrates:

> *"When I tune in to my body, it feels like there's a tight wire vibrating down the center of it. And I feel my heart beating—like it's working too hard."* Nadine had been diagnosed as hyperthyroid. She had been told by a spiritual counselor that she was holding back her ambi-

tion for fear that excelling in her field would destroy her relationship with her husband. So she had ventured to write and teach, taking Larch and Trumpet Vine flower essences as well as a high-potency homeopathic remedy—and her condition had improved. But the "hyper" feeling was still a constant irritation. "I don't know whether I need to control this—bring it down—or bring me up to match it!"

I thought for a moment. "After you've given a presentation, and felt really 'on,' is it easier to relax the 'taut wire' inside?" It definitely was, she felt. "So maybe you're bimodal," I suggested. "One gear for rising to that level of energy to lecture, and the other for 'chilling.'" And then, thinking aloud, I went on, "So, when the tightness builds up, maybe it just means that it's time to do more teaching." Her face brightened. "So it's a signal, an indication of what I need to do, not a problem at all. It's just reminding me of a part of who I am!"

Though the dynamics of thyroid disease may be different in men, I find this sort of thwarted creativity manifesting as hyperthyroidism quite common in women in their thirties and forties. They have absorbed the message that it is not appropriate for them to be powerfully creative. If the resistance to expressing the energy is fierce enough, the immune system may actually begin to attack the gland, creating the condition known as Hashimoto's thyroiditis, which eventually disables the thyroid and leaves it *hypo*active.

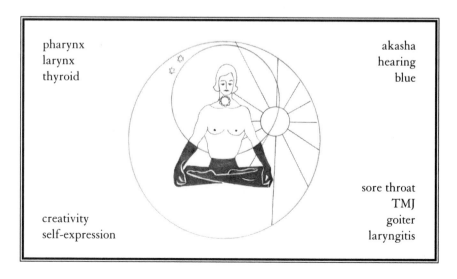

pharynx
larynx
thyroid

akasha
hearing
blue

creativity
self-expression

sore throat
TMJ
goiter
laryngitis

FIGURE 133

6. INTUITION AND THE THIRD-EYE CHAKRA

There's no element to go with the sixth center—though there is a subtle flame often depicted here, meant to light the inner world seen by this other, inward-looking eye. While fire at the third chakra denotes sharpness of outer vision, the domain of this sixth chakra is seeing within. This is the center of intuition, of inner knowledge.

By trying to limit this capacity for knowing to the world of material phenomena we do energetic violence to this area. We suffer accordingly from sinusitis, visual problems, and sleep disturbances. This is the home base of the intellect, but its proper role is that of assistant to the strong currents of inner-based perception, the *gnosis* that comes from a connection to the Infinite. It's not really meant to shoulder the burden of existential knowledge supported only by the limited world of physical phenomena.

The appropriate function of this center is seeing by allowing, not by manipulation of the endless minutiae that we regard as "intellectual." Unfortunately, unresolved issues associated with the chakras below pull energy here out into thoughts and behavior and into involvement with the world in ways that drag the intellect along. This obscures the otherwise clear vision of the third eye, and if there is a heavy emotional charge attached to these interactions with the world, they may color even our most intuitive perceptions.

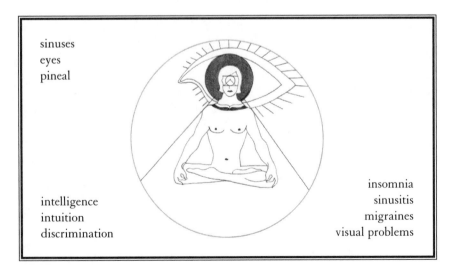

FIGURE 134

If the intuitive process is consciously brought into play at all, the result can be a less-than-accurate "psychic" reading on the situation. Only when the lower chakra issues are brought fully into awareness and to resolution—"lived through," when necessary—does the vision of the third eye clear. Barbara Brennan, whose healing work with energy is widely known and respected, tells of her experience with this process:

> *Just as she was beginning to access intuitive information about other people and enjoy the status of being "a psychic," her teacher, Eva Pierrakos, told her that she was too angry inside to handle the challenge. "You need to close your channel," she said. Barbara realized she was using the psychic work to avoid dealing with important issues in her own life, and that the only really appropriate use of her intuitive ability at that point was for her own personal work. So she limited it to that. "My psychic gifts were a lot to give up," she remembers, but she focused for the next six years on her own transformation. When she was finally ready to reopen access to it, her intuition was much clearer and freer.*[14]

Lifting and lowering your eyebrows repeatedly is a physical maneuver that helps to activate the sixth chakra. A more refined and elegant technique is to close your eyes and imagine that your inhalation is moving up to the point between the eyebrows. Focus your attention at that spot and imagine a tiny flame there. As you succeed in concentrating energy at the third eye, you may begin to catch fleeting glimpses of scenes, objects, and so on. Some of these are old stuff, stored away in your memory records. Others may be current events seen as a brief snapshots. Occasionally there's a very steady, clear seeing that must have given rise to the expression "clairvoyance":

> *Joanna was lying on her back in the large room with its vaulted ceiling, which felt at that moment like a cathedral. I was one of two masseurs working on her body while she breathed her energy up into the higher centers. She lay peacefully, a blissful expression on her face. As the session ended, she opened her eyes cautiously, squinting. Then she smiled and shook her head. "I knew they were closed!" she exclaimed. "What do you mean?" I asked. "I knew my eyes were shut, but I didn't believe it because I was seeing the ceiling and the shadows of the rafters, just as clearly as if they were open."*

If you are overly intellectual, practice sitting with eyes closed and focusing attention on this chakra. This helps to retrain the mind to use the faculties here for reconnecting internally and to break the habit of obsessive preoccupation with external busyness. Awakening the capacity for inner vision, or in more familiar psychologically oriented terms, introspection and insight, is crucial for the understanding and reorganizing needed for fundamental, radical healing.

The most transformative healing is based on insight, understanding, and the thorough reorganization that follows. Even when it might appear that healing is merely physical, if a truly curative process is taking place, a shift to seeing things differently and a reconfiguring of your energy structure and consciousness are going on somewhere underneath, out of sight. But to muster that critical insight and understanding, we must allocate sufficient energy to the chakras above the diaphragmatic horizon.

This becomes a challenge when a huge proportion of that energy is tied up in the lower centers, bound to instinctual biological drives or locked into a dysfunctional pattern of disease. There's a sort of catch-22 dilemma here: without the perspective to see what's going on, you can't choose to focus some of that energy higher. And with very little energy higher up, it's difficult to gain the perspective needed to make that choice. This is a tough one!

The wizards of energy management in various traditions have come up with some clever strategies for tackling this sticky problem. The central principle they employ is a sort of alchemy of energy transmutation, as we will see in the chapter that follows.

Healing as
Transformation

W e have all acquired deeply rooted habits of energy deployment. Since, for the most part, our use of energy is not conscious, neither are those habits. The whole matter is managed outside awareness—automatically, so to speak. This can sometimes make our emotional and energetic patterns seem inevitable. We say, "That's just the way I am." While self-acceptance is often the hallmark of maturity and wisdom, there are certain habits that cause so much grief and suffering they merit a different attitude.

This is a case where I defer to the insight and skill of traditions such as the Tantric, which have made an intensive study of energy dynamics and have distilled techniques for breaking out of confining habit patterns. The core maneuver here is based on an appreciation of the nature of energy and its characteristic tendencies—specifically, what it will do if not automatically expended.

Tantric masters observed that if you let the urge to act build, it gathers more and more intensity and energy. If not able to express in its usual way, it will eventually "explode"—burst out of the confines of the habit pattern. There's a lot of power in this explosion, and like the combustion of vaporized gasoline in the cylinder of an automobile engine it can be harnessed. I'd heard about this, but grasped its full import only when I stumbled on the phenomenon during meditation:

I was in Lucknow, in northern India, living in the household of a professor at the Ayurvedic College. Sitting cross-legged for my evening practice, I had adjusted my posture so that I was upright, and

*would not require effort to maintain the position, aside from a mini-
mal exertion of the muscles along the spine—which was fine, since
that brought my attention to the central axis of my body. I went
through my program of systematic relaxation, releasing, as much as I
could, the tension in all the other muscles. Then I regulated my breath
so that it was essentially diaphragmatic and smooth. Then I turned
my attention to my mind.*

*It was not quiet, the way it should be after all that laborious prepa-
ration. In fact, it was fit to be tied. It assailed me mercilessly. "What
is the point of this? How can you be so stupid? Can't you see the
absurdity of sitting here like an inanimate object? Are you going to let
yourself be talked into self-torture? Just get up and forget about this
nonsense!"*

*The urge to move was like a physical irritation. The building
crescendo of voices was overwhelming. Doggedly I focused on relaxing my body, which had begun to tense up again. I tried to quiet my
tightening breath. Like the parent of restless, screaming kids, I rushed
about, calming, soothing. But the rising tension was undeniable. I felt
hot, almost on fire. I was sure something would burst. And then it did.*

*After what seemed like an explosion in my head, I suddenly found
myself in a quiet place. A wave of tranquillity and bliss lifted me to a
place where I could see myself more clearly. My body was at peace. I
was amazed by what had happened. In a fraction of a second, everything had shifted.*

What I had experienced was a taste of *tapas*.[1] *Tapas* involves arousing
play an energy-invested impulse, in this case the urge to move, and then
electing not to express it in routine or habitual fashion. *Tapas* is not suppression or denial, which are ways to avoid experiencing the urgency of the
impulse. You experience it fully and powerfully and yet—despite the discomfort of its urgency—you choose not to act on it. You pass. You simply
decline to be moved by it. You intentionally contain and accept the discomfort of the building energy/impulse and wait for it to find a new course.

The Tantric Key to Transmuting Energy

It's like an internal version of Gandhi's passive resistance strategy. You
refuse to be moved, and the immense power that is mobilized around

that refusal tends to get transmuted. Only here, it's all playing out inside you. Your past actions are prompting for continuation, but you're declining to cooperate, to accede to the impulse. All the force connected with that behavior, and more, builds and builds the longer you decline. Finally it turns into liquid fire—a potent stream of powerful energy.

At some point the energy you're choosing not to express finds another route. What typically happens is that you feel a sudden heat. It's like a fire. The word *tapas* carries the connotation of burning, and it's perhaps from the use of this technique that we get the idea of "burning off karma." Your past actions, or karma, are pushing for control and you're blowing their circuits. It may be a sexual feeling that is arising, or it could be hunger, or anger, or anything surrounded by a significant charge of energy.

So, once more in a nutshell, here's how it works: You feel the energy, you contain the energy, consciously and deliberately choosing not to express it in the customary way. When it attempts to move through its habitual channel, toward its usual goal, you say, "No, I don't think so . . ." and you wait. It boils. It rattles its cage and gets furious. Finally it explodes upward to find another outlet. If a bit of a foundation has been laid, for example, by practicing breathing up the spine (as you learned to do in Chapter 10), its movement will be in that direction, bumping the energy up to a higher chakra. It's an exhilarating and empowering experience (see Fig. 135).

When I describe the containment aspect of *tapas*, audiences are often skeptical. "Isn't this just repression?" I'm asked. "Denying your impulses can't be healthy." But the energy isn't denied here—or the action it's trying to push. You've just made a conscious decision to deactivate a particular habit. And the energy is contained, amplified, and allowed to force open a new pathway.

By contrast, when you repress or deny, you simply shove the impulse out of your awareness. It keeps trying to express itself, and if you refuse to let it have its usual way, it will find another indirect way. That expression may look different on the surface, but it's really only a new version of the same old behavior. You don't notice that because you've turned a blind eye to the whole matter.

The energy transmutation of *tapas,* on the other hand, demands total awareness. You are very conscious of the impulse and your usual response to it. You simply choose not to let it move into expression. This choice brings your inner impulse back to life. The *spanda* you learned to listen to in your exercise sessions, the innermost spark of creative movement, is

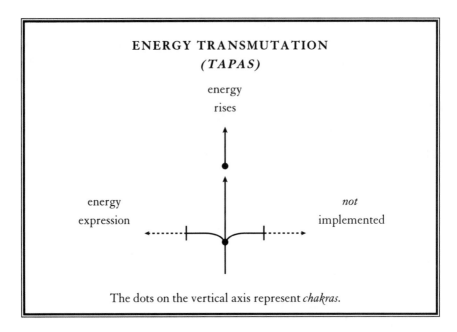

ENERGY TRANSMUTATION
(*TAPAS*)

energy
rises

energy   *not*
expression   implemented

The dots on the vertical axis represent *chakras*.

FIGURE 135

revived and empowered. The energy it needs for expression is rescued from its circular trap. You contain the building energy and allow it to move you *only* when your sharpest discrimination senses that it is ready to burst forth into a course of action or thought that is not only authentic and fulfilling but is also one that will propel you into a new way of being.

As a result, your actions will enjoy a freshness and genuine spontaneity that makes each moment surprising for you.[2] Without this, what passes for spontaneity is only a counterfeit. It's not the adventurous creativity that is the essence of life, but is instead the dull routine of ingrained habit carrying you toward ennui and loss of vitality.

Although even your most genuinely spontaneous response is to some degree a reflection of your unresolved issues, what is creative about it is the way it contributes to living through the experiences needed to move past those issues. Without employing some version of *tapas,* you remain prey to habits you wish you could change because they carry you nowhere. Without some radical measure, those habitual patterns, rooted in the unconscious, are continually reinforced by the actions they prompt, so that the lion's share of your energy is tied up in a circular chain of action, reaction, frustration, and resentment. Breaking out of this requires only a bit of skillful attention.

TAPAS IN LIFE AND IN HEALING

Energy moves where you have created a groove for it. Breathwork establishes pathways that are familiar and well traveled. The movement of energy up the axis, the central *nadi,* becomes freer as you lend the sweep of your attention to sharpen and accentuate its flow. What interrupts that current is diverting energy out into issues related to a specific chakra. For example, you may decide to contain the energy at the second chakra, and not to expend it through habitual, no-longer-satisfying sexual activity, when suddenly you notice a lot of activity one stop up, at the solar plexus. At that point you begin to feel aggressive, irritable, fiery, and want to hit your roommate over the head.

That doesn't mean you've somehow failed. Maybe you *need* to hit your roommate over the head—figuratively if not literally. Maybe expressing the assertive energy of the third chakra is the next item on your life's agenda. But at some point that, too, begins to get old. So you say to yourself, "Hmm, I've run through three roommates now, and this is a bit of a drag." What was an exploration has become a self-defeating habit. At that juncture, you may choose to haul out the tool we've called *tapas* and jack up the energy another notch. Now you're set to deal with the matter of compassion and nurturance (fourth-chakra issues) in your life.

Of course this is a cartoonlike oversimplification of a sequence of events that will be much more complex, and therefore considerably less obvious, in a real person's life. Boredom is not always conscious, and not every transmutation moves up to the next chakra. There will be multiple challenges at each, and they mesh and interdigitate in intricate ways, so that any given crisis or struggle may reflect issues that stem from several centers. Sometimes the shift has a more global feel, and often it's an illness that provides the occasion for it. This was true when Sky, my eldest son, came down with a severe case of chicken pox.

> He was just hitting his teens and was discovering his considerable magnetism. Classmates adored him, and a movie talent scout invited him for an audition. He was especially attentive to his complexion— teenage zits were anathema. Then the chicken pox hit, and he was told that if he scratched the sores that covered his face, he would have scars. That was the last thing he wanted.
>
> But Sky was not used to restraining himself. His desires were generally not unreasonable, but when he wanted something, he didn't

take no for an answer. And he was a very physical type—athletic and always on the move. So, lying in bed, wanting desperately to scratch the intensely itchy chicken-pox pustules on his face, was torture. It could not have been more perfectly designed to arouse powerful impulses, with equally strong motives to resist them—a match, as it turned out, made in heaven.

Sky lay in bed for ten days, and he did not scratch. "I knew every movement of the leaves on the oak tree outside my window," he said, "and there was one branch, the closest, that became my friend." He had never had the experience of being so quiet and reflective for so long.

"It was the hardest thing I ever did," he observed afterward. But he did it. The urge to scratch, and the energy that powered it, were contained, and rechanneled. And the effect was transformative. He became more thoughtful, more responsible. On every front, at school and at home, he matured in visible ways.

The atypical and unsuspected situations one is thrust into during illness can provide opportunities for significant developmental leaps. Moreover, often the disease itself is an expression of the habits in which you are stuck. The symptoms may represent repetitive, unconscious-driven, counterproductive patterns, evidence of stagnation and thwarted growth.

Simply staying with the discomfort unleashes all the impatience, the urge to escape, and the inner voices that demand quick-fix medications and an immediate way out. Containing and transmuting the energy beneath those impulses provides the heat, the fire that powers the healing crisis. It may be only a shift in consciousness that lifts you out of the illness, or it may involve an actual fever that "cooks the disordered humors" or annihilates the microbes associated with disease.

We might say that disease is *tapas* thrust upon us when we have put it off endlessly. We have turned away the opportunity when it was optional, and now it's become mandatory. Of course, we can use suppressive medications to postpone it yet again. But each time it returns, it comes back with more insistence, with less room to escape.

In any case, it's the transmutational process of *tapas* that is the essence of the healing experience, whether it's the transformation and healing of a psychological disorder or the resolution of a physical illness. A magical confluence of polar opposites mix together here to create the mystery of healing. The process hinges on your being fully in control, totally able to make a choice about how you deal with the crisis; at the same time, illness gives you the gift of helplessness—the overwhelming awareness that your way of being has, at least in some respects, failed.

You have pushed to your limits and you have come up empty-handed. This creates a moment when you are receptive to a spontaneous response from a much deeper level of being—what one might call grace, an inspired vision of the heretofore unimagined. It seems necessary to experience a certain sense of giving up, of surrender, in order to discover a totally new way of being and functioning. A homeopathic remedy—even the most skillfully chosen and deepest acting—cannot replace or obviate this process. Neither can the best acupuncture. But they can help you move through it more expeditiously and more gracefully.

Cleansing can remove obstacles to this process, too, and breathwork can prepare you to let go more skillfully of the obstacles you might throw up that prevent energy from shifting and refocusing. Meditation allows you to discover the transmutation that can occur, and to taste a more encompassing consciousness. But for the transformation to happen, the energy needed to power it—to push through to a new place—must be accessible.

Kundalini and Transformation

The energy needed for healing won't be available if it's constantly expended before it can build. Deep-seated habits organized around fear and insecurity can keep energy flowing out at the first chakra. For example, your eating habits may fall into this category. They may be based on attempts to feel cozy, to reward yourself, or to calm down. Or perhaps you work compulsively to feel as if you've "been good," or drink to blot out anxiety, or use sexual release to relax.

Drained off in these ways, the energy can't gather enough force to move up. From the point of view of creativity or healing, you might say that your vitality, your life force, is being bled away—absorbed by intoxication with creature comforts, reassurances, and a preoccupation with the consumption of "stuff."[3]

Potentially, that life energy is a powerful, serpentlike force that can ascend the chain of chakras, bringing more and more expanded consciousness and, as a result, healing—as suggested by the two snakes winding up the medical caduceus. But instead it lies dormant, coiled at the base of the spine, its power dissipated in desperate efforts to blot out fear. The Tantrists called this serpentine force *kundalini shakti,* the transformative power or creative force inside you. It is your individual manifestation of the larger Shakti, which is the creative force of the universe (counterpart to the cosmic consciousness identified with Shiva).

This power can seem frightening to the more limited ego, whose consciousness is stuck at the base chakra and preoccupied with shoring up its security and keeping threats to survival at bay. For *kundalini* is the ultimate shaker and mover. When uncoiled, she will force her way upward, bursting through barriers to stir up feelings, emotion, and creativity and to give life. She shatters the established order with her thrust toward evolution. These qualities make her seem dangerous, subversive, a threat to the status quo and to external authority. She obeys only the law of *spanda,* and, as she ascends above the diaphragmatic horizon and comes into her own, the power of love (fourth chakra) and the love of creativity (fifth).

Individual fears, social forces, and economic interests converge in an unconscious conspiracy to keep this *kundalini shakti* pacified, plugged into intoxicating consumerism, drugs, and workaholism, undermining the ecstatic electricity of her unleashed power.

For example, what would otherwise be a pure expression of sensual merging at the second chakra is often so distorted by unresolved first-chakra existential insecurities—fear of death and a lack of spiritual grounding—that sexual energies are easy to control with tribal taboos. One who is shaky about his footing is easily intimidated by threats of being made an outcast. In this way, constrained sexual energy can be exploited, and the natural, playful celebration of sexuality, which would provide the opportunity to discover how to use that energy creatively, is forbidden.

The "off limits" sign posted over sexuality makes it an area we are afraid to enter in a fully conscious way, and a prime target for forces of greed and social control. Like the Mafia moving into a neighborhood where the local boss has died, advertising mavens seize upon it to serve their ends. This creates a constant source of stimulation, so that sexual urges are continually stirred up, but with little of the self-awareness that might make it possible to deal in a constructive, growth-inducing way with the energy thus aroused. It instead ends up fueling consumerism and contributing to sexual disorders and diseases.

Freeing *kundalini* from these paralyzing involvements allows her to move up from the first chakra and freely explore the expression of *spanda* through the second.

FEAR OF THE FEMININE

Kundalini shakti is a manifestation of the feminine force in the universe, not just the nurturing and receptive aspect of the feminine, but the destructive and creative part, that which tears open and gives birth. She is connected with feelings, she empowers intuition, she is the life-giver. Shakti wants you to *move*. She wants you to express yourself. "Don't just sit there like a stone. *Say* something, for God's sake!" she demands. "Don't you have any *feelings?*" Shakti pushes for action.[4]

Many of those aspects of our civilization that create and sustain disease are bastions of resistance to the evolutionary impulse of this active femininity. Women are kept in their passive roles as nurturing containers. They can receive, they can be soft, but they are not to embody the active power of the feminine. Increasingly they aren't even allowed the assertiveness of giving birth; instead, the baby is surgically removed from them. When recognized at all, this feminine power has been cast as demonic, Dionysian, savage, uncivilized.

There's a telling scene in Kevin Costner's celebrated film, *Dances with Wolves,* where an infantryman discovers the protagonist dressed in the manner of the Lakota Sioux. He looks at him with utter horror and contempt. "You've turned injun!" he spits. The most repulsive thing he could imagine was that a white man would lower himself to embrace the savage life of the uncivilized, who were attuned to the earth's rhythms and lived a life that pulsed with her primal energies. These "savages" spoke to the spirits of animals and embraced their sexuality with a frankness and openness that scandalized the Europeans.[5] For example, in many tribes the medicine men were *winktes,* men who dressed like women and sometimes slept with other men.

Fear of the feminine has given rise to a complex set of gender and sexual roles that not only serve to keep us away from the awesome power of the feminine force, but also in effect lock us into the linear thinking and reductionism that characterize what we think of as rational, responsible (i.e., male) thought. Limiting consciousness in this way prevents us from engaging the other aspects of ourselves that may be crucial for the healing process. Most important, we cut ourselves off from the assertive feminine energy that is necessary to "birth" a genuinely new way of being. This is what has been called the uterine aspect of the feminine. The uterus "knows" when the time has come to end the nurturing of gestation and thrust forward with a new life, and it does so decisively and uncompromisingly. We don't say, "Yes, I know you want to have the baby, but perhaps tomorrow would be a better time." Instead, we drop everything and pitch in to help when this uterine power takes charge. Neither masculine energy nor the passive feminine are capable of the unerring sense of timing, the unhesitating willingness to destroy the old in order to bring into being the new that is the dynamic power of the assertive uterine energy. And without that push from old to new, the effort to heal is doomed to fizzle.

To the "civilized" mind, however, unearthing the feminine power is forbidden. It would mean breaking down fear-based, first-chakra controls on the expression of energy and would undermine the rigid control of the narrow ego with its monopoly on defining "reality." It would also mean releasing the *kundalini* energy to be available sexually and freely exploring the expression of *spanda* through the second chakra. This is where the serpent power of *kundalini* first bursts into full manifestation, as suggested by the ancient name of the second chakra, *svadisthana,* which means "her own home."

The serpent was a sacred symbol in most ancient cultures, especially those that were "sex positive." In the Judeo-Christian tradition, however, the serpent is feared and maligned, since it represents that knowledge of Good and Evil that Eve gained by eating forbidden fruit, thereby ending her privilege of paradise.

Bringing assertive feminine energy into consciousness is terrifying—especially to the male, where it arouses many fears, most notably homophobia. If a man allows himself to embody that feminine power—the radical, destructive, and creative force—what will happen to his orderly world and his ego-oriented goals, and what will it do to his sexual impulses? Will he turn into a wild woman and find himself lusting for other men?

RADICAL SEXUALITY

For the macho male, phallic energy is the only possibility that is compatible with his self-image.[6] He shuns and cannot "own" his own feminine instinctual energy, particularly the aggressive power of his own *shakti*. Instead, he projects this power onto the woman, whom he secretly fears, and requires her to hide it too, and to show only her more nurturing, passive side. Yet he is uneasy, knowing she holds the potential for destruction, for breaking down the rigid world he struggles to maintain.

In some cases the pressure of his fear and loathing pushes him to attack his projection, so he feels compelled to abuse women, either mentally or physically. His agony can erupt as violence, or, when turned inward, as ulcers, heart attacks, or high blood pressure.

A woman, on the other hand, deprived of her feminine power, may try to make a place for herself by adopting the phallic aggressiveness of the man, moving as he does in the world of business or politics. But often in doing so, she becomes increasingly uncomfortable with herself. Her energy wanes and she begins to suffer from a chronic and baffling fatigue. Like her male counterpart, she has turned her back on the feminine force, and she needs, perhaps even more than he does, to acknowledge, honor, and embody it. I saw a patient whose plight underscored this point.

> *Alexis is an artist, tall and powerfully built, with straight blond hair, strong features, and deep eyes. But she sits in the waiting room looking dazed and numb. In fact, those are some of the words she uses to describe her condition, along with others, such as queasy, nauseated, shaky, and weak. "I feel ill, as though I had the flu and I can't think, reason, or find words." After high titers of Epstein-Barr virus antibodies were found in her blood, she was told she had chronic fatigue syndrome.*
>
> *Alexis had called it depression, and it had gotten worse when her father died, after not speaking to her the last time she visited. She seemed ambivalent about her marriage, though she loved her husband. A regular sort of guy, he seemed baffled by her condition, and just wanted her to do what wives are supposed to do and to "get over this." He dismissed her interest in holistic medicine and insisted on her seeing a psychiatrist and taking the antidepressant prescribed by him.*
>
> *The medication made her feel worse, and though acupuncture helped some, she seemed stuck, confused about her marriage, unable to untangle the feelings for her father and husband or to see her way toward a role that would allow her to use her creativity and be fulfilled as a person.*

Though Alexis's dilemma is not unusual, change is in the air. An increasing number of women refuse to play opposite the archaic male lead and are rebelling. Yet they often remain ambivalent. Not having reclaimed the *shakti* within themselves, they continue to look to the macho male as the sole source of power. Divested of power themselves, they feel drawn to him as a romantic partner, though more often than not they are unhappy with the relationship that results.

Therefore, the shell of the old pattern persists, a sort of rote repetition of what is familiar but obsolete. Many women accept a subordinate role, as an exclusively passive caricature of womanhood, at least long enough to have their children and get them off to school. But after a while they get fed up and demand a divorce. My wife did, and I don't blame her. As we men become more insecure, as we more rigidly assert our "manhood," we grow increasingly distant, withdrawn, and less emotional.

At present, it seems that both men and women are struggling with issues of gender and sexuality. We are each searching for a way to embrace and integrate not only the masculine and feminine principles, but both the active and receptive versions of each. Any experience that can contribute to attaining that wholeness is a healing one.

BODY ELECTRIC AND THE RAISING OF EROTIC ENERGY

For me the first step was a weekend with the Body Electric School. I was terrified. When I hadn't exited this life with the racking cough I had had for three months, I had come to feel, through a series of insights, that my reason for hanging around on this physical plane had to do with reconnecting with the sexual energy that I had abandoned in the final phases of my dying marriage. I had no idea how to go about that, but I was willing to try anything, even a course of instruction in a school called Body Electric.

The school was founded by a gay Jesuit priest, Joe Kramer. He had made it his ministry to help men reconnect their hearts with their genitals. It was an ambitious undertaking, especially in a time when men aren't comfortable exploring their feelings, their hearts are often shut down, and sex is commonly a matter of getting rid of energy that has built up at the second chakra. Kramer's approach was based on Taoist and Tantric principles. It centered around stimulating erotic energy through sexually explicit genital massage and breathing to move the energy created up the spine to the higher centers, especially to the heart chakra. Ejaculation was strongly discouraged. The idea was to conserve that energy and use it to open the heart. It worked. Men wept and had visions. They rediscovered their feelings and their connection with other human beings.

After Joe turned his school over to one of its young teachers, Collin Brown, Body Electric extended its message to women. Collin developed coed workshops, and at one of these he met Sellah, now his partner and the mother of his daughter. The teaching had evolved through a sort of cycle, from same-sex work to a rediscovery of the opposite sex. My first workshop was all men. "When I do this weekend in Europe," Matthew, our leader, commented, "eighty percent of the men are straight-identified. In the U.S., there seems to be more anxiety about working sexually with a group of other men, so the majority of the participants are those who think of themselves as gay."

While I couldn't quite think of myself as "gay"—like "straight," the label felt confining—I knew that I had a longing for a tender, intimate connection with other men. But I wasn't sure that was possible. I was nervous and uptight. When I saw the group sitting naked in the hot tub, talking openly and confidently, I decided I didn't belong there. I wasn't one of *them,* meaning homosexuals. It was only later that I could see how much my own homophobia had locked me into a place of isolation, of fear of my feelings, my vulnerability, and even my intuition.

But at that moment I was only aware that I was cut off from others. I was convinced I was a rather cold and unfeeling person. My ex-wife had told me so, with the authority of twelve years of increasingly painful experience. I had no doubt that it was true. The next morning, however, when I stood in a circle of men, facing one after another, putting my hand on their hearts or giving them full-body hugs, tears came into my eyes. I realized that there was, deep beneath my desperate male image, a capacity for warmth and affection. It was a life-changing insight, one I don't think I could have had with women, who in me called forth instead the need to play the dogged, determined patriarch.

As the experience continued, I was introduced to the power of mobilizing erotic energy and of the incredible healing that could result. Had my own sexual energy remained locked away in forbidden zones, the *shakti* that can transform would have been inaccessible and I would have forfeited the possibility of uncovering and resolving a number of deep and crippling conflicts.

Homophobia was the wall I had to break through, and it is a common obstacle to healing, especially in men. Not only is the assertive (uterine) feminine necessary for bringing into being a radically new internal organizational pattern, the passive feminine is what makes it possible for us to love and nurture ourselves. When men are cut off from these feminine aspects of themselves, they are severely handicapped in their efforts to heal themselves or others, or for that matter, to participate effectively in the healing of the planet.

FREE TO GROW

The beauty of the Tantric use of sexual energy is that it is judgment-free. It lifts you out of the worry about what sort of sexual activity is "normal" or "healthy" and what is not. It allows you to be honest and accepting of the sexual inclinations you feel at the moment and to celebrate the energy they stir up. In a sense, all fuel is the same in this work. Anything that creates erotic arousal is valuable, because the energy so produced can be raised, transmuted, and used to flip the switches at the higher centers and to brighten the compassion, creativity, and insight that they can offer.

You don't have to worry, "Oh God! Is this what turns me on? I must be really sick!" It doesn't matter. If it turns you on, that is, by definition, great, for the energy generated will be used to transform you and your relationships with others. So everyone is going to grow and evolve. Better be ready (if you were aiming to hide in a stagnant, repetitive relationship, watch out!)

But this Tantric approach to sexuality works only if there is a containment of the energy generated. Simply "having sex," whatever the trappings, is hardly Tantra if the energy is not gathered and transmuted. The critical capacity to hold the energy might be best thought of as an aspect of the masculine, though one distinct from the stereotype of phallic/aggressive masculinity.

Just as feminine energy has its assertive side, in addition to its more conventional passive/receptive one, aggressive masculine energy has its other side, too, a more passive one that contains, conserves, and protects. Oriental sages like to say that within every *yin* there is a *yang,* and within every *yang* a *yin* (see Fig. 136). The more obvious nurturing *yin* nature of the woman harbors a capacity for *shakti*'s assertion and vitalizing push, which, though more *yang,* is still decidedly feminine. Similarly, the phallic activity of the man obscures his capacity for a peculiarly male ability to keep safe, to hold in readiness. This is the provider's nest egg, the farmer's granary, the investor's reserves.

Holographically this dual capacity is depicted by the anatomy of the male. While the penis points outward and is the instrument of penetration, the testicle is a container. The word *testis* comes from a Latin root that means "earthen vessel." It is this aspect of the masculine energy that needs to be brought to bear to use *tapas* effectively. This is the knowledge of when to wait, when not to expend energy, but to hold it and allow it to build.

While it is the woman's challenge to integrate her *shakti,* the more *yang* aspect of the feminine, men must honor the more holding, containing, *yin* aspect of the masculine. In fact, there are four of us in here. Inside me, besides the more apparent phallic/assertive masculine, there is also the more *yin* testicular. But that's just my first foot forward, my obvious persona, as Jung called our more surface identity. There's also my anima, my feminine side, and it has two aspects, too, the *yin* passive and nurturing, and the *yang shakti.* Somehow I have to integrate and coordinate all four. No wonder there is so much confusion about gender roles and sexual identities!

To be whole and to heal, we need to learn to call on all four of these energies, using each when it is what is needed. Just as men must learn to draw on the feminine, so women will need to tap their capacity for the masculine energies at times. Phallic male energy should not be off-limits to the woman. It is an indispensable part of her repertoire, too, even though it is not a substitute for the feminine version of the assertive. Nor is it for a man either. There are occasions when he, too, needs to dip into his *anima* and come up with the uterine exertional impulse with its relentless capacity to destroy the old and to bring into being something totally new, with its sense of timing, its clarity on the rightness of this moment to act. If we are to produce leaders who can redirect the world, who can divert it from its catastrophic course and give birth to a new consciousness, they will need, first and foremost, to embody this assertive feminine power.

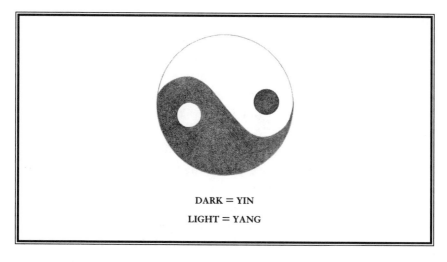

DARK = YIN
LIGHT = YANG

FIGURE 136

The next most grievously neglected energy is the more passive or *yin* masculine. Without cultivating the capacity to contain and conserve, the *kundalini shakti* cannot be accumulated sufficiently to be redirected through the technique of *tapas* so it can power deep healing. Again, both men and women need to develop this capability. Practicing the containment of energy, so that it can be moved upward, is most often done with a partner. But that can be confusing at the beginning, because of all the intricate interpersonal interactions going on between the eight (!) of you. For this reason some teachers recommend that initially the techniques be mastered solo, so that you can concentrate more singlemindedly on what you're doing.[7]

Holistic Mindwork

If we can do bodywork and energy work, then why not "mindwork"? Actually the foundation we've just laid, in our discussion of *tapas,* opens just this possibility. Bumping energy up to activate higher chakras and to raise consciousness to a more encompassing level gives you new leverage in working with the mind. Now you are not limited to being caught up in your own mental processes or on relying on another person, such as a psychotherapist, to take you through the psychological changes you need to undergo. Instead, you have the option to bring into play a different level of awareness within yourself. Stepping back into this "consciousness outside the mental field" allows it to refocus your mind. This supramental consciousness can also, when appropriate, revamp the mind's habitual response patterns, eliminating rote interference mental habits might otherwise offer to personal transformation and spiritual evolution.

The assumption that we as humans are evolving spiritually is an ancient and universal one—a basic part of what Aldous Huxley called "the perennial philosophy." But it's new to much of psychology and medicine.

Psychologists have talked rather glibly about "growth," especially during the 1970s, when we were entering the peak of the humanistic movement. But exactly where this growth was to take us was not clear. With the influx of Eastern influences and the increasing emergence of holistic perspectives, however, the concept has evolved into one that carries more spiritual overtones. This not only allows, but actually requires, that we begin to talk about a more encompassing, unifying consciousness or "Spirit" as a context for working therapeutically with the mind, and to integrate into our thinking an acknowledgment of our strivings toward connection to that Spirit.

Meanwhile, as the holistic movement struggles to integrate its various parts, this perspective of "spiritual growth" has moved into the treatment of purely physical problems, so that we begin to see a widespread acceptance of the idea that physical symptoms may be a result of one's resistance to the expansion of consciousness and one's hesitance to move toward a more universal connection to an encompassing Spirit.

Throughout our tour of holistic medicine we have repeatedly seen that the greatest leverage for healing is found at the subtlest levels of function. If the specifics of physical ailments are expressions of a hitch in a process of moving along life's path, which is ultimately about the flowering of consciousness, then the mind can either contribute to or sabotage this movement. If we can go directly to the mind and deconstruct those automatic sequences that interfere with that movement, and enhance those that are freeing, we will have a most effective and efficient tool for healing.

But first it's necessary to learn to step free of the sort of narrow identification with the mind that plagued the following person:

> "If the bank comes through with the loan in time, I'll be able to salvage the deal," Barton sighed, his brow wrinkled and his eyes tense with the signs of insomnia and constant obsessive worry. "But there's only another twenty-three days before the offer expires." He was fifty-six years old, and caught in a business transaction that threatened to ruin him financially. His anxiety prevented him from taking the steps he might have to negotiate a new mortgage, and so matters, he noted, had continued to deteriorate. Barton's psychotherapist had suggested he see a psychopharmacologist for medication, but he was hesitant. "It's my attitude: 'Poor me, I'm a victim. I'll be a failure forever.' That's how I think, even though I know I have a lot of talent and intelligence and creative ability."

Barton could see that his repetitive thoughts were at the root of his problem, but he couldn't entertain the possibility that he could alter them. Like Dr. Cottle, the breath researcher in Chapter 5, who saw his respiratory pattern and resigned himself to a heart attack, Barton felt at the mercy of his mind. The first step toward freeing yourself from the tyranny of mental habits is to realize that you are not limited to your mind. Without an experience such as meditation to familiarize you with consciousness beyond the mental, it is difficult to envisage the potential for "mindwork."

Contemporary man operates from such a firm assumption that he *is* his mind, that he is hard pressed to conceive of himself as distinct from it. Perhaps the biggest challenge for teachers from the East has been to address this issue effectively. A student with serious psychiatric problems once approached Swami Muktananda:

> "I've been hospitalized three times," she explained. "The diagnosis is schizophrenia or manic psychosis, they can't be sure. But I just lose it. My husband found me in the bus station at 4:00 A.M. It made sense to me at the time—going there, I mean. But then I was so upset when he tried to take me home that he had to call an ambulance and they put me in restraints." She stopped, out of breath. "I guess I'm a mess," she said plaintively, expecting, it seemed, for the Indian teacher to either deny that or to share her hopelessness. But he did neither.
>
> Instead, he nodded his head in agreement. "It's true," he said. "Your mind is crazy." Then he paused for emphasis and added, "But you're *not*."

Muktananda was inserting a wedge between the mind and its owner. Instead of being dragged back and forth by the mind's currents and cross-currents and acting or reacting to them, by simply entertaining the possibility of a consciousness broader than that busy activity, you open new doors. But this possibility hinges on your ability to maintain a clear distinction between the limited, ego-dominated *mind* and the larger, more encompassing *consciousness,* of which this mind is only a small part.[8] Beginning meditators often express frustration at their inability to "empty the mind." But emptying the mind is not necessary. Simply sitting and beginning to experience the functioning of the mind from a larger awareness is the revolutionary move. If you can envision the mind as something to embrace and relate to, you can work with it the way you did with the body, or with energy.

I struggle with words to communicate this sense of a consciousness that *includes the mind, but does not separate itself from it.* Some traditions speak of a "witness," and that term captures one aspect of the encompassing consciousness—that it can grasp the mind without being confined to it. But, like the notion of the "observer," it is tricky and can lead you off on a tangent. It is of very limited use to withdraw from the mind, create a new—and again separate—consciousness that "sees" the mind, but only from outside.

Such splitting is contrary to the principle of healing as reconnection and making whole. In this case, separating off an observer may result in a detachment that undermines your capacity to experience fully, or to absorb in an integrated way, the impact of your emotional experiences. In other words, you may end up "in your head," and not entirely present to life's lessons. What is needed is a "relationship with the mind" that subsumes it at the same time it goes beyond it.

Should we call this new, more encompassing awareness "the witness," "the observer," "the expanded ego which is no longer egotistical," or what? Each one fails us in some significant way. Confusion stems from the fact that your sense of "I" is constantly evolving during healing work. Always seeking to disentangle yourself from a more limited identity, to contain it, and yet be larger than that, you will forever be discarding one label after another.[9]

In any case the limited mind is the part of you that gathers and collates information, and it may misrepresent or distort that data according to its idiosyncrasies and disorders. Because of its potential for distortion and confusion, your limited mind has become an obstacle to your growth and evolution, leading you off on tangents and creating unnecessary crises and conflicts that drain your energy. But, running well and cleared of glitches, it can be a vital asset, for the mind also serves as a gatekeeper for the vaster consciousness that lies beyond it. Since it can choose to take in information, or turn away from it, it can be a valuable filter. If garbage is let in, it not only comes out later as speech and behavior, but also clogs the inner world with distractions and impediments. The mind can learn to function as an efficient checkpoint officer—letting in only what might be of benefit and screening out what would not.

You're already familiar with this principle. When physical dross obstructs the connective tissue spaces, the subtle currents of ch'i can be impeded. Just as you learn to pick and choose what you eat, you can train your mind to pick and choose what it takes in. When you move on to explore the inner recesses of the world of consciousness, much of what you will stumble over is what you carelessly put in.

Besides discriminating nourishment the mind also needs cleansing, exercise, and rest. But it needs these in the lighter, less effortful mode of releasing negativity, and of being allowed to find its natural rhythms of dance and rest. Once the mind is in reasonable condition, functioning well, without chaos and crises to preempt your attention, you will find it easier to allow your awareness to shift out of the mental field, to cease identifying with it, and to establish your consciousness in a position from which much healing integration can be accomplished. This shift results from movement to a more inclusive perspective.

OUT OF YOUR MIND

To extricate your identity from the chatter and busyness of the mental field requires a new "relationship with yourself." Though you cannot will it into existence, you can create the conditions that will encourage that to happen:

First, eliminate distractions. Sit quietly, relax your muscles—at least the surface muscles. A position that will allow you to align your head, neck, and trunk comfortably will prove most effective. The core or intrinsic muscles along the spine will need to be exerted a bit to hold you in that erect posture that encourages the energy to move up—and, of course, using them tends to bring your consciousness to the axis of your being. This is the central *nadi* (neither right nor left) that supports an integrated consciousness—one that will help you rise above the apparent contradictions of polarities.

Next, regulate your breath. Make sure it's diaphragmatic—this is a time when a calming breath is essential. Focus at a point between the nostrils, to equalize their flow as much as possible. Then breathe up the spine on inhalation, feeling the higher centers wake up a bit. Once your physical body is at ease, and your energy body is humming along rhythmically and comfortably, you might focus your attention on a mental sound, or *mantra*. If you've never been given one, use the universal mantra *so hum,* thinking *so* on inhalation and *hum* on exhalation.[10] This draws your point of orientation upward and inward, so that your ability to be conscious of the inner world is enhanced. If you wish, you can also rest your attention on the space between the eyebrows, the area of the sixth chakra, to support your ability to see clearly within (see Fig. 137).

Once all that is in place, your posture, breathing, sound, and point of orientation established, you are well positioned to fully experience the inner you. You may survey your body—is it calm and relaxed? What's going on with your heart, your intestinal tract, and your breath? What is happening with the currents of energy that we've explored? Is there a

---

THE MEDITATIVE SHIFT
"Embracing the mind"
and how to invite that to happen:

1.

Eliminate distractions:
find a quiet place, sit comfortably,
relax all muscles not needed to
maintain an upright posture.

2.

Allow the breath to become regular
and diaphragmatic
with both nostrils open,
inhaling up, exhaling down.

3.

Encompass thoughts,
but don't identify with them;
use a mantra as an anchor
(e.g., "so" on inhalation, "hum" on exhalation).

FIGURE 137

perceptible upwelling of energy when you inhale? If not, can you "allow" it to happen more? And finally, check out your mind. What's it up to?

Chances are, it will be chattering away. Your job, remember, is simply to be with it—as though you flipped channels and happened to tune in to your own mental process. The more you are free from *doing,* the more is revealed to you. This non-doing establishes a beachhead beyond the mind on the shores of a vast inner consciousness that remains to be explored. Already, from this new vantage point, you can begin to assimilate the simple but revolutionary fact that your mind is *not you.* Your mind may be an instrument, but it is not who you are. Its faults and foibles may be silly or endearing; they can be seen through or appreciated, as you might appreciate a drama acted out before you, or the squalls and storms, sunrises, and cloud formations of the weather's spectacle.

Declining to operate from the usual, ego-related, "busy doing," kind of awareness allows another to "flow in" and replace it. This is *tapas* in action: a limited consciousness gives way to one that is more encompassing. If you stick with this inner exploration, you will increasingly discover a new identity—one that is less separate because it's more connected to a pervasive Spirit, to a buoying matrix of universal and unconditional love. This discovery is at the core of your radical healing.

MONKS WITHOUT MONASTERIES

Such work represents a coming together of two ways of living that were traditionally kept quite separate. In the spiritual traditions, monastic life was devoted to contemplation and meditation—the cultivation of an all-embracing consciousness. This was accomplished by surrender of the self to the Divine. Life in the world, on the other hand, was accepted as immersion in the busy details of practical matters with the aim of developing the individual self. This was the self that worked to earn a living or to make its mark, the self that plunged into relationships and the drama of life. In more recent times, our notion of the worldly life has been extended to include the analysis and understanding of this self. During lunch hour we see our therapists; personal growth has become one more responsibility of being in the world. But the study of the self, if pursued earnestly and sincerely (not as another ego ornamentation), will open awareness toward an ever-more-inclusive consciousness until eventually it approaches that territory historically reserved for the monk and the mystic. The two paths begin to merge.

One might argue that this is a relatively new phenomenon, in the West at least, these seekers not in monasteries—both surrendering the ego and yet developing it to function creatively in the world.[11] Yet this is the logical outcome of our holistic effort. The circle, which is the involvement of the self with the world, is attended to and refined even as the axis, the vertical arrangement of the centers of consciousness, is scaled to bring higher and higher integrative awareness to bear. The synergy of the two accelerates healing transformation.

REPAIR WORK

Besides the maintenance work that comes from applying foundation-stone principles to the mental field, there is also "repair work," that which is done to help the mind move through issues where it might be stuck. The mind is often caught up in polarization of energy at a certain chakra, obscuring a more integrated vision. The resolution of that polarity frees the trapped energy to move on in a more evolutionary direction.

The flower essence is the perfect remedy for such polarization:

> *Joyce is irritable and in a hurry. She has a million things to do, all of which are important. The people around her are inept and, if she were to be frank, a bit dull-witted. They simply can't keep up with her, and what's worse, they create obstacles to accomplishing what needs to be done. What has been created within her is a polarity: the hyper-efficient versus the stupid dullard.*
>
> *During Joyce's childhood her mother had called her stupid and lazy at times when Joyce just wanted to have fun. So she learned to project laziness onto others and she played the other pole, that of super-woman. Most of the energy fueling this scenario is related to the third chakra. The essence of the Impatiens flower does much to help melt this polarization. Joyce begins to feel less rushed, less like her agenda is critical for the survival of mankind. She is more understanding of the desires of others to relax and enjoy the simple pleasures of life. The energy tied up in that polarity comes back to center, brings her a sense of being both calm and dynamic, and begins to move up to open her heart to more compassion and caring.*

As you move away from center, you create polarities by accentuating the left or the right, the active or the passive version of an issue or characteristic. The movement into polarization, the holding on to one side, always calls into being its opposite—whether you feel that pole, too, or whether you project it onto another person. It's the obsessive restricting of consciousness to movement from one extreme to the other, from positive to negative, that establishes the world of manifestation and the energy used for that is not available to illuminate a more evolved or encompassing consciousness (see Fig. 138).[12]

Polarities seduce you, drawing you out of an inclusive consciousness. The issues we associate with the chakras are all polarity issues: domination/submission, taking in/releasing, masculine/feminine. There are innumerable variations and spin-offs from these basic polarities, and they combine to form an amazing array of complex hybrids. Fortunately, there exists in nature an equally staggering array of flowers—each embodying

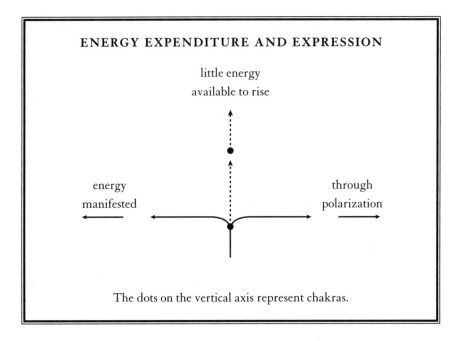

FIGURE 138

the informational message needed to trigger to unifying consciousness that will resolve and transcend some peculiar polarization that the human gets lost in. Not that immersion in the vibratory activity of polar alternation is a bad thing. It is, in fact, the very stuff of life. It's the experience we came here to learn from and delight in.

Healing doesn't mean losing the capacity to dance the polarities. It just means opening to a bridging consciousness that encompasses *both* poles. Then you are able to appreciate your mind taking on one side without feeling trapped in it. Thus equipped, you can play with polarities rather than be swept back and forth by them. It's the difference between having fun in the surf and being terrified by the waves.

GETTING HELP

When you can't manage your diet successfully, see a nutritionist. When you have trouble with your energy body, see an energy worker. When you struggle to do this "mindwork" and run into snags, get help from a professional. Conventional psychotherapy can sometimes fit the bill, but it may also take you off track. Just as conventional medications sometimes add biochemical clutter and confusion, conventional psychotherapy may unwittingly impede your mind's movement to clarity and higher consciousness by adding more cumbersome bulk to it.

What you want is someone who can help you sharpen the skills you need to perform your own mindwork without creating more repetitive intellectual and emotional entanglements.[13] You want someone who can get you through a present crisis, help you see clearly what you're not bringing into focus at the moment, and model the integrative approach—pulling the physical, mental, and energetic into a comprehensible package. A holistic approach might read the body to decipher the mind, as we see in the following example:

> *Melinda entered the office with her head hanging so that her hair covered most of her face. When she sat down and looked at me, I saw why. Her features, usually strikingly attractive, were distorted by swelling that extended across her brow and around her eyes. She was embarrassed to be out in public. But there was something else, too, that was different about Melinda today. Her previously childlike posture and bearing had given way to an aura of maturity and decisiveness that was evident despite her concern about her appearance.*
>
> *Sitting with me was Joseph Aldo, a medical intuitive who had developed his ability to sense energy around chakras in a way that allowed him to contribute to understanding disease. "There seems to be a conflict going on," he said, "between the fifth and sixth chakra." This was the first time he had seen Melinda, and he knew nothing about her history. "It's as though," he said, "you see what you need to do with the third eye, but you're holding back in the area of the throat." Then he looked at me. "Do you see the tightness around her throat?" It was true. She also nodded in agreement. "There's something you need to say to someone," he said, "in order to take the next step that you see so clearly is required." She smiled sheepishly. "I knew that," she said. I explained to Joseph what she was referring to.*
>
> *Melinda had been living for years with an ambitious businessman who had made her a mere appendage to his life. An artist, she had contented herself with gardening, creating a palette of color in the flower beds surrounding his country house. But she knew her own work required that she free herself. She had hinted for some time that she wanted a separation, to find a place of her own, but he seemed not to hear. This present situation represented a crucial turning point in*

Melinda's life. And it was more than a situational challenge. It re-created the theme of her struggles up to this point.

Her father had also insisted on treating Melinda like a little girl, and yet, to support her painting, she had found it necessary to cater to his whims, to show up in his office periodically and play the obedient daughter. If she pleased him, he would send her away with enough money to keep her studio and her artwork going. Fairy Lantern flower essence had helped her step out of her little-girl posture, and Walnut flower essence had helped her move toward breaking the link with the patterns of her past. But now, on the threshold of taking the step, she was clutching, her hesitation expressed in the tension of her throat—where mobilizing energy for creative action is the theme.

After the three of us sat silent for a moment, Melinda looked up and said, "So, can you give me something for the swelling?" Her bid for a prescription was rote. "What will eliminate the swelling, I think, is saying what you need to say." "But I look so ugly," she responded. I laughed. "Maybe what you have to say isn't so pretty." She stood up. "So, you mean all I need to do is talk to my boyfriend?" "I think that's the remedy," I said. She shuddered as she put on her coat. "It's a scary thought." But as she strode out of my office, I knew she was ready.

Here the practitioner functions as *seer*. He looks at the body and at the energy to understand what is going on in the mind. He offers his observations to the patient, but not to the patient's mind so much as to her larger awareness—that aspect of her consciousness which is joining him in looking down at the interplay of mind, energy, and body.

The holistic psychotherapist, or "mindworker," will be inclined to relate to the mind less from an egocentric perspective than from a holographic point of view—employing a variety of complementary skills to round out their psychological understanding and to support it with clues from other aspects of your holographic nature. One possibility is to read the body.

I stood naked while John Pierrakos walked around me, cocking his head, moving an arm or a leg a bit to get a better sense of it. He studied my body as a botanist might scrutinize a field specimen—absorbed, thoughtful. Then he began to tell me about my life, my experiences with my mother, my strengths, my weaknesses. "You're very creative," he said, looking at my hands and forearms. I smiled.

Then, "Your long neck shows you live in your head and try to keep it away from your feeling centers." I quit smiling and pulled my head down a bit, turtle-like.

Besides the body, there's the whole of surrounding nature, which we connect to holographically. The sum total of our symptoms, both physical and mental, may point to a homeopathic remedy—the natural substance with which our present state resonates. This also allows the wealth of information about that plant or mineral to enrich the practitioner's view of you and your mental state.

Homeopathic remedies represent personality types and miasmatic positions because they bring out the subtle patterns that underlie the external features of the earth. Similarly, the basic components of consciousness and its strategies for evolution are reflected in the heavens. Some mindworkers may use your birth chart to decipher your mental and emotional tendencies. Just as Paracelsus saw the herbs as the "external organs," so the astrologically inclined mindworker will see the planets as the mind turned inside out, and the constellations of stars whose energy impacts them at birth suggesting evolutionary strategies that each aspect of your mind will pursue to contribute to your movement along your path in life.

If all pieces of the puzzle—your body, your energy, and your mind—are dealt with holistically, opening to other parts of your self and with the larger whole of which you are a reflection, then a healing reunion is inevitable. Fear of disease has less and less place here, as we fix our sights on the exhilaration of discovery and reconnection and the recovery of a secure place in the matrix of love that we call Spirit. In Chapter 12 we will discover how the spiritual dimension of holistic medicine provides its ultimate payoff and synchronizes your efforts for personal healing with the larger goal of healing the planet's pressing ecological and social disorders.

Reweaving

Only the inner sanctum of the Cathedral was lit. Though not an initiate, I was invited. Sitting among the disciples of the Q'ero—a surviving line of ancient Incan shamans—on a hard pew in the dank grandeur of St. John the Divine, I watched slides of the high Andes.

Five hundred years ago the Q'ero had left Machu Picchu to escape the Conquistadors, fleeing another fifteen hundred feet up into the snow-covered peaks of the surrounding wilderness. Virtually forgotten, they had lived since on the tiny potatoes that could be cultivated during the short growing season there, and had preserved the ancient teachings along with their related techniques of shamanic journeying. But in the 1950s they had descended, proclaiming to a waiting audience that they had been instructed to return to the world—to bring the wisdom and prophecies of old to a planet about to be shaken into a new order.

Now I watched as the Q'ero elders filed in. Wearing the brilliantly colored caps and ponchos of their tradition, they seated themselves on the stone floor of the inner sanctum and set about assembling ritual bundles of stones, shells, flowers, and herbs. Bound into tight little packages, these mesas were laid on our heads in a ceremony of cleansing, healing, and awakening. These bundles are thought to be imbued with great power, since they are created to be a physical expression of the reintegration of the many threads of our lives and consciousness that extend to all corners of the universe.

I felt exquisitely alive, yet not totally there. During a pause in the ceremony I wandered, in a daze, to the cathedral rest room. As I stood before a huge stone urinal, I was overwhelmed by some undefinable feeling that I was a child again, dreaming I was wetting my bed. The sensation was unforgettable, unmistakable. Was I here or there? Was I asleep or awake? Time and all its dimensions seemed to be collapsing around me. . . .

The Q'ero insist that the Earth is in the beginning stages of another *pacchacuti,* or major upheaval. The last was when the Europeans eradicated the indigenous cultures of much of the world, beginning about half a millennium ago. This time, they say, the pendulum will swing back, bringing an end to what they call "the white man's paradigm." We will, they predict, recover our sense of wholeness, our connection to the earth and to our "star brothers," beings from other dimensions of existence. What lends power to their pronouncements is its unanimity. Representatives of indigenous traditions from around the world have begun to meet and discover that this message is a common theme of their spiritual teachings—one that, in virtually every case, specifies that the time for that monumental shift is in the very near future.[1]

With only a little bit of a stretch, we can see that the paradigm that these keepers of the ancient wisdom are describing to replace our reductionistic, patriarchal one bears a striking resemblance to what we have been referring to as the holographic. To say that this is earth-shaking is not an exaggeration. At least when it comes to healing, shifting to a holistic or holographic model is not a trivial change. Genuine holistic medicine is not merely a cosmetically altered form of conventional medicine, embellished with exotic terminology and herbal formulas. Rather, it represents a fundamental shift in thinking, a return to, and a revisioning of, the universal spiritual underpinnings of the great world traditions. Here, sharpened by the discrimination of the truly scientific mind, those ancient teachings take on a renewed clarity and an expanded significance. It's both new *and* old, traditional and yet radical.

The Emerging Paradigm

During the course of this book, a new way of looking at health and healing has been steadily taking shape. It has shown itself in practically every chapter, and we have taken note of the differences between the conventional and the more holistic perspectives with regard to each issue. Now we are at a point where we can step back and look at the totality of what has emerged.

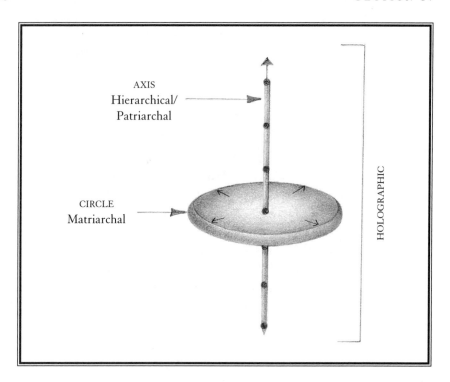

FIGURE 139

The new paradigm is not merely a reversion to ancient thought, to a time when health was a matter of being well knit into the order of nature, when mankind sat in a circle of sharing, like the council of a Native American tribe. But it *is* a recovery of that awareness of natural forces and a synthesis of it with the more linear precision of the modern age.

The hologram is a perfect prototype for this new synthesis, because the gestalt it creates is made possible by harnessing the focused intensity of the laser. The unidirectional power of the laser beam might be taken as a symbol of the accomplishments of the reductionistic mind. It permits penetrating examination as well as the surgical excision of specific pieces, and yet its piercing nature can be harnessed to create the three-dimensionality of the holographic image. The hologram, as model for the new paradigm, moves beyond the tribal circle of prehistory and beyond the vertical line of later hierarchies.[2] It might be thought of as a solid form produced by the combination of the two—like the shape created in Chapter 10 when you turned in a circle with your arms out. The circumference describes your points of interaction with the world, and the axis and your spine your path to a more expanded consciousness (see Fig. 140).

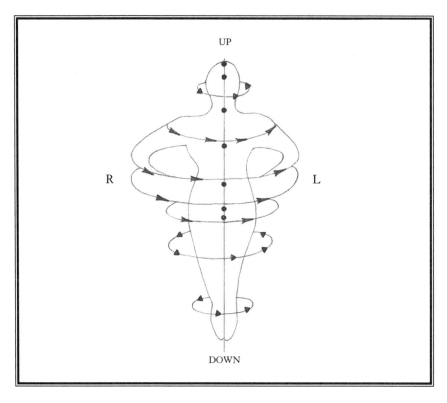

FIGURE 140

In fact, the body might be the perfect example of the holographic image. Like the Incan ritual bundle, it comprises numerous bits and pieces, each being a thread of the universal, woven together into an eloquent depiction of the whole. When we struggle with its feelings, its rhythms, its gurglings and movements, we are seeing our own glimmerings of shifting stars, hearing our own echoes of thunder in the clouds. All our intricate interconnections with the life of the planet and of the universe are expressed here, ingeniously coordinated to create a functioning holographic representation of the macrocosm. And it's not a static image, because the universe it reflects is not static. Your body is constantly in flux, its changes reflecting your own journey toward comprehension of the whole, your progressive opening to something larger, and your gradual recognition that *that* is you. So healing is the reweaving of the holographic image, connecting and reconnecting, picking up lost threads and reintegrating them into the multicolored splendor of your own individual existence, finding that your piece of the pattern is only one small part of a greater Oneness.

That existence involves your living through the experiences that carry you along your path of personal discovery, evolving step by step as those life experiences resolve issues at each center, releasing energy to move up to activate a more encompassing consciousness. When you're stuck, illness ensues. When you withdraw your energy from the process, more serious disease of a deeper, miasmatic nature follows. That deeper disease is your individual expression of the larger, planetary withdrawal of energy from collective evolution. The dark and destructive structures—ecologically unsound cities, stifling institutions, and greedy corporate giants—growing out of that withdrawal both reflect you and offer you an opportunity to contribute to a greater healing.

The Soul's Journey

If healing is reconnection, and we are suffering because of our separation from the nurturing matrix of a more encompassing consciousness, we might wonder what's stopping us from reestablishing that connection. To get some perspective on this question, we can look at the story of the Fall, a common theme in most of what we would call civilized traditions— especially those of the West. Man is seen as suffering from isolation and alienation, a fall from grace. Spirituality here concerns itself with *salvation,* a return to a state of connection with the Divine. But most indigenous spiritual traditions do not have a concept of salvation, nor do they tell the story of a fall. They still "live in the Garden." Their spirituality antedates the alienation of the reductionistic era. They still feel themselves part of, and shaped by, a more encompassing Whole.

While the surviving traces of indigenous systems are a valuable touchstone for us, clues to a dimension of existence that we long to recover, we are treading a different path. We are, for the most part, struggling with the isolation of the materialistic ego, the journey of the hero who has chosen separation and must now wander through the wilderness of alienation until he discovers a way to a new union—one that honors his individuality at the same time as it celebrates his oneness with the universal. This will yield a new human consciousness, one that reveres the Earth but *also* embraces the stars.

What we can do to help this struggling hero is to offer him or her the best that our wisdom has developed in the way of maps of the territory in which he or she is lost. Such maps must cover our fusion with nurturing figures in early life and extend through the rigors of separation and our futile efforts to recapture the bliss of that initial passive dependence. If she can negotiate all these dangers and resist their allure, our hero can discover that she is guided in her journey by inner voices that are part of a vast realm of power and consciousness—one that is, in fact, the essence of who she is herself. Then she knows that she is utterly safe and cared for, and that her every spontaneous movement is an expression of the Divine, and is perfect and right.

But for those who have not yet reached that epic goal, who see themselves as separate and vulnerable, life is still dominated by fear and anxiety. And if we are to subscribe faithfully to the concept that consciousness is the most powerful causative level of our being, then this conviction of separation has far-reaching consequences.

A DRAMA OF NECESSARY FOLLIES

Separation and isolation are the great adventures of that hero we might call "the soul." I'm always hesitant to drag out a term like that, which may call forth so many associations for so many people. But what intrigues me about the idea of soul is that it can be contrasted with spirit—especially Spirit with a capital *S*.

Sometimes it's the very experience of confusion, depression, or isolation that the soul needs to go through in order to get more in touch with the Universal or the Spirit. Those experiences define what I've been calling "your own path," "the agenda for your life," circumlocutions intended to hint at the wanderings—the deeds and misdeeds—that constitute the journey of the soul. The guru might say, "Where do you need to go? You are already one with the Universe!" And of course that is true in a sense. But what you have to go through to *realize* that—that is the long and arduous odyssey of the soul. It is true that some of the things you put yourself through are not necessary. Some can be accelerated or done more efficiently. But others are trials that you simply have to pass through. They are necessary for your learning.

There are times when there is value in feeling the downside of life's experiences—savoring the bitter taste, as we've put it. My daughter went through a dark period during her adolescence, turning tragic and depressed. She lived for the gray, rainy days and sat, miserable, writing grim poetry with dark, sinister images. I tried to draw her out, to cheer her up, but to no avail. Finally she'd say, "Leave me alone, Dad. I'm depressed. I *need* to be depressed." My ten-year-old son put it even more succinctly one evening. Distraught by his sadness, I was searching desperately for a way to turn it around. He kept pushing me away and I kept coming back. Finally he lost his patience and said disgustedly, "Stop trying to *fix* it, Dad!"

The Greek word *psyche* means both "soul" and "butterfly." The image it offers suggests that the soul is capable of metamorphosis from earthbound caterpillar to chrysalis to a winged, heaven-bound creature. The soul is the intermediary, the transformed being in progress, struggling to escape its cocoon. Its arena is the sphere of experimentation, its challenge is to disentangle itself from materialistic consciousness, and its joy is the dance of liberation. The soul is closely connected to, and intermeshed with, the energy body and the emotions.[3] Its life lies between body and spirit. It involves the mind and subtle energy, and it unfurls a long series of scenarios, its own agenda of experiences that it is intent on living through.

As Thomas Moore says in his book *Care of the Soul,* working with this part of yourself allows you to take back what has been disowned. The soul's struggle involves dirtying yourself by plunging into those thoughts and feelings you have avoided and disowned. This doesn't mean that you have to abandon that consciousness that encompasses and accepts. On the contrary, just being aware of where you are lifts you out of your misery in some subtle way. Nevertheless, there remains a part of you that will say, "Yes, but I'm still depressed." And that's okay.

Go ahead. Be depressed. You can do it better, more thoroughly—and certainly more effectively—because you are larger than this drama. Containing it within a larger, encompassing consciousness means you learn about it more quickly and have to repeat it less. This embracing consciousness shepherds the soul through its journey. This larger awareness, which was born when it discovered it could stand back from and yet contain the mind, is very allied with—and becomes increasingly synchronous with—the Spirit. As it expands and matures, and as it allows more and more of that universal consciousness in, it moves toward becoming one with it. Meanwhile the soul is going through its journey on earth as it needs to, the very journey that moves it toward the greater wisdom and further evolution of the more inclusive Self.

Thomas Moore says that observing yourself nonjudgmentally is homeopathic in its workings rather than allopathic. That is to say it befriends a problem instead of making an enemy of it. The homeopathic remedy builds on the transformational crisis, making of it an asset rather than a disaster to be averted or denied. It is embraced as an opportunity for learning, for reorganization. The homeopathic remedy, the flower essence, the well-placed acupuncture needle, or the psychotherapeutic insight can lift us over the bump in the road so we see it clearly, help us regain our footing, and set us on our path again, a bit farther along, a bit more aware.

FROM PARANOIA TO DEPRESSION

In the cultural context in which most of us exist, the soul's journey is a passage through the experience of separation. This is the challenge of a patriarchal, materialistic age. It is a tortuous path through states that we have come to describe in the reductionistic language of pathology and alienation. It starts with, and is grounded in, the process of projection, since that process is the root of splitting—of disconnection and separation from the matrix of love that would sustain us. We are whole until we project a part of ourselves outside. On entering this life, we initiate this separation by dividing the chaotic world that surrounds us (and ourselves) into two simple components, the Good and the Bad.[4]

Some things make us feel good: kind words, food when hungry, a quiet place when tired. Others cause suffering and pain: physical trauma, cold indifference, an angry scowl. All the good, psychologists have observed, tends to be grouped together and identified with some idealized parent or partner—the perfect mother or the dream lover. The other forces, those that leave you cold or hungry and bristle with frustration, anger or rejection, are pinned on some negative figure in your world—the difficult boss, the nasty cabdriver, the guy who cut you out of a lucrative financial deal. That is a different, darker image, one that inspires fear—and may even take on demonic dimensions.

How to handle life at this point seems obvious. Stay as close to the Good as possible, and as far away from the Bad as you can. This turns out to be a pretty neat trick: everything good is here;[5] everything bad is out there and I simply need to give it wide berth. Welcome to the world of projection and paranoia. A basic approach to the unpleasant aspects of life has been established. Whatever I feel that is troublesome must be coming from outside. If I can stay away from it I'll feel fine; if I can't, then I just may be forced to attack it and try to destroy it.

Though the paranoid game keeps us flirting with the illusion of connection, of oneness with a powerful (if unpredictable) being, it's not a very happy place to be. There's always something dark and menacing out there. The tragedy of projection is that the more of ourselves we split off from the whole and project outward, the more we feel incomplete and afraid. The fear that follows leads to the urge to attack. If attack is felt to be unacceptable, it gets projected, too, and the fear intensifies. This reaction to fear—the attempt to overcome it rather than to embrace it and operate from a consciousness larger than it is—is the unconscious basis of most of the physical and mental diseases that plague us.

Panic attacks are a hint that one might still be heavily invested in this position, as are feelings of rage or persecution. "I'd be doing great, but my boss is constantly on my case, and she makes my life miserable. Everything would be fine if it weren't for *her.*" Convenient as the projection may be, it may also be sufficiently uncomfortable to nudge us toward hazarding another step on our journey through the desert of separation.

Right in the middle of the terrain the soul must traverse is a bleak place called Depression. Much of the hero's challenge is to find her or his way across this wasteland (see Fig. 141).[6] The emptiness of depression comes from losing the buoyant nurturing of the idealized other. She or he—mother, father, lover, best friend, or whoever—is the source of all that makes you feel warm, secure, and happy. Losing her or him leaves you desolate.

We all work through this loss to some extent in early childhood, but it is seldom totally resolved. Since, in this present era, our inner life is so separate from the Spirit that sustains us, we return repeatedly to this "depressive position," baffled by the profound sense of isolation and loneliness that plagues us. We struggle to hang on to the narrow identity of the ego and still find a way to feel connected to something larger, and the impossibility of that effort doesn't stop us from trying again and again. We resort to desperate measures to recapture the bliss of union with the perfect partner. Alcohol is a common strategy, and it works to a degree. After a few drinks we are enveloped in the warm, rosy glow of security and comfort. We are back, or at least have the feeling that we are, in Ultimate Mother's safe embrace.

Or it may be a shot or a pill, a double chocolate cheesecake, or even a computer game. The addictive mode has many faces—all look great at the outset, but fail to hold up. There's always the next morning, when we find ourselves back in the bleak cold of the depressive dilemma, one more attempt at reunion having failed. But when you're hovering on the edge of depression, the addictive tactic is well-nigh irresistible. Another com-

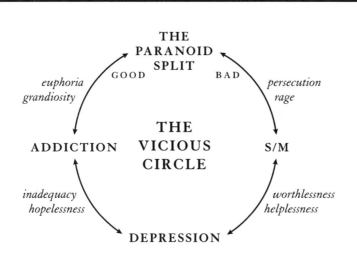

Arrows show possible movements around the circle, e.g., from the depressive to the addictive modes of function. Moving back and forth in that territory usually involves feelings of inadequacy and hopelessness. While addiction is an illusory reunion with a good parent or object, shifting up toward more paranoid thinking may intensify that illusion, with resulting euphoria and grandiose self-concepts.

FIGURE 141

mon example is the allure of the antidepressant drug. It promises respite and creates the illusion that all is well. But when it's discontinued, the feelings reemerge because the drug has failed to move us through the expansion of consciousness that would ultimately bring us out of this circular impasse.

THE VICIOUS CIRCLE AND HOW TO GET OUT OF IT

Another desperate tactic to escape depression is to deal with the negative pole of what has been projected and take on the Bad Guys—simply quit running away and face their wrath. Deep down, those fearful forces are connected with primal guilt.[7] Submit to their punishment and surely you will be forgiven, nurturance and bliss once more bestowed upon you. This sadomasochistic maneuver may involve a relationship of domination and abuse, or the dynamic may be staged internally, with suffering and pain created physiologically, sometimes becoming a full-blown illness. Lurking in the back of the mind is the conviction that clemency will be granted if the suffering is severe enough.

A great deal of life can be spent going round and round this Vicious Circle,[8] creating new versions of old strategies—from addiction to depression, from depression to guilt and pain, and back to a place of paranoia and suspicion. We emerge from it when we decide to cease the circular movement, contain the energy we've been investing in it, and through some *tapas*-like maneuver hoist ourselves up where we can see better. Moving up the chakras, we discover a different quality of sustenance, one that makes the fuzzy, warm feeling that we were seeking before look like the funky sofa of a couch potato.

We are unconsciously struggling with a choice between union with Spirit and union with "other"—the stubbornly persistent, though doomed, effort to fuse with another person or thing in order to attain the security, tranquillity, and bliss that would attend an awareness of our oneness with the Universal Matrix of nurturing love. This is not to imply that there is no evolutionary value in our one-on-one relationships. If, through our effort to make contact, our heart chakra opens a bit more, and some degree of love prevails, we give up a bit of our ego rigidity and take one more step toward acknowledging our identity with the Whole.

This sort of discovery occurs when we keep the dynamism of *spanda* alive. If, on the contrary, we stop basing our actions on *spanda,* then we stagnate and disconnect from the aliveness that our adventure in this life would otherwise provide. When the soul stops its journey to Spirit, it loses contact with its source of energy and motivation, and the body falls into disease.

The 3-D World: Digression, Disconnection, and Disease

In the course of this book, in order to understand the complexities of sickness and health and the principles of healing, we have established a multilevel model of your being. Besides your physical body, there is an "energy body," a network of chakras and energy pathways that has a shape or form that corresponds to that of the physical body. There's a "mental body" of sorts, also, with its conscious and unconscious components and

COPING WITH DEPRESSION

Movement

Moving is key. Exercise is a must. Aerobics is the first step, but movement therapies are also of great value.

Cleansing

You can't move on if you're hanging on to the residues of the past. A thorough detox program can dislodge many a stuck soul.

Breathing

Kappalbhati is a cleansing breath. Your breath is your anchor in an independent and "separate"—but still joyful and secure—existence because it's also your connection to the nurturing matrix which is your *real* "Good Mother."

Remedies

St. John's wort is getting a lot of press, and sure beats the pharmaceutical antidepressants, but the high-potency homeopathic that fits your whole picture is the ultimate. Flower essences can often be helpful until that perfect remedy comes along.

Psychotherapy

Go for the body-oriented type. Work with what you're holding in the muscles and tissues of the physical body. Pure talk can bog down.

Meditation

Identify rote habits that you know are dead-end. Sit with the anxiety and watch the energy burst into new options.

FIGURE 142

its territories of memories and associations that flood into your awareness as you work with specific areas through massage or yoga. The functioning of these three bodies is intricately intertwined.

Although conventional medical science has made us most aware of the impact of what goes on in the physical body—how physiology or biochemistry affect your mind, for example—in this book we have emphasized causality that moves in the opposite direction, from the subtle down to the physical. This perspective—a key one in the holistic approach, and a legacy of the more ancient medical traditions—suggests that the mind shapes the flow of energy, which in turn determines what happens on the physical level. It is the composite of these effects expressed in all three bodies that we see as disease.

Although, from this perspective, mind plays an important role, it is not the ultimate causal force in creating health and illness. In these last chapters we have seen that there is something beyond the limited mind, which shapes it. This is a larger, more encompassing consciousness—one that shades into the realm of the spiritual. Strictures on this larger consciousness—impediments that prevent the soul from fully identifying with the Universal Matrix that sustains us—cause the larger consciousness to have a distorting influence on the mind. This triggers a chain of events that runs down from the mental to the energetic and finally to the physical, creating the conditions for disease.

Therefore, although the larger consciousness that can observe and embrace the mind can be your instrument of healing, to the extent that it is still constricted and separate from the Whole—from Spirit with a capital S—it can also be the agent of suffering. The distortions in this larger consciousness that cause suffering are belief systems and unconscious archetypes that we don't see because they are so much a part of our way of being in the world. Separation, fear, guilt, and projection are manifestations of these distortions.

Such distortions of consciousness constrain our thoughts and actions. As a result, the full expression of our unique individual *spanda* is inhibited, and we are prevented from living fully as co-creators and powerful spiritual beings—a way of living that would completely activate our minds, energize our bodies, and create a state of dynamic health and maximal vitality. We have referred to such distortions of consciousness generically as *miasms*. Exactly how they produce disorder and disease can be traced in detail.

DIGRESSION FROM *SPANDA*

As we have noted, your three-body, physical/mental/energetic composite is a holographic representation of your experience of life, and a map for your soul's journey. Your central axis is the line along which the chakras are located (see Fig. 143), and moving energy up that line activates higher centers, bringing into play a progressively expanded, com-

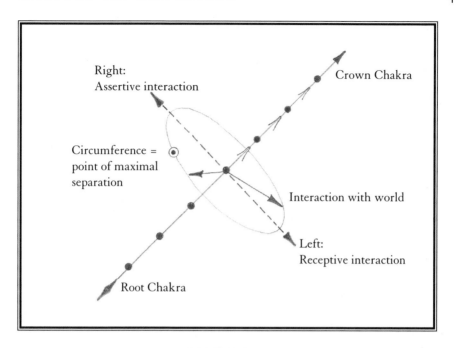

Right:
Assertive interaction

Crown Chakra

Circumference =
point of maximal
separation

Interaction with world

Left:
Receptive interaction

Root Chakra

FIGURE 143

prehensive, and reconnected consciousness. At each station along this line, energy can be pulled out into form and manifestation. This happens through polarization, with polarities tending to coalesce around fundamental dichotomies such as positive and negative, male and female, or assertive and receptive. Such polarities are the language of separation and disconnection from the more encompassing consciousness, and their resolution through integration is an increment of reconnection with it.

The circle, your point of contact with the world around you, is where you interact with other separated entities. Your circumference, the surface of your body, is, in fact, the point at which you experience maximal separation. Going inside far enough takes you to the center of your being, which is the universal. This is reconnection. Going outside takes you to the grandeur of nature and your oneness with it, and beyond that to the stars. But at your skin you are most conscious of borders, separateness. What we think of as our "intimate encounters" are moments when we struggle, by bringing our bodies together, to overcome the loneliness of our isolation.

Bringing energy out to the surface for interaction with the world of separateness is an effort to live through the dilemma, to come to terms with the sense of being closed off, to reach a resolution and thereby experience a measure of healing reconnection. So each of the dramas you stage in your life, each time you take the energy of one or more chakras and throw it out into manifestation—physically as actions, mentally as thoughts, or energetically as pranic interplay—there is some healing intent.

Perhaps you've wondered what effect an antidepressant drug would have. You've read about it, you've talked about it with practitioners, and now you feel impatient. You just want to try it. So you take the medication. You feel calmer, more peaceful—maybe even complacent. You have a sense that everything is okay, though nothing has changed. Things that might have moved you to action, don't. Times when you might have stood up for what was important to you are allowed to slide by. It's as though Mother were there and approving, though she's not.

The experience is, in effect, an experiment, driven by your spontaneous inner urge. By interacting with the world around you, you experience sensations and feelings, you have reactions, and all of this is feedback on how the medication has affected you. These are the results of your experiment. If you take that data, integrate it into your being, and go to the next experiment, your soul moves along its path. But if you do the experiment and don't absorb the feedback, you are shying away from your next step, safeguarding the willful ignorance that will allow you to repeat the same behavior again—and yet again. *Spanda* is no longer engaged. Vitality stagnates, and disease will eventually follow.

The process described can take place on any one of the three levels: mental, energetic, or physical. When there's an issue you've not yet worked through, it demands energy. That energy spins out from the chakra in question, like something popping out to the surface. An issue that moves from the center out to manifestation at the surface, where it can be accessed with a needle, for example, is ready for a stab at resolution. If an expert acupuncturist places a needle in precisely the right point, presto! Everything begins to shift.

Or the issue may move out from the center on the mental level, reverberating into polarization and expressing as an interpersonal conflict, an emotional storm, or a vivid fantasy. The mental body also has its axis and its "surface." Moving out to the surface of the mental body means taking on the form of ideas, images, interactions with other people. In any case, movement to the outer surface—whether physically, energetically, or psychologically—indicates a readiness for being dealt with. You might say it's like a pustule or boil. But it's not *like* that; it *is* that: a boil is an example of exactly that process on the physical level.

Any one of these scenarios, physical, energetic, or mental, has the potential to be meaningful—even if it involves "getting sick." It can be an example of successfully living through the experience needed to come to terms with, and resolve, an issue that previously has tied up some bit of your energy and limited your consciousness. But such a happy outcome is not automatic. The scenario created may fail to lead to insight and reorganization.

If an impulse to integration has been launched into action, giving rise to an interpersonal experience, for instance, but does so outside an integrating awareness, then it may keep spinning on, creating a repetitive pattern of behavior or thought or feeling, and not lead to any resolution at all. Then it ceases to be an experiment—for example with how a drug effect mimics the state of feeling loved—and, by falling into repetition, becomes an addiction. Or it expresses physiologically as a cyst, a tumor, or asthma. These are all chronic disorders. The impulse is out there, doing its thing, but it is not accessible; it has lost contact with the integrating thread of consciousness that would be able to explore, understand, integrate.[9]

For example, I'm eating supper with my youngest son. He's ten and he has a vigorous appetite. What's more, he truly enjoys his food. He takes his time and savors each bite. I admire his *kaphic* contentment, and I am tempted to eat more along with him, to share in the obvious pleasure he is deriving from the spaghetti and seitan balls with tomato sauce. It tastes good. But I've had enough. The center inside of me that determines just what I need says "no more." I decide to ignore it, however, and have more anyway.

But it no longer tastes as good as it did, and besides, I know I'm skating on thin ice. It doesn't take many such "crimes against wisdom," as the Ayurvedists like to phrase it, before you lose touch with your inner sense of what's right for you and begin to function on the basis of other cues. Soon you are eating uncontrollably. The action spins on and on, since you've lost touch with the inner signals that would tell you when to stop. At that point you have taken a giant step toward the eventual development of chronic disease.

There are many such chronic diseases, each involving energy radiating out from some chakra or combination of chakras that was intended to activate a growthful experience, but has gotten stuck like a broken record. Each might be thought of as having become an avoidance of what you are really here to experience, of what feels alive and authentic to you, a departure from the genuine spontaneous expression of your soul's journey. Each such disease began with actions that were no longer on track—that were not satisfying—like the food that my body says no to, but I eat anyway.

When you become disconnected from creative, spontaneous living, then stale, confining habits increasingly direct the course of events. As it deepens and progresses, this miasmatic reshaping of the mind goes through a series of stages. These steps were studied by homeopaths who found that how far a patient had moved along such a course could be determined by mental and physical signs and symptoms. This perspective is useful in healing work because what we are faced with depends on how far that miasmatic process has gone, how far habits have taken you from authentically spontaneous exploration that is enlivening, how disconnected your actions are from the guiding influence of *spanda*.

In the first degree, for example, your sense of what is relevant to you is still intact. You realize you're about to step out of what is "really you," but hesitate. Though you avoid taking the step, energy is tied up in that desire to move out into digression, as the following case illustrates.

> *Hugh consulted me because of headaches, feverishness, anxiety, weakness, and "an itchy psychosomatic rash." Though treated with anti-anxiety medications, his symptoms had gotten progressively worse, so that now his work was jeopardized. When I asked what had changed in his life in the last year, he became agitated, confused, and more anxious.*
>
> *Finally it emerged that during that time he had become increasingly friendly with his assistant. She was a young woman who was from the same strict Christian sect as he, and who was also, like him, married. Of very rigid religious upbringing, he found it difficult to bring to consciousness the intensity of affection he felt for her, or to acknowledge that she was his nearly constant preoccupation. He suspected that she had feelings for him, too, but they had not discussed the matter.*
>
> *It was my impression that although he was very deeply involved with his wife, he had been having trouble responding honestly and firmly to her frustration and anger, had become more withdrawn from her, and was living with a subconscious fantasy of a made-for-TV romance with his young helper. Only when she was transferred by their company to another job did his symptoms slowly begin to abate.*

The energy used to resist an impulse like this is unavailable, and its loss is disruptive to your function. As a result, you are not fully you; some substantial part of your vital energy is trapped in the unexpressed urge. This is distracting, and it undermines your sense of well-being. If you *consciously* sit with the urge and raise the energy, you have accomplished a transmutation of that energy, *tapas*. If you work it through physically— as with a fever—it's a healing crisis. But if it's denied and suppressed, by drugs, for example, it begins to affect your life adversely. According to the classical homeopathic texts, this initial distraction of energy corresponds to the *psoric* miasm.[10]

The process takes a deeper turn when the impulse to act on outer cues is no longer resisted.

> *Ethel has a strong feeling that it's time to move on from the job she's had for fifteen years, which has stagnated. What was originally something of a challenge is now routine, despite repeated promotions. Her children are finishing school, and she no longer needs the level of income that was required to see them through. But giving up the familiarity of the office and the position of responsibility she earned is difficult for her. And to do what she wants, to try making it as a free-lance photographer, would mean cutting expenses and moving out of the fashionable three-bedroom apartment she's lived in for decades. So she has stayed.*
>
> *Ethel's complaints—fatigue, sinusitis, joint pain, and mild asthma—all express her dilemma: the wheezing her sense of smothering where she is, her joint pain her feeling confined, and her post-nasal drip her internalized grief over waiving the opportunity to live fully. When asked, she believes her fatigue comes from bicoastal meetings, entertaining at home, and going out too many nights, all the enviable fruits of her "excellent job," rewards she is determined to enjoy—even if she has to push herself to do so.*

Overdoing is the key word for this second step of digression. It's overdoing because it's a course of action that is *not* exploratory—it does not move you farther down your path to the resolution of your life's issues. This could easily be the *kaphic* type wallowing in heavy foods and vegetating in front of the tube, or the *pittic* type launching into predictable fits of ire. Such *sycotic* indulgence is a distraction, a repetitious pattern that no longer has any real significance for you.

The diseases that cluster around this underlying dynamic are those that in some way express overdoing. Disorders of the mucous membranes are the most common: the linings of the nose, throat, bronchi, ears, vagina, urethra, and rectum, which are the points of contact with the external world. They secrete in order to accommodate traffic with the world—taking in, putting out. The impulse to overdo, to indulge pointlessly, may manifest as a constant oozing from those areas where you might interface with the objects of your indulgence—as if each surface were screaming "More! More! More!" Tumors and cysts are also classic examples of disorders stemming from this second degree of digression. They are overgrowths, another physiologic manifestation of overdoing. *Sycotic* patients are often overweight, too—and struggle with it endlessly.

Warts, little outgrowths of tissue overproduction, considered by the homeopaths the hallmark of *sycosis,* are a visible declaration of your tendency to overdo, and are a physical sign of shame. If the itchy urge to step off your path is the keynote of *psora,* the shame of having done so is the mindset of this second miasmatic position, *sycosis.*

On some level you recognize hiding in repetitive behaviors as a failure to live fully, which generates, even though it may be unconscious, a sense of shame. Shame springs from the knowledge that this is *not* going to give you what you desire from the deepest center of your being.[11] But, at the same time, shame is also a remaining thread of connection. It says, "I know I should stop this, it's the obstacle to my feeling thoroughly alive." Like the string reeled out by a spelunker to help him find his way back out of a cave, the sense of shame is a reminder of how to get back to where you know you profoundly need and want to be (see Fig. 144).

THE EROSIVE DISORDERS AND THE CRUMBLING OF STRUCTURE

With further disconnection, the habit of acting without taking your cue from authentic inner guidance becomes so ingrained that it is now your modus operandi. By this time you have lost touch with the genuine spark within. Shame is no longer felt. You have moved past the point of compulsive indulgence to a sort of boredom and indifference. That doesn't mean the behavior or the thought pattern stops. On the contrary, now it has its own momentum. There's simply no longer any conflict over it. You do it because you see no reason *not* to. The adjective that fits here is *jaded.*

THE SIGNIFICANCE OF CLASSIC HOMEOPATHIC
MIASMS IN AN INTEGRATED HOLISTIC CONTEXT

Miasm	1	2	3
Pathologic process	Deficiency	Excess	Erosion
Prevailing mentality	Suppressed desire	Overdoing/ shame	Disconnection/ terror
Element/chakra	Fire/third	Water/second	Earth/first
Classic symptoms	Itch	Catarrhal discharges, warts	Ulceration
Prime target area/ prototypical disease	Skin, scabies	Mucous membranes, gonorrhea	Nervous system, syphilis
Major remedies	Sulfur (Psorinum)*	Thuja, Medorrhinum	Mercurius, Syphilinum
Hahnemannian name	*Psora*	*Sycosis*	*Syphilis*

*Not purely a *psoric* remedy, though classically considered to be such.

FIGURE 144

This has a very different quality from mere overdoing, where there was always a subliminal comparison going on between what you were doing and what you *should* be doing. Now, that is lost. There is no longer any sense of where you should be. You've let go the reference point. You are adrift with no land in sight, without even the memory that such a thing as land existed. Without awareness of your original intention, with no thread of connection to your purpose or raison d'être, there's no organizing energy to hold your physical vehicle in form. When you withdraw your intention to be in this life, the instrument of that intent, your body, is no longer relevant. Disconnected from its intent, it begins to deteriorate.

There is little pain or discomfort because there's no struggle here. The conflict—the feeling of being torn between two impulses, between the desire to indulge and the urge to do what is authentically you—is gone. Only the rote habit of indulgence remains, and it has lost its excitement without the "straight and narrow" to compare itself with. The fun of rebelling, of "transgressing," has faded away.

It's very tricky to talk about this process without falling into moralistic thinking. But this is not about morality—or at least not about social mores. One can be totally compliant with all the moral laws of religion and culture and yet thoroughly lost. I struggled with this dilemma for many years when dealing with the homeopathic concept of miasms. I was sure that it held some of the most valuable secrets of how illness and spirituality fit together, yet I was repelled by the judgmental tone of what little was written on the subject. It especially bothered me that this erosive class of disorders was termed *syphilitic*. It seemed that they were being regarded as some sort of retribution for failure to conform to religious precepts. Then I noticed that there were two distinct types of patients that developed erosive diseases.

With the first, the derelict, the alcoholic living on the street, careless about who uses his or her body, or for what, the disconnection and erosion seemed obvious. But the second type, of which the following case is an example, was a surprise.

Bernice is fifty-two. She had polio as a girl, but recovered with only a slight weakness in her left leg. She has been able to function normally, and has two grown daughters. Now she comes in because of a numbness and tingling in the affected leg, and a sense of weakness that troubles her. A neurologist called it "post-polio syndrome."

She is a very proper and somewhat compulsive person. Her hair is carefully coiffed, and her clothes look as though just pressed. While she is almost ingratiatingly polite, there is some undefinable lack of warmth in her presence. She seems a bit stiff, stilted. Her friends say she is a "neat freak." In fact, she is a meticulous house cleaner, and puts a great deal of effort into making sure that everything is spotless. She complains of dry skin on her hands, but realizes that it's due at least in part to the fact that she washes them so frequently. She smiles and says that everything in her family life is "fine," but she does acknowledge that she sometimes sleeps fitfully, worrying about tragedies that might befall her children or grandchildren.

Though she has scrupulously done everything "properly," Bernice has lost all touch with the sense of authentic spontaneity in her life, with her inner intent and fire. As a result, her nervous system staggered and nearly fell earlier in life, and now that the enlivening demands of child-rearing and family life have let up, that disease has resumed, and she is losing sensation and strength. At night her mind sinks into despair and terror of separation from purpose and support—her husband, her children, those she relies on for some sense of security and reassurance. Though she holds tightly to her routines and etiquettes, her world is surrounded by a dark frame of the most bone-rending fear and terror.

Subtler versions of this process will be even less obvious, but are often so deeply embedded in the infrastructure of consciousness and the basic functioning of a person that they are still insidious and seriously damaging. Such miasmatic digressions from the soul's journey are rooted in the delicate matter of how closely you adhere to the inner impulse, the central energy of the core of yourself that prompts and guides you along your path of unfoldment. If you ignore that innermost impulse, no matter how superficially ideal your life may look, your body is not properly vitalized by the use it requires (*your* body is designed for *your* path), and where the energy doesn't flow, deterioration begins. It may take years or even decades to reach the point where it is recognized as disease. In fact, it may not express fully until the next generation.

BEYOND GENETIC DETERMINANTS?

There are generational trends in diseases that reveal miasmatic threads running through a family (see Fig. 145). The erosive tendency manifests as the more severe structural abnormalities and degenerations—especially of the nervous system. Birth defects, alcoholism, Parkinson's disease, and strokes are seen, and generally males are more severely affected.[12] In the genealogy characterized by the overdoing disorders, the *sycotic* miasm of homeopathy, you're more likely to find asthma, arthritis, prostate disease, cysts, and tumors. A purely *psoric* family may have, for example, eczema, anxiety, and only functional disorders of the heart, its structure not being affected. Of course, it's rare to see one miasm in isolation, and most of us exhibit some mixture of two of them or of all three.

Understanding the miasmatic nature of these deeper, generational disorders is especially rewarding when treating children. My own son was an excellent example. I was very concerned about the history of heart attacks in my family, because both grandfathers, my father, and most of my uncles had died from them. My teacher understood my apprehension and said, "Let me remove this."

I wasn't quite sure what he meant, but when he instructed me to give a dose of *Thuja* in high potency to the child I did so. A few weeks later I was horrified to observe a huge wart, the size of the end of his four-year-old thumb, appear on his chest, just to the left of his sternum—directly over the heart. I told Swami Rama about it, and he smiled. "That's what I wanted," he said. "Now give him *Medorrhinum* 10M." I did that, too, and a few weeks later the wart simply fell off. "Now he is free!" Swamiji grinned with a gleam in his eye. "That problem will stop here."

The fact that familial trends can be identified does not mean that some families are inferior to others, or that some are "sicker." We might surmise that part of your soul's orienting itself in this confusing world is to wander in those spots where it can get lost. That way you get clear on what is progress and movement—discovery and aliveness—and what is stagnation and inertia. You learn what it's like to be far off the track and, knowing that territory better, how to step around it and get back on.

GENERATIONAL DISORDERS

Psora	*Sycosis*	*Syphilis*
Eczema	Ear problems	Strokes
Anxiety	Moderate obesity	Alcoholism
Functional heart	Hirsutism	Polio
problems	Asthma	Weak or absent
	Manic disorders	male offspring
	Arthritis	Miscarriages
	Tumors	(especially repeated)
	Prostatism	Suicide
	Cystic diseases	Autism
		Infant deaths
		Parkinson's disease
		Alzheimer's
		Multiple sclerosis

FIGURE 145

We might then conceive of a family as an impromptu workshop set up by a group of souls, each wanting to sample that same quality of experience. What we do with our experience, and where we are in our individual evolution, might vary widely, but for a moment we share a taste of life and perhaps a turn in the murky backwaters of miasmatic torpor.

Planetary Miasms

It's a stretch to encompass birth defects, digressions from one's spiritual path, warts, and shame all in one coherent discussion. That's why the miasmatic perspective is so mind-boggling and, at the same time, so intriguing for those of us who are reaching for an integrative vision. And it can be extended even further. According to homeopaths who think in such terms, not only does the effect of miasms span generations, but an understanding of them promises to offer some insight into the relationship between our diseases, our mindset, and our social and environmental disorders.

From this point of view, it is a limited and distorted consciousness that produces disease through how it shapes the mind/energy/body complex (see Fig. 146). That potentially all-embracing consciousness is limited and constrained by belief systems and archetypes that are unspoken and usually unconscious. The mind/energy/body distortions that result are varied and therefore produce a whole spectrum of diseases. Hahnemann, however, identified three *groups* of disorders. He seemed to sense that these three groups of disorders, his three miasmatic classifications, corresponded to three degrees of disconnection of awareness from what we have been calling *spanda*. I'll briefly review below the characteristic mindset of each of the three. We'll also look at how the collective expression (as social and economic problems) of the last two miasms echoes their expression in the individual person.

- The first level of miasmatic distortion is captured in the picture of the *psoric* patient. His attention drawn away from where *spanda* might lead him, he nevertheless manages to hold back from taking action. But he depletes his energy with his constant longing. His fire is expended in subconscious fantasies of forbidden transgressions, and in the effort to restrain himself. He assimilates poorly because the solar plexus power he might use to digest his food is instead diverted into this struggle to control himself. As a

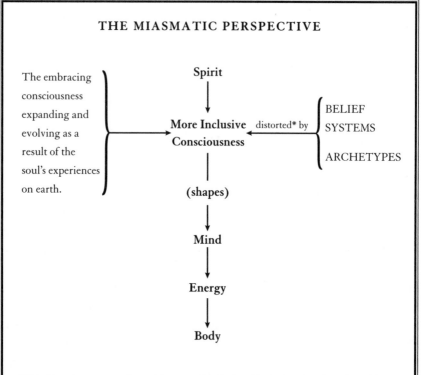

THE MIASMATIC PERSPECTIVE

The embracing
consciousness
expanding and
evolving as a
result of the
soul's experiences
on earth.

Spirit

More Inclusive   distorted* by
Consciousness

BELIEF
SYSTEMS

ARCHETYPES

(shapes)

Mind

Energy

Body

*This distortion prevents the soul from moving freely with the impulse of *spanda* and living fully. Without that distortion, consciousness (fully identified with Spirit) and *spanda* could cocreate our lives. Distortions in the way consciousness shapes mind/energy/body create a spectrum of diseases. The miasm is the *type* of distortion—homeopaths classically distinguished three patterns of distortion, i.e., three miasms.

FIGURE 146

result, he develops deficiencies. His pent-up passion, his itching to step over the line, may express as other symptoms—for example, fiery, itchy eruptions on the skin.

• The next step further into miasmatic disconnection from spiritual moorings is an escape from this self-imposed restraint. In this second miasm, which homeopaths have called *sycosis,* one has had enough of holding back. He's decided to give in to the impulse and *do it!* But without a connection to authentic *spanda* or genuine need, there's no sense of fulfillment from what's done, and no clear end point, no way to know when you've had enough. The result is constant overdoing and pointless repetition. Everything's in excess not only behaviorally but physiologically, too, with tumors, obesity, and overproduction of mucusy discharges.

This stance is more than an individual one. The *Zeitgeist* that supports it has built a society around this pattern of overdoing. Much of modern urban life is a frantic rush of excess activity. Many of us are running about madly, doing twice as much as any human could reasonably be expected to manage—and will try to do three times as much, unless our immune systems collapse first. The physical level of life mirrors our madness: too many possessions, too many books—we've got more words on paper than our ancestors could ever have imagined. We are smothering under mountains of assorted types of garbage, and we have constructed an economy that will collapse unless the production of goods continues to increase. Clogged with surplus, we can't keep up with the necessary cleaning out. We have created a world that expresses the essence of excess: our basements and attics are filled with junk, our bodies with chemicals, and our minds with the chaotic images of the media.

Unfortunately, that may be only the most superficial layer of the miasmatic distortions that have crept into our group psyche. Again following the classical homeopathic model, *pseudosycosis* indicates a stance that displays the signs and symptoms of overdoing, while beneath that apparent disorder is a more severe disconnection. It seems to me that our social confusion is more of this sort. Beneath the busyness of our excesses is a more gnawing sense of emptiness and alienation that would correspond to the third miasm of the homeopath:

- The third or *syphilitic* miasm is a muck where there's no footing. It is the "eating away," destructuring level of disconnection. Here, even the pain that reminds you that you're missing a more alive and authentic existence is lost. With the absence of awareness that there's a contract and purpose for your life, the *intent* that holds the Earth Element in form is missing. Without that spirit to vitalize the physical body, it begins to crumble and erode, like an abandoned adobe village.

A CRUMBLING SOCIAL ORDER

A flavor of the Kafkaesque dissociation from life that this latter stance involves is seen in the homeopathic cases that respond to the miasmatic remedies geared to it. For example, Dr. Philip Bailey describes a case he once treated: "As a child she was so fascinated with death that she would keep the bodies of dead animals in a drawer, so that she could look at them from time to time. She buried her pet cat in the garden, but would repeatedly dig it up to examine the remains . . . and felt no sadness, but only fascination with the process of decay." The problem she had consulted him for, a fear of being in unfamiliar open spaces, responded very well to *Syphilinum* in high potency, a primary remedy for the erosive miasm. Others of the patients he'd seen, who later improved with the same remedy, he notes, "have something of a sadistic streak, in that they enjoy watching animals die, and will find themselves stepping on insects, or putting them in water and watching them drown."[13]

Though we may find these descriptions bizarre or repugnant, the attitude they represent is not as alien to our lives as we would like to think. As a society we have come to feel it's normal to gaze indifferently as blood, violence, and murder are splashed across our television and movie screens. On a larger scale, there's a similar flavor to our attitude toward social issues. As multinational corporations move to destroy ecosystems—eradicating tribal cultures and endangered species, or polluting the rivers and air with toxic substances that cause wide-scale suffering and death—those of us who man their offices and factories comment blankly, "It's just a job, you know. It's a good job, in fact. It pays well, and the benefits are great." Even those of us who wouldn't work there casually buy stock funds invested in the same firms, offering our life savings to finance activities we say we don't believe in.

In this way our social structures, even as they begin to erode and crumble, mirror the miasmatic afflictions we suffer as individuals. We wander about numbly, feeling more emptiness than pain, decrying the demise of the environment, yet contributing to it with each day's purchases, activities, or thoughts. That mentality conjures up for me the image of a nursing home where my aunt and uncle were domiciled. A few years ago my daughter and I visited them there.

It was a new facility, built to serve the rural community I had grown up in. Though it seemed large for such a population, it had been expanded not long after it was opened. Now it housed hundreds of the disabled elderly, most of whom, in this building, suffered from chronic dementia, various versions of severe senility such as Alzheimer's disease. As I walked down the long halls, I recognized on the doors names of the families of childhood friends. Though many of these people were quite old, a large percentage weren't; some were still in their sixties.

My aunt had not opened her eyes in years, and often cried out as though experiencing some unspeakable terror. Her brother, my uncle, now in his late seventies, did not recognize me. It was not clear whether he knew his wife or his daughter when they visited. The attendants were, for the most part, considerate and gentle, but there was little they could offer to many of the patients, who wandered about, confused and troubled. One old lady took my daughter's hand and asked repeatedly, "Can you help me?" The answers she received seemed not to alter the words or the inflection of the question. But her grip was tight and she would not let go. Finally her fingers had to be pried loose. As we walked away, we could hear her question, fainter but unchanged: "Can you help me?"

Hahnemann expressed his insight into the deep roots of chronic illness through the language of disease classification. As a psychiatrist, my attention is more on the warping of consciousness that creates those diseases. Hahnemann was not a psychologist or philosopher by training, and did not have the jargon of those disciplines at his disposal. But it appears to me that behind the miasmatic distortions of function and structure that he highlighted, we can glimpse the outlines of vast realms of commonly held ideas, assumptions, and mental constructs. They are significant because they are so ingrained that they constitute a sort of planetary ceiling to what can be accomplished therapeutically.[14]

MIASMATIC CAGES

If we apply uncompromisingly the paradigm that has been taking shape through the course of this book, we will have to conclude that most, if not all, illness can be resolved by a realignment and reorganization of consciousness, a reconnection of individual consciousness with its sustaining Matrix, and a resulting shift in attitudes and thought patterns. This should redirect the flow of subtle energy and reshape the course of physiologic events so that we are able to handle most problems with ease. Let's take a viral infection as an example of how this might work, since viruses are an object of growing concern.

A virus is literally a fragment of DNA or RNA. DNA is the stuff of chromosomes—encoded information that can direct the cell's functioning.

(RNA is a messenger form of the same molecular sequences.) If you were living in a fully conscious way, grounded in the Universal Matrix of love that holds you, attentive to the spark of *spanda,* and allowing the interplay of the two to focus and direct your energy systems, the appearance of a virus on the scene, with its instructions for disrupting healthy cellular activity, would be of little consequence. It would be dispatched briskly and matter-of-factly by an efficient immune system.

The organizational information the virus might bring to bear would simply be ignored, because the operation of the organism would be managed in a different way by the conscious inflow of intent and spontaneity. The virus would then be nothing more than a bit of clutter to be swept away as you work—like a memorandum from someone whose input you don't care for.

But if you have chosen to operate unconsciously, or if you have bought into the belief that you are controlled by external agents, the situation is dramatically different. In that case management is out, and there is a risk that directives from the least qualified will be followed. In other words, the virus has free rein to dictate a course of events. If consciousness itself is focused narrowly on the world of matter, invested in the conviction that causality resides in the physical and that it cannot itself prevail, then it will not use its power, and that belief becomes a "reality." In that case the virus's coded instructions are treated as ultimate destiny. What could have been a faint message, easily dismissed, instead becomes a mandate.

What makes this unfortunate scenario possible is a complex web of beliefs and assumptions about human nature and how body and mind function. In this case it's the conviction that disease is caused physically— by germs, for example. Major support for this belief comes from a series of interlocking archetypal images that define the roles we and those around us must play—villain and victim, judge and transgressor, and so on. Like the extrinsic muscles and fascial sheaths that restrict the body's motion, they hold our minds prisoner. Yet, also like those muscles and connective-tissue structures, they allow us to function in the world as it is. At this point our archetypes are grounded in the hierarchical notion that we are powerless, and they are strongly rooted in a structure of reality that derives from projection.

Our power is projected outward. We become the passive recipients of help or persecution. The multiplicity of archetypal constructs elaborated on this pattern trap us in certain confines of thought and belief—ranging from the general (I am separate from the Divine, matter controls consciousness) to the specific (microbes cause disease). The total complex of such belief systems places a stringent limitation on our options for healing reorganization.

When these limiting structures are systematically identified and broken, "spontaneous healings" can occur.

> *Martin comes to his appointment uncharacteristically enthused: "I have some wonderful news!" He'd been swimming when a young girl sitting on the edge of the pool asked why he didn't turn his head. Prompted by her query, he tried it and soon found himself both kicking and turning his head with each stroke. And the next day he did it again.*
>
> *This was cause for celebration because Martin had Parkinson's disease. Though he had persisted in his swimming, his movements had become increasingly limited and he had not been able to kick for many months. That day was a turning point, and marked the beginning of a remarkable period of improvement. I was thrilled, too, as I had watched him deteriorate over a period of years, all my efforts to help having been of little use.*

I asked Martin what he thought had made the difference. He felt it was his diligent study of *A Course in Miracles*. "It's very radical in its effect," he said. That made sense to me. The attitude underlying Parkinson's disease is said to be "fear and an intense desire to control everything and everyone."[15] The fear and need to control, we can now see, comes from the alienation of the ego from the Spirit which would nurture it, and also comes from the ego's effort to protect itself by controlling all the menacing projections it has thrown out into the world. Physically, Parkinson's disease is a deterioration of the basal ganglia, structures deep in the brain that mediate balance and coordination or movement. The basal ganglia, small in the human, make up the bulk of the brain in birds and enable them to flow easily with forces larger than themselves, so that they can defy gravity and soar into the heavens.

Perhaps the *Course in Miracles* was helping Martin let go of the ego and reconnect with a larger identity. But that's always a tall order and filling it a radical step. I knew that the *Course* was extreme in its critique of our reality, and had heard reports of some who began its study rebelling, throwing the book off a bridge. Its insistence on letting go our death-grip on the stubbornly constricted and separated world of ego consciousness, and on allowing reconnection with a transpersonal, encompassing Spirit, had threatened their hold on their reality. They felt it might drive them crazy. I suspected it might have "driven them sane"—or at least positioned them to heal themselves more effectively.

It is only, I believe, through revolutionary change on some fundamental level of consciousness that a disease such as Parkinson's can be stopped or reversed. The disease is, I feel, so much an outcome of a way of being that is normal in our society that it remains "incurable" as long as those accepted ways of thinking go unchallenged. Of course, it's not an easy matter to change such deeply embedded beliefs, and the attempt to do so can leave you feeling that the very foundation of your existence is being ripped apart.

Martin's challenge might be seen as a metaphor for a larger one. We are struggling on a large scale to extricate ourselves from a "reality" that involves rigid egos and an intense need to control the natural world. Perhaps in this setting the process of disease has some evolutionary utility. At this time, when we have painted ourselves into a corner by creating a huge superstructure of patriarchally based institutions, attitudes, and beliefs that have become destructive, we may find it necessary at times to simply sit with the agony of their insanity as they begin to crumble. This is a healing crisis on a planetary scale. All you can do to prevent yourself from being carried down with the collapse is to begin the process of allowing your own consciousness to be reconfigured, inviting a radical deconstruction and rebuilding of the mind of the sort that Martin had begun with his study of *A Course in Miracles*.

Breaking out of our belief systems, or "miasmatic cages," may be the major challenge that we face in the coming years as we strive to foster individual and collective healing. Part of planetary healing is rediscovering our capacity for a fuller consciousness. That larger consciousness *can* reshape the physical (via the energetic). But we operate under the constraints of a mindset that denies this possibility, that isolates us from that larger Self, or Spirit, which has the power to heal. That denial has a powerful effect. So planetary healing is not merely cleaning up the environment or getting our ecological priorities straight. It's reshaping belief systems—reconfiguring the fabric of our collective mind. The results of this will, I suspect, go far beyond anything we can presently imagine.

But change of this magnitude is no small order. We need to scramble high enough up the hill to be able to look down and *see* the network of limiting mindsets from which we want to disentangle ourselves. This involves stepping out of the limited ego, but it also means probing deep into other unconscious parts of the inner world.

The Innermost Frontiers of Healing

The last frontier in our healing journey is a vast territory within that we don't consciously visit. That's where our miasmatic constrictions and our unspoken beliefs are rooted. Here the tendrils that choke the spirit flourish and grow. Psychologists call this realm the unconscious. It is kept unconscious because we can't deal with it, and because social organizations depend on its silent support. Western psychoanalysis and psychology have respected the "No Admittance" sign on the door to this area, maintaining that the unconscious could never be entered.[16] Though such a belief may enable one to live more comfortably in a society organized around a limited consciousness, it is often at odds with efforts at personal or group healing. The broader integrating consciousness necessary for healing in a deeper way can only be reached by moving through those forbidden zones.

Meanwhile, renegade yogis have provided a different and in some ways more inspiring model.[17] By separating themselves from society, they were able to ignore its insistence on keeping the unconscious off limits. They developed the simple principles of "mindwork," applying to the mind the same techniques that have proved effective in caring for the body—nourishing, cleansing, exercise, and rest. They cleaned out its garbage, fed it empowering images and ideas, trained it to be supple and strong, and regularly let it have periods of rest, when it could find its source of inspiration.

Unencumbered by the mind's distractions and sabotage, they could push on where others had been unable to go—venturing into and beyond the forbidden zones, violating taboos and moving past that part of consciousness which is bound by the rules of time, space, and causality. This meant going beyond the ego—that part of our consciousness which follows those rules of thought with which we reinforce our concept of reality, the ego which is the reductionistic, linear agent within, which stubbornly and insistently identifies itself as separate and cut off from the nurturing matrix of loving support provided by the Spirit.

Moving beyond this ego-dominated consciousness is accomplished by an extension of the basic meditative maneuver described in Chapter 11 (Fig. 147). By going a step further, you fully release the ego and embrace its

EXPLORING THE UNKNOWN MIND
(extending the meditative shift)

1.

Sit quietly and
comfortably with head, neck,
and trunk straight.

2.

Breathe
diaphragmatically.

3.

Embrace mind,
"see" it, own it, "contain" it.
Use a mantra to create largeness.

4.

Follow the ascending energy.
Don't be afraid to let go of the ego.
Hold on to the breath and the sound.
Enjoy the sense of expansion.

5.

Open to view
the forbidden impulses,
and feel the vastness and peace
of what lies beyond.

FIGURE 147

counterparts, aspects of yourself you have never accepted because they are the antithesis of the ego's image of itself. That done, you are able to relax in some deep and profound way, and feel yourself flooded by a larger identity. Rather than something you "do," this is the relief and release of *ceasing to do* what had been seen as necessary to protect the ego from certain thoughts and feelings. That is what makes for the joy and serenity of this process.

What lies outside the realm of the limited ego, the unconscious that includes all those aspects of yourself that your ego manages not to see, might be divided into two parts. The first is that which contains the mass of polarizations and conflicts, some of which you must live out in the course of your journey if you are to untangle them. This is what might be called the "personal unconscious." The other part encompasses your areas of connection with the Whole, your access to a more universal awareness, your holographic linkage to other components of the universe. This latter part of the unconscious is where you go at night when you sink into dreamless sleep, the universal Self you secretly visit to replenish yourself.[18] It might be called the "superconscious." It's what you need to bring into play in order to more easily implement major healing reorganization.

But the personal unconscious functions as a sort of barrier to this superconscious realm. When you try to approach the Universal, the personal unconscious scares you off because it's full of all the dirt you swept under the rug, the unpleasant things about yourself that you didn't want to face, and the many aspects of your being that don't fit into the ego's self-concept. The roadblock formed by the personal unconscious can be whittled away by cultivating the habit of patient, neutral observing. This is what allows you to incorporate, bit by bit, pieces of this unconscious territory into the gradually expanding conscious mind.[19] That won't work, though, if you slip back into an ego posture and pass judgment on what you find. And much of what you will encounter will not be pretty.

THE SHADOW

In the personal unconscious you will find the destructive beliefs and assumptions that paralyze you and frighten you away from spontaneity and joy. Poke at them, and they snarl and snap at you. This is the dark side of the inner world. These are the taproots of the miasmatic creepers that choke and bind. You will not be able to explore this territory without trying on the black outfits of the villainous characters who lurk there. Here is where you experience the intensity of the darkest miasmatic thinking and suffering.

For example, when you step into the space where vitality is withdrawn and erosion is allowed to occur—what Hahnemann would have called the *syphilitic miasm*—you are testing the territory of extreme disconnection. But even this darkness and the destruction it can produce have value, since we all embody, to some extent, the dark miasmatic forces of the planet, and since there are structures they have produced—external institutions and internal belief systems—that need to crumble. Playing with the destructive process allows you to learn how it can operate in some cosmically purposeful manner, rather than merely occur as personal pathological deterioration.

Before we can see with total clarity the holism of health, we may need to plumb the holistic nature of illness. We are each taking on some part of the darkness of the whole. There is a net that strangles us, a net of miasmatic distortion and ignorance that holds us captive and prevents us from being free to use our incredible power as spiritual beings. Though we fear death, we must befriend it and make it our ally, because what needs to die is this dark net. It will do so through the collective effect of letting it crumble and die in each of us.

Our experimentation with the deeper miasms is like the yogi dancing on the burning *ghat* where corpses are cremated—it's playing with death. It seems to me that has been happening frequently with AIDS, which pushes young people to delve consciously into the process of dying. By looking death in the face, by teasing and taunting it, by testing the waters and ultimately plunging in, they have shifted the group consciousness around death. In terms of classic homeopathic miasms, AIDS is *syphilitic,* but here it's done as though it were a necessary exploration into the intricacies of destruction, erosion, and death. It's confronting the planetary shadow—and experimenting with the means that might be used to be rid of it once and for all.

When we finally comprehend that process clearly, then we will know exactly how to let the dark net that's holding us in its grip disintegrate and die. The notion that you can hold on to the Spirit—that you can operate from light and clarity—and still play with the darkness and learn to bring it to heel like a pit bull is very much in the spirit of the Radical Healing that this book aims to convey. But you can't do that until you learn how those darker forces work, and probably until you have embodied them—at least in the private recesses of your inner world.

Carlene is in my office because she has a kidney problem. It's hard for me to attend to the details of her symptoms because I am so taken by how different she looks now from the picture she presented when she first came to see me over ten years ago. At that time she was a rather meek, hesitant young woman, a secretary in the corporate world who seemed apologetic and uncertain.

Now she's finished training as a flower essence prescriber and is leading tours to Peru that provide an experience of native shamanic healing. Her tentative manner has been replaced with an aura of confidence. She is also organizing initiatives to preserve rain forest habitats, and has already had one run-in with oil company executives who commandeered the airplane she was about to use to return with her group from the jungle.

As she finishes describing the pain in the small of her back, she mentions that she had recently cut off communication with her mother. "At first I was afraid to do it, fearful that she'd retaliate somehow, be really nasty to me." She saw her mother as cruel, and had been dealing in therapy with memories of abuse by her. In Chinese medicine, the kidneys relate to fear. Carlene's focus on that part of her body at this moment might be seen as recoiling in fear from her mother, stepping "backward into her kidneys" to protect herself.

But the kidney problem brings up in my mind the issue of poisoning. When kidneys fail, filtration falls off and poisons build up in the blood; you become poisoned by negativity that you can't acknowledge and release.

"Why don't you take Black Cohosh flower essence?" I suggested. Black cohosh is a beautiful plant that hides a horrible smell. The flower essence is said to help "wrestle with the shadow parts in the self and in others." "Your mother represents a part of yourself that you have projected and need to reclaim."

She looked at me intently for a moment. "Tell me more," she said.

"You have to recover the power you've given over to your mother. It's a part of you that is split off and projected. The power is you, but the negative use of it is not. You are afraid of the power because you are afraid you can't use it constructively. Your first step may be to feel it inside you in its negative form. This may scare you, but you have to hold it before you can transmute it."

Her pensive face lit up with a sudden smile. "That's already begun! A man came up to me in my parking garage yesterday and told me to move my car. I turned around and let him know in no uncertain terms that he could wait his turn. He just backed away.

"And that's not all," she went on, putting the pieces together excitedly. "Last week, my dog was attacked in the park. A big Irish wolfhound, hunting, came after her, grabbed her in his jaws. I knew that with a toss of the head a wolfhound can break the neck of a small

animal. I leapt on top of him and had the huge animal in a headlock.
Onlookers were terrified and shocked. I put my head against that of
the wolfhound, and my spirit said to his, 'No, you will not break my
dog's neck.' He let go. I gathered my dog up, ran to the street, got a
cab, and took her to the vet. She's fine now."

As she told her story, I saw a different person. Her hair was flying,
her eyes flashing, and she loomed powerful in the room. "You began
to feel your strength," I observed.

"Yes, I was huge!*" I recalled stories of shamanic healing, where*
the shaman had traveled through the whirlwinds and darkness of
other realities and other dimensions to grasp and retrieve a soul in dis-
tress. She had done it in the wilds of Central Park.

"You've hardly begun." I laughed. "When you reclaim all your
shakti, your full power, you will pick up bulldozers from the banks
of the Amazon and throw them into the Pacific." As I looked at her, I
felt that was no exaggeration.

Learning the purpose of the dark, destructive forces and how to harness them is the last and perhaps the greatest healing adventure. It is what
transforms the pervasive miasmatic foundations of illness from a dis-
heartening fate into a challenge that is exciting and filled with the
promise of revolutionary change and the joy of liberation.

If you use the principles of *tapas* and the other keys offered in this
book, you will realize that your healing is part of some larger process of
healing. As you bump consciousness up to the higher chakras, you move
out of the perception of individual pathology and the isolation of personal
suffering into the appreciation of the transpersonal nature of your struggles. What you are dealing with, then, is not just your own illness; your
suffering is global suffering. You have taken on some piece of it—a piece
that only you can handle. You are not alone, it's all taking place on a
grander scale. That lifts your struggle out of private anguish and into cosmic evolution.

AND FINALLY, BACK TO THE BODY

Reintegrating all these seemingly disparate facets of healing may
bring us the coherence and scope of vision we need to transcend the narrow concepts and values responsible for individual and planetary illness.
As we face this challenge, as we stretch in an effort to envision a new sci-

ence of consciousness, we might take inspiration from the sacred art of Incan weaving. For the Incas, weaving is symbolic of pulling back together the pieces of ourselves. They employ this principle in their spiritual rituals and in the making of the *mesa,* where many substances—representative of the various facets of the natural world—are put together into one package. The *mesa* could be seen as the reintegrated human.

The ancient Incas used colored, knotted threads to record and inventory the items of their world. Anthropologists regarded this as curious, but when we see their weaving, the intermingling of all the brightly hued threads that represented the objects of their experience, we might conclude that it speaks of the reconvergence of those disparate pieces of reality. It might express, for example, their shamanic travel into different realms—the journeys that reconnected them to their many selves on multiple dimensions.

Similarly, a new science of healing will need to focus on reweaving the estranged parts of ourselves. Weaving is endlessly creative. Though we may all use the same colors, the way each of us does it creates a pattern that is uniquely ours, that has a beauty to be found nowhere else, that is an indispensable piece of the holographic composition that constitutes the cosmic Whole. As we have seen repeatedly, every little ailment is evidence of some disconnected aspect of yourself and an opportunity to further the process of reweaving and reuniting the scattered fragments to create a new, reorganized, and more complete self. In fact, these "little" opportunities are, in a way, the most significant, because they are "bite-sized"—manageable, easy to assimilate.

Development unfolds through meeting the tiny challenges posed by the experiences we are drawn into as we express our genuinely spontaneous urges and inclinations. And many of these little hurdles have to do with the health of the body.

By overlaying our different aspects like a series of transparencies depicting different facets of the same figure—the physiological, the microbial, the energetic, the environmental, the psychological, the spiritual—we finally see the beautiful complexity of the gestalt. We grasp how all the threads weave together to express our multifaceted existence, and see how their interrelations are profoundly meaningful.

The radical healing we are searching for will lift us out of our suffering and return us to a harmonious blending of our personal soul's journey with the unfolding of planetary destiny. Though leaving our state of dis-ease is a radical departure for us, a step out of our familiar world, it may actually be a step back into a "reality more real," a movement from digression, disconnection, and disease to reconnection, coherence, and an encompassing consciousness.

That shift, the magnitude and miracle of it, is held quietly in the easily overlooked, but awesomely powerful informational content of the plant, of the flower, or of the crystalline structure of a stone. An herb or a homeopathic remedy can shatter and reconfigure the subtlest and most basic patterns that govern our existence, bringing us back into fulfilling engagement with the world around us, reconnecting us with all the other dimensions of existence to which the Earth is holographically linked.

> *I stop along my usual jogging path to catch the fall sun, trapped by a stone wall. Just above eye level is a vine whose exotic habit looks strangely out of place in the Bronx. It hangs over my head, heavy with strange spiked fruit and dusky, drooping leaves that seem a bit tired in the November chill, but still thick and substantial. This plant, like most, when I look carefully, has a personality, a way of being, that is clear and definite—unique, I'd be tempted to say, but then I feel its similarity to people I've known, or diseases they've had.*
>
> *This correspondence is not merely a poetic one, a quaint symbolism that the mind might toy with; there's an awesome intensity contained in the plant's peculiarity that holds me spellbound. I know that the formative forces implicit in it could reshape the merely physical, and that when the curative sweep of such power is harnessed, it will make the awkward machinations of chemical drugs and surgical excision look cumbersome, off-target, and embarrassingly primitive.*

Just as the complete healing we are seeking for a chronic or "incurable" disease might seem radical in the terms of the reality we live in, the plant I stare at seems strangely at odds with the world of pavement and chain-link fences. Yet its way of being, alien though it may appear, is quite comfortably integrated into the reality of Gaia, the Earth, which is, in turn, firmly and coherently interconnected with the cosmos and its inherent interlocking structures and interdependent realities.

Unable to identify the plant, I went back and picked one of its strange fruits and put it in my pocket. I came home to a meeting with Linda, my illustrator, who is a botanical artist, and when I put it in front of her she said, "Oh, it's a thornapple." I had not recognized the plant without its flowers, but knew it as jimsonweed or *Stramonium,* the name used by homeopaths. "I just finished two days of intensive silverpoint, drawing this plant!" Linda exclaimed, struck by the coincidence. Meanwhile, I had recently received a book on the use of homeopathic *Stramonium* from Dr. Paul Herscu, and a few days before had given the remedy in potency to my son. It had thrown him into a paroxysm of coughing mucus release and behavioral change. Now he was coming out of his adolescent fog and asserting his individuality.

This confluence of events was too much for notions of probability and coincidence to accommodate. Yet at the heart of several days of experience for three people was this plant, which had stopped me on my walk. Will we ever learn to think in these terms? Can we acknowledge and accept the succinct power of the plant's organizational message? Can we see why a skilled shaman might have brought the plant into a sweat lodge with the three of us? Is the use of the remedy shamanism? Is such thinking strange, or is it just more real than what we're accustomed to?

Concluding Thoughts on

Energy and Consciousness

The reconnection that is the essence of healing is a process that reaches deeper and deeper, reshaping your consciousness and redirecting your energy so that your body is brought into greater and greater synchrony with the pulsing of the larger wholes of which you are a part. The farthest reaches of healing stretch the mind and stagger the imagination. It is a matter of cosmic proportions. The journey you have embarked upon by reading this book is an epic one, and not one that you will complete soon. Your healing is a process that will extend far into the future, bringing you to realizations and transformations that you cannot now imagine.

But at the same time, this business of healing is not something abstract and otherworldly. It is firmly anchored in the practical. Your healing may be important to the universe, but it is also a matter of simple and concrete urgency for you personally. It is what is required to address the aches and pains in your body, the fears and anxieties of your everyday world. Healing is the natural and necessary response to the issues at hand. Despite our unfortunate habit of considering our illnesses and disorders obstacles to living, that is not what they are. They are instead, as we have seen, opportunities. The secret of fulfillment in your life is dealing with the problems that seem to plague you and prevent you from moving forward. Whatever is "in your way" *is* your way.

The key to your personal transformation is the thorn in your side. You need not wax philosophical, or lose yourself in conjecture and speculation. Address whatever bothers you most, and you will be on the track of personal evolution and your contribution to the struggles of mankind. Your body will tell you what to deal with, or, failing that, your mental or emotional issues will do so. But for this to work, you cannot deal with your crises and challenges suppressively. You must use the tools and techniques of a truly holistic medicine.

Listen to the eloquent language of the body, of the emotions; step back and see what are the knots that the mind gnaws on. To be of value, what you notice doesn't have to be a grave disorder. If you don't have a major health challenge, start with the little ailments and problems that seem insignificant. Whether large or small, use your symptoms as clues to the steps you need to take at this moment. Look up the problems you have in the Self-Help Index in the following section, and check the general index so you can reread the applicable passages from the first four sections. Ask yourself what cleansing needs to be done, what you need to let go from the past.

Allow yourself to see your "defects" more clearly, own them, value their utility for you. They unlock mysteries, open doors. Don't hide from them. If you feel trapped in mental attitudes, hung up in a position of polarity that blocks your awareness, read up on the flower essences and use them. If you don't find the remedies you need described in this text, go to the Guide to Further Study, also in the next section, and order the book you need. If you feel that the complex of physical and emotional problems is too big to get a fix on, look for a homeopathic remedy that fits the whole pattern, and if you can't find it, but feel that homeopathy is the answer, look in the listing of Products and Services and get the help of a practitioner.

Explore, experiment, use your body as a laboratory. Make learning from your body and from your mental and emotional challenges your modus operandi. Rejoice in the challenge of this moment, this sensation, this opportunity. Make a habit of letting go the old and moving into the new. Let your journey be a constant delight, a daring dance. Make radical healing a way of life, a celebration of your presence on this earth.

RESOURCES

Here are the tools you need to implement Radical Healing. The Self-Help Index will get you started with suggestions on how to address some of the more common health challenges you are likely to face. At the end of the Index is a list you can use to assemble your own home medicine chest. Though it cannot contain all the possible remedies you will find mentioned in the index, it will include the most common ones.

When you need to go more into depth on an illness or a therapeutic approach, flip over to the Guide to Further Study. Here you will find brief descriptions of some of the important books to turn to when you want more information on a subject. The descriptions should allow you to find the book that fits your needs. Many books are now available, and more coming out every day. The fact that a book is not listed does not indicate that I consider it inferior. Rather, I have selected the books to fit with and flow from your reading of this text. Though it is important to follow your curiosity, random reading can sometimes lead to confusion, since authors vary so widely in perspective, conceptual frame of reference, and language. The books listed here should rest relatively comfortably on the foundation you establish through your reading and use of *Radical Healing,* and will often be the best first step, preparing you to branch out to others later.

The third part of this section is a listing of sources for Products and Services. Space limitations require that this be selective, and so I have concentrated on what you may not readily find through more common channels.

Self-Help Index
and Home Medicine Kit

Introduction

I had great fun doing this. For nearly thirty years I've scanned everything written on holistic therapies, to find what might benefit the patient at hand. But there was always an urgency about it, because someone was waiting for help. This time it was different. Though I already knew the territory, I could take my time and return to all the little corners, pull it all together, rank each therapeutic possibility against the others, and consider how they best combine or might be tried in sequence.

The result is, I think, a uniquely integrative, highly refined, and methodically honed guide, concise and yet broad in its scope. Nothing here is gratuitous. Every little detail has been considered carefully and weighed against decades of experience and study. Each entry may be only a few lines, but if you take the trouble to "decode" it, I think you will find the information you need to tackle the problems facing you and start the process that can uncover the secrets they hold for your growth and evolution.

How to Use This Index

Order: Recommendations are listed in descending order of importance—i.e., based on clinical experience, those listed first are the ones I expect to be the most likely, in general, to be helpful. So if the homeopathic suggestions come last, that means that in my experience, homeopathy has not been as effective for this disorder as have other measures.

Missing items: If a category is missing, that's because I haven't found it effective or relevant for that disorder. For example, in my experience, homeopathic remedies don't offer much for baldness or emphysema; tissue salts are not of much use for obesity or Lyme disease; herbs really shine for some problems and are relatively ineffective for others—though reference books will list a homeopathic remedy or an herb for everything. The beauty of integrating all these is that we can begin to refine our treatments, choosing the tool most likely to be helpful for the complaint in question.

Individualizing: Please realize this is being done "blind"—I know nothing about the person, and am basing the recommendations on a single complaint. You can rectify this by using what you've learned about constitutional types and other approaches to individualizing (Section II), more accurately choosing which interventions are most likely to help you. If a flower essence is listed, read about it in Chapter 3 or in a reference book on flower essences, and see if it fits the person with the problem. Of course, treating the underlying constitution or the overall symptom picture with homeopathy, acupuncture, or a properly formulated herbal remedy may result in clearing any number of specific complaints. That is always the most ideal approach.

Getting best results: The best results will come when these specific measures are applied in the context of following the total approach that the book lays out. If you are working on your diet, detoxing, exercising, organizing your life with your constitution in mind, and tuning in to your energy and mind, then these tips will see you through many, if not most, bumps in the road. If you're not working with yourself in a more general way, their effectiveness will be more limited.

Dosages: For vitamins and herbs, I have given dosages when they are specific to this disorder. When no dosage is listed, use your own judgment, following usual recommendations and your knowledge of what you have responded to in the past. For herbal tinctures, see also explanation of the abbreviation *dpl,* below. For homeopathic remedies, the classical method is to be followed (see pages 88–92) unless otherwise indicated. Chinese patent medicines come with dosages on the label.

Combinations: I have avoided mentioning proprietary preparations such as combination homeopathic and herbal preparations. This doesn't mean that I think they're inferior; sometimes they combine a spectrum of useful natural agents in a way that not only simplifies treatment for the user, but also may create an effective synergism. The downside of such products is that they are notoriously ephemeral, coming and going in the blink of an eye. It is my hope that by being alerted to the usefulness of several single nutrients, herbs, and/or homeopathics you will be able to intelligently assess the latest combination products and decide whether they are a good bet or not. You can also put together your own combinations. Though technically also proprietary combinations, I consider the Chinese patent medicines a separate category—the formulas are for the most part well established, enduring, and consistently available, often from more than one manufacturer. Moreover, their effects are most often a result of the synergism of the individual ingredients, and may not be obvious from looking at those ingredients separately.

Special entries: A few disorders (those marked with an asterisk) are too complex to deal with fully in this format. In such cases the reader will be referred to a separate listing in the Guide to Further Study (which follows) dedicated to a selection of books recommended on the subject.

Definitions: If you run into something you don't understand, e.g., "nasal wash" under Hay Fever, look it up in the general index of this book and go to the appropriate pages and read about it. (Page numbers in boldface in the index are where the basic definition or description of the term will be found.) If it's not there, you should find it in the Glossary.

Abbreviations used in the Index:
AA's: Amino acids taken therapeutically
acmpd by: Accompanied by (seen along with—a second symptom or disorder that helps to characterize which variation of this disorder we are dealing with)
AV: Ayurvedic
ck: Check—test for
combn: Combination (of herbs, e.g.)
CPM: Chinese Patent Medicine—usually herbal; when a medicine contains animal products, it will be marked *NV* (not vegan).
cstl: Constitutional (homeopathic) remedy

dpl: "dose per label." For tinctures especially, this means you should follow the dose recommended on the label. Often there will be a range (e.g., 20–40 drops, 2 to 4 times a day). If you are an adult of average weight, take the middle range of this (30 drops), and if your illness is moderately severe, the intermediate frequency (e.g., 3 times a day).

elim: Eliminate, elimination

EPO: Evening Primrose Oil

ERx: Exercise techniques for this problem

FE: Flower essence

Hmp: Homeopathic; when potencies below 200C are recommended, the potency will usually be given. When no potency is given, this means the higher potencies may be used. (See Chapter 2 for frequency of doses in such cases.)

Hrbl: Herbal

hx: History—has had in past

mdcl sprv: Requires medical supervision

MT: Mother Tincture—a homeopathic term. Homeopathic medicines are sometimes used as tinctures—these will often be similar to the tinctures used by herbalists and used in the same way. The significance of this term is that you may most easily find the remedy through homeopathic supply houses. Also, the name used may be different from that used by herbalists. (Note that homeopathic MT's are usually a 1:10 strength, while ordinary herbal tinctures are 1:5.)

NV: Not vegan (contains animal products)

Rprtz/esp: Repertorize (see pages 78–85), but especially consider the following (for homeopathic remedies and flower essences)

Rx: Prescription or treatment

RxFs: Therapeutic foods

tbt: "to bowel tolerance" of vitamin C. Vitamin C will, when given in doses beyond what can be absorbed, cause loose bowel movements. In order to give the maximum dose possible, it is sometimes given in ascending doses until the stool becomes loose.

TS: Tissue salt (cell salt); see page 55 for names and abbreviations

YRx: Yoga postures and techniques for this problem

< = Worse from

> = Better from

↑ = Increase (intake of food or water)

The 100+ Common Complaints

Abnormal Pap Smear (see Cervical Dysplasia).

Abscess (see Boil).

Acne: Dislike of yourself.[1] Avoid fats, oils, chocolate, sugar; zinc, up to 100mg and/or vit A up to 20,000 IU a day for up to a month; FE: Crabapple; work on self-acceptance; Hrbl: Red Clover tea, 3 times daily; CPM: Margarite Acne Pills (NV).

*AIDS (see page 568).

Alcoholism: Sugar-free (yeast control) diet; high doses of B vits esp. during detox; Hmp: cstl: rprtz/esp: *Nux v,* or *Sulph,* sometimes *Lach;* when familial, may need repeated doses of *Syphilinum.* Need to open to a higher power/purpose. AV: Liv 52 to support/regenerate the liver; FE: rprtz/esp: Chaparral, Milkweed, Mountain Pennyroyal.

Alopecia (see Hair Loss).

Alzheimer's: Opting out of the game. Milder versions may be deficiency disorders, e.g., B vits, esp. B_{12}; NADH 10 mg a day; chelation therapy; pycnogenol in high doses as an antioxidant and to help detoxify the myriad of chemicals that are thought to contribute to nervous system deterioration.[2] Early Rx/prevention critical.

Anemia: Full range of trace minerals as well as iron; combine iron with vit C; use cast-iron cookware; TS: *FP;* when iron is low but supplement not effective, take Loha Bhasma (AV); often B_{12}, esp. in vegans. Fear of, or not feeling worthy of, engaging fully in life.

Angina, Acute: Hmp: *Cactus g* 30C can abort viselike chest pain; meanwhile, transport to ER and give O_2. Chronic: Hmp: *Cactus g* 30C 1–2 times daily; fear of opening heart to others. Hawthorn Berry tinct; CoQ10 and carnitine (see also ASCVD, on page 508, if applicable).

Anorexia Nervosa: Test for zinc def. Must work on feeling of not having the right to nurture oneself—or even to live. Hmp: rprtz/esp: *Natrum mur, Medor* (sometimes *Thuja*), *Ignatia, Sepia;* FE: rprtz/esp: Cherry Plum, Chestnut Bud, Fairy Lantern, Pretty Face.

Anxiety: Not trusting the Universe's plan. B vits, esp B_1; FE: Aspen; diaphragmatic breathing; acupuncture; TS: *KP* or combo of 5 Phoses; Hmp: rprtz/esp: *Ars a, Sepia, Medor, Syph;* Hrbl: Kava kava; most Nervine herbs (Skullcap, Hops, Passaflora) are bitter, cooling and/or drying and may work well to calm *pitta* types, but can aggravate *vata* unless combined with others that are nourishing and grounding; CPM (which combine calming and grounding herbs): An Mian Pian, Ding Xin Wan, and Emperor's Tea (pills).

Arrhythmias, Cardiac: Elim wheat, caffeine; magnesium 400 mg twice daily (IV in ER for crises); Hbl: To calm a *vatic*/irregular heart, a combn of Skullcap and Ashwagandha; Hawthorn berry tincture when acmpd by high blood pressure and/or congestive failure, also, CoQ10; ck potassium levels and food/chemical sensitivities. Lack of joy/caught up in stress and strain.

Arthritis, osteo-: Unable to move with changes. Cleansing diet, distilled water, whey; watch calc/phos ratios and vit D intake; exercise and heat; ginger (topically and by mouth); Hmp: *Bryonia* 30C vs *Rhus tox* 30C; Hrbl: Devil's Claw, Yucca, Tahitian Noni; RxFs: cherries/cherry juice, cod liver oil, avocado; vit B_6, proanthocyanidins; chondroitin sulfate, glucosamine; citrus/cider vinegar may cause pain but help dissolve deposits.

Arthritis, rheumatoid: Feeling trapped, unloved, resentful, and critical. Hmp: *Rhus tox* 30C, 200C of *Strep* or other initiating microbes (ck titers); MSM cetyl myristoleate; Hrbl: Devil's Claw, Yucca, Chaparral; Vits: Pantothenic acid 1g, C; Copper sebacate or even salicylate (60 mg twice daily), or even a copper bracelet! (Monitor zinc levels—copper may suppress); Bromelain; avoid nightshade vegs and ck other food sensitivities if hx of heavy use of NSAIDs.

*ASCVD (Arteriosclerotic Cardiovascular Disease): A set negativity in the mind that manifests as plaque in the arteries; alter that and change lifestyle and it can melt. ERx: jogging (start slowly); YRx: head and shoulder stands, peacock; cleansing diet; RxFs: Legumes (beans and peas); Hrbl: Gugulu, Hawthorne; chelation Rx and TS: *CF* for calcified plaque; vits C, B_6, chromium, copper, and zinc (see page 569).

Asthma: Feeling smothered. Hmp: Acute: *Ars a* 30C and/or *Blatta O* MT when acmpd by obesity; chronic: rptx/esp: *Nat Sulph, Medor, Syph, Nat mur;* Vit B_6, molybdenum (children B_{12}); TS: *NS* (if < humidity) and *MP;* YRx: upper (stomach) wash; avoid dairy, peanuts, nuts, wheat, aged cheese; Hrbl: Wild Plum Bark Tea. Acute: Coleus forskohlii. Chronic: Aloe vera gel; FE: Yerba santa; CPM: Ping Chuan Wan (NV) or Chi Kuan Yen Wan.

Athlete's foot: Itching to step forward. Sycosis; avoid sweets—often related to widespread yeast/fungal overgrowth; urine topically, or diluted vinegar; keep feet dry (cotton socks, shoes that "breathe"); Pau D'arco tea.

Attention Deficit Disorder: Desire to bring feeling and body into learning—look for school/work that honors your learning/operating style. Hmp: *Tuberc, Medor, Stram, Lyc, Tarent, Hyoscam;* the Dx is often an expression of the frustration of those trying to deal with a child (or themselves); elim sweets and chemicals in foods; avoid fluorescent lighting; proanthocyanidins; FE: rprtz/esp Impatiens, Chamomile, Clematis; TS: *KP* or combo of 5 Phoses.

Backache (see Low Back Pain).

Baldness (see Hair Loss).

Bedwetting: Hmp: reprtz/esp *Medor, Puls, Tuberc, Lyc, Sycotic co.* Fear of parent, usually father. FE: St. John's Wort, Sunflower; trial elim of dairy products; Hrbl: Cinnamon oil, Agrimony tea. Poor bladder tone: *NP* 3x (TS in special potency) and magnesium suppl.; vits A, D, C, and E.

Bee Stings: "Epipen" (and ER) for severe reactions; otherwise or meanwhile: *Ledum* 30C, sometimes *Apis* 1M; FE: Rescue Remedy (Five Flower); open cigarette and moisten (e.g., saliva) tobacco, apply wad topically (with tape or Band-Aid).

Bipolar Disorder: B_6 200mg a day with AA: L-phenylalanine in ascending doses (500 mg, > 3g a day) for depressive phases (2–6 month trial); also, for manic phases, L-tryptophan (6–12 g a day) or lecithin, 15–20 g a day;[3] careful repertorization to find homeopathic remedy, esp. consider: *Calc c, Lach, Medor, Nat s, Anac.*

Bladder Infection: Anxious fear of letting go; "pissed off." Increase fluids, whey; Dolomite; *NS* (or *NS/KM* combination); moxibustion, acupuncture; Acute: Hmp: *Cantharis, Cann ind* or *sat,* or *Sepia,* all 30C; Hrbl: Buchu, Juniper berry, Marshmallow, and/or Uva ursi (try combn tea); FRx: cranberry, grapefruit, and/or cherry juices. Chronic, prevention (females): cotton pants, frequent urination.

Boil/Abscess: Anger popping out. Acute: *Sil* 6x (TS) until it "gathers" (comes to a head), then *Sil* 1M ("homeopathic scalpel") once, to open it and initiate drainage. *CS* 6x (TS) until drainage finishes. *Consult professional* if you note 1) lymphangitis (red line extending toward heart) Hmp: *Pyrogenium* 30C or 2) cellutitis (red inflamed area surrounding) Hmp *Strep* 200C—both signs of bacterial spread. Chronic/recurrent: Anti-*pitta* Rx; Hrbl: blood cleansers like Chaparral, Echinacea, Indigo, Pokeroot, Red Clover, Yellow Dock. Hmp: *Staphylococcus* 200C, or *Arn, Sul,* or *Hepar* 3x.

Bone Loss (see Osteoporosis).

Bone Spurs: Monitor carefully calcium/phosphorus ratio of diet; TS: *CF* distilled water, whey; may be due to excess vit D, def magnesium, or gout; cod liver oil and B_{12} may relieve pain (B_{12} injections, 1,000 mcg daily, have been reported to dissolve bone spurs); topical castor oil packs overnight.

Bronchitis: Inflamed interpersonal environment. Vit C, also zinc and vit A; acupuncture; TS: *KM, CS;* Hrbl: Echinacea, Usnea, Goldenseal, Osha; Mustard plaster (powdered mustard seed: flour: : 1 : 4 mixed with water, spread paste on thin cloth, fold and place on chest, ck freq to avoid blistering). Chronic: postural drainage for excess mucus; *quasa;*[4] to liquify stubborn mucus: AA: N-acetylcystein 250–1500 mg daily or Myrrh; Hmp: rprtz/esp: *Acon, Bry, Ant t, Ipec, Kali b, Puls;* chronic/recurrent: rprtz/esp: *Tub, Ant t, Calc c, Puls, Kali bi;* FE Yerba Santa; CPM: Hsiao Keh Chuan. See also Cough, on page 512.

Bursitis: Who do you want to hit? Hmp: *Bry* 30C, *Ruta* 30C, *Sil;* vit C with bioflvns, 1 g, thrice daily; esp when calcified, B_{12} injections (as under Bone Spurs).

*Cancer (see page 570)

Candidiasis: No sugar (includes "natural sugars," sweet fruit, etc.). Scattered, frustrated—not engaging third-chakra fire in life (so gut "molds"). Martial arts, career/relationship changes. Hmp: *Candida* 30C plus cstl; Hrbl: Citrus Seed Extract, Garlic (perles), Pau D'arco (tea); caprylic acid, acidophilus; Avoid refined CHO's, yeasted/fermented foods, and dairy products; in stubborn cases, address immune weakness.

Carpal tunnel syndrome: Feeling victimized—hand(s) tied. B_6 50–100 mg thrice daily, reduce dose when symptoms clear; acupuncture; deep tissue massage/release wrist, arm and armpit; Hmp: *Ruta* and or *Hypericum* in 12x or 30C.

Cataracts: Not wanting to see the future—esp elderly who have materialistic concepts of death. *Cineraria m* eye drops (need Rx from M.D.); TS: *CF;* AV: Yellow Mustard Oil or Lotus Honey, a drop in each eye twice daily (Such Rx's may burn as they bring circulation to the eye); also Dr. Christopher's herbal eyewash (Bayberry bark, Euphrasia, Raspberry, Goldenseal in equal parts with ⅛ as much cayenne—or amount tolerated; steep 1 tsp in 1 cup boiling distilled water, decant, cool, and use in glass eye cup 2–5 times a day; should bring mucus discharge).

Cervical Dysplasia (abnormal Pap smear): vit A and zinc, also vit C and, after pregnancy or BC pills, folic acid (in high doses—e.g., 15 mg qd, with mcdl sprv.); yogurt douches; Hmp: *Thuja/Medor,* also *Ars a* 30C or *Kreos* 6x if acmpd by irritating discharge.

Chicken Pox: Vit E oil topically on itchy spots; Vit C tbt; TS: *KM* throughout, *FP* when fever; to ease itching, oatmeal or baking soda bath; when itching unbearable, FE: Sweet Chestnut, or try a drop of patient's blood potentized to 7C and given every 2 hours; Hmp: may help when symptoms fit, consider: *Ant tart* or *crud, Rhus tox, Puls, Sulph,* all in 30C; thymus extr, maybe B_{12}.

Cholesterol, High (see Hyperlipidemia).

*Chronic Fatigue Syndrome: Find out why you're here. Thorough detox is essential; ck for ELF (see page 559); magnesium; NADH 10 mg a day Hmp: Rprtz/esp: *Scuttelaria;* Hrbl: Lomatium diss. isolate, 4 days on, 4 off, in altn with Dioxychlor D3 also 4 days on, 4 off (latter in ascending doses); eliminate any candidiasis; and address "leaky gut"; elim aspartame sweetners, Stevia is okay; see also page 571.

Colic (infants): Impatience, annoyance in caregivers. TS: *NP, MP;* Hmp: *Cham* 30C; FE: Chamomile, Dill Water; in newborns, increase water intake and "burp" thoroughly when nursing; watch mother's diet: most common offending foods: onions/garlic, cabbage fam., veggies, beans, dairy, raw foods.

Colitis: Fear of letting go. Acupuncture; rice-based diet—avoid raw foods and sugar, sometimes dairy and/or wheat; acidophilus; Aloe gel, 2 oz. three times a day; ck for parasites; Hmp: *Aloe s* 6x when acmpd by mucus and explosive gas, *China* 6x when bleeding predominates; vit A and zinc; *TS: CS, NM, KM* combined.

Common Cold: Often a cleansing process—facilitate mucus discharge. TS: *KM, CS* if mucus yellow; take warming herbs: Ginger, Garlic, also Echinacea, Goldenseal, Myrrh, Astragalus. Cold with fever: CPM: Sang Ju Gan Mao Pian, with muscle ache and dry cough: Yin Qiao Jie Du Pian, or, if more severe, Zhong Gan Ling; vit C tbt (e.g., 1g every 2 hrs); nasal wash.

Congestive Heart Failure: *Requires close medical supervision.* CoQ10, 30–90 mg daily; cardiotonics: *Cactus g* MT, or match symptoms to: *Crataegus* (hawthorn), *Convallaria, Arjuna, Adonis, Oleander, Digitalis Strophanthus, Spartium,* or, *Scilla*—in MT or low potencies and *carefully adjusted doses,* since some of these can be toxic in excess; AA:

Taurine 2g, 2 or 3 times daily; CPM: Duzhong Bu Tian Su, 2 to 4 tablets twice daily; magnesium, potassium, and/or calcium supplementation (ck levels first).

Conjunctivitis: TS: *FP, CS* when yellow discharge; Angry and frustrated by what you see. Hrbl: Eyebright (eye wash, compress, and/or by mouth); vit D and calcium, also vit A; wash with boric acid solution. If chronic or recurrent and due to liver heat: CPM: Long Dan Xie Gan Wan.

Constipation: Reluctance to "let go the residue of the past." Acute: 6–8 hr fast. Chronic: lemon/honey/salt/hot water drink on arising in a.m.; trifala; avoid cheese, rice, white flour, meat; chew 1–2 T flaxseed after each meal; a 40-min brisk walk or 20 mins aerobics each day (stubborn cases may be due to medications that can disturb the downward-moving flow of energy that moves the bowels); CPM: Run Chang Wan (when due to heat, or def. of fluid or chi'i).

*Coronary Heart Disease (see ASCVD)

Cough: Preemptive demand to be heard (feeling suffocated)—this must be addressed. Meanwhile herbs, homeopathics may palliate. If dry, irritated, use demulcents like slippery elm, mullein; if congested with stubborn mucus, use expectorants like ginger, NAC (AA)—Coltsfoot *(Tussilago)*, Horehound, Momordica fruit (Lo Han Kuo—available as syrup with Fritillaria) do both. If triggered by tickle in throat: Rumex 12x–30C; see page 210; see also Bronchitis.

Crohn's Disease (see Colitis and Irritable Bowel Syndrome).

Cystitis (see Bladder Infection).

Depression: Aerobic exercise. *(Move!)* "Spirit is trying to move you through a change, and you are resisting." Thorough detox; 5 HTP 100 mg thrice daily; Hrbl: St. John's Wort 30–60 drops twice daily (allow one month to see full effect); Liver treatment; FE: Mustard (cf. Borage, Gentian); vit B_6 and zinc, folic acid; body-oriented psychotherapy; Hmp rprtz/esp: *Natr mur, Sepia, Ignatia, Aurum.*

Diabetes Mellitus: No sugar or simple CHO's; diet: high-fiber, low-fat complex CHO, rich in legumes. Juvenile: detox solvents, metals and chems; clear foci of infection/parasites in pancreas; Hmp constitutional. Adult onset: All the sweetness gone. Aerobic exercise; periodontal program—blotting and massage; RxF: karela (bitter melon); chromium and often zinc, manganese; vits C, E, biotin, maybe B_6; Hmp: *Uranium nit* low; intestinal cleansing; Hrbl: Syzygium jambolum, Fenugreek, and Blueberry leaf.

Diarrhea: Fear. RxFs: Carrot soup, carob powder, rice and yogurt; Elim: sugars, milk, coffee, meat; psyllium husks with yogurt (allow to sit overnight); Hrbl: Meadowsweet (mild but cooling), Blackberry, Oakbark; Hmp: rprtz/esp: *Ars a, Podoph, Sulf, Cupr ars, Veratrum alb* usually all in 30C; acidophilus; Goldenseal or Berberine to treat or prevent microbe-related diarrhea; barley or rice water as needed to replace lost fluids.

Diverticulitis: Avoid both low-residue and mechanically harsh foods; use foods high in soft fiber (= indigestible carbohydrate): peeled fruits, vegetables, whole grains (cooked soft), legumes, and/or oat bran; Esp avoid: animal foods, cheese, sugar, white flour, coffee and alcohol; drink aloe gel; colon cleansing when not acute; acidophilus; Pycnogenol and *CF.* When acute: *MP, FP,* and/or tea of wild yam, chamomile, marshmallow, and comfrey thrice daily.

Dry Skin: Anti-*vata* regimen; minimize soaps, detergents, and baths/showers that deplete skin's oils; Urine topically daily to problem areas; increase water intake; mustard oil massage (then sweat to open pores and towel off excess) weekly; vits A and E, cod liver oil (may also use vit E and/or CLO topically).

Dysmenorrhea: Conflict over expressing the *yang* (assertive) side of the feminine. Acupuncture; TS: MP; Hmp: *Coloc* 30C (> bending double), *Bell* 30C (flushed, restless), *Puls* 30C (weepy); Hrbl: Cramp Bark, Squaw Vine, with headache: Jonosia Asoka; niacin, B_6, magnesium, vit E and sometimes iron, vit C and calcium (or use dolomite); EPO; CPM: Dang Gui, add Butiao to warm cold uterus; with clots and irregular periods: Tong Jing Wan; detox with proanthocyanidins; sometimes chiropractic; see also Muscle Cramps.

Earache, Middle Ear Infection: Angry refusal to hear (in children: parents' arguing). Acute: Mullein oil (warm) in affected ear; Hmp: rprtz/esp: Bell, Cham, Puls, Hep, Mer C all in 30C; screaming with pain *Ferrium phos* 30 or 200C; Chronic: Hmp: rprtz/esp: *Sil* 1M, sometimes *Calc c* or *Thuja;* Reduce dairy, white flour; TS: *KM, CP.*

Eczema: Eliminate wheat, eggs, and dairy—sometimes soy, peanut, chocolate; Hmp: often *Graph (*use 200C every fifth day); EPO, 500 mg thrice daily; zinc 1 mg/lb until improved (max 2 months), also vits C, A, E; topically: ointment of licorice root extract; cleansing herbs: Burdock, Red clover, Turmeric, Forsythia, Bupleurum.

Edema: Holding on. Avoid salt; TS: *NS* (often with *KM*); whey; vit B_6; juice: grapefruit/cucumber/lettuce; watermelon; CPM: Golden

Book Tea (Rehmannia/Wild Yam formula); ERx: rebounder to stimulate lymphatic drainage.

Emphysema: Breathing retraining; Feeling unworthy of inhaling life. vit C in megadoses (to prevent respiratory infections, which would cause progression of the disease), also vit A 25–50,000 IU (mdcl sprv), vit E 400–1200 IU, and B complex; FE: Yerba Santa, Pine.

Endometriosis: Natural progesterone cream—a 2-oz jar used over day 10 to day 28 of each cycle; acupuncture; elim sugar and treat any coexisting candidiasis; vit B complex with extra B_6, selenium, magnesium, zinc, vit C, EPO; castor oil packs to abdomen; Hmp: rprtz/esp: *Calc c, Puls, Medor.*

Enuresis (see Bedwetting).

Environmental Illness (see Multiple Chemical Sensitivities).

Epilepsy: Hmp: *Arnica* high for birth trauma (or *Sulph,* then *Arnica*); Violent struggle against persecution. Hmp rptx/esp: *Calcarea carb* (often), also *Artemisia v, Absinthium, Cuprum;* craniosacral osteop; detox chemicals and metals; vits B_6, also A and E, calcium, magnesium, manganese, and zinc.

Epistaxis (see Nosebleed).

Fibrocystic Breast Disease: Avoid coffee, tea, chocolate, and colas; vit E 400–800 IU daily, vit A; acupuncture; EPO, 1,500 mg twice daily; TS: *CF* and *KM* if hard and fibrous, *CP, KM,* and *NP* if softer cysts predominate.

Fibroids, uterine: Reproductive equipment in knots. TS: *CF* and *KM;* avoid dairy and wheat; Hmp rptx/esp: *Calc c, Nat m, Sepia, Ustilago;* clear stagnant pelvic blood with acupuncture; CPM: Fu Ke Zhong Zi Wan or Hrbl mix: Turmeric (1 part), Licorice (1) and Peach pits (4), plus Cinnamon (4) if no excess heat; FE: Quince.

Flatulence (see Gas, intestinal).

Flu (see Influenza).

Fractures: *Arnica* 200C three times a day for at least 10 days; *calc, magnesium, zinc,* and full range of trace minerals; *Symphytum* 12x; vits D and C; avoid high phosphorus foods (e.g., meat, poultry, fish, and cola drinks).

Gallstones: Bitter, haughty and hard. Low-fat, high-fiber diet; gallbladder flush with lemon juice and olive oil; granular lecithin, 1 T with each meal (warning: high in phosphorus, so may provoke bone loss with prolonged use). For lodged stone with acute pain: *Berberis v* (Barberry) tincture, 8 drops in 2T water every 2–6 hours as needed will usually allow it to pass—use 1–2 times a day over longer period to help stones dissolve and pass; CPM to dissolve stones: Li Dan Pian.

Gas, Intestinal: Hallmark of *vatic* disorders—soothe, ground, and nurture; avoid large amounts of cabbage family vegs, legumes, raw foods; chew carefully; *TS: NP;* charcoal capsules acutely or, if severe, *Colocynth* 30C. Foul gas: *Carbo veg* 30C. Chronic problem suggests intestinal yeast overgrowth (see Candidiasis); Hrbl: digestive teas after meals: esp ginger, fennel (unless *pitta* problematic); generally: *vata* pacifying regimen.

Gout: No meat (esp organ meats) or alcohol, also avoid refined CHO's; Angry need to dominate. Cherries 1–2 cups per day or concentrate 1T thrice daily—also, though less potent, blueberries; EPA (fish oil) 1.5 g a day; plentiful water intake; Hmp rptz/esp: *Bryonia, Ledum, Benz ac, Colchicum* 12x, *Uric acid;* Hrbl: Burdock, Celery or Wild Carrot seed, Devil's claw.

Graves' Disease (see Hyperthyroidism).

Hair Loss (Baldness): scalp massage with mustard or emu (NV) oil or crude petroleum; Tightening of scalp due to effort to control the flow of life. Massage and brush to loosen and relax; YRx: inverted postures (subordinate the ego); correct hypothyroidism with iodine, shoulder stand, glandular preparations (NV); avoid excess salt, sugar, meat; electrical stimulation through hands or with appropriate devices (mdcl sprv); B complex with extra biotin and inositol, also l-cysteine; Hmp rprtz/esp: *Medor, Calc mur;* Rosemary oil topically; FE Red Carnation; *pitta* pacifying regimen.

Hay Fever: Guilty relationship with Mother Nature. TS: *KM* and *NM;* Hmp: *Penthorum* 6 thrice daily for 3 days, then, on fourth day, one dose of *Kali iod* 200C (esp in spring), in ragweed season try *Ambrosia* 30C three times a day, Cnstl: often *Tuberc* 1M; acupuncture; CPM: Bi Yan Pian; FE: Green Rose; raw thymus (NV) 0.5 gm twice daily. Prevention (start 6–12 wks before season): nasal wash with decreasing salt and temperature till using cold water; raw local honey—but only after clearing up any systemic yeast (see below).

Headache, Tension: Yoga, systematic relaxation; biofeedback: EMG trainer; scalp, gum massage, and fix TMJ; acupuncture; Hmp: Rprtz/esp: gastric *Nux v* 30C, weepy, *Puls* 30C, < eyestrain *Nat m,* needlelike on left, *Spig;* massage thumb, finger reflex points or, if gastric, stomach area in palm. If pressure focused in sinus area, see Sinusitis, on page 524.

Headache, Vascular (Migraine): Resistance to the flow of life and/or sexual energy. Biofeedback: temp. trainer; Hmp: for acute headache, right-sided, with nausea: *Sang* 200C; explosive, < bending over, *Glonoine* 30C; flushed, *Bell* 30C, also *Iris v* 30C; miasmatic: often *Syphilinum* 1M; elim coffee, meat, and sugar, also aspartame, nitrates/ites, red wine, cheese, and chocolate; Feverfew as herb or FE, also FE Green Rose; try Magnesium 200–400 mg a day, fish oil.

Heartburn: Fear. AV: *pitta*-calming regimen (esp elim coffee, alcohol, sugar, and fried and acid foods) and meditate on solar plexus to focus fire there; TS: combn *FP, KM,* and, if gassy, *NP;* ↑water; Hrbl: aloe vera gel 1 oz every 4–6 h; deglycyrrhizinated licorice; cabbage juice; Hmp rprtz/esp: *Nux v* 30C; CPM: Wei Te Ling (NV).

Heart Disease (see Congestive Heart Failure, ASCVD and page 569).

Heavy Periods (see Menstrual Bleeding, Excessive).

Hemorrhoids: Figure out what's "a pain in the butt." TS: combn *CF, KM,* and, if bleeding, *FP; Rutin* 50 mg 3 times a day and/or mixed bioflavonoids 100 mg–1 g a day; Hrbl: topical Aesculus ointment, if bleeding, add Hamamelis (witch hazel)—in a pinch, moisten cotton ball with witch hazel, and leave in anus on going to bed; Lesser Celandine ("pilewort") esp fresh root; wash anus thoroughly after bowel movement; warm sitz bath; attend to liver; acupuncture.

Hepatitis: Angry, rageful resistance to change. No alcohol, sugar, or grease. Hmp: *Chel* 12x twice daily, or *Thorazine* 30C once or twice a day; vit C megadoses have been used with success (40–100 *grams* a day); Hrbl: Milk thistle (75–200 mg silymarin 3 times daily), Dandelion (250–500 mg 4:1 extract 3 times daily), and Licorice; CPM: Ji Gu Cao Wan plus Li Gan Pian (both NV).

Hernia: Strained expression, relating. YRx: *uddiyana bandha,* inverted postures; Hmp: *Cocculus* 3x or 3D 3 times daily; TS: *CF;* Copper and vit C are important for elastic fibers of connective tissue; CPM: Bu Zhong Yi Qi Wan.

Herpes Genitalis (Herpes Simplex on genitals): Burning with guilty sexual urges. Same Rx's as for H. Labialis plus: Hmp: *Merc sol* 200C plus TS: *CS; Syph* 1M alternating with *Thuja;* or *Hepar sulph;* FE: Basil, Easter Lily, Crabapple, or Pine.

Herpes Labialis ("cold sores" or Herpes Simplex around mouth): Burning and itching to bitch. Lysine 2g a day, vit C, zinc, vit E;

Lactobacillus acidophilus 3 times a day; Hmp: *Psor* 6x; TS: *KM* for at least 6 mos; Thymus extract (NV).

Herpes Zoster: Vit B_{12} 1,000 mcg twice daily sublingually or (better) 500 mcg by injection daily; vit C in megadoses orally or (better) IV, if medical help available; vit E topically and 1,200–1,600 IU daily for post-herpetic pain; Hmp: rprtz/esp *Ars a*—also for persisting pain.

High Blood Pressure (see Hypertension).

Hives: Elim chemicals, additives, drugs; Making mountains out of mole-hills (fear). Hmp: acute: *Apis* 30C; recurrent: *Kali iod* 200C, consider *Calc c* as cstl; CPM: Chuan Shan Jia Qu Shi Qing Du Wan (NV); if due to "sun allergy," try vit B_6 up to 600 mg a day (mdcl sprv); if acute, severe, and acmpd by respiratory distress, get to an emergency room!

Hot Flashes (menopausal): Energy previously reserved for reproduction is now available and needs to be harnessed or else will hit in these "power surges." Acupuncture; elim: alcohol, chocolate, caffeine, sugar, tobacco; vit E 400–800 IU daily; if acmpd by anger, irritability: *pitta* pacifying regimen; natural progesterone, sometimes low doses of testosterone (both three weeks on, one off); FE: Walnut, sometimes Pomegranate; maca Hrbl: Motherwort tincture, also Shatavari, Dang Gui, Chasteberry, Wild Yam, and Black Cohosh; CPM: Da Bu Yin Wan (NV); Hmp: Rprtz/esp: *Lach, Sepia, Sulphur,* maybe *Ustilago* or *Sumbul* in low potencies.

Hyperlipidemia: Low fat *and* oil diet; Hmp: Rprtz/esp: *Nat m;* see also ASCVD and page 569.

Hypertension (High Blood Pressure): "Holding in" something. Return *pitta* from surface to solar plexus by moving *from* and meditating *on* that point; Hrbl: Garlic, Viscum album (mistletoe), Olive leaves (with meals), if acpd by ASCVD: Hawthorn berry; with mdcl sprv: Rauwolfia in very low doses; YRx: systematic relaxation and diaphragm breathing 10 mins twice daily, for last 3 mins inhale through nose, exhale through mouth; biofeedback: temp trainer; ↑ water to 8 oz/20 lbs. body wt.; ERx: at least 4 times per wk, e.g., 45 min brisk walk; CoQ10 60–90 mg daily, fish oil, sometimes calcium; diet: high fiber, low fat, low salt, no meat; TS: *NS*.

Hyperthyroidism (Graves' Disease, Thyrotoxicosis): Rage at being held down, overlooked—harness your creativity! Hmp: *Natrum mur, Iodum,* or *Thyroidinum;* acupuncture; Hrbl: Lycopus virg (Bugleweed), Leonurus card (Motherwort), or combn—takes about a

month for full effect; CPM: Long Dan Xie Gan Wan or Tian Wang
Bu Xin Wan.

Hypoglycemia: Too dispirited to supply oneself fuel—find your passion!
Elim: all simple (sugars), refined carbohydrates (e.g., white flour),
alcohol; when acmpd by systemic yeast overgrowth (often) also elim:
yeasted and fermented foods; chromium 200 mcg daily, magnesium
400 mg daily.

Hypothyroidism: Giving up, feeling hopelessly stifled. Acupuncture;
elim: (esp raw or undercooked) turnips, cabbage, mustard greens,
soybeans, peanuts, pine nuts, and millet; iodine (small doses intermittently), plus tyrosine 250 mg daily; see Ch. 8, page 276, and n. 5
to that discussion; ck zinc status and try vits A, B complex, and C;
YRx: shoulder stand and fish; FE: Trumpet Vine, Larch, Mountain
Pride.

Immune Weakness: Giving up, self-condemnation.[5] Acupuncture;
Hrbl: Echinacea, Astragalus, Ginseng, Siberian Ginseng; Elim:
sugar, white flour; lactoferrin; Thymic Protein A; CPM: Shen Qi
Da Bu Wan; YRx: balanced program of yoga postures; AV: regimen
for your constitution; thymus extract (NV); FE: rprtz/esp *Pine*.

Impetigo: Hmp: *Staphylococcus* 200C, sometimes *Dioxychlor* D3 also
rprtz/esp: *Antim crud* 30C; elim: all sweets—even fruit; vits A and
C, high doses, short term (mdcl sprv) and zinc; Hrbl: Echinacea;
Topical: scrub off scabs with tincture of green soap, flush with
hydrogen peroxide, and apply gentian violet or tea tree oil.

Impotence: Ck for vascular insufficiency by urologist—if positive, see
ASCVD, on page 508; otherwise: pressure to perform, guilt, fear of
women. Acupuncture; elim: alcohol, tobacco, drugs, and medications; learn to enjoy sex without ejaculation; zinc 50 mg daily; Hrbl:
Ginkgo biloba 60 mg daily (of extract containing 24%
ginkgoflavonglycosides); also Yohimbine and Muira pauma; FE:
Larch, also: Basil, Hibiscus, Sticky or Pink Monkeyflower; progesterone cream or oil; CPM: Kang Wei Ling (NV), Nan Bao (NV), or,
if acmpd by cold hands and feet, low-back pain and weak digestion,
Jin Kui Shen Qi Wan.

Infertility: Is there room in your life for a child? Is parenting really your
path? If so: Hmp: rprtz/esp: *Nat mur, Medor, Syph;* Elim: coffee,
tobacco, alcohol, drugs; full-spectrum trace mineral supplement,
men add extra selenium and zinc; women: FE: rprtz/esp
Pomegranate; CPM: Shou Wu Zhi, and for women: Fu Ke Zhong

Zi Wan (NV) or Women's Precious Pill; AV: ashwagandha and shatavari, and, for men, chavanprash.

Influenza: Caught up in mass negativity, fears, and beliefs. CPM: Gan Mao Ling or, if more severe, Zhong Gan Ling; Russian Bath; Hmp: *Oscillococcinum,* aching in bones: *Eupator,* rprtz/esp: *Bry, Ars a, Gels;* TS: *KM,* also *FP* if fever; vit C tbt; Hrbl: tea of Honeysuckle, Chrysanthemum, and Forsythia, also for *cold* flu: Bayberry and Cinnamon or Ginger, acmpd by mucusy cough: add Angelica; for a hotter, feverish flu: Yarrow, add Boneset or Black Willow for achiness, Pleurisy Root and Elder for cough, and Raspberry Leaf or Catnip for intestinal symptoms.

Injuries (see Trauma, Fractures, Lacerations, etc.).

Insect Bites: Hmp: *Ledum* 30C, sometimes *Apis mel;* FE: Rescue Remedy (5-flower formula); CPM: Yunnan Paiyao; topically, ledum ointment or tincture; if signs of allergic reaction, start to emergency room while giving remedies, and administer "Epipen" (injection of adrenalin); prevention: vit B_1 100 mg three times daily and/or *Staphys* 6x three times a day; see also Bee Stings.

Insomnia: Fear and guilt. Hmp: *Coffea crud* 200C; TS: *FP.* Acmpd by irritability, (fiery, bilious): *pitta* calming regimen plus Hrbl: Skullcap, Passaflora, Jatamamsi, or CPM: Eight Flavor Tea (pills) perhaps *Nux v* 30C. Congestive, phlegmatic type: anti-*kapha* regimen plus CPM: Xiao Yao Wan, or Myrrh and Cinnamon. If windy, nervous, *vatic* (most common type): calming yoga, a warm bath, and oil massage to feet, also Passaflora, Valerian, and a CPM tonic of fo ti and ginseng or AV of ashwagandha. General (all types): elim caffeine; tryptophan 1 g, 30 mins before bed; melatonin 3 mg time-release; calcium/magnesium.

Irritable Bowel Syndrome: Holding on to outmoded phases of development. YRx: balanced program of postures, diaphragm breathing, systematic relaxation; usually *vata*-calming regimen; acupuncture; elim: nicotine, caffeine, sugar, artificial sweeteners (Stevia is okay), and sometimes dairy; ↑soft fiber (vegetables, grains, fruits); ck for specific food sensitivities; peppermint oil, enteric-coated, 0.2–0.5 ml thrice daily; acidophilus (and other probiotics); TS: *CF, MP,* add *NP* if gas; ERx: walk outdoors 45 mins four times a wk.

Kidney Stones: Crystals of poisonous thought and feeling. ↑water intake; vit B_6 and magnesium; elim: foods high in calcium, protein, or oxalic acid, depending on type of stone; in acute attack: *Berb v*

MT, 8 drops in 2 T water every 2–6 hrs as needed, also *Khella;* CPM: Te Xiao Pai Shi Wan; potassium citrate 60 mEq daily (mdcl sprv); Hrbl: Eupator purp, Collinsonia, Desmodium, Madder root; Hmp: *Sarsaparilla* 1–3C.

Lacerations: Calendula ointment; Hmp: *Calendula* 30C; Hrbl: Plantain leaf topically, Yarrow leaf chewed and applied for pain and bleeding.

Laryngitis: Too angry and/or fearful to speak up. Hmp: *Causticum* 30C; Hrbl: Echinacea, also gargle with Balm of Gilead (or Sage or Thyme) tea; FE: Trumpet Vine.

Leukorrhea (see Vaginal Discharge).

Low Back Pain: Financial fears. Read Dr. Sarno's book.[6] Acupuncture. Acute: DMSO topically, followed after one min by *Arnica* gel; *Arnica* 200C thrice daily; TS: *MP, CF;* ck water intake (sensitive kidneys underlie much back trouble). Chronic: YRx: folded leaf (child's pose) *not* when pain acute, and/or find a Pilates instructor; CPM: "Specific Lumbaglin" (not during preg) also Shou Wu Zhi or Yao Tong Pian to strengthen kidneys and back. Prevention: regular yoga; elim: wheat.

Lumbago (see Low Back Pain).

Lyme Disease: A non-venereal expression of the *syphilitic* miasm. For involvement of the central nervous system, IV hydrogen peroxide therapy (mdcl sprv); Hmp: *Dioxychlor* D3, *Syphilinum.*

Macular degeneration: Not wanting to see, forcing *in*sight. Reduced glutathione up to 500 mg thrice daily. Proanthocyanidins ("pycnogenol") 60–120 mg thrice daily; elim: smoking, vegetable oils; zinc; Ginkgo biloba extract (24% ginkgo heterosides) 40 mg thrice daily and Blueberry extract (25% anthocyanidins) 100–150 mg thrice daily; Beta carotene, vits C, E, and selenium, and lutein; antioxidant enzymes (SOD, glutathione, etc); Hmp: *Syphilinum.*

Manic Depressive Disorder (see Bipolar Disorder).

Mastitis: Continue nursing, or pump breast; Hmp: *Phytolac* 30C or 200C, sometimes *Belladonna* 30C; Hrbl: also Phytolac (Poke Root) as poultice or internally in *small* doses (e.g., MT 10–20 drops 3–6 times daily) plus Echinacea 20 drops every 4 hrs; CPM: Chuan Xin Lian Kang Yan; prevention: prenatal prep and proper nursing technique.

Menopausal problems (See Hot Flashes, etc.).

Menstrual Bleeding, Excessive: Physical expression of thwarted yang femininity.[7] Vit A 50,000–75,000 IU a day for 2–4 wks, then half that for 2 mos (mdcl sprv); vit C with bioflavonoids 250 mg thrice daily; Hrbl: Shepherd's Purse (esp if associated with fibroids), Amaranth, Senecio aureus, also Trillium or Cramp Bark (both esp. effective at menopause); Hmp: rprtz for cstl/esp *Calc carb;* CPM: for acute bleeding: Yunnan Paiyao, chronic: Butiao Tablets (NV) and/or Dang Gui Pills (*Chinese* Angelica).

Migraine (see Headache, Vascular).

Mitral Valve Prolapse: Lack of confidence in what you have to give. Magnesium 250 mg 2–3 times a day; CoQ10 (at least in children).

Mononucleosis: Angry at not being valued, but participating in the attitude (i.e., self-depreciation). Hmp: Usually *Carcinosin* 200C, sometimes *Cistus canad* 30–200C; TS: *KM, NP;* FE: Buttercup, Fuchsia; if lingering weakness follows: Dioxychlor D3 and Lomatium dissect tincture (isolate) in alternation, each four days; See also Immune Weakness.

Morning Sickness: Hyperprogesteronism; guilty effort to give too much. Acupuncture; don't let blood sugar drop, or get dehydrated (lots of water and regular eating *prevents* nausea)—take honey and water with a pinch of salt if necessary; vits B_6, K (not synthetic) and C, maybe zinc; Hrbl: Ginger caps 2 thrice daily; Hmp: *Symphoricarpus* 200C or rprtz/esp *Cocculus* 6C; acupressure to Neiguan points inside surface of wrist, 3 finger breadths toward elbow.

Motion Sickness: Fear of not being in control. Ginger caps 2 one hr before and every 3–4 hrs during motion; Hmp: *Cocculus,* if acmpd by reaction to gasoline fumes: *Petr;* acupressure as under Morning Sickness.

Multiple Chemical Sensitivities: Stuck in the paranoid position. Focus efforts on detox and change of mindset; FE: Yarrow or Special Yarrow Formula (Cal FE).

Multiple Sclerosis: Inflexibility and fear. Acupuncture; Ck for heavy-metal toxicity and food sensitivities (latter by ELISA/ACT, or ck pulse—elevation after food suggests reaction); often elim: gluten, animal fat; sunflower seed oil 2T a day; Russian baths (hyperthermia); Deep Muscle Therapy[8] and thorough detox.

Muscle Cramps: "Holding on for dear life." TS: *MP,* 20 tabs in $\frac{1}{4}$ glass of warm water sip every 5 mins; calcium/magnesium; for nocturnal leg and foot cramps: vit E 400–800 IU a day. For "growing pains" in children, use both vit E and calcium/magnesium.

Nosebleed: Feeling unnoticed, crying for love. Acute: Yunnan Paiyao (see pages 67–68). Chronic, prevention: natural (not synthetic) vit K (esp in those who eat no green vegs); vit C with bioflavonoids; Hmp: rprtz/esp: *Medor* (craves citrus, chews ice), *Phos* (bright red, almost gushing), *Puls* (blood dark, clotted), or *Sulph* (messy, dirty in personal habits).

Obesity: Has two roots: (1) fake fulfillment from fake food (2) provides a layer of insulation protecting from exposure and feelings. Write down everything you put in your mouth; eat only sitting down in your dining area at regular times, and chew each bite 32 times; 30 mins of aerobic exercise 4 times wk, plus yoga; drink at least 32 oz water a day; ck basal body temp, if low, see Hypothyroidism above; regulate diet with "One Bowl Approach" (see pages 256–57). If progress stalls, try elim *all* sugar and white flour and, if necessary, all wheat, too; also alcohol and *television;* Hmp: rprtz/esp: *Calc c, Medor, Syph;* FE: rprtz/esp: Black-eyed Susan, Cherry Plum, Chestnut Bud, Morning Glory; Hrbl stims: green tea (not if *vatic*), Guarana, Gotu kola, Ginseng, Malabar Tamarind (in food).

Osteoporosis: Dismantling the framework for life. Elim: coffee, meat, sugar, and high-phosphorus foods[9] (e.g., cola drinks); Exercise 1 hr four times a week, e.g., walking; ipriflavone 600 mg daily, calcium, magnesium, B_6, folic acid, B_{12}, vit K, boron, vit D, strontium, manganese, and a full range of trace minerals; proanthocyanidins;[10] progesterone may be more helpful than estrogen; also DHEA, and sometimes calcitonin (mdcl sprv).

Otitis Externa (see Swimmer's Ear).

Otitis Media (see Earache).

Parkinson's Disease: Fearful need to control; study the *Course in Miracles.* Thorough detox; NADH 10 mg daily; Proanthocyanidins 60–100 mg thrice daily; Hmp: if assocd with head trauma: *Nat s* 200C every 4 days; craniosacral osteopathic treatment.

Peptic Ulcer: Overanxious to please (see also Heartburn). 2 qts water daily; cabbage juice 1 qt. total daily for 10 days (mix with other vegs for palatability) or glutamine 400 mg 4 times daily 1 hr before meals and before bed; high-fiber diet; zinc 75 mg daily; ck for food sensitivities;[11] sometimes helpful to eradicate associated *H. pylori* with bismuth preps;[12] Hrbl: deglycerrhizinated liquorice (DGL) 0.5–1 g a half hour before meals, also Slippery Elm and/or Comfrey tea; if bleeding, take CPM: Yunnan Paiyao on the way to emergency room.

Periodontal Disease: Anger at inability to make and/or back up decisions. Blotting toothbrush;[13] vit C 1–3 g a day; vit A 10,000 IU a day;

CoQ10 60–90 mg a day; also calcium 1 g a day, magnesium 500 mg; rinse mouth with dilute hydrogen peroxide (1 part 3% H_2O_2 to 4 parts water) and massage gums with fingertips; Elim: sugar, white flour, smoking.

PMS: Anger at being caught in a mess made by men (see pages 293–94). Acupuncture; high complex carbohydrate, low-fat diet without sugar or white flour; zinc, vit B_6 100–300 mg a day and/or vit A 100,000–300,000 IU daily for 2 wks preceding period (mdcl sprv); vit E 300–600 IU daily, magnesium 400 mg daily, and Evening Primrose Oil 1.5 g daily; natural progesterone cream in ascending doses for the ten days before menstrual period; thorough detox; aerobic exercise; full-spectrum light 2 hrs daily;[14] FE: rprtz esp.: Pomegranate, Quince, Tiger Lily.

Poison Ivy/Oak: Wash with oil-removing detergent;[15] Hmp: when severe with edema and dark scabs: *Ars a* 200C.

Pre-eclampsia (see Toxemia of Pregnancy).

Pregnancy (see Morning Sickness, Threatened Miscarriage, Toxemia of Pregnancy).

Premature Ventricular Contractions (see Arrhythmias).

Prostate Enlargement/Inflammation: Giving in to your belief in aging. Acupuncture; zinc 50 mg daily, vit B_6 100–250 mg daily; Hrbl: Saw Palmetto berries (liposterolic extract containing 85–95% fatty acids and sterols) 160 mg twice daily, also pollen extract[16] or Pygeum or Equisetum and Hydrangea root; CPM: Qian Lie Xian or Jie Jie Wan; Deep Muscle Release of perineum; AAs: Glycine, Glutamic acid, and Alanine 200 mg each a day; pumpkin seed ⅓ cup a day; YRx: *mula bandha*;[17] avoid alcohol, esp beer; Evening Primrose or Linseed oil; TS: *NS;* Hmp: esp *Thuja* and *Staphys*.

Pruritis Ani (itchy butt): Ck for pinworms; Elim: sugar, coffee, sometimes chocolate, beer, tomatoes; Hmp: Rprtz/esp: *Sulphur, Medor;* wear white cotton underwear; clean (pref *wash*) anus carefully after b.m., also may rinse with dilute vinegar.

Psoriasis: Deadening the sense of self. Colonic irrigation; ck for food sensitivities/allergies, often wheat and dairy; sunlight to affected areas; vit D_3 topically, also capsaicin; fish oil (eg., MAXEPA or Cod Liver Oil); elim: alcohol; Hmp: *Hydrocotyl* 6x, *Syph;* FE: rprtz; general detox and fresh veg juices; Hrbl: Sarsaparilla, Milk Thistle; vit A, B complex, zinc.

Respiratory Infection (see Bronchitis, Pneumonia, Sore throat, Common Cold, Flu, etc.).

Reynaud's Syndrome: Biofeedback (temp trainer); acupuncture; elim: alcohol, tobacco, and coffee, all of which can cause vasoconstriction; Vit E 400–800 IU daily; fish oil or EPO; magnesium 200 mg and taurine 250 mg thrice daily; Hmp: rprtz/esp *Sepia, Secale;* Hrbl: Ginkgo.

Sciatica: Fear/first-chakra issues. Acupuncture; YRx: posterior stretch, child's pose; TS: *CF, MP;* Soothe *vata* with oil massage of feet; CPM: when cold extremities, Guan Jie Yan Wan; vit C, B_1, B_{12}; Hmp: *Colocynth* 30C, pain hip to knee in elderly: *Kali carb;* see also Low Back Pain.

Seasickness (see Motion Sickness).

Shingles (see Herpes Zoster).

Sinusitis: Tension around eyes; irritated by someone close or "over-intentional living." Postnasal drip = internal crying. Nasal wash (*neti*[18]); Hmp: *Kali bichrome* 200C every 4 days, sometimes *Puls;* TS: *KM, CS* if mucus yellow; acupuncture; elim: foods causing reactions, often wheat and dairy; vit C 1–3 g daily, Vit A 10,000 IU daily; CPM: Bi Yan Pian, Pe Min Kan; YRx: Brahmari; Hrbl: Goldenseal, also to reduce congestion: Tulsi, Bayberry, Mullein or 1–3 g Ajwain seeds powdered, thrice daily before meals.

Smoking Habit: A way of controlling impulses and moods. Learn to regulate energy with breathing; the irritation that leads to a cigarette may be due to dehydration, dropping blood sugar, lack of exercise, food or chemical reactions, nutritional deficiencies, as well as emotional issues—identify cause and take care of it; TS: *NM* 3x.

Sore Throat: Holding in anger, not expressing yourself; often first sign of immune system being unable to keep up. Zinc lozenges (25 mg, every 2–4 hrs, no more than 4–5 days); YRx: Lion's pose; FE: Trumpet Vine, Mountain Pride; cold, wet cloth around neck, wrap with a towel and go to bed; Hrbl: Goldenseal if mucusy; Slippery Elm lozenges if raw.

Stasis Ulcers: Folic Acid, vit C, vit E, zinc, also vit E topically; Hrbl: Comfrey[19] (best is to wrap crushed fresh leaf in gauze and apply twice daily), also topical Goldenseal; Hmp: rptrz; usually due to poor circulation; if arterial, consider IV chelation and/or H_2O_2 therapy and see ASCVD above; if venous, see Varicose Veins, on page 526.

Stroke: "Rather die than change." Rejection of life. For post-stroke paralysis: Deep Muscle Therapy (see note 8) and thorough detox; CPM: Tsai Tsao Wan; Hrbl: Vinca minor extract (vincamine—

mdcl sprv); immediately after stroke, to avoid disability, give CPM: Yan Shen Jai Jao or Xi Huang Wan (both NV and not during pregnancy) on the way to ER; prevention: CPM: Mao Dong Qing; Hmp: *Syph,* also *Lyc* if symptoms or previous strokes on right side, *Lach* if on left; see also ASCVD.

Sunburn: Free-radical damage triggered by excess sunlight. *Pitta* types especially susceptible. Antioxidants: vit E in megadoses: 800–1,600 IU (no more than a few days), also topically, esp micelized form; proanthocyanidins 60–120 mg thrice daily; both of these, taken before exposure to the sun, reduce susceptibility to burning; topically for burn: CPM: Jing Wan Hong.

Surgery (recovery from): Zinc to support wound healing; *Arnica* 200C thrice daily for 7–10 days; calendula ointment may help wounds; *Ledum* for tenderness and discomfort from injections or IVs; diaphragmatic breathing post-op prevents many complications; detox from anesthetics and drugs; for fatigue and weakness following: CPM: Dan Gui Gin Gao, Hai Long Bu Wan, or Quan Lu Wan (all 3 NV).

Swimmer's Ear: Several drops of a solution of one part vinegar to four parts water, then plug with cotton; avoid sweets.

Tendonitis ("tennis elbow"): *Bryonia* 30C; see also Bursitis.

Threatened Miscarriage: Hmp: rprtz/esp: dark spotting: *Secale* 200C, bright red blood: *Sabina* 6C, also *Viburnum op* (Cramp Bark tincture or very low potencies); Hrbl: tea of Blue Cohosh: False Unicorn root : Cramp Bark :: 2:2:1 thrice daily; CPM: An Tai Wan.

Thrush: Elim: sweets; *Borax* 3x thrice daily; acidophilus; often a sign that the immune system can't keep up (see also Immune Weakness).

Toxemia of Pregnancy: Most often due to protein malnutrition;[20] legume/grain combos, tofu, low-fat cheeses, eggs, and/or fish; megadoses (with mdcl sprv) of magnesium and vit B_6: 200–800 mg B_6 and 400–1500 mg magnesium daily; if edema and blood pressure already up, give both B_6 and magnesium IV; TS: *NS, KM, MP.*

Trauma (see Chapter 2, pages 65–70).

Ulcers, Leg (see Stasis Ulcers).

Ulcers, Stomach/Duodenal (see Peptic Ulcer).

Urinary Incontinence: Emotional overflow. Years of controlling the emotions. TS: *CF, NP;* YRx: practice *mula bandha;* Hrbl: tea of Horsetail, Agrimony, and/or Sweet Sumac (root bark); sometimes acupuncture; in children at night, see Bedwetting.

Urticaria (see Hives).

Vaginal Discharge: Anger at partner and/or guilt about sex. Avoid synthetic underwear, chemical irritants, tampons with perfumes or deodorants, and antibiotics; if discharge yeasty, elim sugar and all sweets and start with vinegar douche (2T in 1 qt water); Goldenseal tea and (live) yogurt douches in alternation. Chronic recurrent: Hmp: reprtz/esp: if discharge greenish, *Medor;* if itchy and irritated, *Kreos* 6x thrice daily; CPM: Qian Jin Zhi Dai Wan.

Varicose Veins: Standing on, not with, your legs because you're in a situation you hate. TS: *CF;* proanthocyanidins 60–120 mg thrice daily; Hrbl: Gotu kola extract (70% triterperic acid) 30 mg thrice daily; Aesculus hipp (root bark .5 g thrice daily); Butcher's Broom (extract 10% ruscogenin, 60–120 mg thrice daily); YRx: inverted postures; keep legs alive and in motion while standing; ten minutes twice a day on a slantboard at 10–15° incline; witch hazel topically.

Warts: Feeling hateful and ugly because of indulging in what you don't really want. Hmp: *Thuja* first, if symptoms fit, but if no results give *Sulph,* then repeat, also consider *Staphys,* sometimes *Causticum* (near tip of finger and painful) or *Nitric Acid* (sticking pain, bleeds); Hrbl: topically Ficus carica or Podophylum tinctures or Noni juice.

Water Retention (see Edema).

Worms: Inhabited by alien entities. Elim: sugar and white flour; Hmp: *Cina* 1M once weekly for 3 doses; to set the stage for natural agents to work, a semi-fast or light diet for a few days, including foods that "worms don't like," e.g., onions, garlic, shredded coconut or carrot, pumpkin seeds, rhubarb, pomegranate; then a cup of strong Wormwood tea A.M. and P.M.; or 3–10 drops of Wormseed oil with honey thrice daily for 3 days; on the fourth day Senna tea or epsom salts to clean dead worms from the bowel; also Pinkroot, Male Fern, or Pomegrate root bark can be used.[21]

Yeast Infection, Vaginal (see Vaginal Discharge).

Yeast Infection, Systemic (see Candidiasis).

A Simple Home Medicine Kit

The full kit is 50 items. Asterisked items are the most essential. Each category and/or item will be found listed in the General Index of this book, which will guide you to the passages where it is introduced and discussed.

Cell Salts: *Kali mur* 6x,* *Ferrum phos* 6x,* *Mag phos* 6x,* *Calc sulph* 6x,* *Natrum sulph* 6x, *Natrum phos* 6x, *Calc fluor* 6x, *Kali phos* 6x, *Calc phos* 6x

Homeopathic Remedies: *Aconitum* 30C,* *Arnica* 200C,* *Arsenicum alb* 30C,* *Belladonna* 30C,* *Bryonia* 30C,* *Cactus g* 30C,* *Carbo veg* 30C, *Coffea cruda* 200C,* *Colocynth* 30C,* *Hypericum* 30C,* *Kali bichrome* 200C, *Ledum* 30C,* *Merc sol* 30C, *Nux vom* 30C,* *Pulsatilla* 30C,* *Rhus tox* 30C, *Rumex* 30C, *Sanguinaria* 200C

Herbs (in tincture): *Astragalus, Berberis vulgaris* (Barberry)*, Cat's Claw, *Echinacea,** *Goldenseal,* Osha

Chinese Remedies: Gan Mao Ling,* Zhong Gan Ling,* Yunnan Pai Yao*, Po Chai, or Pill Curing.[a]

Topicals: Calendula,* Arnica gel,* Tea Tree oil

Flower Essences: Rescue Remedy*

Supplements: Zinc Lozenges, vit C,* High-potency vit E*, calcium/magnesium

Miscellaneous: Charcoal capsules, Melatonin (sustained release) 2–3 mg, colloidal silver, Gold Drops (if you can get them),[b] mullein oil (ear drops)

This entire kit, either the 26- or 50-item version, can be ordered, already assembled, from Wellspring Pharmacy (see page 572).

a. For general upset stomach.
b. See Chapter 1, page 40.

Guide to the Further Study of
Holistic Medicine

This book list will offer backup information for each chapter as well as help you to find more to read on the subjects that interest you. I've included brief descriptions and critiques of each book to help you decide which ones fit your needs and interests. There are few if any bookstores or libraries where you will find this selection of books available to flip through and evaluate. Nothing is more frustrating than ordering a book and discovering that it was not at all what you had expected or wanted.

I apologize to the many authors whose books I have not included, but whose contributions have been invaluable and have served as a foundation for my work and that of so many others in this field.

Chapter 1. HERBAL TRADITIONS

The Book of Herbal Wisdom: Using Plants as Medicines, Matthew Wood, North Atlantic Books, Berkeley, Calif., 1997. Perhaps the first book to attempt a full integration of so many traditionally different approaches to herbal medicine—e.g., Native American, Chinese, and homeopathic. It deliberately aims to bring together the spiritual significance of the plant along with its energetic message and its effect on the Five Elements. Unfortunately only a limited number of herbs are covered, but the 64 introductory pages alone are worth the cost of the book. Highly recommended.

Herbal Medicine, Rudolph Fritz Weiss, M.D., Beaconsfield Publishers, Beaconsfield, England, 1988. This much-touted book is a translation of the sixth German edition of the standard work on phytotherapy in Germany. It is rigorous, and includes only those herbal medicines well documented by scientific research. It is, as a result, somewhat restricted in scope.

Of Man and Plants, Maurice Messegue, Macmillan, New York, 1973. A fascinating anecdotal biography of France's most famous unschooled herbalists. Messegue learned his art from his father, and, applying it skillfully and intuitively, he became a minor celebrity, summoned to treat the famous in France and abroad. An appendix includes recipes for his treatments, many of which were administered as foot or hand baths. The drawback for many readers will be that the application of this technique requires ample quantities of the plants used; some must be fresh, and though others can be dried, they must have been properly gathered and be available in quantity.

A Modern Herbal, 2 vols., Mrs. Grieve, Dover, New York, 1971. Mrs. Grieve is the twentieth century's answer to Culpeper. In two volumes, her work is possibly the most encyclopedic and scholarly collection of herbal lore available in the English language. Though it draws extensively from the homeopathic Materia Medica and some continental sources, it is preeminently a British perspective on herbalism, but that means colonial Britain, and there are plants from all the corners of the Empire, presented with the precision, good taste, and aplomb we associate with the best of that era.

American Indian Medicine, Virgil J. Vogel, University of Oklahoma Press, 1970. More anthropological than medical in its perspective, this book remains the single best work on Native American medicinal plants. Though unfortunately not arranged in such a way as to be very useful to the practicing clinician, it is nevertheless a valuable reference work.

Planetary Herbology, Michael Tierra, Lotus Press, Santa Fe, N.M., 1988. An inspiring attempt to integrate the four major herbal medicine traditions of the world: Ayurvedic, Chinese, European, and Native American. Though one would need some passing knowledge of each of these systems to be able to use this book to greatest advantage, it remains unique and stimulating.

American Medicinal Plants, Charles F. Millspaugh, Dover, N.Y., 1974. Originally published in the nineteenth century, this is the classic Materia

Medica of American plants used in homeopathy. The line drawings are beautiful and helpful for plant identification. Many if not most of these plants are familiar to Americans.

How to Be Your Own Herbal Pharmacist, Linda Rector-Page, Ph.D., Crystal Star Herbs, Sonora, Calif., 1991; new edition, 1997. This is an easy-to-use guide to putting together your own herbal combination remedies. Grouped by system or complaint (Circulatory, Respiratory, Infection, etc.), with charts showing groups of herbs that have varying actions on that system. Useful, but the new edition has almost too much detail and information to deal with.

Botanical Influences on Illness: A Sourcebook of Clinical Research, Melvyn R. Werbach, M.D., and Michael T. Murray, N.D., Third Line Press, Tarzana, Calif., 1994. An authoritative, if limited, presentation of the best documented herbal treatments for common problems.

The Yoga of Herbs, Dr. David Frawley and Dr. Vasant Lad, Lotus Press, Santa Fe, N.M., 1986. One wishes this book were more extensive. It discusses a limited number of Eastern and Western herbs from an Ayurvedic perspective.

The New Holistic Herbal, David Hoffmann, Element, Inc., Rockport, Mass., 1992. By a well-known and respected contemporary herbalist, this is a compilation of information on American and European herbs from the perspective and in the terminology of the modern European herbal tradition.

Healing Wise: The Wise Woman Herbal, Susun S. Weed, Ash Tree Publishing, Woodstock, N.Y., 1989. A powerful encouragement for a woman to reclaim her relationship to nature and plants, and a very folksy, hands-on treatment of seven herbs you can find around you and use.

Creating Your Herbal Profile, Dorothy Hall, Keats Publishing, New Canaan, Conn., 1988. Though it may try to take the use of herbs to places homeopathic potencies work much better, this book is nevertheless wonderful in its probing into the resonance of the personality of the human and that of the plant.

Sacred Plant Medicine, Stephen Harrod Buhner, Roberts Rinehart, Boulder, Colo., 1996. This is the book quoted so extensively in Chapter 1 of the present work, and the most successful work so far, I think, in capturing the spirit of what plants have meant in the Native American tradition.

Chapter 2. HOMEOPATHIC REMEDIES AND CELL SALTS

Cell Salts

An Abridged Therapy: Manual for the Biochemical Treatment of Disease, 25th edition (1897), W. H. Schuessler, M.D., Haren & Brother, Calcutta (first Indian edition), 1960. This is the last edition done by the author and founder of the system of cell salts or tissue salts. It's a short little book and gives succinct information on how to use the remedies. The reader might note that in it the author acknowledges that *Calcarea sulph* seems effective, but with no evidence of its constant presence in the body, he excluded it from his system. It is currently considered one of the basic twelve.

The Twelve Tissue Remedies of Schuessler, W. Boericke, M.D., and W. A. Dewey, M.D., Aperture, New York, 1911. A classic work on the tissue salts, this book, by two prominent homeopaths of the Golden Era of homeopathy in America, compares the usage of the remedies in the system of Schuessler with their use in homeopathic medicine.

Dr. Schuessler's Biochemistry: A Natural Method of Healing, J. B. Chapman, M.D., Thorsons Publishing, Rochester, Vt., 1973. One of the few contemporary treatments of cell salts, with a materia medica and repertory.

Guide to the Twelve Tissue Remedies of Biochemistry, E. P. Anshutz, M.D., Boericke and Tafel, Philadelphia, 1927. Homeopaths in recent decades have ignored or dismissed the Biochemic system of therapy. But Dr. Anshutz, a well-known homeopath and author of his era, says of the tissue salts: "The brilliant success that has attended their use lends colour to the claims of Schuessler; whether they are 'all-sufficient' therapeutically is a question that must remain open. Their value is, however, so marked that every physician would do well to familiarize himself with them."

Homeopathy

Materia Medica with Repertory, William Boericke, M.D., Boericke and Runyon, Philadelphia, 1927. The *Merck Manual* of homeopaths. Portable yet encyclopedic, it includes both a concise materia medica (symptoms listed under remedies) and a condensed repertory (remedies listed under symptoms).

Homeopathy as Art and Science, Elizabeth Wright Hubbard, M.D., edited by M. Panos, M.D., Beaconsfield Publishers, Beaconsfield, England, 1990.

The "Brief Study Course" (pp. 262–341) is a classic. Elegant and concise, it has been reprinted endlessly and is alone worth the price of the book. It is a good way to get the rudiments of practice—but don't miss the articles on the mental portraits of remedies, and the one on *Thuja*.

Homeopathy, a Frontier in Medical Science: Experimental Studies and Theoretical Foundations, Paolo Bellavite, M.D., and Andrea Signorini, M.D., North Atlantic Books, Berkeley, Calif., 1995. On the back cover of this volume, Marvin McMillen, M.D., of the Yale University School of Medicine, notes: "The concepts of microdoses and the principle of similars have often been discussed by academic physicians and scientists in terms more reminiscent of the religious wars of the sixteenth century than respectful academic discourse. We live in an era where an investigator who transposes a rabbit cardiac calcium channel into a frog egg . . . is allowed to extrapolate his finding to the sick human heart, but investigating microdose effects in patients . . . or the concept of similars is sure academic suicide." This book, the joint effort of a medical school professor and a homeopathic physician, finally treats the subject of homeopathy with both academic respect and clinical curiosity. The result, appearing two hundred years after Hahnemann's first book on his work, is rigorous and groundbreaking.

Divided Legacy: A History of the Schism in Medical Thought, 4 vols., Harris Livermore Coulter, Ph.D., Wehawken Books, Washington, D.C., 1973, 1988, 1994. The "schism" of the title is that between the empirical (Platonic) and rational (Aristotelian) points of view. Coulter traces that conflict through the history of medicine, starting with Hippocrates and ending in twentieth-century America. Coulter's book is extremely scholarly and meticulously researched, though not yet the final word in the history of medicine. His primary interest is in homeopathy, and this book is probably best viewed as the tracing of the roots of the conflict between homeopathy and allopathy as it finally emerged in its definitive form in the late 1800s in America. If this is what you want to know about, you won't find it better described. On the downside, it is strongly Eurocentric and mid-twentieth-century academic. There is nothing mentioned before the Greeks, and the enormous debt that Greek medicine and alchemy owe to Ayurveda is not even footnoted. Volume One covers Hippocrates to Paracelsus; Volume Two contains an excellent section on Hahnemann and the history of homeopathy; and Volume Three traces the struggles in American medicine from 1800 to 1914 between the Thomsonians and other herbalists, the homeopaths, and the allopaths.

Volume Three is probably the most readable and relevant to under-standing current holistic medicine.

The Principles and Art of Cure in Homeopathy: A Modern Textbook, Herbert Roberts, M.D., Health Science Press, Rustington, England, 1942. First published in 1936, this remains one of the best introductions to home-opathy for the practitioner. It goes step by step in a cogent, leisurely way through the basic principles and how to apply them. Chapters 22 through 31 are an excellent introduction to the miasms. Recommended.

The Science of Homeopathy, George Vithoulkas, Grove Press, New York, 1980. A major and influential attempt to bring the theory of homeo-pathic practice into the language and conceptual framework of late-twentieth-century thought. Vithoulkas was an engineer who was bitten by the homeopathy bug, went to India from his native Greece to study, and by virtue of diligent effort and a brilliant mind made himself one of the prime exponents of homeopathy in the world today. He has trained a whole generation of European and American practitioners, and had his intuitive process enshrined in AI software (The Vithoulkas Expert System).

Portraits of Homeopathic Medicines: Psychophysical Analyses of Selected Constitutional Types, 3 vols., Catherine R. Coulter, North Atlantic Books, Berkeley, Calif., 1988, 1998. A rich and detailed analysis of the personal-ities of some of the most commonly indicated homeopathic constitu-tional remedies. Ms. Coulter, a lay prescriber and wife of medical historian Harris Coulter, has written a classic book that will set a stan-dard for many years to come.

Homeopathic Psychology: Personality Profiles of the Major Constitutional Remedies, Philip M. Bailey, M.D., North Atlantic Books, Berkeley, Calif., 1995. This newest addition to the emerging psychologically oriented lit-erature on homeopathy covers a much wider spectrum of remedies than does Catherine Coulter's work, though in less depth and detail. Its author, a homeopathic physician, trained in England and Greece, now practices in Australia.

The Homeopathic Treatment of Children: Pediatric Constitutional Types, Paul Herscu, N.D., North Atlantic Books, Berkeley, Calif., 1991. To neglect to offer a needed homeopathic constitutional remedy to a growing child is a tragic oversight. Besides curing and preventing diseases, the remedy can, in a profound and life-changing way, ensure a balanced process of matu-ration and a full realization of the child's potential. I can imagine the day when it will be considered serious malpractice and the highest breach of medical ethics to fail to provide such a deeply helpful intervention. This is perhaps the best of the newer books on prescribing for children.

Homeopathy: Medicine for the New Man, George Vithoulkas, ARCO Publishing, New York, 1979. A short, popular, exciting introduction to homeopathy for the health professional or patient. Though written some years ago, it is still one of the best short primers.

Psyche and Substance: Essays on Homeopathy in the Light of Jungian Psychology, Edward Whitmont, M.D., North Atlantic Books, Berkeley, Calif., 1982. These are largely reprints of the excellent articles on materia medica published by Dr. Whitmont over the course of a long and distinguished career as a Jungian analyst and homeopath. Included are his conceptualizations of how the homeopathic remedy operates to reorganize the morphogenic fields (as described by Rupert Sheldrake). This is an excellent book.

The Magic of the Minimum Dose, Dr. Dorothy Shepherd, Health Science Press, Hengiscote, England, 1964. A series of narrative vignettes that are wonderfully entertaining and yet educational, written by one of England's great homeopaths. A good way to approach the subject gently.

Homeopathic Remedies for Health Professionals and Laypeople, Dale Buegel, M.D., Blair Lewis, P.A., and Dennis Chernin, M.D., Himalayan Publishers, Honesdale, Pa., 1991. A very simple handbook for home use of basic remedies for minor ailments and injuries. Limited to a manageable number of remedies.

Homeopathic Medicine at Home, Maesimund Panos, M.D., J. P. Tarcher, Los Angeles, 1980. Another good home care handbook. With more remedies covered; for those who have a source of homeopathic remedies at hand.

Everybody's Guide to Homeopathic Medicines, Stephen Cummings, M.D., and Dana Ullman M.P.H., North Atlantic Books, Berkeley, Calif., 1997. Even more extensive, this is the top-selling family homeopathic guidebook. It takes you stepwise through the selection of the correct remedy for common ailments and injuries.

Chapter 3. FLOWER REMEDIES

Flower Essence Repertory, Patricia Kaminski and Richard Katz, The Flower Essence Society, Nevada City, Calif., 1994. Actually, this is both a repertory and a materia medica of flower remedies. That is, it has a section that lists the remedies under complaints for which they might be prescribed (a repertory) as well as a detailed description of each remedy and what its used for (a materia medica). Though, as the title suggests, the book is marketed as a reference work, very useful in selecting the essence you need, it also contains a lengthy and very valuable introductory section. This is the most complete exposition of the concept of flower essences, how they work, and the philosophy behind their use that I have seen. The only shortcoming of this book is that it covers only the English (Bach) and California essences.

Handbook of the Bach Flower Remedies, Philip Chancellor, C. W. Daniel, London, 1971. Probably out of print by now, this well-worn volume is still my favorite reference for the English essences. It accurately reflects the "generic" nature of the Bach remedies, whose scope seems to be broader than the many more specific remedies now available. At least that's the tone of Edward Bach's descriptions of the indications for his preparations, which this little book faithfully conveys.

The Encyclopaedia of Flower Remedies, Clare Harvey and Amanda Cochrane, Thorsons, London and San Francisco, 1995. This volume has a much scantier introduction to use of the remedies than the *FES Repertory,* and much shorter descriptions of the remedies. But it covers flower essences from all over the world: Europe, Africa, North America, Japan, Australia, and India. It offers separate (though brief) repertories for physical, psychological, and spiritual ailments. It also has an interesting section of case histories at the end, as well as a list of telephone numbers and addresses for sources of the various remedies and for information on course work and instruction.

Flower Essences: Reordering Our Understanding and Approach to Illness and Health, Machaelle Small Wright, Perelandra, Jeffersonton, Va., 1988. Besides describing her own unique lines of vegetable flower essences and of rose essences (the latter are used primarily to ease the experience of dying), the author explains her system of using a simplified form of kinesiology (muscle testing) to confirm your choice of remedy. But the beauty of this book is the sense it gives of how the healing power of the flowers is communicated to the receptive person by the forces of nature.

Flower Power: Flower Remedies for Healing Body and Soul Through Herbalism, Homeopathy, Aromatherapy, and Flower Essences, Anne McIntyre, Henry Holt, New York, 1996. With ofttimes breathtaking color illustrations, this beautiful book explores one plant at a time, giving a bit of history on its use and then comparing the therapeutics of herbal and homeopathic preparations made from it with those of its flower essence and aromatherapy oil. A wonderful way to get to know the plants in depth.

Earth: Pleiadian Keys to the Living Library, Barbara Marciniak, Bear & Company, Santa Fe, N.M., 1995. This book will help you grasp how much crucial information is encoded in each and every one of the life forms that fill the living library we call Earth. Each is an indispensable piece of the holographic message that this planet presents to those who choose to study here. Once you get the picture, the way in which herbal and homeopathic remedies work becomes much more understandable.

Care of the Soul: A Guide for Cultivating Depth and Sacredness in Everyday Life, Thomas Moore, HarperCollins, New York, 1992. The Flower Essence Society in California speaks of flower remedies as "soul therapy." We must have patience with the need of the soul to make its slow, deliberate, and sometimes painfully winding journey. This book helps us do that.

Chapter 4. THE MEANING OF DIAGNOSIS

The Holistic Paradigm

A Practical Guide to Holistic Health, Swami Rama, Himalayan Publishers, Honesdale, Pa., 1980. A short, succinct, and very readable introduction to the timeless principles of health that underlie and unite yoga and Ayurveda, written by the man who guided my learning. The fundamental elements of nourishing, cleansing, exercising, stillness, and self-training emerge in this book with clarity and elegance. These concepts are basic to the holistic paradigm.

Lectures on Yoga, Swami Rama, Himalayan Publishers, Honesdale, Pa., 1979. A straightforward introduction to the eight basic aspects of the physical/mental/spiritual system of self-development that is a nearly universal foundation for the world's great systems of healing and self-development.

The Alchemy of Healing, Psyche, and Soma, Edward C. Whitmont, M.D., North Atlantic Books, Berkeley, Calif., 1993. "The paradigm proposed here views illness and healing as a dramatic staging of conflict and conflict resolution by virtue of interplay of polarizing forms which are always prior to the material shapes in which they manifest. This dramatic play serves the goal of eventual resolution through a discovery of ever more differentiated forms of consciousness. . . . In reconciling or bridging polarities, this lineage of healing-creating appears to be of major significance for the evolution of mankind as well as the organism of our planet" (From the Introduction). Perhaps more than any other, the work of Whitmont (who is highly regarded both as a homeopath and a Jungian analyst) articulates the philosophical/spiritual and psychological underpinnings of the new paradigm in the terms of classic Western thought. (See also his *Psyche and Substance*.)

Encyclopedia of Natural Medicine, Michael T. Murray, N.D. and Joseph E. Pizzorno, N.D., Prima, Rocklin, Calif., 1991 (new edition, 1997). This is a comprehensive textbook of naturopathic medicine as it is (at its best) practiced today. It's probably the closest thing to an outline of holistic medicine published, but still falls far short of the ideal. It's strong on commonsensical physiology, nutrition, detoxification, and a down-to-earth approach to such issues as immune function and liver support. Its weaknesses are in the areas of mind and energy, which will have to play a central role in holistic medical concepts. The best part of the book is 430 pages devoted to a natural (nutrition and herbs, especially) approach to sixty-two common disorders. Keep it on your desk. (The new edition seems to have more entries, but less depth for each.)

The Complete Encyclopedia of Natural Healing: A Comprehensive A–Z Listing of Common and Chronic Illnesses and Their Proven Natural Treatments, Gary Null, Ph.D., Kensington Books, New York, 1998. In a fashion similar to that of the first edition of the book above by Murray and Pizzorno, Null discusses causes and symptoms of each of seventy-two major (mostly chronic and severe) disorders. He then offers what his research suggests are the best therapies for each, including diet, herbs, supplements, bodywork, homeopathy, acupuncture, psycho-spiritual practice, and exercise. In Section II, he discusses the rationale of each of twenty-five major holistic therapeutic approaches, such as chiropractic, colon therapy, and chelation, and gives a number of case histories of patients who have benefited from each. The book is a labor of love, and besides its usefulness as a reference work, taken as a whole, it is a fairly accurate representation of what holistic medicine is at the moment "out in the trenches."

Holistic Medicine: From Stress to Optimum Health, Kenneth R. Pelletier, Ph.D., Delacorte Press, New York, 1979. Pelletier speaks eloquently yet calmly to the many social and economic issues that surround the attempt to move from a conventional to a holistic approach to medical care. He is very knowledgable yet not polemical, the kind who can and does speak to corporate heads and get a sympathetic hearing.

Quantum Healing: Exploring the Frontiers of Mind/Body Medicine, Deepak Chopra, M.D., Bantam Books, New York, 1989. The book that put Deepak Chopra on the map (and TM in the limelight again), this was a best-seller. For those of us who have not yet totally extricated ourselves from conventional thinking about health and illness, reading it is an enlightening experience.

The Holographic Universe, Michael Talbot, HarperPerennial, New York, 1991. An easy-to-read introduction to the revolutionary import of the holographic model. This book, written by someone who has a knack for putting complex scientific principles into simple terms, will help you see how thinking holographically will make the world look like a different place.

Wholeness and the Implicate Order, David Bohm, Ark Paperbacks, London, 1983. Bohm is the physicist who blazed a trail many others have followed in recent years. He revived the Platonic idea of the *eidos,* and planted it firmly in the center of modern science.

A New Science of Life: The Hypothesis of Formative Causation, Rupert Sheldrake, Ph.D., J. P. Tarcher, Los Angeles, 1981. After a stint in India, where, he notes, that he "had many valuable discussions" and completed the first draft of this book, Sheldrake returned to England and completed his treatise on how something subtler shapes the physical manifestations of living beings. This subtler influence he terms a "morphogenetic field," and proposes that such fields are molded by the form and behavior of past organisms of the same species through direct connections across both *space* and *time,* what he calls "morphic resonance." In articulating this idea, he did for biology what Bohm did for physics, and this book stirs hope that Western science might at last outgrow its naive materialism. Not without resistance, however. *Nature,* one of Britain's most influential scientific periodicals, called this book "the best candidate for burning there has been for many years." Meanwhile, the equally prestigious *New Scientist* stated, "It is quite clear that one is dealing here with an important scientific inquiry into the nature of biological and physical reality."

Spontaneous Healing, Andrew Weil, M.D., Fawcett, New York, 1995. A best-seller, Weil's book is engaging and persuasive. It establishes many of the basic principles of holistic medicine which this present book is built on.

Meaning and Medicine, Larry Dossey, M.D., Bantam Books, New York, 1991. Dr. Dossey eloquently argues that illness is not an experience that is accidental, statistical, or a mere matter of the mechanical unfoldment of physical causality, but that it has meaning and significance in your life. This is a crucial concept, and he demonstrates it convincingly.

Anthroposophical Medicine, Victor Bott, M.D., Healing Arts Press, Rochester, Vt., 1984. A concise summary of the medical system established by Rudolf Steiner, called anthroposophical medicine. Steiner, initially absorbed in the theosophical school (a syncretism of Christianity and Indian Vedanta), combined this background with a careful study of the writings of Goethe to establish a uniquely German/European spirituality. The concept of Elements is recognizable here, and basic to his thinking, though modified from the classic Asian form.

The Healing Power of Illness: The Meaning of Symptoms and How to Interpret Them, Thorwald Dethlefsen and Rudiger Dahlke, M.D., Element Books, Rockport, Mass., 1991. Exploring the psychological and spiritual significance of symptoms and illnesses, rather more European than Asian in its consciousness, this fascinating book will sometimes be at variance with what is presented in *Radical Healing,* but will offer an interesting and stimulating contrast.

A Holistic Critique of Medical History, Philosophy, and Practice

Divided Legacy: A History of the Schism in Medical Thought. 4 vols., Harris Livermore Coulter, Ph.D., Wehawken Books, Washington, D.C., 1973, 1988, 1994. See description under Chapter 2. Volume Three is the most relevant to understanding current holistic medicine.

Medical Nemesis: The Expropriation of Health, Ivan Illich, Pantheon Books, New York, 1976. One of the earliest contemporary critiques of current medical practice, this book is astute, incisive, and acerbic. The author, a radical Jesuit priest, argues with endless documentation that modern medicine is not only largely ineffective but harmful, undermining the average person's sense of self-reliance, self-exploration, and self-direction.

Medicine on Trial: The Appalling Story of Ineptitude, Malfeasance, Neglect, and Arrogance, Charles B. Inlander, Lowell S. Levin, and Ed Weiner, Prentice-Hall, New York, 1988. As the title says, this book is an expose of medical incompetence, a detailed documentation of the abuses, ineptitudes, and bungling that characterize modern medicine. All this is useful and important to have on record, but the book fails to address causes. In other words, the underlying approach to health and illness that allows this climate of abuse and mistreatment to develop is not discussed.

The Social Transformation of American Medicine: The Rise of a Sovereign Profession and the Making of a Vast Industry, Paul Starr, Basic Books, New York, 1982. Conventional medicine of two decades ago, at its peak of prestige, is examined as a sociological phenomenon. The author made no attempt to critique medicine's philosophy or therapeutic methods, but simply studied the institution, as sociologists might study any other. What emerged was a rather startling portrait of an institution that had acquired inordinate power and influence.

When Antibiotics Fail: Restoring the Ecology of the Body, Marc Lappé, North Atlantic Books, Berkeley, Calif., 1986. This book is included in this section because it may serve as a prototype for critiquing the basic therapeutic tools of conventional medicine. In this case it is antibiotics that get the spotlight: their shortcomings and side effects, and the growing problem of resistant organisms are discussed at length, as well as alternative approaches to controlling infections.

Chapter 5. BODY MAPS: TECHNIQUES FOR SELF-DIAGNOSIS

Psychosomatic Medicine, Franz Alexander, M.D., W. W. Norton, New York, 1950. This may not be the original book on psychosomatics, but it's the most classic. First published in 1950, it reflects the collective work of a group of psychoanalysts at the Chicago Institute. Seventeen years of observation and collaboration went into the still fascinating and incisive formulations of the mental and emotional aspects of the commonly recognized psychosomatic diseases: peptic ulcer, hypertension, hyperthyroidism, asthma, and arthritis. Though the psychoanalytic point of view may be an obstacle for some readers, the book remains a gold mine of ideas and a foundation for much of the mind-body work going on today.

Deceits of the Mind and Their Effects on the Body, Jane G. Goldberg, Ph.D., Transaction Publishers, New Brunswick, N.J., 1991. An update of psychosomatic psychoanalysis. Especially recommended is the chapter on Psychosis of the Body—Cancer of the Mind (The Isomorphic Relation Between Cancer and Schizophrenia).

Yoga and Psychotherapy: The Evolution of Consciousness, Swami Rama, Rudolph Ballentine, M.D., and Swami Ajaya, Ph.D., Himalayan Publishers, Honesdale, Pa., 1976. How mental, emotional, and physical functions interrelate as understood within the framework of yoga. (See fuller description under Chapter 11 below.)

Body/Mind, Ken Dychwald, J. P. Tarcher, Los Angeles, 1979. Not a new book, either, but one of the most readable and enjoyable introductions to the relationship of the mental and the physical. Very helpful for those who want to learn to infer the psychological from observation of physical structure, habits of movement, and posture.

Who Gets Sick? Thinking and Health, Blair Justice, Peak Press, Houston, Tex., 1987. A wide-ranging introduction to new concepts of mind-body interactions, the immune system, and how attitudes and psychological postures affect health. Chatty and written as though for the best-seller list, the book is extremely well documented, with hundreds of references to scientific literature.

Will to Be Well, The Real Alternative Medicine, Neville Hodgkinson, Samuel Weiser, York Beach, Maine, 1986. This is a book for doctors and patients. The bulk of it is devoted to dealing with specific medical illnesses and talking about the real psychological issues that underlie them. It is fresh and bold, nonacademic, and usually right on the mark.

The Creation of Health: Merging Traditional Medicine with Intuitive Diagnosis, Norman Shealy, M.D., Ph.D., and Caroline Myss, Stillpoint Publishing, Walpole, N.H., 1988. As much as any other, this book marked the beginning of a new kind of medicine in the West. It involved what was at the time a rather daring collaboration between Norman Shealy, M.D., the founder of the American Holistic Medical Association, and Caroline Myss, a former journalist with a master's degree in religious studies. Myss managed to develop skills in intuitive diagnosis which she carried out on several patients of Shealy's; she never saw the patients in person, but diagnosed them by telephone. The book first documents her accuracy, next goes on to discuss the system of chakras around which she organizes her discussions, and finally offers comments by both authors on how her formulations relate to the patients' specific diseases.

Life Energy: Using the Meridians to Unlock the Hidden Power of Your Emotions, John Diamond, M.D., Paragon House, New York, 1985. This book may be compared to the Shealy and Myss one described above. In this case,

John Diamond, the physician who took George Goodheart Jr.'s Applied Kinesiology and developed from it what he came to call Behavioral Kinesiology, focuses on meridians rather than on chakras. As with Shealy and Myss, the emphasis here is on diagnosis: clarifying the relationship between the mental and the physical by using "muscle testing" to identify the meridian that is "weak." One can then relate that finding to Diamond's observations on the mental and emotional issues associated with that meridian and to the organs with which it is connected. The weakness of the book is that it is based primarily on the observations of one clinician. Nevertheless, it is fascinating and useful.

Heal Your Body, Louise L. Hay, Hay House, Santa Monica, Calif., 1988. The famous "little blue book" (mentioned in Chapter 4, page 147). It would appear that one either likes Louise Hay or doesn't. Some people dismiss this book with a smirk; others carry it around in their purse or pocket, to refer to constantly. According to the introduction, the author has based these formulations on the experience of a number of clinicians as well as her own observations. All I can say is that at times I find it uncannily accurate.

How to See Your Health: Book of Oriental Diagnosis, Michio Kushi, Japan Publications, Tokyo, 1980. Face maps, tongue maps, the meaning of different-shaped eyes, nose, mouth, ears—all by the major exponent of macrobiotics in the West.

Reading the Body: Ohashi's Book of Oriental Diagnosis, Wataru Ohashi with Tom Monte, Penguin, New York, 1991. Another version of body reading, this time more aligned with meridian maps as taught by Wataru Ohashi, the master who has trained a generation of shiatsu therapists in the West.

Indications of Miasm, Dr. Harimohon Choudhury, Jain Publishers, New Delhi, 1988. Exhaustive detail on the signs and symptoms of each miasm by a contemporary Indian homeopath who has focused on the subject of miasms.

Chapter 6. MULTILEVEL DIAGNOSIS AND CONSTITUTION: WHAT'S YOUR MIND-BODY TYPE?

Ayurveda

Ayurvedic Healing: A Comprehensive Guide, David Frawley, O.M.D., Passage Press, Salt Lake City, Utah, 1989. Vedic scholar and teacher David

Frawley, who is trained in both Ayurveda and Traditional Ci
Medicine, examines the basic concepts of Ayurveda. There are also secti̤
on the treatment of specific diseases, and a materia medica of both classic̤
and modern Ayurvedic formulas. From time to time, Frawley draws parallels and connections between Ayurvedic and Chinese approaches.

Charaka Samhita, 3 vols., Ram K. Sharma and Vaidya B. Dash, eds.,
Jamnagar, 1949. The classic reference work in three volumes. This most
complete and authoritative exposition, dating back over a thousand
years, is still used as a textbook in Ayurvedic medical colleges in India.

Fundamentals of Ayurvedic Medicine, Vaidya Bhagavan Dash, Bansal and
Company, New Delhi, 1982. An outline of basic principles. One of the
most concise and authentic of the modern books, though somewhat dry
and academic.

A Handbook of Ayurveda, Vaidya Bhagavan Dash and Acarya M. Junius,
Concept Publishing, New Delhi, 1983. A companion volume to Dash's
Fundamentals of Ayurvedic Medicine. Some repetitions in the first part,
but over half of this volume is a materia medica of basic Ayurvedic plant
remedies and a guide to treatment of specific disorders.

Introduction to Ayurveda, the Science of Life, Dr. Chandrashekhar Thakkur,
ASI Publishers, New York, 1974. This remains one of the best, most
complete, readable, and authentic books on Ayurveda in the English
language. Unfortunately, it is not easy to find nowadays.

Perfect Health: The Complete Mind/Body Guide, Deepak Chopra, M.D.,
Harmony Books, New York, 1990. Perhaps the best of the recent
attempts to adapt Ayurveda to Western needs. Enjoyable and inspiring,
though with some deviations from the strictly traditional Ayurvedic
teachings. Like all of Chopra's books, the writing is eloquent and a pleasure to read; therefore, this is a good way to begin learning about the
subject of Ayurveda.

Prakruti: Your Ayurvedic Constitution, Robert Svoboda, Geocom, Albuquerque, N.M., 1988. Written by an American who graduated from an
Ayurvedic medical school in India, this book is well done. Though its
focus is ostensibly rather narrow (constitution or "type"), it ends up covering a wide spectrum of Ayurvedic concepts intelligently and accurately. It is unique among the books in English in that it consistently
reflects the way in which authentic Ayurvedic principles cut across
Western conceptual boundaries and unify the physical, nutritional, men-

hical. It even succeeds at times in bringing out the sheer
the Ayurvedic teachings. Though I recommend this
t the best for beginners.

of Self-Healing, Vasant Lad, Lotus Press, Santa Fe,
. A pioneering attempt to make Ayurveda understandable to
ern readers, this is simple and clear, though there are elements of
other traditions added without always identifying them as such. An easy
way to introduce yourself to Ayurveda.

Diet and Nutrition: A Holistic Approach, Rudolph Ballentine, M.D.,
Himalayan Publishers, Honesdale, Pa., 1978. Although this is a book on
nutrition, it's based on an Ayurvedic conceptual framework. If you use it
enough, you'll find you have a grasp on some basic Ayurvedic principles.

Traditional Chinese Medicine

Asian Health Secrets: The Complete Guide to Asian Herbal Medicine, Letha
Hadady, D.Ac., Crown, New York, 1996. A substantial and practical
guide to using available patent Chinese and other common remedies for
the garden-variety problems of daily life: depression, overweight, PMS,
etc. Hadady ventures into the realm of integration by juxtaposing
Chinese and Tibetan (which is basically Ayurvedic) approaches to diagnosis. A hands-on, user-friendly book.

Between Heaven and Earth: A Guide to Chinese Medicine, Harriet Beinfield,
L.Ac., and Efrem Korngold, O.M.D., Ballantine Books, New York,
1991. This book is based on nearly two decades of clinical experience.
This husband-and-wife team has produced what is, at this point, the
most understandable and comprehensive view of the Western practice of
Traditional Chinese Medicine. Excellent sections on the Five Phases or
Elements, on acupuncture, on herbs, and on the TCM approach to diet.
Highly recommended.

The Essential Book of Chinese Traditional Medicine. 2 vols., Liu Yan Chi,
Columbia University Press, New York, 1988. The most authoritative,
comprehensive, and well-organized book by a respected leader of traditional medicine in China that will be found in English. It is in two volumes, the first having to do with theory and the second with practice.

The Web That Has No Weaver, Ted J. Kaptchuk, O.M.D., Congdon & Weed,
New York, 1983. This was, for a long time, the most comprehensive and
readable book on Chinese traditional medicine available to the American

reader. It is long and detailed and one needs patience to immerse oneself in the system and gradually understand it, but it is well worth the effort.

Dragon Rises Red Bird Flies: Psychology and Chinese Medicine, Leon Hammer, M.D., Station Hill Press, New York, 1990. For those who wish to approach Traditional Chinese Medicine in terms of the Five Elements and to probe the subtler psychological aspects of the system, this book is unique. Thoughtful, philosophical, and poetic, it is written by an American psychoanalyst with decades of experience in acupuncture. The understanding of the Five Elements that emerges from this book can be applied to Ayurvedic as well as Chinese medicine.

Chinese Herbal Patent Formulas, Jake Fratkin, Institute of Traditional Medicine, Portland, Ore., 1986. This may not be ivory-tower Traditional Chinese Medicine, but it's what you find in shops and homes, and what millions of people rely on. It's also a good way to get started. Most of the Chinese Patent Medicines listed in the Self-Help Index will be found described in the book.

Zang Fu: The Organ Systems of Traditional Chinese Medicine, Jeremy Ross, D.Ac., Churchill Livingstone, New York, 1985. Quite technical and textbookish, this is nevertheless a valuable reference work. It has detailed sections on each of the organ systems, with clinical signs and symptoms of each pattern of disharmony that can affect it.

Chapter 7. NUTRITION

Diet and Nutrition: A Holistic Approach, Rudolph Ballentine, M.D., Himalayan Publishers, Honesdale, Pa., 1978. A comprehensive textbook of nutrition covering agricultural, biochemical, physiological, psychological, and philosophical aspects of nutrition (also see description under Ayurveda).

Nutritional Influences on Illness, Melvyn Werbach, M.D., Third Line Press, Tarzana, Calif., 1987. An indispensable desk reference. Organized by diseases, abstracts of research papers on the relationship between specific nutrients and their role in the cause and treatment of those diseases are given. Strongly recommended.

Prescription for Nutritional Healing, James Balch, M.D., and Phyllis Balch, Avery Publishing, Garden City Park, N.Y., 1997. A book organized similarly to *Nutritional Influences* (see above), but without documentation. It

does, however, cover more disorders and a wider spectrum of supplements, herbs, etc. It also gives dosages. Useful.

*The Clinician's Handbook of Natural Healing: The First Comprehensive Guide
to Scientific Peer Review Studies of Natural Supplements and Their Proven
Treatment Values,* Gary Null, Ph.D., Kensington Books, New York,
1997. This huge volume follows a format similar to that of Werbach's
above. The jacket flap says it covers more than 1.3 million studies. Null
has been a tireless advocate of healthy living and the informed use of
nutritional therapies and is something of a folk hero to many New
Yorkers. He spent years and much money to put this information into
the hands of the consumer.

Transition to Vegetarianism: An Evolutionary Step, Rudolph Ballentine, M.D.,
Himalayan Publishers, Honesdale, Pa., 1987. Based on sound medical
and scientific findings, in an easy-to-read format. It approaches becoming a vegetarian in stages, and concludes with a chapter on how to refine
a vegetarian diet.

Himalayan Mountain Cookery, Martha Ballentine, Himalayan Publishers,
Honesdale, Pa., 1976. These are the recipes taught to me by Swami
Rama during more than two years of our cooking two meals a day
together. They are the traditional recipes of the yogis who raised him,
and who designed their diet to balance the *doshas* and promote clarity of
mind and health of body. (My rough notes were translated into precise
measurements, kitchen-tested, and written up by my mother, Martha.)

Guide to Healing with Nutrition, Jonathan V. Wright, M.D., Rodale Press,
Emmaus, Pa., 1984. Dr. Wright is one of the foremost nutrition-oriented
physicians today, and this book is a series of cases that show, in readable
and entertaining style, how many common problems can be successfully
addressed through working with diet and supplements.

Eating for A's, Alexander Schauss, Barbara Friedlander Meyer, and Arnold
Meyer, Pocket Books, New York, 1991. How diet affects the academic
performance of kids. A must for all parents and teachers.

For Tomorrow's Children: A Manual for Future Parents, Preconception Care,
Blooming Glen, Pa., 1990. A summary of research on how preconception and prenatal nutrition dramatically cut the incidence of birth
defects in Britain. This book is sobering, and should be required reading for all couples who are considering having a child.

Food and Healing, Annemarie Colbin, Ballantine Books, New York, 1986. A classic book, this volume covers the practical use of foods and home remedies to deal with common ailments. It is written from a largely macrobiotic point of view, and backed up by the author's many years of experience.

Healing with Whole Foods: Oriental Traditions and Modern Nutrition, Paul Pitchford, North Atlantic Books, Berkeley, Calif., 1993. This huge, awe-inspiring tome covers the subtleties of dietary regulation from the point of view of Traditional Chinese Medicine concepts (yin and yang, and the Five Elements or Phases). It is carefully and thoughtfully done, and many practitioners I know turn to it first for helping themselves.

Mad Cow USA: Could the Nightmare Happen Here?, Sheldon Rampton and John Stauber, Common Courage Press, Monroe, Maine, 1997. Read this book to find out why it's not smart to eat commercial meat, but, more important, read it to understand how information is distorted and hidden from the public on issues that affect your health in profound and critical ways. This book should be required reading in every school.

Chapter 8. DETOX: A LIGHTER AND CLEARER YOU

Our Stolen Future: Are We Threatening Our Fertility, Intelligence, and Survival?—A Scientific Detective Story, Theo Colborn, Dianne Dumanoski, and John Peterson Myers, Penguin, New York, 1997. The foreword by Vice President Al Gore compares this to the classic *Silent Spring* of thirty years ago. This book brings the awareness of pollution to a new level by showing that toxins present in the environment at concentrations one thousandth of what we thought was safe are having a profoundly destructive impact on hormonal systems. Indispensable.

Beating Alzheimer's: A Step Towards Unlocking the Mysteries of Brain Diseases, Tom Warren, Avery Publishing, Garden City Park, N.Y., 1991. The cover calls this, "The remarkable story of how one man reversed the devastating symptoms of Alzheimer's disease." In 1983, the author was exhausted, cantankerous, confused, and rapidly losing his memory. A CAT scan showed atrophy of the brain and he was diagnosed as suffering from Alzheimer's. After four years of struggle, involving research (at first difficult because his mind was impaired), nutritional work, and detox (especially removal of heavy metals), he was fit, energetic, actively writing and teaching, and his CAT scan was normal.

It's All in Your Head: The Link Between Mercury Amalgams and Illness, Hal A. Huggins, D.D.S., Avery Publishing, Garden City Park, N.Y., 1993. The National Association of Dental Surgeons banned dentists who placed mercury, a known toxin, in the mouth. In 1840, the professional organization crumbled because so many dentists were using the cheap and easy-to-use amalgam. They formed the American Dental Association, which, not surprisingly has maintained ever since that mercury is safe. The dean of mercury-free dentistry, Dr. Huggins has spearheaded the movement against this orthodoxy and describes the improvements in such chronic diseases as MS, Parkinson's, arthritis, lupus, and ALS that have followed the removal of mercury fillings.

The Superhormone Promise: Nature's Antidote to Aging, William Regelson, M.D., and Carol Colman, Simon & Schuster, New York, 1996. The latest information on DHEA, testosterone, estrogen and progesterone, thyroid and growth hormones, and melatonin, with advice on dosages and sources.

Homotoxicology: The Core of a Probiotic and Holistic Approach to Medicine, Claus F. Claussen, M.D., Aurelia Verlag, Baden-Baden, Germany, 1991. A concise summary of the concepts of homotoxicology, which is a modern extension and refinement of some aspects of Herring's Law of Cure (homeopathy). Useful concepts and illustrated with helpful diagrams, but difficult to read nonetheless.

Your Body's Many Cries for Water: You Are Not Sick, You Are Thirsty!, F. Batmanghelidj, M.D., Global Health Solutions, Falls Church, Va., 1995. A political prisoner awaiting trial in an Iranian prison, Dr. Batmanghelidj was left to care for the ill around him without medications. When a young man developed severe peptic ulcer pain, having nothing else to offer, he gave him two glasses of water and within eight minutes the pain disappeared. He went on to treat other ulcer patients similarly, and his work resulted in his release from prison and a path of research that also identified dehydration as a major factor in many cases of colitis, arthritis, headaches, high blood pressure, obesity, asthma, diabetes, and depression. Dr. Batmanghelidj's work goes beyond the importance of dehydration; in later articles, he speaks of a paradigm shift: attention to the role of the dynamics of the solvent (field) rather than an exclusive focus on the solute.

Elixir of the Ageless: You Are What You Drink, Patrick Flanagan, M.D., Ph.D., and Gael Crystal Flanagan, M.D., Vortex Press, San Francisco, 1986.

Cutting-edge ideas (and beyond?) on water structure and its effects on health and consciousness.

The Colon Health Handbook: New Health Through Colon Rejuvenation, Robert Gray, Emerald Publishing, Reno, Nev., 1981. Gray's program uses herbal combinations to loosen bowel accretions and gradually expel them. Weekly colonics are recommended, and the process takes at least three months. An intelligently written little handbook.

Tissue Cleansing Through Bowel Management, Bernard Jensen, D.C., Bernard Jensen Enterprises, Escondido, Calif., 1981. You can't look at the photos of what came out of people's colons without becoming motivated to do some cleaning out yourself. (Though part of what comes out is the bulking agent that is put in.) This is an enzyme, volcanic ash, colema program, seven days with fasting. Quick, dramatic, if a bit drastic.

You Can Regain the Vitality of Your Youth: Colon Health, the Key to a Vibrant Life, Norman W. Walker, D.Sc., Norwalk Press, Prescott, Ariz., 1979. Another colon-cleansing guide, this one by "the Juice Doctor" (see page 551). Much information on the relation between colon toxicity and its effects on disorders of other organs.

The Science of Facial Expression, Louis Kuhne, Benedict Lust, Butler, N.J., 1917, (Facsimile edition: Health Research, Mokelume Hill, Calif., 1970). The illustrations of "encumbrances" (accumulated wastes) and the descriptions of his system of diagnosing the parts of the body affected by the physiognomy are fascinating and still useful today.

Drainage in Homeopathy, Dr. E. A. Maury, Health Science Press, Rustington, England, 1965. A brief introduction to the concept of Vannier and the French School on the use of low-potency remedies to facilitate the expulsion of wastes and thereby prepare for and support the action of high-potency and deeper-acting remedies.

Hathapradipika of Svatmarama, S.M.Y.M. Samiti, Kaivalyadhama, Lonavla, India, 1970. The most authoritative source of yoga teachings on cleansing and health.

Panchakarma Therapy in Ayurveda, Divakar Ojha, Ph.D., and Ashok Kumar, D.Ay.M., Chaukhamba Amarabharati Prakashan, Varanasi, India, 1978. Though this book is in English, it is very difficult for the Western readers to understand; nevertheless, it is included here because it is one of the most extensive and authoritative scriptures on *panchakarma* therapy, the most classic and sophisticated system of medical cleansing.

Matrix and Matrix Regulation: Basis for a Holistic Therapy in Medicine, A. Pischinger, M.D., Edition Hary International, Brussels, 1991 (original German edition, 1975). Very detailed and technical treatment of the biochemic structure of the connective tissue: how it functions as a storage site as well as a major physiological integrator, and how it is accessed and altered by acupuncture.

Health Through Inner Body Cleansing, Erich Rauch, M.D., Haug Publishers, Heidelberg, Germany, 1986. The famous Mayr Intestinal Therapy, a modified fast with mild laxatives (a very popular semi-spa treatment in Europe), followed by a healthier diet and exercise. Of special interest are Mayr's observations on the relation between postural habits and the condition of the intestinal tract.

Tattva Shuddhi: The Tantric Practice of Inner Purification, Swami Satyasanganananda Saraswati, Bihar School of Yoga, Munger, India, 1984. An example of inner (psychological, emotional, and spiritual) cleansing techniques, as used in the Tantric tradition.

The Essene Gospel of Peace, Book One, Edmond Bordeaux Szekely, International Biogenic Society, Cartago, Costa Rica, 1981 (originally published, 1928). A lyrical, and apparently authentic, excerpt from early Christian teachings on the importance of cleansing to spiritual life. The title page says, "The Third Century Aramaic Manuscript and Old Slavonic Texts Compared," edited and translated by Szekely, who was a remarkable scholar and revered spiritual teacher. His widow established the Golden Door, perhaps the most refined (and expensive) spa in the world today.

Textbook of Dr. Vodder's Manual Lymph Drainage, H. and G. Wittlinger, Haug Publishers, Heidelberg, Germany (third English edition, 1990). This husband-and-wife team have carried on the work of Dr. Vodder and his wife, who discovered that many, if not most, disorders would respond dramatically to skillful massage techniques they developed to encourage more efficient lymph drainage from the areas of the body that were sick. This book, which includes a fascinating foreword by Dr. Vodder, is half theory and rationale and half technique.

The Golden Seven Plus One, Conquer Disease With Eight Keys to Health, Beauty, and Peace, C. Samuel West, N.D., Samuel Publications, Orem, Utah, 1981. In its fifteenth printing, this book is a pastiche of largely ignored scientific evidence, evangelistic exhortations, and testimonials—all adding up to emphasize the importance of what Dr. West calls "lymphasizing," i.e., removing the wastes from the extracellular space by promoting lymph flow. There is little doubt that he is an expert on this matter, and that it is every bit as important as he says it is. Chief among his techniques is the minitrampoline or "rebounder."

Water: The Element of Life, Theodor and Wolfram Schwenk, Anthroposophic Press, Hudson, N.Y., 1989. Beautiful photos of a "drop test" developed to show the differences in various kinds of water. The difference between pure and polluted water is striking.

Ayurveda: Life, Health and Longevity, Robert E. Svoboda, Penguin, London, 1992. This book contains a concise description of *panchakarma,* as well as more on *aama.* See also Svovoda's other book under Ayurveda (Chapter 6).

The Nature Doctor: A Manual of Traditional and Complementary Medicine, Dr. H. C. Vogel, Keats Publishing, New Canaan, Conn., 1991. Note especially the section on baths, but the whole book is a gas. A German equivalent of Mao's *Barefoot Doctor's Manual.*

Raw Vegetable Juices: What's Missing in Your Body, Norman W. Walker, D.Sc., Norwalk Press, Phoenix, 1970. Fasting is a basic cleansing technique, but in a population like ours, where there are widespread deficiencies of micronutrients, water fasts are dangerous and ill-advised. In such situations, juice fasts are very valuable. But fresh juices, prepared properly and made from the proper fruits and vegetables, are critical. Dr. Walker was a pioneer in this field, and the juicer he developed, the Norwalk, is the gold standard by which others are judged.

Live Food Juices, H. E. Kirschner, M.D., Kirschner Publications, Monrovia, Calif., 1957. Case histories (and some photos) of patients treated with fresh juices. Very inspiring.

Raw Juice Therapy, John B. Lust, Thorsons Publishers, Wellingborough, England, 1959. A classic.

The Chelation Way: The Complete Book of Chelation Therapy, Morton Walker, D.P.M., Avery Publication Group, Garden City Park, N.Y., 1990. A very comprehensive survey of the subject. Here you will find discussions of both intravenous and oral chelation, as well as a chapter on the politics and economics surrounding its use, as well as a chapter on the research done on its effectiveness, and the struggle to get such studies before the medical profession. See more on chelation under ASCVD (following reading list for Chapter 12).

The New Microbiology

Cell Wall Deficient Forms, Lida H. Mattman, Ph.D., CRC Press, Cleveland, 1974. Though this book is now out of print, it is the authoritative text on cell-wall-deficient bacteria, those that often remain after antibiotic therapy. Cell-wall-deficient bacteria, also called "L-forms," have been seen to reside inside the cell, whence they may emerge and reproduce when resistance is low. The profound implications of Mattman's observations for conventional medicine and its common use of antibiotics have not been acknowledged by conventional medicine.

Cell Wall Deficient Bacteria, Gerald J. Domingue, Ph.D., ed., Addison-Wesley, Reading, Mass., 1982. This is the second most important book on the subject of cell-wall-deficient forms. It is fascinating and encouraging for those dealing with many chronic diseases, where Domingue has found cell-wall-deficient infections that can be cleared to produce cure.

The Rife Report: The Cancer Cure that Worked! Fifty Years of Suppression, Barry Lynes, Marcus Books, Queensville, Ontario, Canada, 1987. Though not well produced, this book provides a fascinating account of the life of Royal Rife, a medical maverick and genius who developed microscopic and electromagnetic techniques for diagnosing and treating the microbial infections he found in chronic diseases such as cancer. Rife produced many documented cures of advanced cancer, and his microscope was put in the Smithsonian. Despite its strident tone, this little volume is an eye-opener.

The Conquest of Cancer: Vaccines and Diet, Virginia Livingston-Wheeler, M.D., Franklin Watts, New York, 1984. The Livingston Clinic still operates in San Diego, where it treats cancer with an immune therapy. This work is based on the research of Virginia Livingstone and her associates, who, along with other workers, documented the presence of microbes in cancerous tissues and felt they satisfied Koch's postulates, thereby demonstrating the microbial etiology of the disease. Though other workers now have a different slant on this research, it remains important and the book is readable and inspiring.

Hidden Killers: The Revolutionary Medical Discoveries of Professor Guenther Enderlein, Erik Enby, M.D., Sheehan Communications, Saratoga, Calif., 1990. As of this writing, this is the only book available in English on the work of Dr. Guenther Enderlein in Germany, who spent decades studying and describing the life cycle of those microbes still not recognized by conventional microbiology. It suggests interesting relationships between cell-wall-deficient bacteria, conventional bacteria, and the yeast and fungal forms often observed in the blood under darkfield examination.

Bakterien-Cyclogenie, G. Enderlein, Semmelweis Institute Publishing, Hoya, Germany, second edition, 1981. (Originally published in 1925. Mention is made in periodicals of that time of an English translation that appeared in the early 1930s, but apparently it is no longer to be found.) This is probably still the most definitive work in existence on the complexities of the cyclic metamorphosis through which microbes can move, and the intricate interplay between cellular and subcellular components and microorganisms. Though additional research has been done since Enderlein's time, his work will probably be studied for many years to come as a model of how to integrate all this data.

The Persecution and Trial of Gaston Naessens (American edition); *The Galileo of the Microscope* (Canadian edition), Christopher Bird, H. J. Kramer, Tiburon, Calif., 1991. The only book in English on the work of another pioneer, Gaston Naessens, whose concepts parallel those of Guenther Enderlein (see page 552). The book is actually an account of the trial of Naessens in Quebec, where he was taken to court by the medical establishment. Nevertheless, a report of the testimony reveals much about Naessens's ideas and work.

The Cancer Biopathy, Wilhelm Reich, Farrar, Straus and Giroux, New York, 1973. Reich was far ahead of his time on many issues, and he observed what he called the "bion," a tiny particle comparable to those mentioned by Béchamps, Enderlein, and Naessens. His concepts on energy, the origin of microbes, and cancer are still radical, refreshing, and intriguing.

A New Bacteriology, Sorin Sonea and Maurice Panisset, Jones and Bartlett, Boston, 1980. Though this book comes from medical academia, it is an attempt to understand the relationship between microbes occupying various niches in the ecological scheme. This idea that microbes communicate, interrelate, and form an underlying or penetrating matrix that is an "organism" of its own is an idea that is beginning to gain some ground among more avant-garde thinkers.

Béchamps or Pasteur? A Lost Chapter in the History of Biology, E. Douglas Hume, C. W. Daniel, London, 1932 (Facsimile edition: Health Research,

Mokelumne Hill, Calif., 1989). Since much of our thinking about infection and disease dates back to Louis Pasteur, this book is valuable. It reexamines Pasteur's career and suggests that many of his "discoveries" were lifted from work of a contemporary, Antoine Béchamps. Béchamps resented not so much Pasteur's stealing the limelight as he did Pasteur's distortion of his observations. Béchamps saw infection as developing in an unhealthy host through a pathological series of changes in tiny particles (microzymas) that were ubiquitous, rather than as a hostile invasion by external agents. On his deathbed, Pasteur is said to have confessed that the *terrain* was everything, the germ nothing.

The Blood and Its Third Anatomical Element, Antoine Béchamps, M.D., D.Sc., John Ouseley, London, 1912 (Facsimile edition: Health Research, Mokelumne Hill, Calif., 1990). The original English translation of Béchamps' work. Useful companion to the above.

Chapter 9. MOVEMENT AND EXERCISE

Hatha Pratipika, Kevin and Venika Kingtsland, Grael Communications, Devon, England, 1977. This is the classic exposition of the system of hatha yoga. A fairly late development, it was an attempt to systematize the physical aspects of yoga as opposed to the meditative aspects that receive most emphasis in the Yoga Sutras. These verses deal with the care and regulation of the physical body, and there are many tie-ins with, and references to, Ayurveda.

Science Studies Yoga, James Funderburk, Ph.D., Himalayan Publishers, Honesdale, Pa., 1977. Though this book is dated, it is an excellent and well-documented survey of research verifying the profound physiologic effects of hatha yoga, breathing, and meditation. Studies showing the effect of postures on autonomic balance, and of breathing techniques on blood pressure, are classic and should be known by all those who are interested in natural medicine.

Hatha Manual I/Hatha Manual II, Samskrti and Veda/Samskrti and Judith Frank, Himalayan Publishers, Honesdale, Pa., 1977, 1978. These spiral-bound books are among the best for learning and refining one's practice of hatha yoga postures.

Exercise Without Movement, as taught by Swami Rama, Himalayan Publishers, Honesdale, Pa., 1984. A system of exercise developed by the yogis who spent years in caves, these techniques are appropriate to those who lead a sedentary life or often find themselves deprived of the opportunity to engage in more conventional forms of exercise.

Discovering the Body's Wisdom: A Comprehensive Guide to More Than Fifty Mind-Body Practices, Mirka Knaster, Bantam Books, New York, 1996. There are a number of such books available now—books that catalog the available body-oriented therapies such as Rolfing, Alexander, Feldenkrais, Pilates, and Trager. But this one impresses me with its breadth—it includes everything I've ever heard of, plus lots I haven't— as well as its depth and detail. It's also easy to read and has an introductory section that explains the general principles of body work. Highly recommended.

Joints and Glands, as taught by Swami Rama, Rudolph Ballentine, M.D., ed., Himalayan Publishers, Honesdale, Pa., 1977. This little book is an excellent summary of exercises that are used to improve the flexibility of the joints and to encourage lymphatic drainage from the tissues.

Self Healing: My Life and Vision, Meir Schneider, Routledge & Kegan Paul, New York, 1987. Considered congenitally blind until a sixteen-year-old high school friend insisted that with exercises he could learn to see, Schneider worked intensively with juices and diet, with massage, movement and imagery, and now reads without glasses. In the process of healing himself, he learned to extend his techniques to others with various disorders, who also benefited dramatically. This inspiring book should be read by all physicians and patients dealing with such diseases as arthritis and multiple sclerosis. It shows what can be accomplished by systematic and persistent use of simple exercises, massage, and a healthful diet.

The Ultimate Athlete, George Leonard, Avon Books, New York, 1975. A useful guide to rethinking your relationship to movement and athletics and their ability to reconnect you to yourself.

The Miracles of Rebound Exercise, Albert E. Carter, Snohomish Publishing, Snohomish, Wash., 1979. A pep talk on the benefits of the mini-trampoline.

Balancing Your Body: A Self-Help Approach to Rolfing Movement, Mary Bond, Healing Arts Press, Rochester, Vt., 1993. How to use Rolfing principles at home to enhance awareness and release your body from its constraints.

The Endless Web, R. Louis Schultz, Ph.D., and Rosemary Feitis, D.O., North Atlantic Books, Berkeley, Calif., 1996. A small but masterful exposition by two of the main teachers of Rolfing today. Beautiful line drawings are juxtaposed with photos of real people to show where "holding" on the muscular level has resulted in connective-tissue bands that constrict and limit movement, breathing, and (I would add) the flow of subtle energy.

Phoenix Rising Yoga Therapy: A Bridge from Body to Soul, Michael Lee, Health Communications, Deerfield Beach, Fla., 1997. This is the story of how Michael Lee, a yoga teacher, helped move the use of hatha yoga postures from its traditional focus on self-training to its flowering as a therapeutic tool.

Meridian Exercises, Shizuto Masunaga, Japan Publications, Tokyo and New York, 1987. By the founder of "Oki yoga" (actually, Iokai, the name Masunaga chose for his teaching center), this book describes the postures its author devised to stretch and activate the meridians. Masunaga was a legendary figure. His students say his knowledge of the meridians and energy was so thorough that he would hurl subjects from the stage where he was lecturing so that they would fall in precisely the right place to open the problematic meridian and cure their ills.

Bone, Breath and Gesture, Don Hanlon Johnson, ed., North Atlantic Books, Berkeley, Calif., 1995. A compilation of interviews and writings of some of the pioneers of breath and body work, such as Ida Rolf, Ilse Middendorf, and Moshe Feldenkrais. A great way to get a feel for the vision that each held.

Body, Mind and Sport, John Douillard, Crown, New York, 1994. Specifics on which sports are most effective for different Ayurvedic types, by one of Chopra's protégés.

The Body Reveals: An Illustrated Guide to the Psychology of the Body, Ron Kurtz and Hector Prestera, M.D., Harper & Row, New York, 1976. A classic book, this is one of the early and still inspiring efforts to learn what the positions and shapes of the body tell us about attitudes and emotions. Kurtz went on to develop the Hakomi Method of Body Centered Psychotherapy.

Iron Shirt Chi Kung I, Mantak Chia, Healing Tao Books, Huntington, N.Y., 1986. A comprehensive explication of how qigong techniques can be used to promote the fuller movement and flow of energy and ensure physical, mental, and spiritual health.

Chapter 10. ENERGY AND BREATH

Science of Breath, Swami Rama, Rudolph Ballentine, M.D., and Alan Hymes, M.D., Himalayan Publishers, Honesdale, Pa., 1979. This book is listed first in this section because the primary obstacle to working with the energy level of functioning in the human being is lack of awareness of it. According to the Eastern disciplines, this level of functioning or "energy body" is observable through introspection. A guide to the relationship between breathing and *prana* that is part of the ancient yogic disciplines, the book includes a final chapter on the science of prana with numerous exercises that can be used to acquaint oneself with the phenomenon.

Nature's Finer Forces: The Science of Breath and the Philosophy of the Tattvas, Rama Prasad, Theosophical Publication Society, London, 1889 (Republished in facsimile edition: Health Research, Mokelumne Hill, Calif., 1969). One of the most authoritative books on the subtleties of breathing and energy. It is theosophically oriented, which causes some degree of confusion for the modern reader. However, the last third of the book is a straight translation of portions of the *Shivagama.* This will be studied with intense interest and amazement by anyone interested in breath and energy.

Blueprint for Immortality: The Electric Patterns of Life, Harold Saxton Burr, Ph.D., Neville Spearman, London, 1972. Though long out of print, this is a landmark book. It was the first acknowledgment by the academic world that subtle, nonphysical forces could shape the material world of biological beings. Dr. Burr was a professor of anatomy at the Yale University School of Medicine.

Encounters with Qi: Exploring Chinese Medicine, David Eisenberg, M.D., W. W. Norton, New York, 1985. Fun to read, this book is the account of a modern physician going to present-day China and observing the many and astounding ways that the Chinese manipulate ch'i for fun, profit, and, often, therapy. A great introduction to the China of acupuncture, qigong, and traditional medicine.

Subtle Energy: Awakening to the Unseen Forces in Our Lives, William Collinge, Ph.D., Warner Books, New York, 1998. If you're still not sure what all this energy stuff is about, this book is a wonderful introduction to the subject. It is an up-to-date compilation of research data and traditional insights that makes accessible and entertaining reading.

Path of Fire and Light. 2 vols., Swami Rama, Himalayan Publishers, Honesdale, Pa., 1986, 1988. These two books offer further introduction to the advanced practices of energy control, by my teacher, one of the few authorities who has chosen to share this knowledge with the public. A great deal of this information is not to be found in English elsewhere.

Energy Fields and Medicine: A Study of Device Technology Based on Acupuncture Meridians and Chi Energy, Fetzer Foundation, Kalamazoo, Mich., 1989. A typewritten, 275-page collection of articles by various authors on subjects that relate to energy fields, meridians, and the recently developed devices that are used to measure and manipulate these phenomena. It is a gold mine of information for those who are interested in things like Motoyama's AMI System for measuring functioning of the meridians and their corresponding internal organs; relationship between acupuncture and homeopathy; laser acupuncture; and electrodermal diagnostic instruments (e.g., the Voll dermaton).

Vibrational Medicine, Richard Gerber, M.D., Bear & Company, Santa Fe, N.M., 1988. An ambitious attempt to pull together all the therapeutic tools that affect energy into one comprehensive composite, from flower remedies and homeopathy to acupuncture and crystals. For people who like to talk in terms of holograms and etheric and astral planes and how they relate to radionics, this is the book.

The Web of Life, John Davidson, C. W. Daniel Co., Essex, England, 1988. A fairly recent and quite comprehensive neo-Vedic treatment of the world of energy phenomena, and the various disciplines and traditions that have explored it. This book is worth studying in depth.

Orgone, Reich and Eros: Wilhelm Reich's Theory of Life Energy, W. Edward Mann, Simon and Schuster, New York, 1973. Still probably the most systematic treatment of the Western tradition of energy exploration. Though the author's orientation is Reichian, I find his historical survey of Reich's predecessors, including such fascinating figures as von Reichenbach and Lakhovsky, especially valuable.

The Creative Use of Emotion, Swami Rama and Swami Ajaya, Ph.D., Himalayan Institute, Honesdale, Pa., 1988. Since emotion and energy are so tied together, it will often be impossible to learn to deal effectively with energy without revising your approach to your emotions. This book helps you to understand the energetic source of emotional streams in the biological urges and to provide for and manage the related needs skillfully so as to defuse and prevent confusing and disabling emotional storms.

Breathing: Expanding Your Power and Energy, Michael Sky, Bear & Company, Santa Fe, N.M., 1990. A simple book, but readable and a good way to get started with the subject. In contrast to many other works on breathing, it is not laden with exotic terms and inscrutable techniques.

Anatomy of the Spirit: The Seven Stages of Power and Healing, Caroline Myss, Ph.D., Harmony Books, New York, 1996. This book has been phenomenally popular, as have the author's audiotapes on the subject. A "medical intuitive," she analyzes the energy systems that underlie the physical body, with a special emphasis on the psychological and emotional issues that relate to each chakra and the challenges each presents to personal evolution.

Awakening Intuition: Using Your Mind-Body Network for Insight and Healing, Mona Lisa Schulz, M.D., Ph.D., Harmony Books, New York, 1998. Dr. Schulz represents a new generation of holistic practitioners: she is academically credentialed to the hilt, genuinely intuitive, spiritually oriented, and she writes well to boot! The appearance of books like this shows that medicine is about to undergo an amazing transformation. Schulz leads us gently into the process of intuition, showing us that we can all use it, and then she deals with each chakra and the diseases related to it. This book is engaging and highly recommended.

Currents of Death: Power Lines, Computer Terminals and the Attempt to Cover Up Their Threat to Your Health, Paul Brodeur, Simon and Schuster, New York, 1989. There is also a downside—energy can also have negative effects, especially that which is generated in the environment without thought to its repercussions in the world of living organisms (e.g., ELF, extra-low frequency radiation). Scary but useful information.

Hands of Light: A Guide to Healing Through the Human Energy Field; Light Emerging: The Journey of Personal Healing, Barbara Ann Brennan, Bantam Books, New York, 1987, 1993. These two large-format, illustrated books are like textbooks on energy healing. The author is a well-known exponent of such energy work, and runs a school in New York that has turned out many healers.

Pranic Healing, Choa Kok Sui, Samuel Weiser, York Beach, Maine, 1990. This is what the Chinese might call *wei qi,* or external qigong, the emanation of energy from the hands to effect healing in another person. Today there are lots of people around doing things like this, and this is probably the most cogent and comprehensive presentation of the theory and techniques.

Your Hands Can Heal: Learn to Channel Healing Energy, Ric A. Weinman, Penguin, New York, 1992. One of a number of simple books now available that put healing in your hands, it demystifies the process and helps you through the simple steps to developing your own innate ability to do hands-on (or -off) healing.

Super Magnetic Field: Prana Science, Sang Myung Lee, Department of Chemistry, Dong Eui University, Pusan, Korea, 1991. A most extraordinary little self-published book, this is a description of laboratory research done in Korea on what the author calls "super space transition": the dematerialization, relocation, and rematerialization of objects. According to my conversations with the author, a number of workers in Korea have succeeded in carrying out this process, and they have established a network of scientists with an interest in the area, but they have not been able to gain entry to Western, English-medium scientific meetings and publications. (Unfortunately, this book doesn't do much to remedy that situation, since its English is almost indecipherable.)

The MORA Concept, Franz Morell, M.D., Karl F. Haug, Heidelberg, Germany, 1990. MORA therapy is a marriage of meridian therapy and high technology with homeopathic theory. Currents from the acupuncture point are measured, reversed, and reintroduced to provide a healing energetic message.

The Golden Fountain: The Complete Guide to Urine Therapy, Coen van der Kroon, Amethyst Books, Oxford, England, 1996. I include this book here since urine therapy is probably best conceptualized as a technique of offering the system an energetic portrait of its functioning in the manner of homeopathic treatment. Of all the books on this fascinating and useful subject, I like this one best. It contains descriptions of various approaches and testimonials from users, as well as a translation of the entirety of a Sanskrit scripture on this method of healing and rejuvenation.

Chapter 11. HEALING AS TRANSFORMATION

Sexuality

Women's Bodies, Women's Wisdom, Christiane Northrup, M.D., Bantam Books, New York, 1994. This book introduced the public (especially the female half) to the concept of listening to what the body tells you about yourself and the issues you need to address to move through an illness. While charting a new territory for women's medicine, it also manages to provide practical information on such topics as the treatment of endometriosis with castor oil packs.

Uniting Sex, Self and Spirit, Genia Pauli Haddon, D.Min., Ph.D., PLUS Publications, Scotland, Conn., 1993. Though published a year before Northrup's book, this smaller volume serves to take her work a step further. It looks at the anatomy and physiology of the genitals and reads their holographic messages about the multifaceted nature of gender. Haddon argues eloquently that there is a *yang* or assertive femininity (that which forces into being, what she calls the *uterine*) just as there is a *yin* or passive/receptive one (that which nurtures). The *yang* femininity has been suppressed not only in women, but any awareness of it as part of the anima of the man has also been ignored and denied. This is of critical importance as we seek urgently to birth the new consciousness that can lift us out of ecological and planetary disaster. By the same token, it's the *yin* masculine that can conserve and hold energy for transmutation, and in our two-dimensional (male is all *yang* and female all *yin*) concept of gender, this has also been lost. This is an important book.

Healing Love Through the Tao: Cultivating Female Sexual Energy, Mantak Chia and Naneewan Chia, Healing Tao Books, Huntington, N.Y., 1986. Mantak Chia and his wife, Naneewan, have traveled the earth giving seminars on the conscious control of sexual energy and its use for healing. They have been at the forefront of bringing the ancient principles of taoism and tantra to the attention of the public.

Taoist Secrets of Love: Cultivating Male Sexual Energy, Mantak Chia with Michael Winn, Aurora Press, Santa Fe, N.M., 1984. A corresponding volume for men to the one above, it provides valuable information on containment and circulation of sexual energy as an alternative to expenditure during ejaculation. The perspective is more Taoist, emphasizing not only the movement of energy up the spine but also back down the front of the body, through what is called in the Chinese traditions "the microcosmic orbit." This is in contradistinction to the more exclusive Tantric aim of moving the energy *up* to higher chakras. Chia explains the "big draw," the method of stimulating oneself to the point of near ejaculation, then using first muscular contraction (and later mental control) to circulate the energy.

The Tao of Sexology, Dr. Stephen T. Chang, Tao Publishing, San Francisco, 1986. Covering territory similar to that covered in the Chias' books, Dr. Chang's work is briefer yet manages to include some interesting material not mentioned in the other two. Like Chia, he details the reflex points on the penis and in the vaginal canal that should be stimulated in a balanced way in order for masturbation or intercourse to energize the body evenly and not cause imbalances. He too emphasizes the Eastern concept that ejaculation can deplete the system and lead to immune deficiency. Adaptations are offered for same sex partners.

Passion Play: Ancient Secrets for a Lifetime of Health and Happiness Through Sensational Sex, Felice Dunas, Ph.D., Penguin, New York, 1997. A modern rendition of traditional Chinese teachings on using sexual activity as a healing modality by a contemporary American acupuncturist. More accessible for the average reader than the books above.

Sexual Peace: Beyond the Cominator Virus, Michael Sky, Bear & Company, Santa Fe, N.M., 1993. This book argues that the attitudes and relationships we inculcate in our children perpetuate a domination/control dynamic that substitutes violence and oppression for the free flow of love and energy that could otherwise prevail. So deeply embedded in the fabric of our being does this become that it is nearly viral or genetic. The attitude "I hate this body and I project the hate I feel onto others," Sky says, "is the energetic core of patriarchy and the root cause of all of the current abuses of dominator reality . . . when we are rendered incapable of feeling a true energetic connection with another, then any chance for a partnership relationship is crippled, if not entirely lost, and we tend instead toward the patriarchal patterns of domination and submission." But we can operate otherwise. "Healing our sexuality involves saying yes to the living current of our sexual energy and at the same time recognizing our ability and responsibility to feel and express it as we choose." A very valuable book.

Aghora: At the Left Hand of God, Robert E. Svoboda, Brotherhood of Life Publishing, Albuquerque, N.M., 1986. An extraordinary and amazing exploration of the life and experiences of a modern-day *Aghori,* practitioner of what is perhaps the most radical of the Tantric paths. The chapter titled "Sex" is especially enlightening, but the whole book delivers a culture shock even as it reads like an adventure novel. Highly recommended.

Aghora II: Kundalini and *Aghora III: The Law of Karma,* Robert E. Svoboda, Brotherhood of Life Publishing, Albuquerque, N.M., 1993, 1998. Not quite as much fun as the first volume in this series, *Aghora II* is still a fascinating and valuable book. It is essentially a verbatim transcript of instructions given to Svoboda by his teacher in the rich and usually secret teachings of Tantra and Kundalini yoga. *Aghora III* continues the account, becoming less didactic and more narrative, and ends with the death of the teacher.

Homophobia: How We All Pay the Price, Warren J. Blumenfeld, ed., Beacon Press, Boston, 1992. An invaluable collection of articles on how to understand and overcome the homophobia that is a major obstacle to honoring and using the critically important feminine energy in each of us.

Tapta Marga: Asceticism and Initiation in Vedic India, Walter O. Kaelber, State University of New York Press, Albany, N.Y., 1989. A contemporary academic treatment of the subject of *tapas,* albeit a highly competent and knowledgeable one. The book underscores the universality and central role of the transformational fire.

Holistic Psychotherapy ("Mindwork")

Yoga and Psychotherapy: The Evolution of Consciousness, Swami Rama, Rudolph Ballentine, M.D., and Swami Ajaya, Ph.D., Himalayan Publishers, Honesdale, Pa., 1976. Using the system of yoga as a philosophical point of departure, this book examines the relationship between body, energy, mind, and spirit and how the psychotherapeutic process involves and alters each of these levels. The closing chapter on the chakras is particularly helpful for those who are trying to integrate concepts of personal evolution and Eastern thought.

Theory and Practice of Meditation, Rudolph Ballentine, M.D., ed., Himalayan Publishers, Honesdale, Pa., 1986. Meditation is psychotherapy done alone; it can either replace conventional psychotherapy or be an adjunct to it. Any system of holistic psychotherapy should prepare one to practice some kind of meditative discipline, so that the process of introspective analysis, exploration, and change can continue after the therapeutic relationship ends.

Atharveda and Ayurveda, V. W. Karambelkar, Ph.D., Usha Karambelkar, Nagpur, India, 1961. The Atharveda is the veda that is most related to traditional medicine. It does not, however, deal exclusively with diet, herbs, and what we would today consider medical interventions. A great deal of it is devoted to the use of mantra and ritual. These techniques, the use of sound to heal and the ritual creation of a healing space, have barely been investigated in the West and remain two of the great frontiers for holistic medicine in the future. An enlightened psychotherapist should learn to harness the power of mantra in multiple strategic ways, and ritual as healing opens the possibility of working with groups in a profoundly powerful and efficient way.

Freedom from the Bondage of Karma, Swami Rama, Himalayan Publishers, Honesdale, Pa., 1977. One of the unique features of any psychotherapy that is based on the yoga system is its clear understanding of the role of karma and of how the patient can extricate himself from its effects. This book is a concise formulation of that understanding.

Psychotherapy East and West: A Unifying Paradigm, Swami Ajaya, Ph.D., Himalayan Publishers, Honesdale, Pa., 1983. This magnum opus is an impressive attempt to synthesize the understandings of the major Western thinkers in the field of psychotherapy within the context of Eastern philosophy and psychology. For the serious psychotherapist or student. A careful study of it can transform one's thinking on the subject.

Yoga Psychology, Swami Ajaya, Ph.D., Himalayan Publishers, Honesdale, Pa., 1976. This simple manual is a nice primer for the practice of meditation, and points out clearly its relationship to the process of making the mind healthier.

Beyond the Brain: Birth, Death and Transcendence in Psychotherapy, Stanislav Grof, SUNY Press, Albany, N.Y., 1985. This brilliant book pioneers the use of the new holographic paradigm to study consciousness and elevate psychotherapy to a new level of spiritual significance. It dares to introduce into psychological discourse the existence of consciousness beyond the confines of time and space. In this context, Grof uses his experience with psychedelics as a springboard to explore the evolutionary intent of medical states psychiatry has heretofore seen as merely pathological. A seminal work.

Psychology: Sanction for Selfishness, the Error of Egoism in Theory and Therapy, Michael Wallach and Lise Wallach, W. H. Freeman, San Francisco, 1983. This book demonstrates the growing awareness that our ideas about psychological theory and psychotherapy are in need of revision, especially as regards their tacit acceptance of our egocentric worldview. The Eastern concepts of *ahimsa* and selfless service, around which many of the basic techniques for self-development and the evolution of consciousness are built, are not compatible with much of modern psychology.

Therapeutic Astrology: Using the Birth Chart in Psychotherapy and Spiritual Counseling, Greg Bogart, Ph.D., Dawn Mountain Press, Berkeley, Calif., 1996. This is the cutting edge of astrology, where it has at last come of age. Now skilled and knowledgeable therapists are realizing that it is irresponsible to ignore the birth chart, with its wealth of information about their client's inclinations, personality makeup, and personal spiritual path. This small book discusses the concept of using astrology in a therapeutic setting, and offers a number of fascinating case histories.

The Inner Sky: The Dynamic New Astrology for Everyone, Steven Forrest, ACS Publishers, San Diego, Calif., 1988. For the novice, this is a must. It starts you off on the right foot: Forrest shows you how each astrological sign represents a distinct evolutionary strategy. Each planet is a faculty of human consciousness, and the houses are the arenas in which that aspect of your personality will pursue the evolutionary strategy indicated by the sign that rules it and the sign in which the planet was situated at the moment your consciousness took shape.

The Development of the Personality: Seminars in Psychological Astrology, Volume I, Liz Greene and Howard Sasportas, Samuel Weiser, York Beach, Maine, 1987. This volume, and those that follow in the series, as well as other works by these authors, represent the best of a new generation of astrologers who have lifted the subject out of the realm of tabloid predictions to a sophisticated tool for profound psychological analysis and spiritually grounded guidance. Though Sasportas has passed on, Greene, a Jungian analyst, continues as co-director of the Centre for Psychological Astrology, the school they founded in England.

Chapter 12. REWEAVING

State of the World: A Worldwatch Institute Report on Progress Toward a Sustainable Society, Worldwatch Institute, W. W. Norton, New York, 1998. From a truly holistic point of view, the healing of the individual cannot be separated from the healing of the larger whole of which he or she is a part. This annual report is a diagnostic assessment of the health of the planet, and the news is not good. The earth's aquifers are being depleted at a rate that far exceeds their recharging capacity so that severe droughts seem imminent. Soils are no longer going into production, but now coming out, because of abuse. Grain reserves have dwindled dramatically, even as populations have soared. In the midst of this building disaster, governments talk of "growth" and support economies built on accelerating the exploitation of natural resources that are no longer there. The data assembled by Worldwatch documents the erosion of the superstructure of life on the planet, the manifestation of the gravest miasmatic disorder in the body of Gaia and in the mindset of her inhabitants.

Chronic Disease: Its Cause and Cure (4th edition), P. N. Banerjee, Banerjee & Company, Gidni, India, 1971. This little volume, originally published in 1931 at the height of the golden age of spiritual homeopathy in Bengal, was my inspiration as I first explored the twisted labyrinths of miasmatic disease. If you can sidestep the heavily moralistic language it is couched in, it is a gold mine of insight.

Notes on the Miasms, or Hahnemann's Chronic Diseases, Dr. Proceso Sanchez Ortega (English translation by Harris Coulter, Ph.D.), National Homeopathic Pharmacy, New Delhi, 1980. By a Mexican master of homeopathy, this volume does much to probe the vast implications of the concept of miasms. Especially see his section on "Miasms in the Structure of Commercial Medical Science" in Chapter 16.

Dance of the Four Winds: Secrets of the Inca Medicine Wheel, Alberto Villoldo and Erik Jendresen, Destiny Books, Rochester, Vt., 1995.
Of Water and the Spirit: Ritual, Magic, and Initiation in the Life of an African Shaman, Malidoma Patrice Some, Putnam, New York, 1994.
A Course in Miracles, Foundation for Inner Peace, Glen Ellen, Calif., 1992.
Mitzvot as Spiritual Practices: A Jewish Guidebook for the Soul, Esther G. Chasin, Jason Aronson, Northvale, N.J., 1997.
Mother Earth Spirituality: Native American Paths to Healing Ourselves and Our World, Ed McGaa and Eagle Man, HarperCollins, San Francisco, 1990.
Voices of the First Day, Awakening in the Aboriginal Dreamtime, Robert Lawlor, Inner Traditions, Rochester, Vt., 1991.
The Heart of the Koran, Lex Hixon, Theosophical Publishing House, Wheaton, Ill., 1988.

These books reframe their respective spiritual traditions (Incan, African, Christian, Orthodox Jewish, Native North American, Australian Aboriginal, and Muslim) in the terms of healing and transformation that are the foundation of *Radical Healing*. Appropriate books from this list might help you integrate the healing of your body and mind with the pursuit of your spiritual path.

Journeys Out of the Body, Far Journeys, Robert A. Monroe, Doubleday, New York, 1977, 1985. These two books reflect the immediate possibilities for exploring the unknown mind. Monroe has documented the inner travels that his trainees have experienced and brings what we might consider exotic and inaccessible—the domain of the shaman—into the realm of the doable.

Astral Travel, Gavin and Yvonne Frost, Samuel Weiser, York Beach, Maine, 1982. The Frosts have established teaching centers in England and the United States where one can learn the techniques of out-of-body journeying.

Regression Therapy: A Handbook for Professionals, Volume I: Past-Life Therapy, Volume II: Special Instances of Altered State Work, Winafred Blake Lucas, Ph.D., Deep Forest Press, Crest Park, Calif., 1993. Healing not only involves reconnection with other lives and dimensions but sometimes establishing (temporary) separation from entities that may overwhelm and obstruct your soul and its movement along its unique path. Dr. Lucas covers in authoritative detail the pioneering work in the fields of past-life regression and what is commonly called "depossession."

The Dark Side of Love: The Positive Role of Our Negative Feelings—Anger, Jealousy, and Hate, Jane G. Goldberg, Ph.D., Putnam, New York, 1993. The nuts and bolts of integrating the Shadow.

Coyote Medicine, Lewis Mehl-Madrona, M.D., Scribner, New York, 1997. The fascinating account of the medical career of a half-Cherokee physician who has dedicated himself to bridging conventional medicine and Native American shamanism. This book will give you much insight into the profundity and beauty—as well as the limitations—of the spirit work of healing ritual. Dr. Mehl-Madrona is honest, open, humble, and uniquely qualified to take us into this world.

Light Years Ahead, Brian Joseph Breiling, Celestial Arts, Berkeley, Calif., 1996. Though there are a number of books available on light and healing, this one, being both recent and a collection of articles by a dozen of those working in the field, is a good way to get a grasp of what is going on in this area of futuristic therapy. Light is energy and energy healing promises to be a major feature of the New Medicine.

Maharaj: A Biography of Shriman Tapasviji Maharaj, a Mahatma Who Lived for 185 Years, T. S. Anantha Murthy, Dawn Horse Press, San Rafael, Calif., 1972. I include this book here because it so charmingly points up the utter arbitrariness of our assumptions about aging, and, by implication, about many aspects of life on this plane.

The Pleiadian Agenda: A New Cosmology for the Age of Light, Barbara Hand Clow, Bear & Company, Santa Fe, N.M., 1995. When I am not feeling sufficiently challenged, I turn to this book. The most sweepingly integrative of the New Age books on spirituality, it amuses, dazzles, and overwhelms. I find it unendingly stimulating and fascinating.

BOOKS ON SPECIFIC DISEASES/DISORDERS AND THEIR HOLISTIC MANAGEMENT

These are the epidemics of our age. We are so immersed in the mindsets that lie at the base of these disorders that we find it very difficult to get a handle on them. For this reason there are many books on each, none very satisfactorily providing a clear and complete understanding. Such diseases will be found to have many "causes"—that is, many facets of our lifestyle and mentality contribute to their development. One who is coping with such a disease will need to survey the best writings and identify which causal threads are most relevant to his or her case. I have selected those books whose perspective is closest to that provided by *Radical Healing*.

AIDS

The Immune Power Personality: Seven Traits You Can Develop to Stay Healthy, Henry Dreher, Dutton, New York, 1995.

Beyond AIDS: A Journey Into Healing, George R. Melton in collaboration with Wil Garcia, Brotherhood Press, Beverly Hills, Calif., 1988.

Healing AIDS Naturally, Laurence E. Badgley, M.D., Human Energy Press, Foster City, Calif., 1987.

AIDS and the Healer Within, Nick Bamforth, Amethyst Books, Emeryville, Calif., 1987.

AIDS: The HIV Myth, Jad Adams, St. Martin's Press, New York, 1989.

Homophobia: How We All Pay the Price, Warren J. Blumenfeld, ed., Beacon Press, Boston, 1992.

Oxygen Therapies: A New Way of Approaching Disease, Ed MacCabe, Energy Publications, Morrisville, N.Y., 1988.

A Holistic Protocol for the Immune System: A Manual for HIV/ARC/AIDS, Candidiasis, Epstein-Barr, Herpes and Other Opportunistic Infections, Scott J. Gregory, O.M.D., Tree of Life Publications, Palm Springs, Calif., 1989.

HEAL: Health Education/Aids Liaison, Information Packet, Tel. 212-674-HOPE.

"AIDS" Myths, Truths, Solutions, Bill Holub, Ph.D., and Claudia Holub, Life Systems Learning Center, Cottage Industry Press, Melville, N.Y., 1993.

Roger's Recovery from AIDS, Bob Owen, Davar, Malibu, Calif., 1987.

Poison by Prescription: The AZT Story, John Lauritsen, Asklepios, New York, 1990.

Infectious AIDS: Have We Been Misled?, Peter H. Duesberg, North Atlantic Books, Berkeley, Calif., 1995.

AIDS and Chinese Medicine, Qingcai Zhang, M.D., and Hong-Yen Hsu, Ph.D., Keats Publishing, New Canaan, Conn., 1990.

AIDS and Syphilis: The Hidden Link, Harris L. Coulter, Ph.D., North Atlantic Books, Berkeley, Calif., 1987.

Nine Ounces: A Nine-Part Program for the Prevention of AIDS in HIV-Positive Persons, Bob Flaws, Blue Poppy Press, Boulder, Colo., 1992.

Syphilis as AIDS, Robert Ben Mitchell, Banned Books, Austin, Tex., 1988.

ASCVD

(Arteriosclerotic Cardiovascular Disease) Includes: Coronary Heart Disease, Strokes, Hypertension and Aneurysms (when based on plaque in arteries)

Questions from the Heart: Answers to 100 Questions About Chelation Therapy, a Safe Alternative to Bypass Surgery, Terry Chappell, M.D., Hampton Roads Publishing, Charlottesville, Va., 1995.

The Homocysteine Revolution, Kilmer S. McCully, M.D., Keats Publishing, New Canaan, Conn., 1997.

Solved: The Riddle of Heart Attacks, Broda O. Barnes, M.D., Ph.D., and Charlotte W. Barnes, Robinson Press, Fort Collins, Colo., 1976.

The Language of the Heart: The Human Body in Dialogue, James J. Lynch, Basic Books, New York, 1985.

Fighting Heart Disease: A Practical Self-Help Guide to Prevention and Treatment, Chandra Patel, M.D., Dorling Kindersley, London, 1987.

Reversing Heart Disease, Julian M. Whitaker, M.D., Warner Books, New York, 1985.

Dr. Dean Ornish's Program for Reversing Heart Disease: The Only System Scientifically Proven to Reverse Heart Disease Without Drugs or Surgery, Dean Ornish, M.D., Ivy Books, New York, 1996.

Love and Survival: The Scientific Basis for the Healing Power of Intimacy, Dean Ornish, M.D., HarperCollins, New York, 1998.

Cancer

Third Opinion: An International Directory to Alternative Therapy Centers for the Treatment and Prevention of Cancer and Other Degenerative Diseases, John M. Fink, Avery Publications, Garden City Park, N.Y., Third Edition, 1997.

An Alternative Medicine Definitive Guide to Cancer, W. John Diamond, MD, W. Lee Cowden, MD, with Burton Goldberg, Future Medicine Publishing, Inc., Tiburon, Calif., 1997.

Psychotherapeutic Treatment of Cancer Patients, Jane Goldberg, Ph.D., ed., Macmillan, New York, 1981.

Laetril Case Histories: The Richardson Cancer Clinic Experience, John A. Richardson, M.D., and Patricia Griffin, Bantam Books, New York, 1977.

The Cancer Syndrome, Ralph W. Moss, Grove Press, New York, 1980.

Cancer and Vitamin C: A Discussion of the Nature, Causes, Prevention and Treatment of Cancer with Special Reference to the Value of Vitamin C, Ewan Cameron and Linus Pauling, The Linus Pauling Institute of Science and Medicine, Menlo Park, Calif., 1979.

Recalled by Life: The Story of My Recovery from Cancer, Anthony J. Sattilaro, M.D., Houghton Mifflin, Boston, 1982.

Love, Medicine and Miracles, Bernie S. Siegel, M.D., Harper & Row, New York, 1986.

Cancer Alternative Therapies, Cure Rates, Ralph Hovanian, Natural Hygiene, Huntington, N.Y., 1985.

The Rife Report: The Cancer Cure That Worked! Fifty Years of Suppression, Barry Lynes, Marcus Books, Queensville, Ontario, Canada, 1987.

Choices: Realistic Alternatives in Cancer Treatment, 3rd ed. Marion Morra and Eva Potts, Avon Books, New York, 1999.

Dr. Anne's Journal, Robert Lloyd, Ph.D., Davar Publishing, Cannon Beach, Ore., 1990.

The Cancer Biopathy, Wilhelm Reich, Farrar, Straus and Giroux, New York, 1973.

Repression and Reform in the Evaluation of Alternative Cancer Therapies, Robert G. Houston, Project Cure, Washington, D.C., 1989.

The Conquest of Cancer: Vaccines and Diet, Virginia Livingston-Wheeler, M.D., Franklin Watts, New York, 1984.

How to Fight Cancer and Win: Scientific Guidelines and Documented Facts for the Successful Treatment and Prevention of Cancer and Other Related Health Problems, William L. Fischer, Fischer Publishing, Canfield, Ohio, 1987.

Chronic Fatigue Syndrome

When Antibiotics Fail, Marc Lappe, North Atlantic Books, Berkeley, Calif., 1986.

Adrenal Syndrome, G. E. Poesnecker, N.D., D.C., Humanitarian Publishing, Quakertown, Pa., 1983.

Chronic Fatigue Syndrome—The Hidden Epidemic, Jesse A. Stoff, M.D., and Charles R. Pellegrino, Ph.D., Harper & Row, New York, 1988.

The Missing Diagnosis, C. Orian Truss, M.D., The Missing Diagnosis, Inc., Birmingham, Ala., 1983.

The Yeast Connection, William G. Crook, M.D., Professional Books, Jackson, Tenn., 1983.

Products and Services

This is a rapidly evolving scene. New schools and businesses are popping up every day. What I have offered here are those that appear to be the most enduring and well-established. I have also selected them because their philosophies and orientations mesh with those of this book.

Natural Medicinals

Radical Healing Store: 212 243-6057
www.radicalhealingstore.com
> Highest quality, personally selected items for transformation used by myself to support health and healing: remedies, flower essences, and supplements, as well as key books, neti pots, rebounders, and more.

Wellspring Pharmacy: 570 253-5650
> A broader selection of Homeopathics, cell salts, herbal remedies, and supplements. This is the pharmacy I helped establish at the Himalayan Institute and its proprietor has made a life's study of making and stocking traditional preparations.

Homeopathy Overnight: 800 ARNICA30
> Fast delivery of homeopathic remedies.

Flower Essence Society: 800 548-0075
> English and California Flower Essences. They will make up combinations.

Elizabeth Herb Medicine: 212 925-7105
> A wide variety of Chinese Patent Medicines.

Hickey Chemists: 800 724-5566
> A broad selection of natural medicinals, including the latest "nutriceuticals."

Courses of Instruction and Practitioners

The Center for Holistic Medicine
(Rudolph Ballentine, M.D., and associates)
> How to start a Radical Healing study group and learn about our
> new group consultations (Radical Healing Circles).
> 212 243-6057

World Health and Healing Collaborative
> Consulting and training by myself (Rudolph Ballentine, M.D.),
> Linda Bark, Ph.D., and Ryma Bielkus; health coaching, etc.
> 877 777-2010   www.worldhealthandhealing.com

National Center for Homeopathy
> Info on their own and other courses. NCH also publishes a
> directory of homeopathic practitioners.
> 703 548-7790

Flower Essence Society
> Courses on the use of Flower Essences
> 800 548-0075

New York Open Center
> In-depth courses and conferences on holistic medicine, yoga,
> astrology, shamanism, and more.
> 212 219-2527   www.opencenter.org

Himalayan Institute
> Weekend seminars on yoga, meditation, Tantra, breathing, and
> holistic health.
> 570 253-5551   www.himalayaninstitute.org

American Institute of Vedic Studies
> Correspondence courses on Ayurveda by Dr. David Frawley.
> 505 983-9385   www.vedanet.com

Clayton College of Natural Health
> Home study of naturopathy, holistic nutrition and natural health.
> 800 659-8274   www.ccnh.edu

Body Electric School
> Seminars and retreats exploring erotic energy through the use
> of Tantric and Taoist techniques. Training in sexual healing.
> 510 653-1594   www.bodyelectric.org

TheSpiritWorks
> Coaching by phone designed to identify core values and to align
> your actions in the world with your inner spark (spanda).
> 877 292-4425   www.TheSpiritWorks.org

Equipment

Radical Healing Store

> Essential tools for health and transformation: Neti pots, blotting brushes, the best (in my opinion) rebounders, and more. We only carry what I've used and recommend. Also remedies and books.
>
> 212 243-6057   www.radicalhealingstore.com

Cutting Edge Catalogue

> Full spectrum lighting, ELF meters (for testing) and devices to protect, air and water purification systems, catalyst water (by Flannagan), magnets, chemical-free cleaners.
>
> Orders: 800 497-9516
>
> Questions: 516 287-3813   www.cutcat.com

Books, Tapes, Videos, Software

Radical Healing Store

> Carefully selected essential books and tapes that I often recommend to patients.
>
> (see above)

Homeopathic Educational Services

> Hard-to-find homeopathic books, tapes, videos, software, and remedies.
>
> Orders: 800 359-9051
>
> Questions: 510 649-0294   www.homeopathic.com

Minimum Price

> Also books, tapes, videos, and software on homeopathy.
>
> Orders: 800 663-8272   www.minimum.com

Himalayan Press

> A sure source of additional copies of *Radical Healing,* they also carry all my earlier books, including *Diet and Nutrition, Science of Breath* and *Yoga and Psychotherapy.*
>
> 800 822-4547   www.himalayaninstitute.org

East West Books

> Hard to find books on Eastern thought, yoga, Tantra, New Age philosophy, and holistic healing.
>
> 212 243-5994

Glossary

This brief glossary is meant to define terms that may be unfamiliar to the average reader. Other expressions not in wide use will be prominently defined in the passages where they are used. If you do not find a word listed here, look in the Index. The page number in bold type will indicate where the term is introduced and explained.

Aama [AH-muh]. Matter that is generated internally and/or results from poor assimilation of food.

Akasha [a-KAHSH-a]. Emptiness or space. The fundamental or first Element in Indian Tantric cosmology.

Allopathic. Operating according to the Law of Contraries or opposites, in contradistinction to those approaches that are based on the Law of Similars, which are referred to as *homeopathic.* Treating a fever with cold, for example, is allopathic.

Anima/animus. The other, less visible and less expressed aspect of the man's or woman's personality. The *anima* is the male's feminine side and vice versa.

Chakra. From Sanskrit for "wheel"—a whirling focus of energy; a point of coordination of energy phenomena with physical and mental functions.

Ch'i [chee]. Subtle energy, the Chinese equivalent of *prana* in the Indian systems.

Dosha [DOE-shuh]. A dynamic factor in human function in the Ayurvedic system of thought. There are three *doshas: vata, pitta,* and *kapha.*

Dysbiosis. Dys = difficult, problematic; *-biosis* = life forms (in the intestine.) A recent term used to indicate disrupted microbial populations in the gastrointestinal tract. The normal flora are critical to healthy digestion and assimilation.

Element. A basic component of reality. Modern materialistic science uses the term to apply to atomic variants. Ancient science used it to designate fundamental building blocks of a multilevel universe—spanning the physical, the energetic, and consciousness.

Ether. See *akasha.*

Fascia. The connective tissue sheets and sheaths that surround and support muscle. The honeycomb-like fascial network is what determines body structure and shape, stores wastes, and transports some subtler electrical currents (see Chapter 8).

Hologram. A recording of an image through a laser technology that allows it to be re-created in three dimensions. Because one of the unique properties of the hologram is that a fragment of it can be used to reproduce the whole, it has become a model for conceptualizing the holistic aspects of interrelated systems.

Holographic. Of or pertaining to a hologram.

Kapha [KAH-fuh]. One of the three *doshas* or dynamic factors in human functioning, as conceptualized in Ayurvedic medicine. It has to do with the more solid and substantial aspects of the person, and is made up of the Elements of Earth *(prithivi)* and Water *(apas).*

Kundalini [KOON-duh-LEE-nee]. The potential energy *(shakti)* available to an individual, often latent because of unconscious conflicts that keep it tied up. It bears a close relationship to what the Western mind might consider erotic energy, and its form and behavior are often experienced as serpentlike.

Mantra [MAHN-tra]. A sound used to direct or reorganize consciousness. See under *Sanskrit.*

Materia Medica. A reference book that groups all the information about a remedy, including the indications for its use, under the name of the remedy.

Matrical. Having to do with a period of prehistory that is prepatriarchal and nonhierarchical. It has been suggested as a replacement for *matriarchal* to apply to that era, since this term suggests a hierarchical ordering of power for which there is little evidence.

Meridian. A pathway through which subtle energy is thought to flow. These are the channels accessible to the exterior—tapped into by the acupuncturist and manually manipulated by the shiatsu therapist.

Miasm [MY-asm]. A basic pattern of dysfunction that underlies and sustains chronic disease or the recurrence of more acute disorders. The miasmatic pattern manifests on physical, energetic, and mental/spiritual levels. As originally formulated by Hahnemann, there are three miasms: *psora, sycosis,* and *syphilis.*

Nadi [NAH-dee]. A pathway through which subtle energy moves. These channels radiate from or connect to the chakras.

Persona. The aspect of the personality that is presented to the world— the conscious and visible parts of the self.

Pitta [PIT-uh]. One of the three *dosha*s or dynamic factors in human functioning, as conceptualized in Ayurvedic medicine. It has to do with the fiery aspects of the human, and is central to digestion, intelligence, and transformation.

Potency. The degree to which a homeopathic preparation has been processed. Higher potencies are reckoned to be more capable of affecting the subtler levels of consciousness and spirit.

Prana [PRAH-nuh]. Subtle energy, the Indian equivalent of *ch'i* in the Chinese system.

Proving. A process of eliciting the symptoms that a substance will produce. The homeopathic method is based on careful (often double-blind) studies that collect such data. The symptom pictures that emerge for the substance are those for which it is prescribed.

Psoric [SO-rick]. Pertaining to the first or fundamental of the three miasms as described by Hahnemann.

Qi. An alternate spelling of *ch'i* (see above).

Qigong [chee-GUNG]. Generic term to denote a variety of Chinese techniques for controlling subtle energy (*qi* = energy, *gong* = control).

Repertory. The homeopathic reference book that lists remedies under symptom headings.

Sanskrit. Root language for most of Europe and South Asia. Sanskrit is to the Indo-European languages as Latin is to the Romance languages. Scholars have suggested that the basic sounds of Sanskrit bear a close intrinsic relationship to the objects, thoughts, and feelings that they stand for. Hence Sanskrit words are often used in meditation or healing (mantras), since the inherent effect of the sound would obtain even for those who don't know the language.

Shakti [SHOCK-tee]. Potential energy or power—usually identified with the feminine principle in the universe.

Shaman. From Tungusu-Manchurian *saman,* which means "to know." One who is skilled in accessing realities not apparent to ordinary people in order to communicate with conscious entities there and/or make adjustments that will result in healing on this plane.

Shiatsu [shee-AHT-soo]. A system of working with subtle energy and the meridians through pressure rather than with needles.

Shiva [SHEE-vuh]. A term with multiple meanings in Indian teachings, it sometimes refers to a specific deity, while at other times it is used to indicate the principle of consciousness usually associated with the masculine principle in the universe. It is considered the counterpart of *shakti,* the feminine energy or power. Both men and women are thought of as embodying both *shiva* and *shakti.*

Spanda [SPAHN-duh]. Tantric term indicating a core impulse or authentic urge to act. Distinguished from habit, unconsciously determined compulsive actions, and reflex, it has the qualities of being both effortless and at the same time voluntary, in that one has the freedom to not do it if he or she so chooses. It flows joyfully.

Sycotic [sy-KOTT-ik]. Of or pertaining to one of the three miasms described by Hahnemann. The prototypical manifestation of sycosis is gonorrhea, though, as a result of the widespread use of antibiotics, the disease is currently absent in most sycotic states.

Syphilitic. Of or pertaining to the most severe of the three miasms described by Hahnemann. The prototypical manifestation of this miasm is infectious syphilis, though it is not now ordinarily present, owing to the use of antibiotics.

Tantra [TAHN-truh]. A body of spiritual teachings that emphasize the involvement of the body and the evolutionary value of its energies and impulses. The Tantric tradition is the root of most of our concepts about chakras, and of much of our appreciation of the relationship of breath and energy to consciousness.

Tapas [TAHP-us]. A core technique in the transformative spiritual traditions that involves transmuting the energy of an impulse so that it will ignite a more illuminating consciousness.

Tridosha. The system of three *dosha*s or functional aspects of human life that provides the foundation for Ayurvedic thinking. The *dosha*s are derived from the Five Elements.

Trituration. A process of grinding (originally with a mortar and pestle) a substance in order to alter it so that it is more suitable for medicinal use.

Vata [VAH-tuh]. One of the three *dosha*s in the Ayurvedic system, *vata* is responsible for motion and is nearly synonymous with *vayu* or "wind." It is made up of the Elements of Air and Ether *(Akasha).*

Vayu [VAH-yoo]. Literally "wind." A very generic term that has entered many of the Indian traditions and disciplines, taking on a slightly different shade of meaning in each. In some contexts it simply means "energy flow." In others it takes on a more precise significance, especially when modified, as in *prana vayu,* a compound of two general terms, which refers to a specific upward-moving, nourishing current (see Chapter 10).

Vital force. The homeopaths' equivalent to the Asian concepts of *ch'i* or *prana.* It is this vital force or pattern of subtle energy that is thought to be the primary target of the action of the homeopathic remedy.

Yang. That which is active, light, and hot. It is usually identified with the masculine principle in the universe.

Yin. That which is receptive, dark, and cold. It is usually identified with the feminine principle in the universe.

Endnotes

When book citations in the Endnotes provide no publisher or date, full information on that book, along with a discussion of its contents, will be found in the Guide to Further Study, Chapter 14. The page on which those descriptions appear can be located by consulting the *General Index* under each author's surname.

Chapter 1

1. Wooster Beach, *The American Practice of Medicine* (New York: Betts and Anstice, 1833), quoted in Harris Coulter, *Divided Legacy: A History of the Schism in Medical Thought,* Vol III, page 88.
2. See Coulter, *Divided Legacy,* vol. 3, ch. 7.
3. In *A New Science of Life,* Rupert Sheldrake calls these *morphogenetic fields.* Edward Whitmont, in *Psyche and Substance,* discusses how this concept clarifies the actions of natural remedies. I have presented a very simplified version of the ground-breaking work of these two authors. (See also David Bohm, *Wholeness and the Implicate Order.*)
4. "Potency" here refers to the homeopathic preparation to be described in the coming chapter. I attribute the success in this case not only to the *Thuja,* which I am sure other homeopaths must have tried, but to several doses of *Sulphur,* also in high potency, given between the doses of *Thuja* on the advice of my teacher.
5. See the discussions of miasms in the next and following chapters. *Thuja* is one of the primary remedies for the *sycotic* miasm.
6. The use of natural remedies, especially homeopathic ones, in acute situations is a complex and challenging field in itself. In the nineteenth century, with no very effective alternatives available, it reached a high level of development. Unfortunately, little of that skill is available today, though I strongly suspect—and fervently hope—that we will recover it in years to come.

7. According to an April 1998 study in the *Journal of the American Medical Association,* adverse reactions to prescription drugs rank somewhere between fourth and sixth as the leading cause of death in the United States. In 1994, more than 100,000 people died from toxic reactions to prescribed medications *that were administered properly.*

8. More than *2 million* people in the United States suffered serious side effects from properly prescribed and administered medications in 1994, according to the study mentioned in the preceding note. (It was in that same year, or thereabouts, that a single case of a patient who developed serious liver disease from *improperly* using an herbal remedy received wide press coverage, and was cited as an indication of the dangers of herbal medicine.)

9. Each of these has been used in a much more reorganizing fashion as an herbal or homeopathic remedy.

10. The illness is seen most often in children under eighteen, but has also been reported in patients in their fifties and sixties. Fatality rates average 21 percent. Using salicylates during an acute flu can increase thirty-five times the odds of coming down with the condition. Because of this, the use of salicylates in persons under eighteen (except for a few specific ill-nesses) is now considered dangerous. (Information from *Merck Manual,* Sixteenth Edition, 1992.)

11. Was it really myrrh, or was it gugulu? Gugulu was from the East, while myrrh came from Africa. Still, it's hard to imagine the Christmas story reading "gold, frankincense, and gugulu."

12. For more on the connections between organs and emotions, see Kenneth Cohen, *The Way of Qi Gong: The Art and Science of Chinese Energy Healing* (New York: Ballantine Books, 1997), Chapter 14.

13. The most notable homeopath to embrace this concept was J. Compton Burnett, M.D., who took his lead from Rademacher. (See A. A. Ramseyer, *Rademacher's Universal and Organ Remedies,* Salt Lake City, 1909). Rademacher, in turn, writing in the mid-1800s, attributed the con-cept to Paracelsus, whence the quote.

14. I have generally tried to capitalize and italicize full scientific names of plants and designations of homeopathic remedies, while giving the com-mon names of herbs in plain type and lowercase. Unfortunately these distinctions are not always as clear as one might wish, since some plants are used in herbal tincture by many homeopaths under a name that is no longer recognized as a scientific term. *Chelidonium* is such a case. I have treated these individually, in whatever way seems least confusing.

15. See Chapter 8 for a description of the many factors that stress the liver.

16. A fuller listing of herbal heart tonics will include *Adonis vernalis, Scilla maritima, Spartium scoparium, Nerium oleander,* and *Strophanthus spp,* in addition to those listed in the text. Each can produce "miraculous" results when correctly matched to the case.

17. See E. Koch and A. Biber, "Pharmacological Effects of Sabal and Urtica Extracts as Basis for a Rational Medication of Benign Prostatic Hyperplasia," *Urologe* 34, no. 2 (1994), 90–95.

18. See also under "Prostate" in the Self-Help Index, Section V.

19. There are a number of lichens that are subsumed under the rubric *usnea.* Most have a hanging habit, like the "Spanish moss" seen in southern climes. See the booklet by Christopher Hobbs, *Usnea: The Herbal Antibiotic* (Capitola, Calif.: Botanica Press, 1990).

20. It has shown activity against staphylococcus, streptococcus, pneumococcus, and the mycobacterium of tuberculosis, as well as against the parasite trichomonas. A topical ointment made in Finland is used for athlete's foot and ringworm. See Hobbs, note 19, above.

21. See his book *Sacred Plant Medicine.*

22. Story adapted from Buhner, pages 131–32.

23. This was a strong cultural current through the Middle Ages in Europe, but was much diminished by the execution of many folk healers during the Inquisition.

24. The *Atharveda,* along with the *Rigveda,* the *Yajurveda,* and the *Samaveda,* constitute what may be the oldest known treatises on philosophy and spirituality.

25. There is much similarity and some overlap between the adaptogens of Chinese medicine and the rejuvenatives of Ayurveda.

Chapter 2

1. Because he considered the list complete, Dr. Schuessler concluded that these minerals were at the heart of human biochemical processes, and called his system "biochemistry," adding yet one more name by which the remedies are sometimes known: "biochemic salts."

2. In fact, the distinction is not so easily drawn. Though cell salts are not prescribed according to the rigorous empirical methodology of homeopathy, they are understood according to a more homeopathic than allopathic line of thought. *Ferrum phos* is iron—that which is responsible for the redness of blood or of red earth—and this is the salt we give for red, inflamed tissues. Moreover, many of the cell-salt compounds, such as

Calcarea fluor and *Natrum mur,* are also used in homeopathy in much higher potencies, though they are chosen in a different way from that used to select remedies in the cell-salt system.

3. For example, of one hundred patients who, according to autopsy, had died of heart attacks, 47 percent had been misdiagnosed. Another study showed that radiologists at Harvard disagreed on the interpretation of chest X rays as much as 56 percent of the time. For a summary of research on this topic, see *Medicine on Trial,* by Inlander, Levin, and Weiner.

4. J. Kleijnen et al., Clinical trials of homeopathy. *British Medical Journal* 302: 316–23, 1991.

5. This is such a strong hallmark of the remedy that in years to come homeopaths would call the *Bryonia* patient "the bear"—leave him alone when he's hibernating, or you'll be sorry!

6. Data quoted from Dr. Dorothy Shepherd, "The Action of the Miminum Dose in Acute Epidemics," in *Magic of the Minimum Dose.*

7. Now a larger group of homeopaths in Germany reported mortality rates in the range of 5–15 percent, while conventional physicians were losing 42 percent of those treated in hospital and 56 percent of those cared for at home. When the regular doctors expressed doubt about these results, one homeopath brought forward 112 officially accredited testimonies for his 148 recovered patients—many of them prominent citizens and clergymen. See Richard Haehl, M.D., *Samuel Hahnemann, His Life and Work, Based on Recently Discovered State Papers, Documents and Letters* vol. 1, reprint of 1922 edition (New Delhi: B. Jain).

8. Dorothy Shepherd, "The Action of the Minimum Dose," cited above, page 13.

9. For an up-to-date summary, see *Homeopathy: A Frontier in Medical Science,* Bellavite and Signorini.

10. Of course, as the previous chapter implies, even the herbal remedy will work best when it's more accurately fitted to the complex, multilevel nature of the person being treated.

11. Classical homeopaths will complain that such remedies can "mix up the case," shifting the symptoms so that it is more difficult to find the correct, deeper-acting remedy. While there is truth in that, my sense is that the confusion is usually short-lived, and if we wait awhile, the less superficial symptoms will generally settle back into the original pattern.

12. According to Hahnemann, suppressive treatment distorts and magnifies miasms so they become both compounded and harder to recognize.

13. Of the three miasms, *psora* was the last to be described by Hahnemann. He relates that it took him many years to discern its presence. Yet he considered it the foundation that made the other two possible. We might hypothesize that it was the most difficult for him to see because it was so close to what was accepted as normal. He did not present the other two as stages of a process, as I have done in this book, but he did consider *syphilis* the most destructive. On this basis, and because it corresponds to nearly universal spiritual teachings, I have adopted this sequential model.

14. The concepts of psychoanalysis (or of Jungian analytic psychology) come the closest, but they approach this domain from a very different angle and generally accept a certain degree of what Hahnemann considered miasmatic as normal socialization. They are not, in any case, tied to medicinals that can efficaciously address those issues, as is miasmatic homeopathy.

Chapter 3

1. This is beginning to change. Information on recent research on the flower essences can be obtained by calling the Flower Essence Society at 800-548-0075.

2. See the *Flower Essence Repertory* by Patricia Kaminski and Richard Katz.

3. This and other descriptions of the California essences in this book come from *Flower Essence Repertory,* cited above.

4. Also sold under such names as "Five-Flower Formula" and "Nature's Rescue."

5. The work of J. Compton Burnett, M.D., in the late 1800s, was often quoted by my teacher as a model of multilevel therapeutics—using herbal tinctures to address dysfunctions of specific organs even as he used high-potency homeopathics to reorganize in a more global fashion. His many monographs on the treatment of various conditions ("Liver," "Enlarged Tonsils," "Stunted Children," etc.) can still be profitably studied by the holistic practitioner of homeopathy.

Chapter 4

1. From a spiritual point of view, healing is establishing union with the universal, but, as we will see later, that involves *transcending* the ego rather than indulging its regressive fantasies. The similarities and differences between pre-ego and post-ego states of fusion or unity are the subject of much confusion and debate in current discourse. See my

(coauthored) earlier book *Yoga and Psychotherapy,* and Swami Ajaya, *Psychotherapy East and West: A Unifying Paradigm.*

2. See the Yoga Sutras of Patanjali, Book 3. On this point I especially recommend the commentary by Swami Hariharananda Aranya, published as *Yoga Philosophy of Patanjali* (University of Calcutta, 1963).

3. See Chapter 7, pages 252–55. I might have used this test for Matthew, to pinpoint foods he might have developed sensitivities to, but for its considerable expense.

4. Dualistic schools of Eastern philosophy attribute causality to both matter and consciousness, but in general, Eastern thought leans toward consciousness as the ultimate cause.

5. See the accounts of Swami Rama's experiments at the Menninger Foundation, described in Chapter 6.

6. See Chapter 2, page 74, and note 4.

7. See Virginia Livingston, M.D. (later Virginia Livingston Wheeler), "Some Cultural, Immunological, and Biochemical Properties of Progenitor Cryptocides," *Trans NY Acad Sci* 36 (1974), 569–82. (See also Section V, New Microbiology, pages 552–4.)

8. See Thomas McPherson Brown, M.D., *The Road Back* (1988), republished and updated as *The Arthritis Breakthrough* (New York: M. Evans and Co., 1993).

9. In a variety of other diseases not usually considered infectious, such as Crohn's disease and sarcoidosis, microbial growth has been identified. See Lida Mattman, *Cell Wall Deficient Forms*, and Gerald Domingue, ed., *Cell Wall-Deficient Bacteria: Basic Principles and Clinical Significance.* To some extent the work cited here, organized around the concept that there are bacterial forms that do not possess the usual cell wall, has been superseded by the rediscovery of the work of Enderlein (see Chapter 8), which puts the matter of "infection" in a larger context. Enderlein's work was a forerunner of that which sees cellular components as combining and recombining in a variety of ways to create a spectrum of functional units—some of which we consider "normal" and others "pathogenic microbes." This more-holographic perspective could revolutionize much of our thinking about disease and the microorganisms associated with it. Mainstream science does not take easily to such major overhauls, however. For example, Lynn Margulis's suggestion that the mitochondrion is an ancient bacterium, recruited eons ago to function symbiotically with our evolving cells (*Science* 252 [1991], 378–81) has met with staunch resistance.

10. It would be more correct to say "a set of energetic derangements that have something in common." Thus there are a number of homeopathic remedies, each representing a somewhat different energetic pattern, that can be used for a specific disease.

Chapter 5

1. Modern techniques have also been developed. Perhaps the most sophisticated and highly evolved system is that originated by Joseph Scogna, which involves an infrared scan of the face. Based on the intensity of blood flow to twenty-three specific areas, computerized correlations with corresponding sets of organs and mental and emotional traits yields a complex personality inventory. After many hours of psychological counseling based on this scan, I was impressed by the profound insights into the relationship between my own bodily functions and psychological and emotional issues that emerged.

2. The right side of the body corresponds to the left half of the brain. The characteristics we mention here are those associated with "left brain" function. Conversely, the left side of the body relates to the right half of the brain.

3. Proceso Sanchez Ortega has classified various malignant conditions by the degree to which each of the three miasms dominates them—those with a preponderance of sycosis showing more proliferation and less invasiveness, those where syphilis is dominant being the most aggressive and destructive. (See his *Notes on the Miasms.*)

4. This relates to the concept of the Five Elements. In Chapter 6 we will see which shapes relate to each Element.

5. Vega Testing, for example, sends a mild electric current through the acupuncture meridian. Abnormal drops in voltage are considered indications of a weakness in the associated organs.

Chapter 6

1. Though there are many schools of Indian philosophy and many variants on their application, my training was based primarily on that which is known as Tantra. Compared to the original Vedas, Tantra represents a later development that extended spiritual practice into the realms of emotion and the body. Free of the caste restrictions of the older tradition and more identified with a reverence for the feminine principle, it was very attuned to the matter of subtle energy. The system of chakras, which will be introduced in this chapter, was largely a product of the

Tantrists. It alone, among the Indian traditions, boldly incorporated the sphere of sexuality into its transformational work. For all these reasons, the Tantric teachings provide an excellent foundation for an integrated approach to healing. (For more detail on the origin and nature of this body of knowledge, see M. P. Pandit, *Lights on the Tantra* [Madras: Ganesh & Co., 1971]).

2. See Doug Boyd, *Swami* (New York: Random House, 1976).

3. Usually the "control cycle" is depicted by the inner arrows and the "generation cycle" by the circle. I have reversed this so the elements can appear in the same order clockwise as they are described in the Tantric writing.

4. Note that the heart is linked to the Element of Fire in the Chinese system, while it is the focus of the fourth chakra and Air Element in the Indian Tantric tradition. The aptness of both these connections is evidenced by the heart's anatomical position—it lies against the diaphragm, which separates the domains of the third (Fire) and fourth (Air or Metal) chakras. Functionally it is both the relayer of energy (oxygen and nutrients) as is emphasized by its connection to Fire, as well as a constant depiction of taking in and releasing—which is the nature of Metal. Its endless giving is also the essence of the compassion associated with the fourth or heart chakra. (See the *Triadic Heart of Shiva* by Paul Eduardo Muller-Ortega, SUNY Press, 1989.) In sum, this apparent contradiction between the two systems is a reflection of the complexity of the human being, and a source of rich detail, with, again, the two traditions providing complementary insights.

5. Fig. 42 indicates that compassion is the emotion associated with the Element of Earth in the Chinese system. The emphasis there is that groundedness is required to be capable of compassion. The Indian tradition instead acknowledges that the compassion is felt in the heart area. This difference points up the distinct stresses of the two perspectives—the Indian organized more around a regional approach (each chakra relating to an area of the body) and the Chinese designed to establish a network of functional components that may be scattered anatomically throughout.

6. See Caroline Myss, *Anatomy of the Spirit* for an excellent discussion of the first chakra and this issue.

7. This is called "Kidney Yin" in Traditional Chinese Medicine, and it is important to note that remedies for that condition will change the associated energies and attitudes as well as strengthening reproductive function. (See the Self-Help Index, under "Infertility.")

8. I am indebted to David Coulter, Ph.D., who co-led workshops with me on Five Element thinking over the course of many years, and helped me immensely in my struggle to understand the common ground between the Chinese and Indian approaches.

9. Metal also relates to the large intestine—but the more hierarchical, vertically regional focus of the chakra perspective ignores this connection. However, the Ayurvedic system, derived, in a sense, from the tantric Five Elements, does connect both lung and large intestine to *vata,* which emcompasses Air and Ether.

10. Actually, the Taoist tradition has a well-developed understanding of the chakras. Though its influence is felt in some aspects of Chinese Medicine, that does not include the Chinese Five Element system.

11. This is a necessarily brief treatment of the relationship of taste to the Five Elements, and focuses on the Ayurvedic concept. The Chinese version is different and provides a valuable complementarity. See Paul Pitchford, *Healing with Whole Foods: Oriental Traditions and Modern Nutrition,* pages 268–76, for a knowledgeable presentation of the Chinese concept of taste and the Elements.

12. See Robert Svoboda's *Prakruti* for a poetic rendering of Ayurvedic taste psychology.

13. See Robert Eliot, M.D., *Is It Worth Dying For?* (New York: Bantam Books, 1989), which describes the "hot reactor" type.

Chapter 7

1. *Diet and Nutrition: A Holistic Approach* (1978) and *Transition to Vegetarianism* (1987).

2. Ballentine, *Diet and Nutrition.*

3. For more information on the politics and economics of meat consumption, see *Diet for a New America* (Walpole, N.H., Stillpoint Publishing, 1987).

4. Ballentine, *Transition to Vegetarianism.*

5. I feel uncertain about the safety of conventionally raised poultry and livestock, since the practice of adding the unused portions of the carcass to the feed of the same animals has become commonplace. The transmission of serious neurological degenerative diseases has been known to occur in such situations. For a balanced and factual treatment of this important issue, see *Mad Cow USA: Could the Nightmare Happen Here?* by Sheldon Rampton and John Stauber.

6. See Peter D'Adamo, *Eat Right for Your Type* (New York: Putnam, 1996). Over many years of clinical work, D'Adamo and his father observed a

correlation between blood type and food intolerances. His thesis is that the lectins of food interact with the cells of your blood to produce clumping and destruction. It will be interesting to see what light food sensitivity testing will throw on this. (See also note 17 for this chapter, below.)

7. This does not mean the impulse was indulged indiscriminately. The ritual act was carried out in a space dedicated to consciousness rather than to mere gratification of impulses. The Tantrists felt it was necessary to "own" that darker part of our individual and collective psyche in order to avoid projecting it. Owning it allows us to move to a point internally from which we can choose not to act on it, but feel instead a clear desire to step around it and let it fade.

8. For a concise guide to the challenges of each of these phases and how to shift back and forth skillfully among them, see Ballentine, *Transition to Vegetarianism.*

9. Ballentine, *Diet and Nutrition,* pages 264–65.

10. Ballentine, *Diet and Nutrition,* pages 95–96, and *Transition to Vegetarianism,* 221–25.

11. Contrary to popular belief, the more unsaturated oils such as safflower or canola may be more problematic because they promote free-radical formation. See Ballentine, *Transition to Vegetarianism,* pages 212–21. Moreover, canola oil is made from a variant of the rapeseed, which contains a toxic substance called erucic acid. Though it has lower levels of the compound than the parent rapeseed, I have not seen convincing evidence of its safety.

12. See Ballentine, *Transition to Vegetarianism.*

13. For a concise explanation of the role of free radicals in disease and the influence of diet, as well as the benefits of butterfat, see Ballentine, *Transition to Vegetarianism,* pages 212–26.

14. This has been traced out in lyric detail in Chapter 4 of *Prakruti, Your Ayurvedic Constitution* by Robert Svoboda.

15. This is an area where research is spotty. This paragraph is more of a summary of my conclusions on the subject than a summary of published findings. For some of the more important data on which it's based, see *Diet and Nutrition,* pages 333–65.

16. This is a controversial subject. Conventional medical thinking runs along the lines I have suggested here. Yet oral enzymes (for bruising), or hormones—both of which are large protein molecules—are routinely administered and apparently absorbed intact. Moreover, some nutritional therapists feel that food enzymes are absorbed and play a vital role

in nutrition. It seems likely that enzyme uptake is accomplished "intentionally" through pinocytosis, while the infiltration of undigested proteins that trigger immune reactions is the involuntary result of a damaged barrier. See W. A. Walker, M.D., "Role of the Mucosal Barrier in Antigen Handling by the Gut," in Brostoff and Challacanke, eds., *Food Allergy and Intolerance* (London/Philadelphia: Balliere Tyndell/W.B. Saunders, 1987).

17. *Lectins* are the compounds often responsible. They are *glycoproteins*—combinations of carbohydrate and protein molecules which bind to cell surfaces. Some of these, for example, will clump red blood cells and are specific to a blood type. (Hence dietary guidelines by blood type.) Others bind to the cells lining the gut, and can cause damage there. Beans and peas are particularly rich in lectins, but cooking or sprouting them reduces their lectin content markedly.

18. Enzyme-linked immuno-sorbent assay/Advanced Cell Test is what he calls his procedure. It measures all delayed sensitivities. The classic allergic reactions, which come on immediately, are picked up by a different test (RAST), but are often so obvious, since their onset is directly after taking in the food, that testing is unnecessary. On the other hand, delayed reactions, which may begin up to forty-eight hours later, are much more difficult to identify without testing.

19. See Anne Marie Colbin, *Food and Healing,* pages 86–87, and *Natural Gourmet* (Ballantine Books, 1989).

20. See *Food and Healing,* pages 63–73. Classic Chinese philosophy and medicine conceptualized the yin as that which was cool, moist, dark, and earthy. This was the feminine principle, and its tendency was to pull in, gather together, build a home, a group, a family. This is the contractive end of the polarity. Yang, the opposite pole, was warm, dry, light, and expansive. Its tendency was to move out, to search and explore. This is the version of yin/yang thought that has come to us through the practitioners of Traditional Chinese Medicine (TCM). Sakurazawa Nyoiti, a Japanese scholar, picked up the term *macrobiotics* from a German physician who combined the Greek *macro* (large or long) and *bios* (life), to convey a sense similar to that of the term *Ayurveda* (which is most accurately translated as "the science of longevity"). Nyoiti, who came to be known as George Ohsawa in the West, taught principles of healthful, spiritually oriented living, and his followers in the United States and Europe established one of the first waves of health-food stores, restaurants, and healing centers. But

Ohsawa altered the basic conceptual scheme of classic Oriental philosophy in one important way. Perhaps feeling that westerners were more focused on the material than the spiritual, he reversed the traditional scheme, and made the Earth the creative yang force and heaven its passive receptive yin counterpart. So, in macrobiotic terms, yin is expansive while in TCM yin is contractive.

21. There is a relationship between the two systems. The *vatic* mind tends to be restless like the *rajasic* state about to be described, and the *kaphic* person will bear some resemblance to *tamas*. But the *pittic* person is also often *rajasic,* or hyperactive, and though the *sattvic* state is transformative, it would be hard to equate with a *pittic* picture.

22. This is an oversimplification, since there is a subtle aspect to the Earth Element as there are grosser aspects to Air or even Ether.

23. This threefold classification of foods and other factors that affect consciousness is called *triguna.*

Chapter 8

1. Most of the data in this discussion comes from *Our Stolen Future: Are We Threatening Our Fertility, Intelligence, and Survival?—A Scientific Detective Story* by Theo Colborn, Dianne Dumanoski, and John Peterson Myers.

2. See my book *Transition to Vegetarianism,* pages 161–64.

3. The toxicity of chemicals and heavy metals is compounded by the presence of solvent residues in our foods. Solvents gravitate toward fats and oils, combining with the lipid membranes of cells and subcellular organelles, and cripple their ability to bring in what is needed or to keep out toxic substances and microbes.

4. This data also comes from Colborn et al., *Our Stolen Future.*

5. I usually start with an iodine preparation, such as *Atomidine,* a drop a day in a glass of water, five days on, five off, or homeopathic thyroid triturates—3x or 6x. If there is no substantial improvement in basal body temperature with these, I'll move to thyroid glandular preparations that have the hormone removed. They should support the strengthening and rebuilding of your own thyroid gland. If that fails, I resort to an animal thyroid preparation. Of course, psychological and spiritual aspects of thyroid function cannot be overlooked.

6. Some writers associate the pineal with the crown, or seventh, chakra and the pituitary with the sixth, though most follow the reverse, which is what I was taught.

7. Most writings on Ayurveda in English have transliterated the Sanskrit word as *ama*. Since the two vowel sounds are represented in Devanagri with two different letters, and since the usual transliteration leads to so many mispronunciations, I have chosen to use a more phonetic spelling.

8. See Chapter 7, pages 250–55.

9. Some researchers have suggested that certain incompletely digested food proteins entering through a "leaky gut" are similar enough to body proteins to result in a cross-reaction in which the antibodies stimulated by the food then attack the body's own tissues. This is in keeping with Ayurvedic contentions that the gut is the source of such problems, and that the source of the substance clogging tissues in autoimmune diseases is incomplete assimilation.

10. Though I have tried to distinguish between wastes that are of exogenous origin and those that are generated internally, distinctions blur. *Aama* is generally considered to be internally generated, but its production is thought of as a result of poor assimilation of food. Poor quality food is more difficult to incorporate and tends to yield *aama*—in this case an accumulation the origin of which would be hard to categorize clearly as either external or internal.

11. The rationale for this is described in detail in Patrick and Gael Crystal Flanagan, *Elixir of the Ageless: You Are What You Drink*.

12. See Lynn Toohey, Ph.D., and Sylvia Kreutle, M.S., *Detox and the Leaky Gut Connection* (Fort Collins, Colo.: Healthquest, Inc., 1997).

13. Clinicians and serious students will want to review carefully Helmut Schimmel and Victor Penzer, *Functional Medicine,* vol. 1, *The Origin and Treatment of Chronic Diseases* (Haug, 1996), especially pages 226–31.

14. For more on how the connective tissue spaces play a key role in the storage of "dross" and the development of chronic disease, see *Homotoxicology: The Core of a Probiotic and Holistic Approach to Medicine,* by Claus-F. Claussen, M.D.

15. See *Matrix and Matrix Regulation: Basis for a Holistic Theory in Medicine,* by Alfred Pischinger, M.D., edited by H. Heine, Ph.D., Ed.

16. A naturopathic perspective on this as it relates to cleansing is summarized in a little booklet, *The Colon Health Handbook,* by Robert Gray.

17. The importance of the blotting brush cannot be overemphasized. It was developed by a Dr. Shipley, who still supplies it. (See page 572.)

18. Dr. Schimmel, in Germany, using electroacupuncture diagnostic techniques, has traced what he calls "causal chains" that seem to connect the various common foci of disease in a network of mutual irritation and

inflammation. Most often involved are the liver, pancreas, kidneys, and sinuses. The pancreas is often stressed by the refined carbohydrates in the diet, as well as by emotional factors. The bile ducts of the liver are thought to be irritated by the saturation of the bile with toxic substances. Dr. Schimmel has suggested that when the energy imbalances resulting from the irritation and stress of these two key organs is shifted to the cranial mucous membranes along the meridian network (the energy channels that run through the connective-tissue matrix) the result is an irritation, then an inflammation of organs there. The end result is sinusitis, recurrent tonsillitis, gingivitis, and/or otitis media. Most common is sinusitis. If you look back at the diagram of the meridians and the face, you will see that many of these energy channels end in the vicinity of the sinuses. This may be one of the factors making sinusitis so common. (See *Functional Medicine*, cited in note 13.)

19. See Robert Svoboda, *Prakruti: Your Ayurvedic Constitution*. It may be helpful, in the effort to understand problems such as schizophrenia, to transpose this mechanism to the psychic level. (See Winifred Lucas *Regression Therapy*, chapters on spirit release work: "depossession.")

20. See the works of Mattman, Livingston, et al., cited in Chapter 4, note 9.

21. See G. Enderlein, *Bakterien-Cyclogenie*.

22. BEV, or BioElectronic Vincent, is a technique developed by French professor Louis-Claude Vincent in Lebanon and later elaborated in Germany by Franz Morell and others, where it has attracted increasing attention as a valuable tool in medicine.

23. This is an excellent example of how reductionistic technology tends to support holistic perspectives. Unfortunately, as of this writing, little is available in English on this remarkable work other than the spiral-bound translation of a brief German introduction by Helmut Elmau, M.D., *Bioelectronics According to Vincent and the Acid-Base Balance in Theory and Practice* (London: East Asia Co., 1987, [101–103 Camden High Street, London NW1 7JN, England]).

24. See Fig. 5, Chapter 1, and the Self-Help Index in Section V for details on dosage, etc.

25. Skin brushes are available in most health-food stores. The skin should be brushed in long strokes, toward the heart, covering the whole surface of the body, for a total of about five minutes, once a day. First thing in the morning is the ideal time.

26. The other two classic modalities were bloodletting and nasal stimulants intended to cause sneezing. I suspect their falling out of favor is less a result of their merit than of the prevailing Western attitudes toward them.

27. There is a set of cleansing techniques in the yoga tradition that parallels those of *panchakarma*. The yogic versions are less invasive, but require more voluntary control. Just as the stomach wash is the yogic equivalent of the Ayurvedic emetic, there is a colon cleanse *(vasti)* done by the yogis that involves squatting in water and, through control of abdominal muscles, drawing it up into the bowel to cleanse it. While most people can easily learn the process of throwing up, this yogic colon cleanse is impractical, so I've stuck with the enema for that purpose.

28. The volume of data amassed on the effectiveness of this technique suggests that it will soon be adopted by conventional cardiologists. For concise information, see *Questions from the Heart: Answers to 100 Questions About Chelation Therapy, a Safe Alternative to Bypass Surgery,* by Terry Chappell, MD., 1995.

29. See Peter R. Rothschild, M.D., Ph.D., *Enzyme Therapy in Immune Complex and Free Radical Contingent Diseases,* University Labs Press, (Honolulu: 1988, pamphlet).

30. Fasting depletes glutathione, one of the major conjugating agents which removes the damaging products of Phase I detoxification pathways. Reduced glutathione or precursors of glutathione can be added to a fresh fruit and vegetable and/or juice regimen to support Phase II clearing of toxic intermediates. (See note 31 below.) Proanthocyanidins (60–120 mg, 1–3 times a day) are also a powerful adjunct. (See note 32 below.)

31. N-acetyl cysteine, L-cysteine, and L-glutamine are glutathione precursors. L-cysteine is thought to have some toxic potential. N-acetyl cysteine is most commonly used to boost glutathione levels. Methionine, taurine, and glycine support other conjugation reactions.

32. Marketed as Pycnogenol or "PCO's." A number of such preparations are on the market. For once, proprietary claims that one delivery system (to enhance absorption) is superior seem to be true of a brand called Kaire, though new products are being developed constantly.

33. These four humors were probably derived from the earlier, neighboring Ayurvedic tradition, and also correspond to the elements of Earth, Fire, Water, and Air.

34. For more on the Greek school and its concept of the healing crisis, see Harris Coulter, *Divided Legacy, Vol IV.*

35. See note 14 above.

36. Such a perspective is more implied than explicit in Ayurvedic medicine as it is practiced currently. Its expression is clearer in the related traditions, such as Tantra, which diverged as Ayurveda became more medical and less spiritual.

37. In the story, which I have abbreviated, there were four stones (which are sprinkled four times). In Native American cosmology this is customarily a reference to the four cardinal points on the compass, representing four Elements, Earth, Water, Fire, and Wind here (Wind, like *Vata*, subsumes both the Air and Ether of the Vedic schema). The story suggests, then, that these Elements are required to reconstitute a life.

38. This story and the information in this passage come from Joseph Bruchac, *The Native American Sweat Lodge: History and Legends* (Freedom, Calif.: The Crossing Press, 1993).

Chapter 9

1. Throughout this book, I have referred to this as Tantra, but a more precise source of the thought represented by this particular discussion is Shaivism—specifically Kashmiri Shaivism, the system that formalized most eloquently such perspectives on healing and spiritual evolution. Technically, a distinction can be made between Tantra and Shaivism, but there are so many schools and offshoots and interminglings that such fine distinctions are often of little practical importance.

2. For a clear explication of *spanda* and its Tantric context, see Kamalakar Mishra, *Significance of the Tantric Tradition* (Varanasi, India: Arddhanarisvara Publications, 1981). As noted there, sometimes the term *kriya* is used synonymously with *spanda*. *Kriya* also carries connotations of cleansing and purifying—removing the obstacles to inspired action. Hence the connection between the process of detoxification as outlined in the preceding chapter, and the issue of authentic movement as presented here.

3. See Mary Bond, *Balancing Your Body: A Self-Help Approach to Rolfing Movement* (Rochester, Vt.: Healing Arts Press, 1993).

4. An outstanding guidebook to the burgeoning spectrum of body-oriented therapies available is Mirka Knaster's *Discovering the Body's Wisdom: A Comprehensive Guide to More Than Fifty Mind-Body Practices That Can Relieve Pain, Reduce Stress, and Foster Health, Spiritual Growth, and Inner Peace*.

5. Some of these insights are taken from the classic book by Ron Kurtz and Hector Prestera, M.D., *The Body Reveals: An Illustrated Guide to the Psychology of the Body*.

6. I am greatly indebted for this understanding to the remarkable book by Meir Schneider, *Self-Healing: My Life and Vision*. Especially persons dealing with arthritis, MS, MD, or visual problems should read this.

7. The armored fishes, or placoderms, are now considered to have been an evolutionary dead end, but heavy scales and other dermal elements in their cousins are thought to have given rise to the shoulder girdle of

mammals, including man. The bones of the skull are also thought to have originated in external plates.

8. In 1975, Horace Dobbs, a former Fellow of England's Royal Society of Medicine and a medical researcher, began the first experiments with using contact with dolphins as a therapy for depression. Today the center of activity in the field is the Florida Keys, the largest program being headquartered in Grassy Key. See David Nathanson, Ph.D., "Long Term Effects of Dolphin Assisted Therapy for Children with Severe Disabilities," *Anthrozoos* 11(1), 1998, pages 22–32.

9. In contrast to the shoulder girdle, the hip girdle and lower extremities are derived entirely from endoskeletal elements.

10. See *Encounters With Qi* by David Eisenberg, M.D., a fascinating and entertaining account of a Western physician who discovers the power of energy in China.

11. See Swami Rama, *Joints and Glands Exercises* for a fuller description of these simple exercises.

12. See *A Practical Guide to Holistic Health* by Swami Rama, Chapter 4, for more details.

13. See John Ott, *Health and Light: The Effects of Natural and Artificial Light on Man and Other Living Things* (New York: Pocket Books, 1973). This book, first published twenty-five years ago, is a classic.

14. Though Gandhi was no authority on matters of health, his views on the subject, like his others, are appealing because of their simplicity and spiritual grounding. My quotes in this chapter come from a small volume of his essays titled *The Health Guide,* published posthumously.

Chapter 10

1. See Ernest Lawrence Rossi, "Altered States of Consciousness in Everyday Life: The Ultradian Rhythms," in *Handbook of States of Consciousness,* edited by Wolman and Ullman (New York: Van Nostrand Reinhold, 1986).

2. The right brain controls the left side of the body and is activated by breathing with the nostril on the left side. The right hand is most often the "active"—that used preferentially to act in the world.

3. Though there is evidence to support this, the observations are based primarily on my own clinical experience.

4. I might never have got it right, had it not been for the work of Jere Mead. See *American Review of Respiratory Disease 119*(2), February 1979 (Supplement) pages 31-32.

5. Another translation of *vayu* is "wind." This carries a sense similar to that of the word *vata*. Wind is the prototype of sweeping currents of subtle energy.

6. This is not to imply that the *hara* and solar plexus are identical. The *hara* is generally located somewhat lower than the third chakra, and seems to be an experiential "center of gravity" for the collective energy of the lower three chakras.

7. Some current writers speak of *udana vayu* as playing the additional role of moving energy up to activate higher consciousness. In my training, the current called *udana* had a more forward and outward motion, tending more toward vocalization and manifestation in the world and less toward activation of centers higher up the axis. That latter function was more related to *prana vayu*. This perspective is also in line with my own experience (or perhaps it is more correct to say that I have organized my experience along those lines).

8. Some traditions term this the "etheric body"; it's subtler than the physical, but very closely related to it. Ted Kaptchuk, in *The Web that Has No Weaver,* suggests that *qi* (*ch'i*) might best be understood as "matter on the verge of becoming energy or energy at the point of materializing."

9. I regret that in order to present a manageable integration, I must sometimes set aside the intriguing complexities that emerge during the comparison of systems. Motoyama, in his thought-provoking book *Theories of the Chakras,* goes through a very knowledgeable and systematic comparison of the *nadis* and the meridians. His work suggests that there are overlaps. For example, there seems to be a close correspondence between the central *nadi,* called *sushumna,* and the "governor vessel," the midline, unpaired, "extraordinary" meridian that is said to govern the six yang meridians. He also thinks that the *yashasvini nadi,* on the right, and the *hastijhiva,* on the left, correspond to the first lines of the urinary bladder meridian and the *pusha* (right) and *ghandhari* (left) to the third. The second lines he likens to *ida* and *pingala*.

10. This includes practitioners trained in the schools of Arnie Mindell, Ilana Rubenfeld, or Dale Cummings (Radix).

11. Caroline Myss's books and tapes are especially helpful in understanding the dynamics of this first center.

12. Sexual energy and the urge to urinate are different. A buildup of wastes in the body creates a pressure for *apana vayu* to flow, which can add to the urgency of urination and be confused with sexual arousal and responded to as a need for sexual release. When a free flow of energy currents is

allowed to expel wastes and negativity regularly through the full and healthy action of *apana vayu,* the more positive sexual energy remains and can be encouraged to move upward as the central *nadi* is opened.

13. An Eastern paradigm would hold that at some theoretical extreme of human perfection, consciousness could easily counter and correct anything that happened on the physical level—but until that point is reached, a neglected body can interfere with the very processes that would make movement toward such perfection possible.

14. See her book *Light Emerging: The Journey of Personal Healing,* pages 266–67.

Chapter 11

1. For a contemporary examination of this complex subject, see *Tapta Marga: Asceticism and Initiation in Vedic India,* by Walter Kaelber.

2. Contemporary students of yoga may find this concept of *tapas* contrary to the more conservative emphasis on control which they have been exposed to. At the other extreme are those who see it as suppressive. The way I understand it, *tapas* is neither, because it leads to a purified (if sometimes socially disruptive) spontaneity.

3. Indian psychology differs from Western in that it attributes to the senses the ability to expend energy. In fact, the term *indriya* includes both the organs of action and the five sensory organs. From this perspective, contact with the world through the sense organs is draining of energy.

4. This is what Genia Pauli Haddon has called the *yang feminine.* She distinguishes it from the more socially condoned *yin* version, which is purely receptive and nurturing. See her book *Uniting Sex, Self and Spirit.*

5. From the perspective of the contemporary phallic masculine consciousness, coming into the body, experiencing its sensations and feelings, is a feminine act. Phallic sexuality at its most limited confines sensation to the penis (or perhaps to the clitoris, in the case of a woman who is operating from this consciousness).

   In many if not most contemporary societies, men lose status by expressing emotions or allowing compassion to rule their actions—behaviors considered feminine. Much of this behavior, activated by the left breath and related to the heart, is suppressed and probably contributes to the high incidence of heart disease. The man instead immerses himself in a rigid, linear consciousness that must deny the intuitive and the receptive.

6. See Haddon, *Uniting Sex, Self and Spirit.*

7. See Mantak Chia and Michael Winn, *Taoist Secrets of Love: Cultivating Male Sexual Energy* and Mantak Chia and Maneewan Chia, *Healing Love Through the Tao: Cultivating Female Sexual Energy.*

8. Of course, contemporary Western writers often use the term *mind* to refer to the totality of consciousness. I am not following that convention, but aiming for a sharp distinction between mind as a limited segment or field of consciousness, and the larger, more encompassing awareness that can embrace it. (See the next chapter for further clarification.)

9. Indian psychology deals with the question of identity very flexibly. *Ahankara* is a term that means "I-ness" and can extend from the sense of self "experienced" by an inanimate object, through the ego identities of the human, all the way to the union with a cosmic, universal Self. See *Yoga and Psychotherapy: The Evolution of Consciousness* by Swami Rama, Rudolph Ballentine, and Swami Ajaya, especially pages 86–94.

10. The sound *so* is an Indo-European root for "that above" while *hum* is related to the roots for *man* and *human.* The sense of the mantra is "as above, so below," or "let me connect the Spirit with the individual man-ifestation." Unlike many mantras that should be individualized, it is appropriate for anyone.

11. For an extensive treatment of this question, see A. H. Almaas, *The Pearl Beyond Price, Integration of Personality into Being: An Object Relations Approach* (Berkeley, Calif.: Diamond Books, 1988). Certainly Indian culture is organized around the idea that nonmonastic life is also a spir-itual path, and such a life was broken down into stages or *ashramas,* moving from childhood and *brahmacharya* to householder, withdrawal to a hermitage, and finally renunciation or *sanyasin.* Even in the West, Judaism has leaned in the same direction, and the more mystical of its traditions have insisted that "living with intense consciousness" can contribute to spiritual progress. See *Mitzvot as Spiritual Practices: A Jewish Guidebook for the Soul* by Esther G. Chasin. Still, it is probably correct to say that in much of the secular West, this attitude has been relatively uncommon.

12. Perhaps the free movement of consciousness, as it shifts more and more rapidly back and forth between—and gradually subsumes—both poles, sets up an accelerating vibration that shatters the structure. If so, zapping a few widely accepted constructs this way just might convince you that our "reality" is, as the yogis put it, merely *maya* or illusion.

13. For a profound analysis of psychotherapy from the holistic perspective, see *Psychotherapy East and West: A Unifying Paradigm,* by Swami Ajaya.

Chapter 12

1. A gathering of Native American, Maori, and Laplander elders with researchers and scientists took place on the Yankton Sioux Reservation in South Dakota in June 1996. Two accounts of this meeting, one by Brian Crissey, Ph.D., and the other by Richard Boylan, Ph.D., appeared in *Sedona, Journal of Emergence,* in November 1996.

2. I am following here the perspective of Genia Pauli Haddon (see Chapter 11, n. 4), who maintains that the pre-patriarchal societies should not be termed *matriarchal,* as they usually are, since even when dominated by women, they were not hierarchical, but tended to operate more as a circle of equal participants. She prefers the term *matrical,* from the same root as *matrix* (uterus).

3. The Eastern traditions do not always emphasize this aspect of experience, but the Vedic term *jivatma* is what corresponds to the Western "soul."

4. If you feel that I have mixed the developmental with the adult, and the physiological with personal and social evolution, you're right. There is a consensus, at least among biologists and developmental psychologists, that "ontogeny recapitulates phylogeny," i.e., that during our individual development we relive the stages that the race as a whole has gone through. For example, the human embryo exhibits gills at earlier stages of gestation, and later loses them. I have extended the concept a bit—in keeping, I hope, with the holographic paradigm, which would suggest that the theme might be repeated on various levels and scales.

5. In me or (as in the case of Good Mother) fused with me and a part of me.

6. Developmentally, this first comes into evidence around eighteen months. Melanie Klein, a pioneering child analyst, called it the "depressive position."

7. Projection inevitably leads to guilt, since the mind, cut off from its Spiritual sustenance (lost as a result of separation from the Whole) can conclude only that it has committed some grievous wrong, and is plagued by its negative projections as retribution. For a fuller explanation of the psychodynamics of guilt, see *A Course in Miracles.*

8. I owe this perspective on development and psychological function to one of my teachers and mentors, John Stocks, M.D., whose masterful integration of a wide spectrum of the most profound ideas in psychotherapy provides one of the foundations for this book.

9. This point of view might bring some clarity to the perplexing issue of defining "mental illness." Most efforts to categorize behavior as pathological have come under justifiable criticism, condemned as imposing

arbitrary values. Evaluating *all* behavior in terms of how it contributes to the "soul's journey" might provide a refreshing alternative.

10. See Chapters 2 (pages 99–104) and 5 (pages 169–73).

11. Shame and the sycotic disorders can also come from buying into social censure. Though you may be right on target with what you do, and though it is an essential part of your soul's journey, if the world around you condemns you, and you have internalized its values and attitudes, you may fall ill. (This is one possible use of the term *pseudosycosis*.)

12. As a general principle, the male will tend to *express* an inherited disorder while the female will, instead, be a *carrier*. It is the nature of woman to *contain;* she is a *vessel*. It is the feminine side of us that has the strength to absorb, hold, and survive even that which is noxious.

13. See Philip M. Bailey, M.D., *Homeopathic Psychology: Personality Profiles of the Major Constitutional Remedies,* pages 368–69.

14. I consider Hahnemann's concept of the three fundamental miasmatic positions elegantly useful as a sort of "meta-schema." See, for example, Proceso Sanchez Ortega's trenchant analysis of organized medicine in classical miasmatic terms in his *Notes on the Miasms*.

15. Louise L. Hay, *Heal Your Body*.

16. Of course, in a sense, this is true. Once it is consciously entered, it ceases to be "unconscious." But the assumption goes further than this. It maintains that the unconscious comprises a body of mental processes the bulk of which by their nature must *remain* outside of awareness.

17. By "renegade yogis" I mean the seekers and daring explorers of the inner world, whatever their culture or nationality. These are the adventurous souls who devoted their lives to this inner journey. Because of the difficulty of this challenge, many of those who have been most successful have had the benefit of the systematic teachings and techniques of yoga. For that reason, as well as because that is my training also, I use the term *yogis,* but with the intent of giving it a more universal flavor.

18. See Swami Rama, et al., *Yoga and Psychotherapy,* Chapter 5: "The Secrets of Sleep."

19. For details on this process see "Meditation and the Unconscious Mind" by Rudolph Ballentine in *The Theory and Practice of Meditation,* Rudolph Ballentine, ed.

Chapter 13

1. Many of these insights into the usual psychological significance of the physical disorder, I owe to Louise Hay, and though in other cases my

interpretation may be somewhat different, the two are usually close enough that her little book *Heal Your Body* can be used as a source of corresponding affirmations to help in getting past the mindset that underlies the present problem.

2. See the book *Beating Alzheimer's,* by Tom Warren.

3. See Melvyn Werbach, M.D., *Nutritional Influences on Illness* for details.

4. Traditional Chinese Medicine technique involving topical applications and frottage.

5. See *Immune Power Personality,* by Henry Dreher.

6. John E. Sarno, MD, *Healing Back Pain, The Mind-Body Connection* (New York, Warner Books, 1991).

7. Read Genia Pauli Haddon, *Uniting Sex, Self, and Spirit,* Chapter 9.

8. To release and reactivate core or intrinsic muscles—especially neck and spine, see Sam Beiser, *Strokes: A Home Treatment that Can Cure Paralysis and Stroke Damage,* by University of Natural Healing, 355 West Rio Road, Charlottesville, Va. (booklet).

9. See Ballentine, *Transition to Vegetarianism,* pages 126–29.

10. Marketed as "Pycnogenol."

11. With ELISA/ACT or with simple pulse test.

12. E.g., Pepto-Bismol.

13. See Chapter 8, pages 297–301, and for how to order, page 572 under Wellspring Pharmacy.

14. Either outdoors or with full-spectrum lighting indoors.

15. One effective preparation available commercially is Technu.

16. Produced in Switzerland as Cernilton.

17. This is the "root lock," also important in developing ejaculatory control. The medical equivalent is the "Kegel" exercise, which involves tightening and releasing the pubococcygeal muscle that forms the floor of the pelvis.

18. See Chapter 8, pages 299–300, and for how to order, page 573 under Equipment.

19. Maggots, which have been used in such ulcers and bedsores, are thought to be effective because they secrete allantoin, of which comfrey is a rich source. Comfrey is very easy to grow—even in a window box.

20. See Gail and Tom Brewer, *What Every Pregnant Woman Should Know* (New York: Random House, 1977), and John Ellis, *Vitamin B_6: The Doctor's Report* (New York: Harper and Row, 1973).

21. See *Planetary Herbology* by Michael Tierra, pages 398–403 for details.

Index

See also alphabetical listings of diseases in Self-Help Index (pp 503–27), which are not repeated here.

ABOUT THE AUTHOR

Rudolph M. Ballentine, M.D., is director of the Center for Holistic Medicine, which he founded twenty-five years ago. He studied psychology at Duke University and the University of Paris (Sorbonne) and received his M.D. from Duke. He was on the faculty of the Louisiana State University School of Medicine, Department of Psychiatry and studied the Ayurvedic and homeopathic systems of medicine in India. For twelve years he served as president of the Himalayan Institute, and for eighteen years as director of its Combined Therapy Program, where he was instrumental in developing models of holistic medical care that have been adopted around the world. Dr. Ballentine has made numerous radio and television appearances. For information on his availability to speak or to participate in special projects, write to:

The Center for Holistic Medicine
P.O. Box 21, Bronx, NY 10471
212 243-6057

or email: Radicalhlg@aol.com

For his schedule of upcoming presentations and for details on his consulting and training services see under Center for Holistic Medicine and World Health and Healing Collaborative, p. 573.